Cytogenetics: Recent Progress

Cytogenetics: Recent Progress

Edited by Clayton Fisher

hayle
medical

New York

Hayle Medical,
750 Third Avenue, 9ᵗʰ Floor,
New York, NY 10017, USA

Visit us on the World Wide Web at:
www.haylemedical.com

ISBN: 978-1-63241-655-1

Cataloging-in-Publication Data

   Cytogenetics : recent progress / edited by Clayton Fisher.
     p. cm.
   Includes bibliographical references and index.
   ISBN 978-1-63241-655-1
   1. Cytogenetics. 2. Medical genetics. 3. Cytology. 4. Genetics. I. Fisher, Clayton.
RB155 .C98 2019
616.042--dc23

Table of Contents

Preface

The study of chromosomes and chromosome abnormalities is encompassed in the branch of cytogenetics. A chromosomal abnormality arises due to a structural abnormality in one or more chromosomes or due to occurrence of atypical number of chromosomes. Structural abnormalities in chromosomes can lead to deletions, duplications, inversions, insertions, translocations, etc. in chromosomes. Some of the disorders arising due to this include Jacobsen syndrome, Wolf-Hirschhorn syndrome, Charcot-Marie-Tooth disease type 1A, etc. Numerical disorders include Down syndrome, Turner syndrome, etc. Some chromosomal abnormalities are chromosomal rearrangements, aneuploidy and genomic deletion/duplication disorders. Microscopy and array comparative genomic hybridization are widely used for cytogenetic studies. This book covers in detail some existing theories and innovative concepts revolving around cytogenetics. Different approaches, evaluations, methodologies and advanced studies on cytogenetics have been included herein. The extensive content of this book provides the readers with a thorough understanding of the subject.

This book unites the global concepts and researches in an organized manner for a comprehensive understanding of the subject. It is a ripe text for all researchers, students, scientists or anyone else who is interested in acquiring a better knowledge of this dynamic field.

I extend my sincere thanks to the contributors for such eloquent research chapters. Finally, I thank my family for being a source of support and help.

Editor

Chromosomal microarray analysis in the genetic evaluation of 279 patients with syndromic obesity

Carla Sustek D'Angelo[1]*, Monica Castro Varela[1], Claudia Irene Emílio de Castro[1], Paulo Alberto Otto[1],
Ana Beatriz Alvarez Perez[2], Charles Marques Lourenço[3], Chong Ae Kim[4], Debora Romeo Bertola[4], Fernando Kok[5],
Luis Garcia-Alonso[2] and Celia Priszkulnik Koiffmann[1]

Abstract

Background: Syndromic obesity is an umbrella term used to describe cases where obesity occurs with additional phenotypes. It often arises as part of a distinct genetic syndrome with Prader-Willi syndrome being a classical example. These rare forms of obesity provide a unique source for identifying obesity-related genetic changes. Chromosomal microarray analysis (CMA) has allowed the characterization of new genetic forms of syndromic obesity, which are due to copy number variants (CNVs); however, CMA in large cohorts requires more study. The aim of this study was to characterize the CNVs detected by CMA in 279 patients with a syndromic obesity phenotype.

Results: Pathogenic CNVs were detected in 61 patients (22%) and, among them, 35 had overlapping/recurrent CNVs. Genomic imbalance disorders known to cause syndromic obesity were found in 8.2% of cases, most commonly deletions of 1p36, 2q37 and 17p11.2 (5.4%), and we also detected deletions at 1p21.3, 2p25.3, 6q16, 9q34, 16p11.2 distal and proximal, as well as an unbalanced translocation resulting in duplication of the *GNB3* gene responsible for a syndromic for of childhood obesity. Deletions of 9p terminal and 22q11.2 proximal/distal were found in 1% and 3% of cases, respectively. They thus emerge as being new putative obesity-susceptibility *loci*. We found additional CNVs in our study that overlapped with CNVs previously reported in cases of syndromic obesity, including a new case of 13q34 deletion (*CHAMP1*), bringing to 7 the number of patients in whom such defects have been described in association with obesity. Our findings implicate many genes previously associated with obesity (e.g. *PTBP2*, *TMEM18*, *MYT1L*, *POU3F2*, *SIM1*, *SH2B1*), and also identified other potentially relevant candidates including *TAS1R3*, *ALOX5AP*, and *GAS6*.

Conclusion: Understanding the genetics of obesity has proven difficult, and considerable insight has been obtained from the study of genomic disorders with obesity associated as part of the phenotype. In our study, CNVs known to be causal for syndromic obesity were detected in 8.2% of patients, but we provide evidence for a genetic basis of obesity in as many as 14% of cases. Overall, our results underscore the genetic heterogeneity in syndromic forms of obesity, which imposes a substantial challenge for diagnosis.

Keywords: Chromosomal microarray analysis (CMA), Copy number variations (CNVs), Body mass index (BMI), Intellectual and developmental disabilities (IDDs), Prader-Willi syndrome (PWS), Syndromic obesity

* Correspondence: cdangelo@ib.usp.br
[1]Human Genome and Stem Cell Research Center (HUG-CELL), Department of Genetics and Evolutionary Biology, Institute of Biosciences, University of Sao Paulo, Rua do Matao no 277, Cidade Universitaria-Butanta, Sao Paulo, SP 05508-090, Brazil
Full list of author information is available at the end of the article

Background

Obesity is a highly heritable multifactorial disorder defined by a body mass index (BMI) of ≥ 30 kg/m^2, which predisposes to many diseases. Rare and common genetic variants associated with obesity identified to date have increased our understanding of the mechanisms by which obesity develops. Copy number variants (CNVs) in a number of chromosomal regions are known to be involved in highly penetrant and individually rare, both isolated and syndromic forms of obesity [1–3]. The latter describes cases where obesity co-occurs with additional phenotypes (e.g., intellectual and developmental disabilities (IDDs), dysmorphism, congenital anomalies) often arising as part of a distinct syndrome, from which Prader-Willi syndrome (PWS; OMIM #176270) is a classical example. Until recently, only a few genomic disorders other than PWS were known to contribute to increased risk of obesity, including the known microdeletion syndromes 1p36 (OMIM #607872), 2q37 (OMIM #600430), 6q16 (*SIM1* gene), 9q34 (OMIM #610253; *EHMT1* gene), 11p14.1 (OMIM #612469), and 17p11.2 (OMIM #182290; *RAI1* gene).

In recent years, however, numerous unique and rare recurring/overlapping CNVs have been associated with a syndromic obesity phenotype in patients through the widespread use of chromosomal microarray analysis (CMA) [4–16]. Examples include deletions of chromosome band 2p25.3 that include the *MYT1L* gene (OMIM #616521), the recurrent 220-kb deletion of distal 16p11.2 including the *SH2B1* gene (OMIM #613444), and the recurrent 600-kb 16p11.2 proximal deletion (OMIM #611913, gene unknown). Also, a novel genomic disorder that causes obesity, ID and seizures has been described in children carrying a recurrent unbalance translocation (8;12)(p23.1;p13.31) that duplicates the *GNB3* gene [17]. Overlapping 1p21.3 deletions comprising the *DPYD* and *MIR137* genes have been detected in patients with a phenotype consisting primarily of obesity, ID, and autism spectrum disorder (ASD) [18, 19]. Small 6q16.1 deletions encompassing the *POU3F2* gene were identified in 10 individuals presenting with obesity, hyperphagia and IDDs [20]. Chromosome 13q34 deletions disrupting the *CHAMP1* gene were linked ID, obesity and mild dysmorphism in five adult individuals [21].

Syndromic obesity is recognized as an etiologically heterogeneous group of disorders for which an obesity-related genetic change can be identified but only a few genetic causes have been identified to date. Only one study has examined the etiology of syndromic obesity with CMA in a cohort of 100 patients specifically selected for obesity [22]. In that study, CNVs were regarded either as pathogenic or potentially pathogenic in 22% of cases, and several novel CNVs for which a defined syndrome has not yet been delineated were uncovered. Herein, we report our experience over the past 5 years using CMA to identify CNVs in 279 patients referred with syndromic obesity. This study adds to the current knowledge of CNVs linked to obesity and provides evidence for association with obesity at new and previously identified candidate *loci*.

Methods

Cohort enrollment and description

Only patients who tested negative for PWS (methylation analysis of *SNURF-SNRPN* exon 1 by our laboratory) were included in our study whether or not they had a positive clinical score for PWS. This test population had a mean age of 9 years (range 8 days to 40 years old), 55% of cases represented by male patients (male/female ratio = 1.2). The 2000 Centers for Disease Control and Prevention (CDC) growth charts (available at https://www.cdc.gov/growthcharts/) were used to plot weight-for-age, height-for-age, weight-for-height, BMI-for-age, and occipito-frontal head circumference (OFC) [23]. We stratified our cohort into 4 age groups: (1) infants ($n = 19$) < 2 years old (mean age 13 months; 9 males and 9 females); (2) children ($n = 153$) aged 2–9 years (mean age 6 years; 80 males and 73 females); (3) adolescents ($n = 98$) aged 10–19 years (mean age 9 years; 61 males and 37 females); (4) adults ($n = 10$) > 20 years old (mean age 27 years; 2 males and 8 females In a majority of patients, recognition of excessive weight gain was based on the following: (1) infants, the standard deviation (SD) of weight-for-height Z-scores > ~1 (mean + 3.23 SD); (2) children and adolescents, BMI-for-age percentiles $\geq$85th (mean 97.4th and 97.9th percentiles, respectively); (3) adults, BMI values $\geq$30 kg/m2 (mean 46.7 kg/m2); In 37 patients, data on weight and/or height were missing but they had a documented diagnosis of overweight or obesity made by attending physicians, and 5 other patients aged < 5 years had hyperphagia with an increase probability of developing obesity. Among a subset of 208 children and adolescents (BMI $\geq$ 95th percentile), we further classified obesity based on the BMI expressed as a percentage above the 95th BMI percentile according to age and sex, as previously described [24, 25]: a BMI 100–119% of the 95th percentile was used to define moderate obesity and a BMI $\geq$120% of the 95th BMI percentile used to define severe obesity. Extreme BMIs were calculated by multiplying the BMI at the 95th percentile by a factor of 1.1 through 1.9 to derive the 110% to 190%, for both genders.

Chromosomal microarray analysis

Any of the following genome-wide array platforms were used according to their availability: CytoSure ISCA v2 4x180K (Oxford Gene Technology, Oxford, UK), SurePrint G3 Human CGH 8x60K (Agilent Technologies, Santa Clara, CA), Affymetrix Mapping 100 K and 500 K arrays (Affymetrix, Santa Clara, CA, USA). Most cases (85%) were investigated using high-density oligonucleotide microarrays

(4x180K OGT platform). DNA was extracted from peripheral blood using Autopure LS® (Gentra Systems, Inc., Minneapolis, MN). Genomic DNA concentration was measured by Nanodrop spectrophotometer (ThermoFisher). Chromosomal microarray testing was performed according to the manufacturers' instructions. In oligonucleotide-based microarrays, two experiments were performed for each patient sample with reversal of the dye labels for the control and test samples, raw data were processed and analyzed using Agilent Feature Extraction and Genomic Workbench software with the statistical algorithm ADM-2 and sensitivity threshold of 6.7. Affymetrix SNP array data was analyzed with the Genotyping Console (GTC) 4.0 software using default settings and a similarly processed reference sample data set. Due to the limited probe coverage, CNVs on chromosome Y were removed from the analysis. We used the American College of Medical Genetics and Genomics (ACMG) 2011 guidelines for variant interpretation to classify variants in 4 categories: pathogenic CNVs (PCNVs), likely PCNVs, variants of uncertain significance (VUS), and likely benign CNVs [26]. Healthy and disease variant databases used included the Database of Genomic Variants (DGV, http://dgv.tcag.ca), the Online Mendelian Inheritance in Man (OMIM, https://www.omim.org/) and the DatabasE of genomiC varIation and Phenotype in Humans using Ensembl Resources (DECIPHER, http://decipher.sanger.ac.uk) [27–29]. All genomic breakpoints were based on the human genome build GRCh37 (hg19) (http://genome.ucsc.cdu/) [30].

Gene prioritization

Genes affected by the detected CNVs were compared to a list of genes related to obesity downloaded from the Text-mined Hypertension, Obesity and Diabetes candidate gene database (T-HOD) [31] and the Human Genome Epidemiology encyclopedia Navigator (HUGE, https://phgkb.cdc.gov/PHGKB) [32]. We specifically searched the term "obesity" and retrieved 835 genes annotated in T-HOD and 1920 genes annotated in the HUGE Phenopedia. We also checked the genes affected by CNVs against a list of 370 genes with evidence for playing a role in obesity curated from literature [33] and a list of 940 genes in the CNV morbidity map for IDDs generated from 29,085 cases and 19,584 controls [34].

Results

Cohort and correlation of PCNVs with specific phenotypes

General clinical findings noted in patients are listed in Table 1 (individual descriptions are provided in Table S1 in Additional file 1). Although patients' records were not always complete and clinical comorbidities could not be fully assessed, the most commonly reported features associated with obesity were IDDs, dysmorphism, behavioral phenotypes, hyperphagia, neonatal hypotonia, and language

Table 1 Additional phenotypes of patients with syndromic obesity

Clinical features	Total cohort (n)	Patients with PCNVs (n)
Intellectual/developmental disabilities	219	55
Craniofacial dysmorphism	149	49
Behavioral problems	132	29
Hyperphagia	112	27
Infantile hypotonia	88	32
Language impairments	80	28
Hands/ft abnormalities	65	21
Abnormal external genitalia	56	20
Eye/vision problems	51	16
Seizures	31	13
Poor motor skills	29	9
Skeletal anomalies	23	9
Brain abnormalities	19	7
Hearing loss	13	6
Cardiac abnormalities	10	4

Prevalence could not be assess as complete phenotypic data was not available

impairments. Hands and feet abnormalities, abnormalities of the external genitalia and eye/vision problems were often reported. Macrocephaly was observed in 92 of 206 (45%) patients, compared to 11 of 206 (5%) patients with microcephaly, and tall stature in 40 of 238 (17%) patients, compared to 22 of 238 (9%) patients with short stature (Z-scores > or < ±2 SD). No association was found between these growth parameters in cases with and without PCNVs using the Fisher's Exact test (Fig. 1).

In an attempt to determine whether there were phenotypic differences associated with the presence of PCNVs, we compared the frequencies of phenotype pairs segregating together in patients with syndromic obesity caused by PCNVs against those without PCNVs. We constructed a matrix representation (heatmap) of the Chi-square p-values between any given pair of phenotypes that co-occurred in patients with and without PCNVs. Out of 133 phenotype pairs that were evaluated (listed in Table S2 in Additional file 2), 12 had significant associations for PCNVs with p-values < 0.05 (Fig. 2a). Next, we constructed using Cytoscape [35] a graphic representation of these phenotype-phenotype associations, where a given pair of phenotype was connected only if they were significant at p < 0.05, to discover the core phenotype variables in the network (those that overlapped most between pairs). The most highly correlated phenotypes are hypotonia, language impairments, abnormalities of the external genitalia, and eye/vision problems. They also correlated with many additional phenotype variables including seizures, sleep problems, tall stature and hands/feet abnormalities (Fig. 2b).

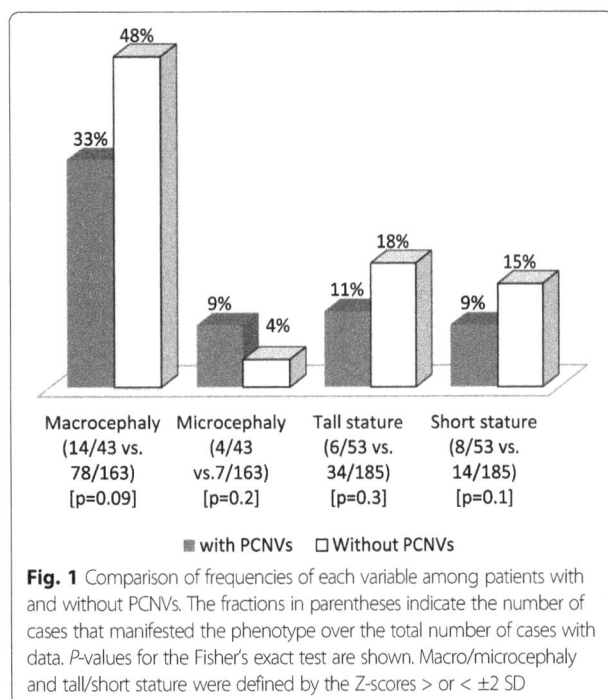

Fig. 1 Comparison of frequencies of each variable among patients with and without PCNVs. The fractions in parentheses indicate the number of cases that manifested the phenotype over the total number of cases with data. *P*-values for the Fisher's exact test are shown. Macro/microcephaly and tall/short stature were defined by the Z-scores > or < ±2 SD

Characterization of CNVs in patients with syndromic obesity

Overall, CMA identified clinically relevant genomic imbalances in 22% of patients, potentially clinically relevant CNVs in 2%, VUS in 5% and likely benign CNVs in 11% (Table 2). All clinically relevant results per individual are listed in Table 3. The genomic regions associated with likely PCNVs, VUS and likely benign CNVs are listed in Additional file 3: Table S3.

Pathogenic CNVs

A total of 68 pathogenic imbalances were detected in 61 patients, the majority of which pathogenic deletions (72%) and rearrangements smaller than 5-Mb (70%). 31 of the patients (6–12, 14, 15, 18, 23, 28, 30–33, 35, 40–43, 46–48, 51, 52, 55, 56, 58–60) had previously been published as separate studies [36–38]. De novo PCNVs were found in 30 patients, whereas only 6 patients inherited a pathogenic deletion or duplication from an apparently unaffected parent, all of which occurring at genomic *loci* which are known *to* have reduced penetrance (16p13.11, 16p11.2, and 22q11.2). The inheritance status could not be determined in 25 cases.

In 47 patients (24 novel cases), the PCNVs overlapped with chromosomal regions associated with known genomic disorders, and, among them, 35 patients were detected with PCNVs at 10 *loci* that were recurrent (same breakpoints) or overlapping in 2 or more unrelated samples (Fig. 3). We found 23 cases with deletions known to cause a syndromic obesity phenotype: 1p36 (n = 5), 1p21.3 (n = 2), 2p25.3 (n = 1), 2q37 (n = 5), 6q16

(n = 1), 9q34.3 (n = 1), 16p11.2 breakpoint (BP) 2–3 (n = 1), 16p11.2 BP 4–5 (n = 1), and 17p11.2 (n = 5). The recurrent translocation t(8;12)(p23.1;p13.31) found in patient 18 is also known to be involved in the pathogenesis of syndromic obesity. In addition, 2 rare deletions at chromosomes 13q12.3 (patient 24) and 19p13.12 (patient 37) overlapped with deletions of different sizes in patients from the literature and the DECIPHER database who were obese (Fig. 4). Mapping of the shortest region of overlap (SRO) in these cases exposed a 660-kb interval at 13q12.3 (chr13:30,880,255–31,540,272 bp, hg19; Fig. 4a) comprising 5 genes (*KATNAL1, LINC00426, HMGB1, USPL1, ALOX5AP*, and *MEDAG*), and a 440-kb interval at 19p13.12 (chr19:15,052,889–15,492,848 bp, hg19; Fig. 4b) comprising 9 genes (*SLC1A6, CCDC105, CASP14, SYDE1, ILVBL NOTCH3, EPHX3, BRD4*, and *AKAP8*).

In other 14 patients, the PCNVs did not overlap with a known genomic imbalance disorder but were de novo in 10 cases or of unknown origin (the remainder), and involved large and complex chromosomal imbalances. Among these, we found 4 PCNVs overlapping with previously identified obesity candidate *loci* (Fig. 5): a novel 22.3-Mb duplication of 3q11.2q13.31 (patient 49), a novel 11.6-Mb duplication of 13q11q12.3 (patient 53), a novel 8.5-Mb deletion of 13q33.2q34 (patient 57), and a 1-Mb duplication of band 14q11.2 (patient 58). Notably, the duplication region at 13q11q12.3 also overlaps with a smaller duplication present in our patient 19, who possessed a second large CNV at the 8p23.1 *locus*. The extent of overlap among our cases with those previously described CNVs is of about 2-Mb in band 3q13.31 (chr3:113,924,534–115,890,384 bp, hg19; Fig. 5a), 1.2-Mb in band 13q12.12 (chr13:23,706,634–24,910,765 bp, hg19; Fig. 5b), 2.4-Mb in band 13q34 (chr13:112,725,394–115,092,648 bp, hg19; Fig. 5c), and 827-kb in band 14q11.2 (chr14:21,424,185–22,250,879 bp, hg19; Fig. 5d). Candidate genes at these intervals are proposed in the discussion.

Likely pathogenic CNVs

CNVs detected in 6 additional patients were classified as potentially clinically significant, including a de novo 340-kb duplication at 16p13.2 comprising the *USP7* gene implicated in a known deletion syndrome (OMIM #616863), a 482-kb paternally inherited duplication of 17q11.2 partially overlapping the gene for neurofibromatosis type I (NF1), and an 1.1-Mb paternally inherited 20q11.2 duplication upstream of the *ASXL1* gene with a likely role in 20q11.2 duplication syndrome [39]. The inheritance of 3 other CNVs could not be determined. The 3 CNVs were a 489-kb duplication in 21q22.13 including the ID gene *DYRK1A* (OMIM #614104), a 703-kb deletion in 7q31.1 affecting the *IMMP2L-DOCK4* gene region implicated in

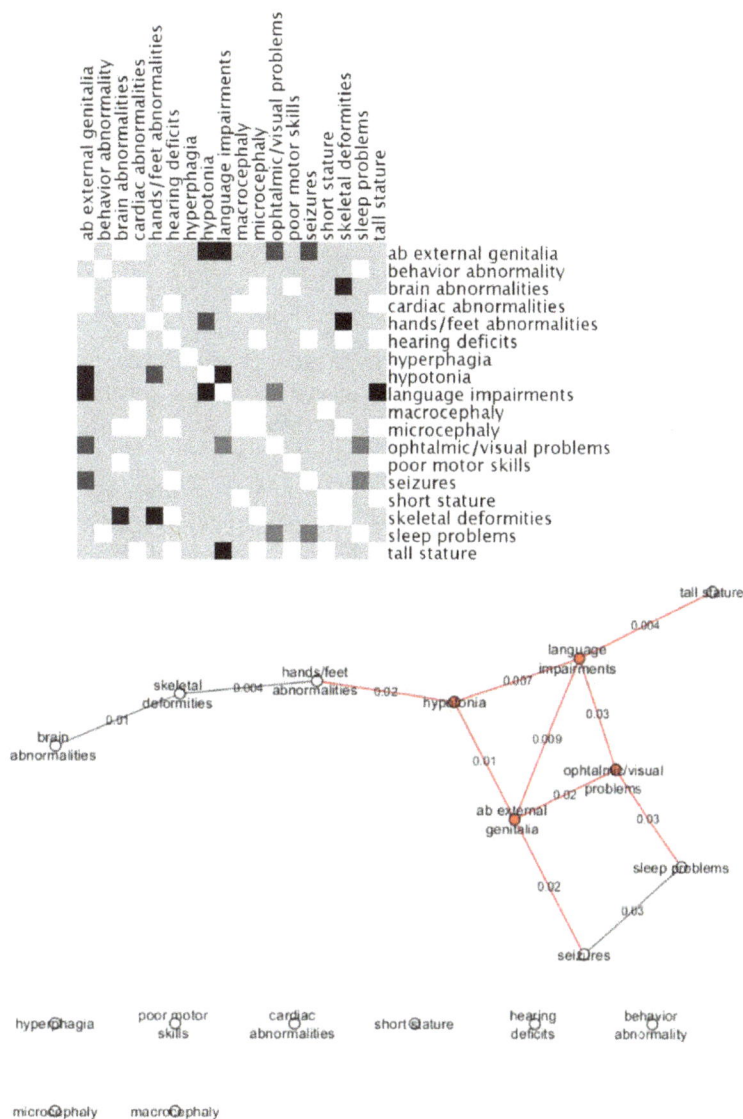

Fig. 2 The heat map constructed from the P-values for the Chi-square statistic test between pairs of phenotypes observed in patients with PCNVs against those without PCNVs is shown at the top, where P-values < 0.05 are represented by small darker gray or black squares and larger values by light gray squares (white squares indicate null values or the absence of association between a given pair of phenotype). Graphical representation of the phenotype network generated using Cytoscape is shown at the bottom, where phenotypes (nodes) are interconnected (edges) if they had significant associations for PCNVs at P < 0.05. The resulting network has 10 interconnected phenotypes and 8 not connected phenotype variables. Red nodes and edges highlight the most highly connected phenotypes and their interactions in the network

IDDs [40], and an intragenic deletion of the *ASTN2* gene at 9q33.1 which has also been implicated in susceptibility to IDDs [41].

Variants of uncertain significance

In 15 patients, we detected CNVs that were classified as VUS. Of these, 2 were de novo events: a 222-kb 12q21.32 duplication including the *CEP290* gene whose mutations cause Bardet-Biedl syndrome (BBS14; OMIM #615991), but which was not associated with previously reported pathogenicity, and a 385-kb 6q27 duplication affecting only

three non-coding RNAs found in a patient who inherited a second large CNV. There were 3 VUS inherited from asymptomatic parents intersecting with genes within CNVs that have previously been implicated with disorders, such as *CACNA2D1* with epilepsy and ID [42], and *MACROD2* and *LINGO2* with autism [43, 44]. Furthermore, 6 VUS (3 inherited and 3 unknown) contained morbid OMIM genes, including *NFIA*, *MPZ*, *PARK2*, *DPP6*, and *KANK1*. Additionally, 3 other cases (2 females and 1 male) inherited large chromosome X duplications from carrier mothers spanning several morbid OMIM genes but with no

Table 2 Overall findings of microarray testing

	Number	%
Total number of cases	279	–
With imbalances	112	40
With pathogenic CNVs	61	22
With Known syndromes	*47*	*17*
Pathogenic imbalances [a]	68	–
Del	49	72
Dup	19	28
> 5 Mb	21	31
De novo	30	49
Inherited	6	10
Unknown	19	31
Not maternal	6	10
With likely pathogenic CNVs	6	2
With CNVs of uncertain significance	15	5
With likely benign CNVs	30	11

[a]Pathogenic imbalances included 45 simple deletions or duplications, 4 unbalanced translocations, an insertional translocation, and 6 other complex rearrangements believed to have been formed from the same rearrangement. In the remaining 5 patients, the rearrangements were associated with a second-site CNV arisen apparently independent which were classified as benign or of uncertain significance

evidence for triplosensitivity phenotypes as determined by the ClinGen Dosage Sensitive Map (http://www.ncbi.nlm.-nih.gov/projects/dbvar/clingen/) [45].

Likely benign CNVs

We also observed 30 patients with CNVs that might represent benign variants. The observed CNVs were most often duplications and < 300-kb in size. In all cases where it was possible to ascertain the parental status, variants were inherited from an asymptomatic parent. We found relevant genes lying within some of these CNVs. Examples of such genes include: *PTEN* in which mutations cause many different disorders including macrocephaly/autism syndrome (OMIM #605309); *VPS13B* whose mutations cause Cohen syndrome characterized by truncal obesity, joint hypermobility and a pigmentary retinopathy (COH1; OMIM #216550); *CIDEA* (OMIM 604440) with a role in regulating energy balance and adiposity; *ULK4* crucial to brain development with CNVs being identified as risk factor in schizophrenia [46]; *KATNAL2* implicated as susceptibility gene of autism [47].

Identification of candidate genes involved in obesity susceptibility

A total of 2684 genes were affected by the detected CNVs. Among these, 234 genes had some previously reported connection to obesity as determined by the overlap with genes from the T-HOD and HUGE database, as well as a gene list

curated from literature [33], and 172 overlapped with genes listed in the CNV morbidity map for IDDs [34] (367 genes in total). Of particular interest are 87 genes that were intersected by different gene sets (Fig. 6). Notably, several known and candidate genes that have previously been implicated in syndromic obesity were retrieved by this candidate gene approach, including *SIM1* [48], *SH2B1* [49], *PTBP2* [38], *PRLH* and *CAPN10* [50], *ACP1* and *TMEM18* [12], *EHMT1* [51], and *GNB3* [17]. Thus, these genes were considered as more likely to have a role in obesity susceptibility. Pathways analysis in Cytoscape using the plugin Reactome FI showed that the majority of these genes were related to metabolic pathways and small molecule metabolic process.

PCNV rates by gender, age and level of obesity in children and adolescents

For the purpose of this study, 208 obese children and adolescents with a BMI ≥95th percentile were considered based on a percentage above the 95th BMI percentile as moderately (< 120% of the 95th percentile) and severely (≥120% of the 95th percentile) obese (Fig. 7a). This sample consisted predominantly of males ($n = 123$ or 59%) and children aged 2–9 years ($n = 125$ or 60%). The majority of patients were classified as severely obese ($n = 160$ or 77%). The prevalence of severe obesity was higher than moderate obesity for both gender and age groups (Fig. 7b) but there were statistically significantly more males than females with severe obesity (105 males, 55 females; Fisher's Exact test, $p < 0.01$); this sex-related difference in obesity was observed in children but not in adolescents aged 10–19 years (Additional file 4: Table S4). Although a higher frequency of PCNVs was observed in females ($n = 23$ or 27%) compared with males ($n = 24$ or 20%), no statistically significantly differences were observed in the frequencies when compared by gender, age at the time of testing, and obesity severity (Fig. 7c and d; Additional file 5: Table S5). In boys, the prevalence of PCNVs was greater in the severe obesity group (20% vs. 17%), particularly among children aged 2–9 years (18% vs. 11%), but was similar at adolescence (22%). In girls, the prevalence of PCNVs was greater among the moderate obesity group (35% vs. 30%), particularly among children aged 2–9 years (35% vs. 25%), and correlated inversely in adolescents (26% severe vs. 20% moderate obesity).

Discussion

This is the second study describing the use of CMA in patients ascertained for syndromic obesity, the largest published to date and also the first in a Brazilian cohort. We identified PCNVs in 22% of patients (68 pathogenic events in 61/279 subjects; Table 3), which is similar to the yield reported by Vuillaume et al. in microarray studies with 100 patients with syndromic obesity [22]. The prevalence of

Table 3 Pathogenic copy number variations (PCNVs) detected in 279 patients with syndromic obesity

Case number	Age	Gender	Weight Status	CNV Type	Cytoband	Genome Coordinate	Size	Origin	Clinical significance	RefSeq genes
Genomic imbalance disorders										
P1	5y	F	Referred as obese	Del	1p36.33	734595-1970865	1236270	Unk	1p36 terminal deletion	**KLHL17**, AGRN, TAS1R3,* **DVL1, VWA1, MMP23B, GABRD**
P2	34y	F	BMI 59.1	Del	1p36.33	734595-2223317	1488722	Unk	1p36 terminal deletion, complex	**KLHL17**, AGRN, TAS1R3,* **DVL1, VWA1, MMP23B, GABRD,** PRKCZ, SKI*
				Dup	1p36.33 p36.32	2225679-2694799	469120			–
P3	14y	F	BMI 26.8 (93.3th)	Del	1p36.33 p36.32	794592-2377269	1582677	De novo	1p36 terminal deletion	**KLHL17**, AGRN, TAS1R3,* **DVL1, VWA1, MMP23B, GABRD,** PRKCZ, SKI*
P4	6y	F	BMI 19.7 (96.8th)	Del	1p36.33 p36.32	734595-3531040	2796445	Unk	1p36 terminal deletion	**KLHL17**, AGRN, TAS1R3,* **DVL1, VWA1, MMP23B, GABRD,** PRKCZ, SKI,* TNFRSF14, PRDM16*
P5	11y	M	BMI 30.8 (99th)	Del	1p36.31 p36.22	6204969-9433118	3228149	Unk	1p36 interstitial deletion	CAMTA1, PER3, UTS2, *RERE*, H6PD*
P6	15y	F	BMI 37.1 (99.1th)	Del	1p22.1 p21.2	93919217-99846176	5926959	De novo	1p21.3 deletion	F3, PTBP2,* **DPYD, MIR137**
P7	8y	F	BMI 33.2 (99.7th)	Del	1p21.3 p13.3	95696444-107755879	12059435	Unk	1p21.3 deletion	PTBP2,* **DPYD, MIR137**, VCAM1,* COL11A1, AMY2B, AMY2A, AMY1A*
P8	6y	M	BMI 28.8 (99.9th)	Dup	1q21.1	146074084-147828029	1753945	Unk	1q21.1 distal duplication	PRKAB2, **CHD1L, GJA5, GJA8**
P9	7y	F	BMI 22.6 (98.2th)	Del	2p25.3	63452-3215593	3152141	De novo	2p25.3 terminal deletion	ACP1,* TMEM18,* **SNTG2**, TPO,* **MYT1L**
P10	8y	F	BMI 29.1 (99.5th)	Del	2q37.2 q37.3	237220842-242995835	5774993	De novo	2q37 terminal deletion	PRLH, LRRFIP1, PER2, **HDAC4**, GPC1,* CAPN10,* GPR35,* **KIF1A**, PASK, STK25*
P11	21y	M	Referred as obese	Del	2q37.2 q37.3	236854160-242995835	6141675	Unk	2q37 terminal deletion	**AGAP1**, PRLH, LRRFIP1, PER2, **HDAC4**, GPC1,* CAPN10,* GPR35,* **KIF1A**, PASK, STK25*
P12	10y	M	BMI 29.8 (99th)	Del	2q37.2 q37.3	236944801-243014630	6069829	De novo	2q37 terminal deletion, complex	**AGAP1**, PRLH, LRRFIP1, PER2, **HDAC4**, GPC1,* CAPN10,* GPR35,* **KIF1A**, PASK, STK25*
				Dup	2q37.1 q37.2	235090417-236802930	1712513			–
P13	9y	F	BMI 24.7 (98.2th)	Del	2q37.1 q37.3	234850276-243028335	8178059	Unk	2q37 terminal deletion, complex	TRPM8, **AGAP1**, PRLH, LRRFIP1, PER2, **HDAC4**, GPC1,* CAPN10,* GPR35,* **KIF1A**, PASK, STK25*
				Dup	2q37.1	233867403-234794816	927413			UTG1A1*
P14	5y	F	BMI 24.0 (99.7th)	Del	2q37.3	240880562-242948060	2067498	Unk	Unbalanced translocation	GPC1,* CAPN10,* GPR35,* **KIF1A**, PASK, STK25*
				Dup	17q25.3	78709250-81036261	2327011			RPTOR, ACTG1, GCGR,* PCYT2, FASN,* CSNK1D, UTS2R
P15	10y	M	BMI 31.0 (99.3th)	Del	6q16.1 q21	95836632-108010940	12174308	De novo	6q16 deletion	KLHL32, *POU3F2*, MCHR2,* SIM1,* **GRIK2**, LIN28B,* ATG5
P16	15y	F	BMI 40.5 (99.4th)	Del	7q11.23	72420782-74985644	2564862	Unk	7q11.23 deletion	**FKBP6, FZD9**, BCL7B, TBL2, MLXIPL, STX1A,* CLDN3, **ELN, LIMK1**, RFC2,* **CLIP2**, GTF2IRD1, GTF2I, NCF1
P17	6y	M	BMI 30.6 (99.9th)	Del	7q11.23	72437606-75053787	2616181	Unk	7q11.23 deletion	**FKBP6, FZD9**, BCL7B, TBL2, MLXIPL, STX1A,* CLDN3, **ELN, LIMK1**, RFC2,* **CLIP2**, GTF2IRD1, GTF2I, NCF1
P18	6y	M	BMI 33.4 (99.9th)	Del	8p23.3 p23.1	176464-7786759	7610295	De novo	Unbalanced translocation	**CLN8**, CSMD1, DEFA1,* **DEFB103A, DEFB103B, DEFB104A, DEFB106A, DEFB105A, DEFB107A, DEFB4A**

Table 3 Pathogenic copy number variations (PCNVs) detected in 279 patients with syndromic obesity *(Continued)*

Case number	Age	Gender	Weight Status	CNV Type	Cytoband	Genome Coordinate	Size	Origin	Clinical significance	RefSeq genes
				Dup	12p13.33 p13.31	204618-8309473	8104855			*SLC6A13*, WNT5B,* ADIPOR2,* *CACNA2D4, CACNA1C*, FOXM1, TEAD4, PARP11, *KCNA1*, NTF3, VWF, TNFRSF1A,* SCNN1A, GAPDH, CD4, GNB3,* CD163, APOBEC1, GDF3, SLC2A14, C3AR1
P19	6y	M	BMI 25.8 (99.8th)	Dup	8p23.1	8054556-11985356	3930800	Not mat	8p23.1 duplication	*CLDN23*, MFHAS1, PPP1R3B, LOC157273, TNKS,* MSRA,* *SOX7*, MTMR9,* BLK, GATA4,* *NEIL2*, FDFT1,* CTSB
				Dup	13q12.12	23706634-24910765	1204131	Not mat	Uncertain	SGCG,¶ *SACS*, MIPEP
P20	11y	F	BMI 26.7 (97.6th)	Del	9p24.3 p22.3	40910-14304973	14264063	De novo	9p terminal deletion	*KANK1, DMRT1*, SMARCA2, VLDLR,* GLIS3, JAK2, *RLN1*, IL33,* KDM4C, PTPRD*
P21	12m	F	Weight-for Height +1sd	Del	9p24.3 p22.3	204149-15260439	15056290	De novo	9p terminal deletion	*KANK1, DMRT1*, SMARCA2, VLDLR,* GLIS3, JAK2, *RLN1*, IL33,* KDM4C, PTPRD,* TTC39B
P22	17y	M	BMI 28.7 (95.7th)	Del	9p24.3 p22.3	201149-8807593	8606444	Unk	9p terminal deletion	*KANK1, DMRT1*, SMARCA2, VLDLR,* GLIS3, JAK2, *RLN1*, IL33,* KDM4C, PTPRD*
P23	9y	F	BMI 31.1 (99.5th)	Del	9q34.3	140665414-141018984	353570	De novo	9q34.3 deletion	EHMT1,* *CACNA1B*
P24	14y	M	BMI 28.7 (97.6th)	Del	13q12.3 q13.1	29081250-33529310	4448060	De novo	13q12.3 deletion	POMP, SLC46A3, MTUS2, SLC7A1, UBL3, KATNAL1, LINC00426, HMGB1, *ALOX5AP,* RXFP2, BRCA2*
P25	8y	M	BMI 25.4 (99.2th)	Del	15q11.2	22729423-23086969	357546	Unk	15q11.2 microdeletion	*NIPA1, NIPA2, CYFIP1*
P26	10y	F	BMI 22.1 (93.4th)	Del	16p13.12 p13.11	14780302-16400774	1620472	Pat	16p13.1 deletion	NDE1, MYH11,* ABCC1, ABCC6
P27	4y	F	Hyperphagia	Dup	16p13.12 p13.11	14796004-16586941	1790937	Pat	16p13.1 duplication	NDE1, MYH11,* ABCC1, ABCC6
P28	7y	F	BMI 20.5 (96.6th)	Del	16p11.2	28843754-29044850	201096	De novo	16p11.2 (BP 2-3) deletion	ATXN2L,* TUFM,* MIR4721, SH2B1,* ATP2A1,* SPNS1
P29	12y	M	BMI 30.4 (98.8th)	Del	16p11.2	29592751-30197466	604715	Not mat	16p11.2 (BP 4-5) deletion	*QPRT, PRRT2, SEZ6L2, DOC2A, ALDOA, TBX6*, MAPK3
P30	8y	M	Referred as obese	Dup	16p11.2	29592751-30197466	604715	Pat	16p11.2 (BP 4-5) duplication	*QPRT, PRRT2, SEZ6L2, DOC2A, ALDOA, TBX6*, MAPK3
P31	11y	M	BMI 42.2 (99.7th)	Del	17p11.2	17006987-20171357	3164370	De novo	17p11.2 deletion	*COPS3, NT5M, MED9*, PEMT,* *RAI1*, SREBF1,* *ATPAF2, DRG2, SMCR8*, MFAP4, SLC47A1, ALDH3A2, *SPECC1*
P32	6y	M	BMI 31.2 (99.9th)	Del	17p11.2	16757563-20395535	3637972	Not mat	17p11.2 deletion	TNFRSF13B, *COPS3, NT5M, MED9*, PEMT,* *RAI1*, SREBF1,* *ATPAF2, DRG2,, SMCR8*, MFAP4, SLC47A1, ALDH3A2, *SPECC1*
P33	7y	F	BMI 21.9 (97.9th)	Del	17p11.2	16603145-20395535	3792390	De novo	17p11.2 deletion	TNFRSF13B, *COPS3, NT5M, MED9*, PEMT,* *RAI1*, SREBF1,* *ATPAF2, DRG2, SMCR8*, MFAP4, SLC47A1, ALDH3A2, *SPECC1*
P34	8y	F	BMI 25.9 (98.9th)	Del	17p11.2	16603145-20395535	3792390	Unk	17p11.2 deletion	TNFRSF13B, *COPS3, NT5M, MED9*, PEMT,* *RAI1*, SREBF1,* *ATPAF2, DRG2, SMCR8*, MFAP4, SLC47A1, ALDH3A2, *SPECC1*
P35	10y	M	BMI 28.1 (99th)	Del	17p11.2	16603145-20463399	3860254	De novo	17p11.2 deletion	TNFRSF13B, *COPS3, NT5M, MED9*, PEMT,* *RAI1*, SREBF1,* *ATPAF2, DRG2, SMCR8*, MFAP4, SLC47A1, ALDH3A2, *SPECC1*
P36	9y	M	BMI 22.2 (96.8th)	Dup	17q21.31 q21.32	40993738-45166786	4173048	De novo	17q21.3 duplication	AOC3, G6PC,* BRCA1,* *SOST,* PPY,* PYY,* TMEM101, HDAC5, ITGA2B,

Table 3 Pathogenic copy number variations (PCNVs) detected in 279 patients with syndromic obesity *(Continued)*

Case number	Age	Gender	Weight Status	CNV Type	Cytoband	Genome Coordinate	Size	Origin	Clinical significance	RefSeq genes
										EFTUD2, PLCD3, CRHR1,* *MAPT*, *KANSL1*
P37	8y	F	BMI 22.3 (97.4th)	Dup	19p13.2	12640509-13231703	591194	Unk	19p13.2 duplication	*MAST1*, *CALR*, **NFIX**
				Dup	9p22.1	19066513-19497724	431211	Unk	Uncertain	PLIN2*
P38	18y	F	BMI 41.5 (99th)	Del	19p13.12	14384925-16034584	1649659	De novo	19p13.12 deletion	*CD97*, *DDX39A*, *PKN1*, *PTGER1*, *GIPC1*, *CASP14*, **NOTCH3**, CYP4F11
P39	8y	F	Referred as obese	Del	22q11.21	18890162-20311554	1421392	De novo	22q11.2 deletion	**PRODH, DGCR2, DGCR14, CDC45, TBX1,** * **GNB1L**, TXNRD2, COMT,* **DGCR8**, ZDHHC8
P40	3y	M	BMI 34.7 (99.9th)	Del	22q11.21	18661758-21684798	3023040	De novo	22q11.2 deletion	**PRODH, DGCR2, DGCR14, CDC45, TBX1,** * **GNB1L**, TXNRD2, COMT,* **DGCR8**, ZDHHC8, **PI4KA**, SLC74A
P41	9y	M	BMI 32.5 (99.6th)	Del	22q11.21	18661758-21684798	3023040	De novo	22q11.2 deletion	**PRODH, DGCR2, DGCR14, CDC45, TBX1,** * **GNB1L**, TXNRD2, COMT,* **DGCR8**, ZDHHC8, **PI4KA**, SLC74A
P42	13m	M	Weight-for Height +1sd	Del	22q11.21	18818429-21661436	2843007	Pat	22q11.2 deletion	**PRODH, DGCR2, DGCR14, CDC45, TBX1,** * **GNB1L**, TXNRD2, COMT,* **DGCR8**, ZDHHC8, **PI4KA**, SLC74A
P43	18y	M	Referred as obese	Dup	22q11.21	18890162-21464056	2573894	Pat	22q11.2 duplication	**PRODH, DGCR2, DGCR14, CDC45, TBX1,** * **GNB1L**, TXNRD2, COMT,* **DGCR8**, ZDHHC8, **PI4KA**, SLC74A
P44	5y	M	BMI 27.9 (99.9th)	Del	22q11.21 q11.23	21759572-23822925	2063353	Unk	22q11.2 deletion, distal	**HIC2**, MAPK1,* **GNAZ, BCR**
P45	7y	F	BMI 24.8 (98.9th)	Del	22q11.21 q11.22	21468437-22959609	1491172	Not mat	22q11.2 deletion, distal	**HIC2**, MAPK1*
				Dup	3p26.3	857110-1414719	557609	Not mat	Uncertain	–
P46	2y	F	BMI 17.7 (85th)	Del	22q11.22 q11.23	23012069-23648827	636758	Mat	22q11.2 deletion, distal	**GNAZ, BCR**
P47	15y	M	BMI 39.5 (99.6th)	Del	22q11.22 q11.23	23063178-23696464	633286	Unk	22q11.2 deletion, distal	**GNAZ, BCR**
Other pathogenic imbalances										
P48	2y	M	BMI 24.4 (99.9th)	Del	3p26.3	73603-1273300	1199697	De novo	Unbalanced translocation	**CHL1**
				Dup	11q22.3 q25	106251478-134668665	28417187			ACAT1, ATM, POU2AF1, IL18,* ANKK1, DRD2,* HTR3B, HTR3A, NNMT, BUD13, APOA5,* APOA4,* APOC3,* APOA1,* BACE1, IL10RA, CD3E, HYOU1, H2AFX, CBL,* USP2, THY1, ARHGEF12, BSX,* HSPA8, CLMP, **NRGN**, SLC37A2, TIRAP, **KCNJ1**, KCNJ5,* OPCML
P49	14y	F	Referred as obese	Del	3p24.1	28719852-30169971	1450119	Unk	Complex rearrangement	LINC00693, RBMS3-AS3, RBMS3, RBMS3-AS1
				Dup	3q11.2 q13.31	93558505-115890384	22331879			EPHA6, ARL6,* STG3GAL6, **COL8A1**, CCDC80, BOC, ZDHHC23, ZBTB20, GAP43, LSAMP, DRD3
P50	10y	M	BMI 30.4 (99.3th)	Del	3q25.33	159252702-160555217	1302515	De novo	Uncertain	IL12A
				Del	13q31.2 q32.1	89522636-95065310	5542674	De novo	Feingold syndrome	**MIR17HG**, GPC5,* **GPC6**
P51	14y	F	BMI 27.9 (95.8th)	Del	7q22.1 q22.3	102358320-105487655	3129335	De novo	Clinically relevant	NAPEPLD, **RELN**, LHFPL3

Table 3 Pathogenic copy number variations (PCNVs) detected in 279 patients with syndromic obesity *(Continued)*

Case number	Age	Gender	Weight Status	CNV Type	Cytoband	Genome Coordinate	Size	Origin	Clinical significance	RefSeq genes
P52	2y	F	BMI 27.0 (99.9th)	Del	10p15.3 p14	269695-11579546	11309851	De novo	Unbalanced translocation	***ZMYND11***, <u>DIP2C</u>,* <u>IDI1</u>, ADRAB2, <u>PFKP</u>,* <u>KLF6</u>, <u>ARK1C1</u>, <u>AKR1C2</u>, <u>ARK1C3</u>, <u>AKR1C4</u>, <u>UCN3</u>, <u>IL15RA</u>, <u>IL2RA</u>,* <u>PFKFB3</u>, <u>PRKCQ</u>, ***GATA3***
				Dup	6q27	169505179-170694486	1189307			*WDR27*
P53	5m	F	Referred as obese	Dup	10p15.3 p12.31	119794-19509585	19389791	Not mat	Complex rearrangement	***ZMYND11***, <u>DIP2C</u>,* <u>IDI1</u>, ADRAB2, <u>PFKP</u>,* <u>KLF6</u>, <u>ARK1C1</u>, <u>AKR1C2</u>, <u>ARK1C3</u>, <u>AKR1C4</u>, <u>UCN3</u>, <u>IL15RA</u>, <u>IL2RA</u>,* <u>PFKFB3</u>, <u>PRKCQ</u>, ***GATA3***, <u>CDC123</u>, <u>CAMK1D</u>, <u>CCDC3</u>, <u>PTER</u>,* <u>CUBN</u>, <u>MRC1</u>, <u>CACNB2</u>
				Dup	13q11 q12.3	19440913-31031907	11590994	Not mat		***TUBA3C***, ***GJB2***, ***CRYL1***, *SGCG*, ***SACS***, *MIPEP*, *GPR12*, *GTF3A*, *MTIF3*,* ***POLR1D***, *PDX1*,* <u>CDX2</u>, *POMP*, *SLC46A3*, *MTUS2*, *SLC7A1*, <u>UBL3</u>, *KATNAL1*, *LINC00426*
P54	9y	F	BMI 34.3 (99.7th)	Dup	10q26.11 q26.3	120306959-135434409	15127450	De novo	10qter duplication	<u>PRLHR</u>,* <u>PRDX3</u>, ***BAG3***, <u>WDR11</u>, <u>FGFR2</u>,* <u>ACADSB</u>, <u>BUB3</u>, <u>OAT</u>, <u>TCERG1L</u>, <u>PRAP1</u>, <u>CYP2E1</u>*
P55	7y	F	BMI 23.6 (98.8th)	Del	12q15 q21.1	70555659-73153191	2597532	De novo	Clinically relevant	<u>PTPRB</u>, <u>TSPAN8</u>,* <u>LGR5</u><u>TPH2</u>
P56	13y	F	BMI 36.8 (99.4th)	Dup	12q21.32 q23.1	88684581-101464859	12780278	De novo	Insertional translocation	<u>KITLG</u>, <u>ATP2B1</u>, <u>SOCS2</u>, <u>LTA4H</u>, <u>RMST</u>, <u>NR1H4</u>*
P57	15y	M	BMI 43.1 (99.7th)	Del	13q33.2 q34	106648660-115105655	8456995	Not mat	13qter deletion	***EFNB2***, *MYO16*, <u>IRS2</u>,* <u>COL4A1</u>, ***ARHGEF7***, <u>F7</u>, <u>GAS6</u>, *CHAMP1*
P58	4y	M	BMI 22.0 (99.9th)	Dup	14q11.2	21244696-22250879	1006183	De novo	14q11.2 microduplication	***SUPT16H***, ***CHD8***
P59	16y	F	BMI 38.5 (99th)	Del	14q12	29781404-30552936	771532	De novo	14q12 deletion, non-critical	<u>PRKD1</u>*
				Dup	4p16.1	10068064-10529023	460959	Mat	Likely benign	***WDR1***
P60	7y	F	BMI 24.8 (99.3th)	Del	Xp22.12 p22.13	18214020-19833634	1619614	Unk	Rett syndrome-like	***CDKL5***, ***RS1***, <u>PHKA2</u>, <u>PDHA1</u>,* <u>SH3KBP1</u>
P61	14y	M	BMI 37.0 (99.5th)	Dup	Xp22.3	75943-2685605	2609662	De novo	Complex rearrangement	***SHOX***, ***ASMTL***, ***ASMT***
				Dup	Xq21.31 q21.32	88489522-92357353	3867831			*TGIF2 LX*, *PABPC5-AS1*, *PABPC5*, *PCDH11X*

Abbreviations: M male, F female, Del deletion, Dup duplication, y years, m months, BMI body mass index, SD standard deviation, unk unknown, mat maternally inherited, pat paternally inherited, not mat not maternally inherited; Genes in bold were listed in the CNV morbidity map of IDDs [34]. Underlined genes were retrieved from the Text-mined Hypertension, Obesity and Diabetes candidate gene database (T-HOD), the Human Genome Epidemiology (HUGE) Phenopedia, and from a list of obesity candidate genes curated from the literature [33]. Genes found at the intersection of at least two gene sets are highlighted (asterisks). Patients 6-12, 14, 15, 18, 23, 28, 30-33, 35, 40-43, 46-48, 51, 52, 55, 56, 58-60) have been published previously as separate studies [36-38]

PCNVs in children and adolescents did not differ significantly between gender and age groups, and obesity severity (Fig. 7). Nevertheless, females had a higher detection rate of PCNVs in comparison to males (27% females and 20% males; overall), with the highest differences (35% females and 11% males) found in the younger age group (2–9 years) with less severe grades of obesity (BMI < 1.2 x 95th percentile). Whilst no single phenotypic feature could be investigated for association with PCNV risk, due to the absence of comprehensively phenotyping of patients, phenotype-phenotype correlation analysis between cases with and without PCNVs identified 12 pairs of phenotypes that were significantly associated with the presence of PCNVs and

combining hypotonia, language impairments, abnormalities of the external genitalia, and eye/vision problems at its core. Of note, patients in our cohort were almost 10 times more likely to manifest macrocephaly as compared to microcephaly. Even though 33% of macrocephalic patients displayed PCNVs, macrocephaly did not associate with the presence of PCNVs.

In the current study, we have identified known genomic imbalance disorders in 47 patients, and, of them, 35 patients (13%) carry overlapping and recurrent CNVs (Table 3; Fig. 3). In our cohort, imbalances that are known to be causal for syndromic obesity were observed in 23 patients (8.2%). The most commonly identified

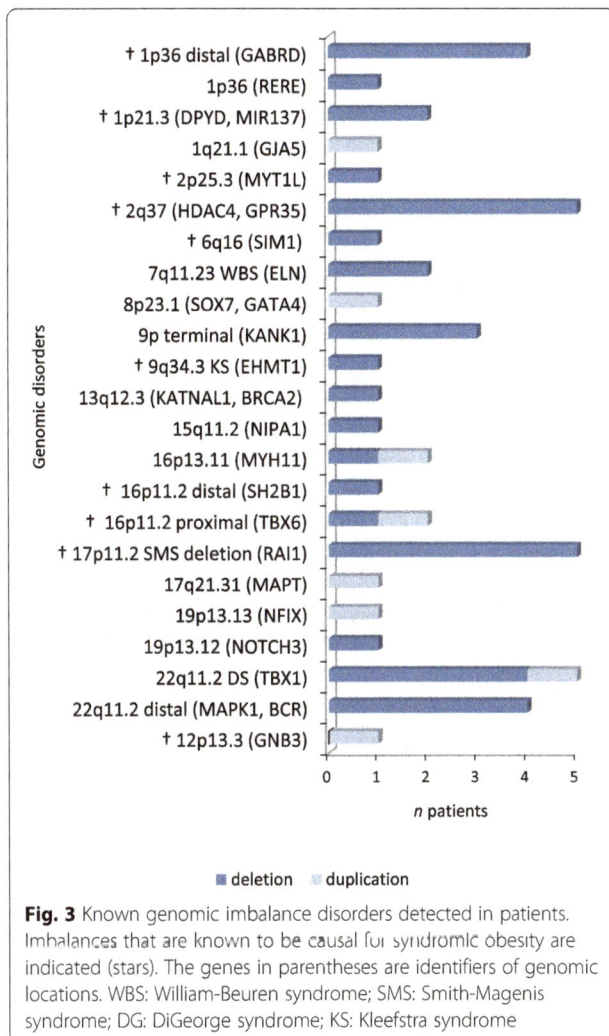

Fig. 3 Known genomic imbalance disorders detected in patients. Imbalances that are known to be causal for syndromic obesity are indicated (stars). The genes in parentheses are identifiers of genomic locations. WBS: William-Beuren syndrome; SMS: Smith-Magenis syndrome; DG: DiGeorge syndrome; KS: Kleefstra syndrome

syndromic forms of obesity were deletions of the chromosomal regions 1p36, 2q37 and 17p11.2, which collectively represented 5.4% of all cases, followed by microdeletions of the 1p21.3 region (2 cases). In 6 other syndromic obesity *loci* (2p25.3, 6q16, 9q34, 16p11.2 proximal and distal, 12p13.31), CNVs were found only in one unrelated individual. The identification of CNVs overlapping *loci* previously shown to be involved in syndromic obesity further implicates them as risk factors for obesity. As previously mentioned, *SH2B1*, *SIM1*, *PTBP2*, *PRLH*, *CAPN10*, *ACP1*, *TMEM18*, *EHMT1*, and *GNB3* are relevant candidate and known genes for obesity within these regions (Fig. 6), and *POU3F2* [20], *HDAC4* [50], *MYT1L* [52], and *RAI1* [53] were also candidate genes identified in these *loci*. Moreover, our gene prioritization analysis identified 20 new genes of interest to obesity overlapping these CNVs, among which we highlight the potential importance of *TAS1R3*, encoding a taste receptor differentially expressed in obese mice

[54]. This gene maps within the common deleted region of patients with distal 1p36 deletion.

In addition to the above, we identified 4 patients with recurrent deletions at the 22q11.2 DiGeorge syndrome (DS) region (we also found a patient with duplication of the same region), 4 patients with distal 22q11.2 recurrent deletions, and 3 patients with overlapping deletions at 9p terminal. As these CNVs arise in more than 2 unrelated individuals, we implicate them as novel *loci* with a potential role in obesity susceptibility. A link between the 22q11.2 region with obesity is also supported by previous works showing that 22q11.2DS deletion carriers have increased rates of obesity [55–57], as well as reports of patients presenting childhood obesity with hyperphagia [58, 59]. Overweight and obesity (with or without hyperphagia) have also been described in a number of patients with distal 22q11.2 deletions [60–63]. We identified 3 genes at 22q11.2 (*TBX1, COMT* and *MAPK1*) that could confer susceptibility to obesity (Fig. 6). Although obesity is not a reported feature of deletion 9p syndrome, weight ≥ 90th percentile at birth or in childhood was documented in 4 of a series of 10 patients with distal deletions of 9p [64], further emphasizing the potential importance of this region. Additionally, we recently detected a deletion at 9p24.3p24.2 in one further patient with syndromic obesity using multiplex ligation-probe amplification (unpublished data from our laboratory). The *VLDLR*, *IL33* and *PTPRD* genes were identified as the most interesting genes for obesity-susceptibility within 9p24 (Fig. 6). Furthermore, we detected 2 patients with Williams-Beuren syndrome (WBS) 7q11.23 deletions. This region was already shown to be associated with several endocrine and metabolic problems including hypothyroidism, hypercalcemia, obesity and diabetes [65, 66]. Two genes related to obesity, *STX1A* and *RFC2*, map to this CNV interval (Fig. 6).

In this study we discovered recurrent CNVs at 1q21.1 and 16p13.1, which are known predisposing factors to IDDs reported sometimes in patients exhibiting obesity [67, 68]. Moreover, CNVs at these *loci* were also documented in a cohort study of syndromic obesity [22]. We also discovered other CNVs overlapping *loci* involved in syndromic obesity cases from the literature and DECIPHER. For instance, patient 24 carry a deletion overlapping the critical region of the 13q12.3 microdeletion syndrome described by Bartholdi et al. in 3 unrelated patients, two of whom with obesity [69]. This deletion was further associated with obesity in a patient from DECHIPER (case 282,282). Five genes map to the common CNV interval (Fig. 4a), among them *ALOX5AP* whose expression was linked to obesity and insulin resistance [70]. Likewise, patient 38 carry a deletion at 19p13.12 partially overlapping with those reported in 3 patients from literature, one of them with obesity [71]. We found 2 other patients in DECIPHER with deletions at this

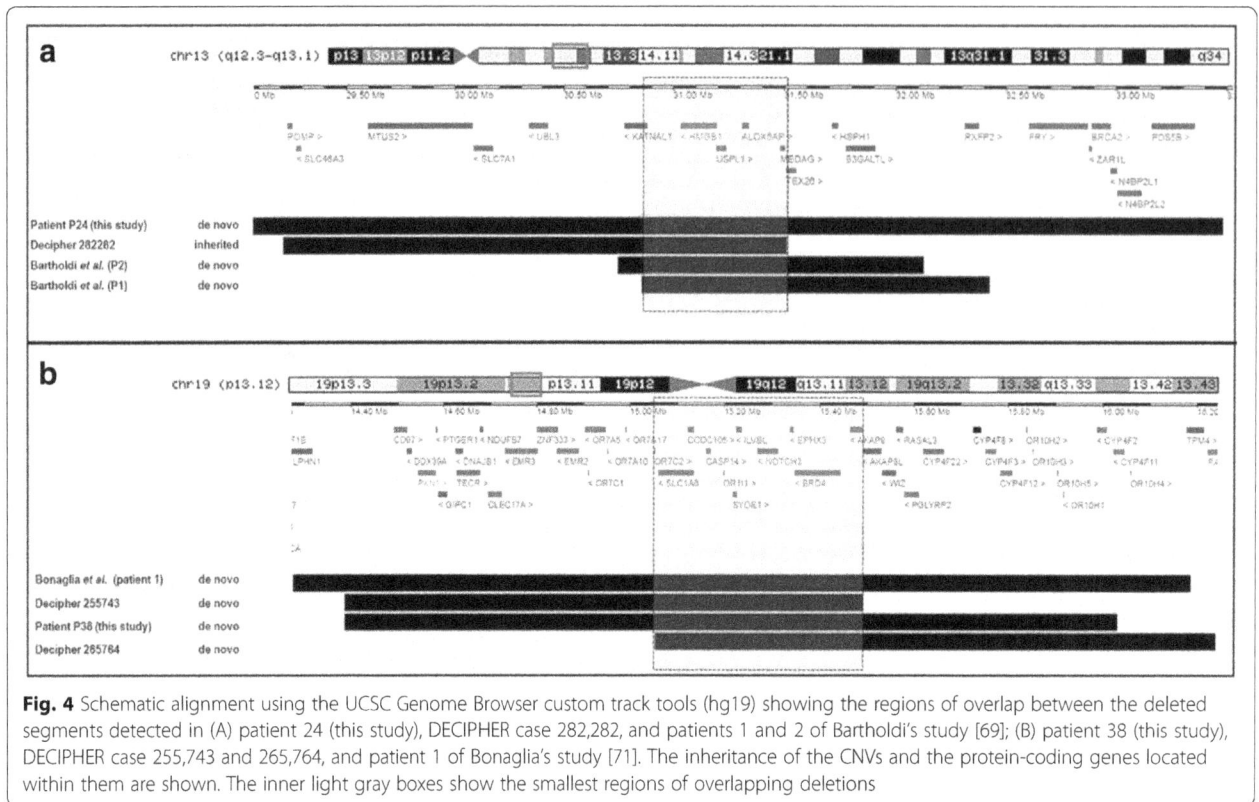

Fig. 4 Schematic alignment using the UCSC Genome Browser custom track tools (hg19) showing the regions of overlap between the deleted segments detected in (A) patient 24 (this study), DECIPHER case 282,282, and patients 1 and 2 of Bartholdi's study [69]; (B) patient 38 (this study), DECIPHER case 255,743 and 265,764, and patient 1 of Bonaglia's study [71]. The inheritance of the CNVs and the protein-coding genes located within them are shown. The inner light gray boxes show the smallest regions of overlapping deletions

locus in addition to obesity (cases 255,743 and 265,764). These cases share a 440-kb SRO encompassing 9 genes, including *NOTCH3* (Fig. 4b). The Notch signaling has recently emerged as a key player in regulating metabolism [72]. We also identified a case of 19p13.2 duplication involving the *NFIX* gene associated with a Sotos syndrome-like phenotype [73]. This CNV was associated with a 430-kb 9p22.1 duplication that encompassed the entire *PLIN2* gene, which is involved in the control of energy balance [74]. Notably, CNV in this gene has previously been identified in a patient with syndromic obesity [22].

Other than CNVs overlapping known genomic disorders *loci*, 14 patients had other chromosomal defects that are known to be clinically relevant, among which 4 overlapped with *loci* previously implicated in obesity. The distal portion of the 3q11.2q13.31 duplication in patient 49 (Fig. 5a) partially overlaps with a 2.76-Mb 3q13.31 duplication found in 2 brothers with syndromic obesity [22], and with a 9.8-Mb 3q13.13q13.32 duplication reported in association with obesity from DECIPHER (case 314,391). The common region of overlap involves 5 genes and among them *ZBTB20* is implicated in Primrose syndrome associated with several endocrine features and obesity (OMIM #259050). The large 13q11q12.3 duplication in our patient 53 (Fig. 5b) overlaps with a 1.2-Mb 13q12.12 duplication also found in our patient 19 and with another 2-Mb 13q12.11q12.12 duplication detected

among cases with moderate and extreme obesity [75]. This region involves the gene *SGCG* with expression in adipose tissues and associated with type 2 diabetes [76]. Patient 57 carry an 8.5-Mb 13q33.2q34 deletion encompassing the ID gene *CHAMP1* (Fig. 5c), which partially overlaps with deletions at 13q34 found in 6 other patients with syndromic obesity reported by Vuillaume et al. [22] and Reinstein et al. [21]. Of interest, the deleted region in each of the 7 cases overlaps the obesity-associated gene *GAS6* [77]. The 14q11.2 microduplication found in our patient 58 (Fig. 5d), including the *SUPT16H* and *CHD8* genes, was also identified in one patient with syndromic obesity reported by Vuillaume et al. [16]. No candidate genes for obesity were associated with this *locus*. Although there is one case of 14q11.2 deletion that was reported with severe obesity, it included a large more proximal segment of 14q11.2, which contains a strong obesity candidate gene [14].

Finally, in a total of 51 patients the CNVs were classified as potentially pathogenic (2.1%), VUS (4.7%) or likely benign variants (11.5%). Overall, a number of interesting genes that could play a role in obesity susceptibility have been identified within these CNVs (e.g. *ASTN2*, *APOA2*, *PARK2*, *LINGO2*, *PLCB1*, *PTEN*, and *CIDEA*). More importantly, we identified a new and de novo 340-kb 16p13.2 duplication that encompasses the entire *USP7* gene. Although its pathogenicity is not certain, since

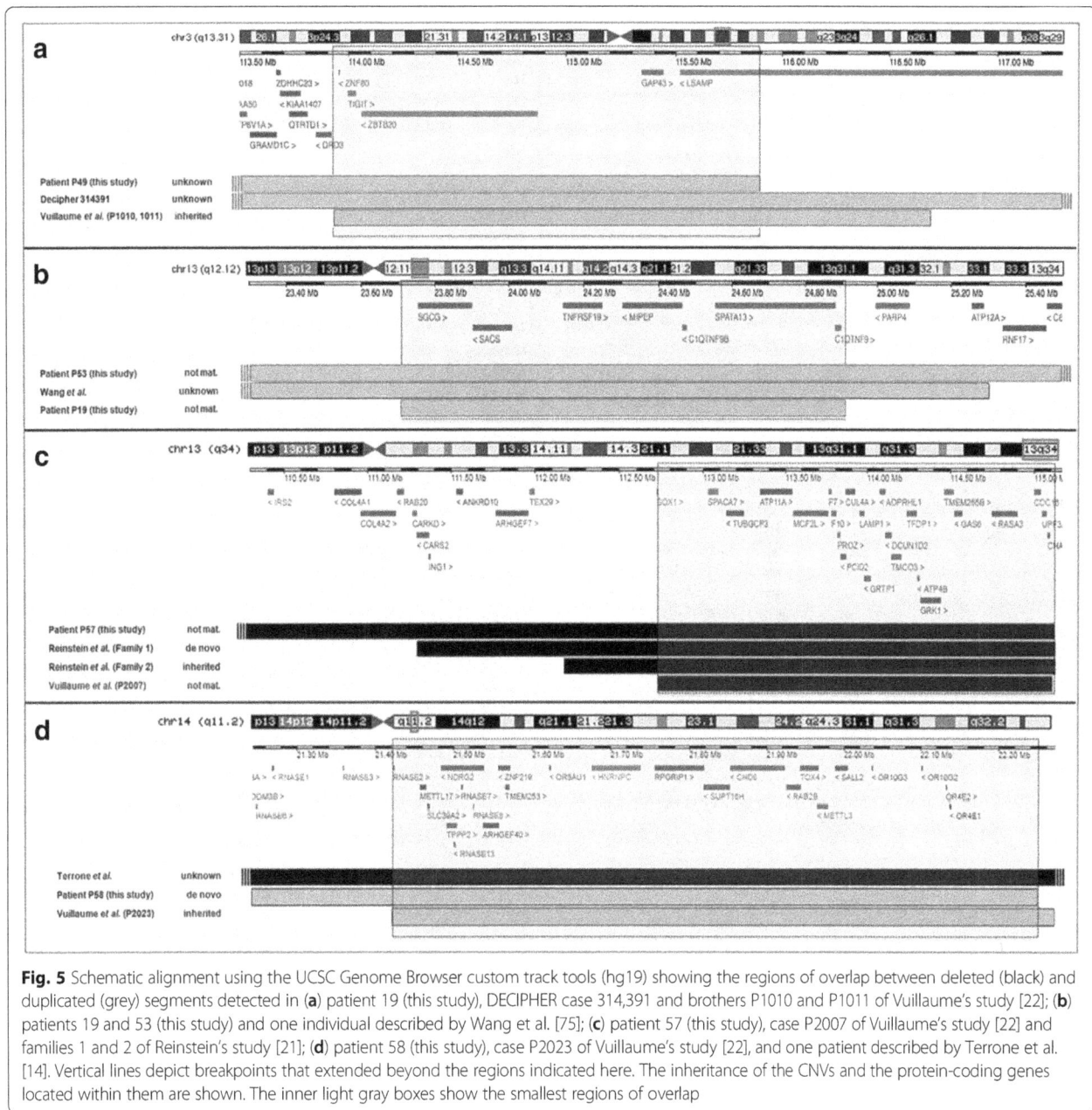

Fig. 5 Schematic alignment using the UCSC Genome Browser custom track tools (hg19) showing the regions of overlap between deleted (black) and duplicated (grey) segments detected in (**a**) patient 19 (this study), DECIPHER case 314,391 and brothers P1010 and P1011 of Vuillaume's study [22]; (**b**) patients 19 and 53 (this study) and one individual described by Wang et al. [75]; (**c**) patient 57 (this study), case P2007 of Vuillaume's study [22] and families 1 and 2 of Reinstein's study [21]; (**d**) patient 58 (this study), case P2023 of Vuillaume's study [22], and one patient described by Terrone et al. [14]. Vertical lines depict breakpoints that extended beyond the regions indicated here. The inheritance of the CNVs and the protein-coding genes located within them are shown. The inner light gray boxes show the smallest regions of overlap

similar duplications have not been reported in the literature, there is one reported patient with larger duplication at the *USP7* locus presenting with severe early-onset obesity and hyperphagia [78]. Of note, USP7 has been identified as an integral component of MAGEL2 and TRIM27 ubiquitin ligase complex, which plays an important role in hypothalamic function [79]. Moreover, deletion or mutation of *USP7* has been shown to result in a neurodevelopmental disorder with overlapping symptoms to Schaaf-Yang syndrome (OMIM #615547), caused by mutations of *MAGEL2* [78]. There are 5 de novo duplication events overlapping *USP7* (400-kb to 1.2-Mb)

reported in DECIPHER with no additional changes detected. These included 3 patients (cases 269,501, 281,449 and 258,037) with delayed speech and language development as common features and 2 patients (cases 254,000 and 267,094) with no phenotypic description. One of the limitations of our study is that additional independent risk factors were not considered, including unidentified genetic factors and those being epigenetic, environmental, or stochastic in origin. Future investigations of genes within disease-specific CNVs detected in the present cohort are also needed. Future directions will involve whole exome sequencing (WES) in patients

Position	Gene		Position	Gene
1p36.33	TAS1R3		11q23.1	IL18
1p36.33	SKI		11q23.2	DRD2
1p36.32	PRDM16		11q23.3	APOA5
1p36.22	H6PD		11q23.3	APOA4
1p21.3	PTBP2		11q23.3	APOC3
1p21.2	VCAM1		11q23.3	APOA1
1p21.1	AMY1A		11q23.3	CBL
1q23.3	APOA2 *		11q24.1	BSX
2p25.3	ACP1		11q24.3	KCNJ5
2p25.3	TMEM18		12p13.33	WNT5B
2p25.3	TPO		12p13.33	ADIPOR2
2q37.1	UGT1A1		12p13.31	TNFRSF1A
2q37.3	GPC1		12p13.31	GNB3
2q37.3	CAPN10		12q21.1	TSPAN8
2q37.3	GPR35		12q23.1	NR1H4
2q37.3	STK25		13q12.2	MTIF3
3q11.2	ARL6		13q12.2	PDX1
6q16.2	MCHR2		13q12.3	ALOX5AP
6q16.3	SIM1		13q13.1	BRCA2
6q16q21	LIN28B		13q31.3	GPC5
6q26	PARK2 *		13q34	IRS2
7q11.23	STX1A		14q12	PRKD1
7q11.23	RFC2		16p13.11	MYH11
8p23.1	DEFA1		16p11.2	ATXN2L
8p23.1	TNKS		16p11.2	TUFM
8p23.1	MSRA		16p11.2	SH2B1
8p23.1	MTMR9		16p11.2	ATP2A1
8p23.1	GATA4		17p11.2	PEMT
8p23.1	FDFT1		17p11.2	SRBEF1
9p22.1	PLIN2		17q21.31	G6PC
9p21	LINGO2 *		17q21.31	BRCA1
9p24.2	VLDLR		17q21.31	SOST
9p24.1	IL33		17q21.31	PPY
9p24p23	PTPRD		17q21.31	PYY
9q33.1	ASTN2 *		17q21.31	CRHR1
9q34.3	EHMT1		17q25.3	GCGR
10p15.3	DIP2C		17q25.3	FASN
10p15.2	PFKP		18p11.21	CIDEA *
10p15.1	IL2RA		20p12.3	PLCB1 *
10p13	PTER		22q11.2	TBX1
10q23.31	PTEN *		22q11.2	COMT
10q26.11	PRLHR		22q11.2	MAPK1
10q26.13	FGFR2		Xp22.12	PDHA1
10q26.3	CYP2E1			

Legend: ■ T-HOD ■ HUGE ■ Literature ■ CNV morbid map

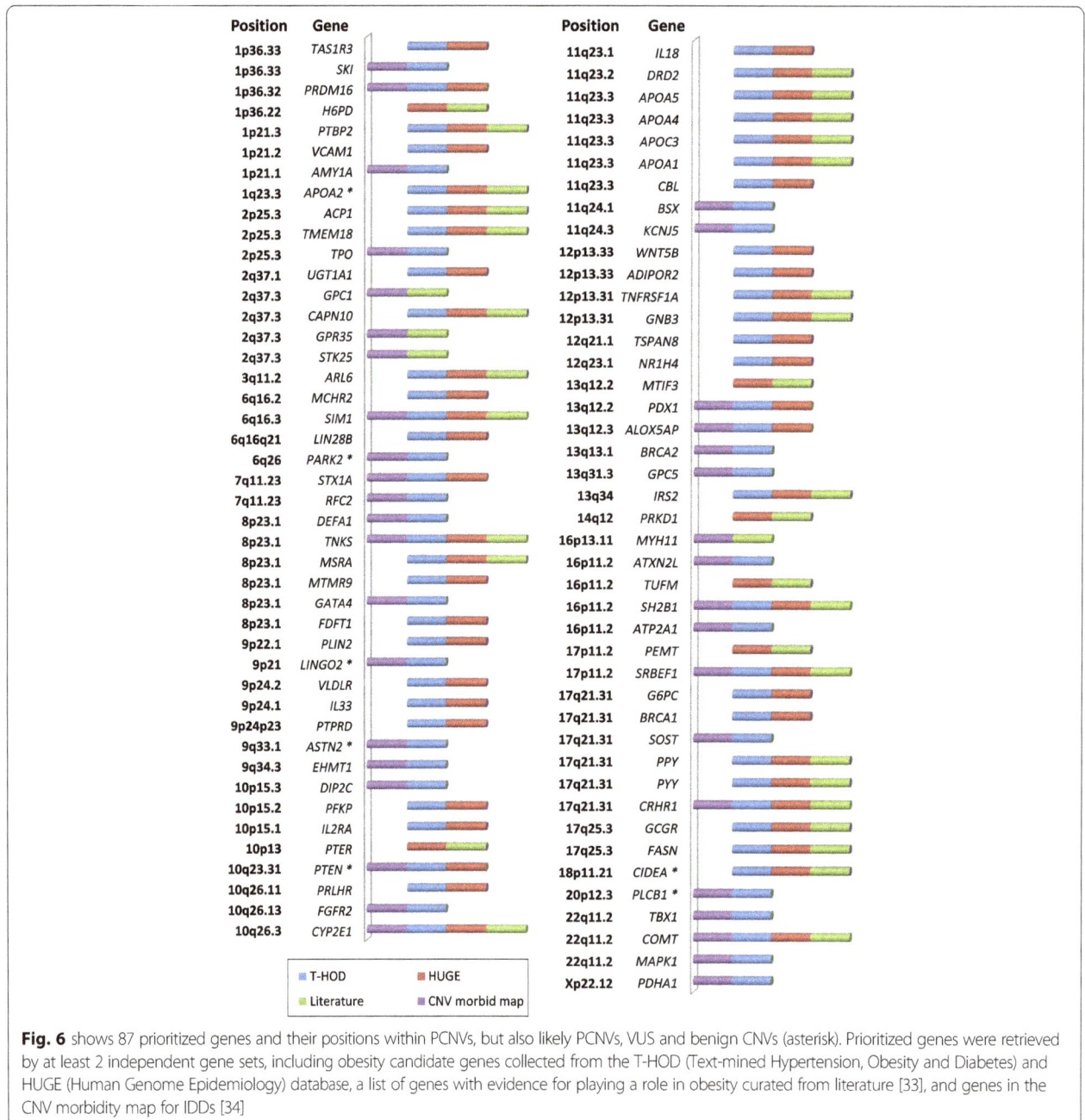

Fig. 6 shows 87 prioritized genes and their positions within PCNVs, but also likely PCNVs, VUS and benign CNVs (asterisk). Prioritized genes were retrieved by at least 2 independent gene sets, including obesity candidate genes collected from the T-HOD (Text-mined Hypertension, Obesity and Diabetes) and HUGE (Human Genome Epidemiology) database, a list of genes with evidence for playing a role in obesity curated from literature [33], and genes in the CNV morbidity map for IDDs [34]

that did not reach a diagnosis to estimate the contribution of single gene mutations in the genetic causation of syndromic obesity. This will allow isolate genes that cause or may affect susceptibility to obesity in humans, advancing our understanding of the molecular mechanisms involved in body weight regulation and provide clues for therapeutic intervention in obesity.

Conclusion
Understanding the genetics of obesity has proven difficult. Although it is likely that not all of the PCNVs

detected in the current study are directly causative of obesity, we found that 23/279 (8.2%) of our patients carried rare CNVs at 10 *loci* already known to increase the risk of obesity. We identified 3 patients with overlapping deletions at 9p terminal, 4 patients with deletions of 22q11.2DS and 4 patients with deletions at distal 22q11.2, which thus emerge as new putative obesity-susceptibility *loci*. In addition, we found that CNVs in at least 6 other cases overlapped with *loci* previously implicated in syndromic obesity, including a new patient with deletion at chromosome 13q34. This

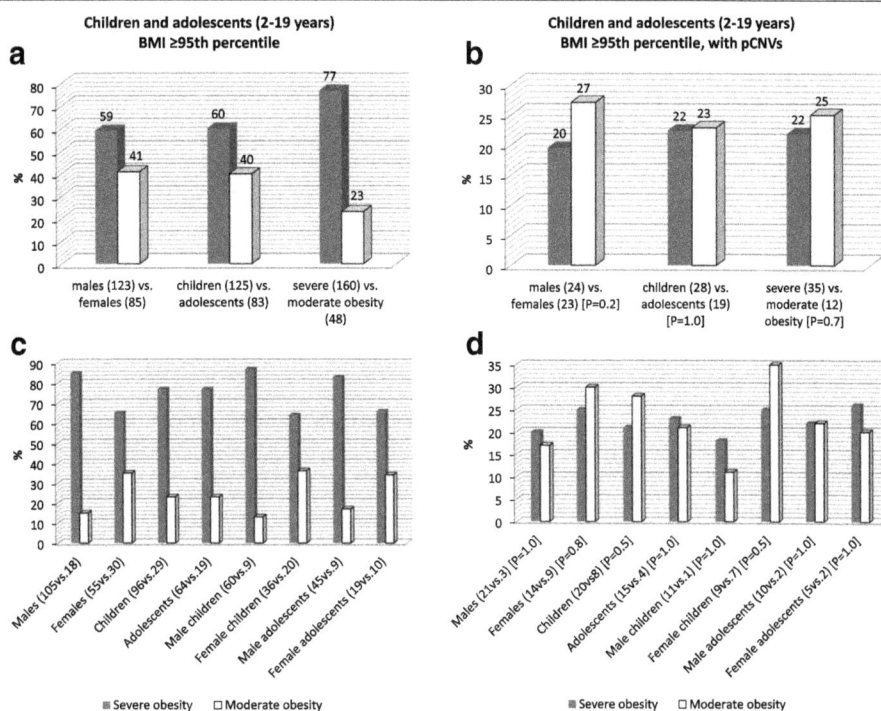

Fig. 7 (A) Frequencies of children and adolescents in the whole cohort with BMI ≥ 95th percentile stratified by gender (males and females), age groups (2–9 years and 10–19 years), and level of obesity (moderate and severe). (B) Sex- and age-related differences of children and adolescents in the whole cohort by level of obesity. (C, D) same comparisons in children and adolescents with PCNVs. The numbers in parentheses indicate the total number of patients in each group. Definition of moderate and severe obesity was based on the BMI below or above 120% of the 95th percentile. P-values for the Fisher's exact test are shown

locus is particularly interesting because our new case brings to 7 the number of patients in whom such defects have been described in association with obesity. Overall, we found CNVs that further implicate genes previously associated with obesity such as *PTBP2*, *TMEM18*, *MYT1L*, *POU3F2*, *SIM1*, *SH2B1* and *GNB3*, and also identified other potentially relevant candidate genes including *TAS1R3*, *ALOX5AP*, and *GAS6*. Our study highlights the significant value of chromosomal microarrays in providing not only a genetic diagnosis for syndromic causes of obesity but in uncovering genes relevant to human obesity.

Additional files

Additional file 1: Table S1. Full description of clinical findings in patients enrolled in this study. (XLSX 71 kb)

Additional file 2: Table S2. Frequencies of phenotypes pairs segregating together in patients with and without pCNVs. (XLSX 18 kb)

Additional file 3: Table S3. Likely PCNVs, VUS and likely benign variants detected in patients with syndromic obesity (XLSX 19 kb)

Additional file 4: Table S4. Evaluation of the level of obesity in 208 children and adolescents with BMI ≥ 95th percentile. (PDF 81 kb)

Additional file 5: Table S5. Comparison of the pCNVs rates for children and adolescents with BMI at or above the 95th percentile by age, sex and level of obesity. (PDF 81 kb)

Abbreviations
ACMG: American college of medical genetics; ASD: Autism spectrum disorder; BBS: Bardet-Biedl Syndrome; BMI: Body mass index; BP: Breakpoint; CDC: Centers for disease control and prevention; ClinGen: Clinical genome resource; CMA: Chromosomal microarray analysis; CNV: Copy number variant; COH1: Cohen syndrome; DECIPHER: DatabasE of genomiC varIation and phenotype in humans using ensembl resources; DG: DiGeorge syndrome; DGV: Database of genomic variants; HUGE: Human genome epidemiology; ID: Intellectual disability; IDD: Intellectual and developmental disabilities; ISCA: International standards for cytogenomic arrays; KS: Kleefstra syndrome; OFC: Occipitofrontal circumference; OMIM: Online mendelian inheritance in man; PCNV: Pathogenic copy number variant; PWS: Prader-Willi syndrome; SD: Standard deviation; SMS: Smith-Magenis syndrome; SRO: Smallest region of overlap; T-HOD: Text-mined hypertension, obesity and diabetes; VUS: Variants of uncertain significance; WBS: Williams-Beuren syndrome; WES: Whole-Exome sequencing

Acknowledgements
We thank the patients and their families for participating in our research studies and other clinicians for referral of patients. This study makes use of data generated by the DECIPHER community. A full list of centres who contributed to the generation of the data is available from http://decipher.sanger.ac.uk and via email from decipher@sanger.ac.uk. Funding for the project was provided by the Wellcome Trust.

Funding
This study was supported by The State of São Paulo Research Foundation, FAPESP (09/52523–1 to C.S.D.), The Centers for Research, Innovation and Diffusion, CEPID-FAPESP (1998/14254–2), and The National Council for Scientific and Technological Development, CNPq (304381/2007–1 to C.P.K.).

Authors' contributions

C.S.D. and C.P.K. designed the study. C.S.D. performed the experiments, analyzed the data and wrote the manuscript. P.A.O. conducted the statistical analyses. A.B.A.P., C.M.L., C.A.K., D.R.B., F.K. and L.G.A. are the main referring clinicians and performed the clinical assessment and physical examination of patients. M.C.V. performed the methylation analysis of the PWS chromosome region. C.S.D. collected anthropometric measurements and phenotypic data with contribution from C.I.E.C. All authors read and approved the final manuscript.

Competing interests

The authors declare that they have no competing interests.

Author details

[1]Human Genome and Stem Cell Research Center (HUG-CELL), Department of Genetics and Evolutionary Biology, Institute of Biosciences, University of Sao Paulo, Rua do Matao no 277, Cidade Universitaria-Butanta, Sao Paulo, SP 05508-090, Brazil. [2]Department of Morphology and Genetics, Paulista School of Medicine, Federal University of Sao Paulo (UNIFESP), Sao Paulo, SP, Brazil. [3]Neurogenetics Unit, Clinics Hospital of Ribeirao Preto, Faculty of Medicine, University of Sao Paulo, FMRP-USP, Ribeirao Preto, SP, Brazil. [4]Genetic Unit, Children's Institute, Faculty of Medicine, University of Sao Paulo, FMUSP, Sao Paulo, SP, Brazil. [5]Department of Neurology, Faculty of Medicine, University of Sao Paulo, FMUSP, Sao Paulo, SP, Brazil.

References

1. D'Angelo CS, Koiffmann CP. Copy Number variants in obesity-related syndromes: review and perspectives on novel molecular approaches. J Obes. 2012;2012:845480.
2. Huvenne H, Dubern B, Clément K, Poitou C. Rare genetic forms of obesity: clinical approach and current treatments in 2016. Obes Facts. 2016;9(3):158–73.
3. Pigeyre M, Yazdi FT, Kaur Y, Meyre D. Recent progress in genetics, epigenetics and metagenomics unveils the pathophysiology of human obesity. Clin Sci (Lond). 2016;130(12):943–86.
4. Davidsson J, Jahnke K, Forsgren M, Collin A, Soller M. Dup(19)(q12q13.2): array-based genotype-phenotype correlation of a new possibly obesity-related syndrome. Obesity (Silver Spring). 2010;18(3):580–7.
5. Wentzel C, Lynch SA, Stattin EL, Sharkey FH, Annerén G, Thuresson AC. Interstitial deletions at 6q14.1-q15 associated with obesity, developmental delay and a distinct clinical phenotype. Mol Syndromol. 2010;1:75–81.
6. Oexle K, Hempel M, Jauch A, Meitinger T, Rivera-Brugués N, Stengel-Rutkowski S, Strom T. 3.7 Mb tandem microduplication in chromosome 5p13.1-p13.2 associated with developmental delay, macrocephaly, obesity, and lymphedema. Further characterization of the dup(5p13) syndrome. Eur J Med Genet. 2011;54(3):225–30.
7. Halgren C, Bache I, Bak M, Myatt MW, Anderson CM, Brøndum-Nielsen K, Tommerup N. Haploinsufficiency of CELF4 at 18q12.2 is associated with developmental and behavioral disorders, seizures, eye manifestations, and obesity. Eur J Hum Genet. 2012;20(12):1315–9.
8. Vergult S, Dauber A, Delle Chiaie B, Van Oudenhove E, Simon M, Rihani A, et al. 17q24.2 microdeletions: a new syndromal entity with intellectual disability, truncal obesity, mood swings and hallucinations. Eur J Hum Genet. 2012;20:534–9.
9. Shichiji M, Ito Y, Shimojima K, Nakamu H, Oguni H, Osawa M, Yamamoto T. A cryptic microdeletion including MBD5 occurring within the breakpoint of a reciprocal translocation between chromosomes 2 and 5 in a patient with developmental delay and obesity. Am J Med Genet A. 2013;161A(4):850–5.
10. Bonaglia MC, Giorda R, Zanini S. A new patient with a terminal de novo 2p25.3 deletion of 1.9 Mb associated with early-onset of obesity, intellectual disabilities and hyperkinetic disorder. Mol Cytogenet. 2014;7:53.
11. Courage C, Houge G, Gallati S, Schjelderup J, Rieubland C. 15q26.1 microdeletion encompassing only CHD2 and RGMA in two adults with moderate intellectual disability, epilepsy and truncal obesity. Eur J Med Genet. 2014;57:520–3.
12. Doco-Fenzy M, Leroy C, Schneider A, Petit F, Delrue MA, Andrieux J, et al. Early-onset obesity and paternal 2pter deletion encompassing the ACP1, TMEM18, and MYT1L genes. Eur J Hum Genet. 2014;22:471–9.
13. Kuroda Y, Ohashi I, Tominaga M, Saito T, Nagai J, Ida K, et al. De novo duplication of 17p13.1-p13.2 in a patient with intellectual disability and obesity. Am J Med Genet A. 2014;164A(6):1550–4.
14. Terrone G, Cappuccio G, Genesio R, Esposito A, Fiorentino V, Riccitelli M, et al. A case of 14q11.2 microdeletion with autistic features, severe obesity and facial dysmorphisms suggestive of wolf-Hirschhorn syndrome. Am J Med Genet A. 2014;164A(1):190–3.
15. Desch L, Marle N, Mosca-Boidron A-L, Faivre L, Eliade M, Payet M, et al. 6q16.3q23.3 duplication associated with Prader-Willi-like syndrome. Mol Cytogenet. 2015;8:42.
16. Biamino E, Di Gregorio E, Belligni EF, Keller R, Riberi E, Gandione M, et al. A novel 3q29 deletion associated with autism, intellectual disability, psychiatric disorders, and obesity. Am J Med Genet B. 2016;171B:290–9.
17. Goldlust IS, Hermetz KE, Catalano LM, Barfield RT, Cozad R, Wynn G, et al. Mouse model implicates GNB3 duplication in a childhood obesity syndrome. Proc Natl Acad Sci U S A. 2013;110:14990–4.
18. Carter MT, Nikkel SM, Fernandez BA, Marshall CR, Noor A, Lionel AC, et al. Hemizygous deletions on chromosome 1p21.3 involving the DPYD gene in individuals with autism spectrum disorder. Clin Genet. 2011;80(5):435–43.
19. Willemsen MH, Valls A, Kirkels LA, Mastebroek M, Loohuis N, Kos A, et al. Chromosome 1p21.3 microdeletions comprising DPYD and MIR137 are associated with intellectual disability. J Med Genet. 2011;48:810–8.
20. Kasher PR, Schertz KE, Thomas M, Jackson A, Annunziata S, Ballesta-Martinez MJ, et al. Small 6q16.1 deletions encompassing POU3F2Cause susceptibility to obesity and variable developmental delay with intellectual disability. Am J Hum Genet. 2016;98(2):363–72.
21. Reinstein E, Liberman M, Feingold-Zadok M, Tenne T, Graham JM Jr. Terminal microdeletions of 13q34 chromosome region in patients with intellectual disability: delineation of an emerging new microdeletion syndrome. Mol Genet Metab. 2016;118(1):60–3.
22. Vuillaume ML, Naudion S, Banneau G, Diene G, Cartault A, Cailley D, et al. New candidate loci identified by array-CGH in a cohort of 100 children presenting with syndromic obesity. Am J Med Genet A. 2014;164A:1965–75.
23. Kuczmarski RJ, Ogden CL, Grummer-Strawn LM, Flegal KM, Guo SS, Wei R, et al. CDC growth charts: United States. Adv Data. 2000;314:1–27.
24. Flegal KM, Wei R, Ogden CL, Freedman DS, Johnson CL, Curtin LR. Characterizing extreme values of body mass index-for-age by using the 2000 Centers for Disease Control and Prevention growth charts. Am J Clin Nutr. 2009;90(5):1314–20.
25. Gulati AK, Kaplan DW, Daniels SR. Clinical tracking of severely obese children: a new growth chart. Pediatrics. 2012;130(6):1136–40.
26. Kearney HM, Thorland EC, Brown KK, Quintero-Rivera F, South ST. American College of Medical Genetics standards and guidelines for interpretation and reporting of postnatal constitutional copy number variants. Genet Med. 2011;13(7):680–5.
27. MacDonald JR, Ziman R, Yuen RK, Feuk L, Scherer SW. The database of genomic variants: a curated collection of structural variation in the human genome. Nucleic Acids Res. 2014;42(Database issue):D986–92.
28. Hamosh A, Scott AF, Amberger J, Valle D, McKusick VA. Online Mendelian inheritance in man (OMIM). Hum Mutat. 2000;15(1):57–61.
29. Firth HV, Richards SM, Bevan AP, Clayton S, Corpas M, Rajan D, et al. DECIPHER: database of chromosomal imbalance and phenotype in humans using Ensembl resources. Am J Hum Genet. 2009;84(4):524–33.
30. Kent WJ, Sugnet CW, Furey TS, Roskin KM, Pringle TH, Zahler AM, Haussler D. The human genome browser at UCSC. Genome Res. 2002;12(6):996–1006.
31. Dai HJ, Wu JC, Tsai RT, Pan WH, Hsu WL. T-HOD: a literature-based candidate gene database for hypertension, database (Oxford) 2013; 2013. p. bas061.
32. Yu W, Clyne M, Khoury MJ, Gwinn M. Phenopedia and Genopedia: disease-centered and gene-centered views of the evolving knowledge of human genetic associations. Bioinformatics. 2010;26(1):145–6.
33. Butler MG, McGuire A, Manzardo AM. Clinically relevant known and candidate genes for obesity and their overlap with human infertility and reproduction. J Assist Reprod Genet. 2015;32(4):495–508.
34. Coe BP, Witherspoon K, Rosenfeld JA, van Bon BW, Vulto-van Silfhout AT, Bosco P, et al. Refining analyses of copy number variation identifies specific genes associated with developmental delay. Nat Genet. 2014;46:1063–71.
35. Lopes CT, Franz M, Kazi F, Donaldson SL, Morris Q, Bader GD. Cytoscape web: an interactive web-based network browser. Bioinformatics. 2010; 15(18)):2347–8.

36. D'Angelo CS, Kohl I, Varela MC, de Castro CI, Kim CA, Bertola DR, et al. Obesity with associated developmental delay and/or learning disability in patients exhibiting additional features: report of novel pathogenic copy number variants. Am J Med Genet A. 2013;161A:479–86.

37. D'Angelo CS, Varela MC, de Castro CI, Kim CA, Bertola DR, Lourenço CM, et al. Investigation of selected genomic deletions and duplications in a cohort of 338 patients presenting with syndromic obesity by multiplex ligation-dependent probe amplification using synthetic probes. Mol Cytogenet. 2014;7:75.

38. D'Angelo CS, Moller dos Santos MF, Alonso LG, Koiffmann CP. Two new cases of 1p21.3 deletions and an unbalanced translocation t(8;12) among individuals with Syndromic obesity. Mol Syndromol. 2015;6(2):63–70.

39. Avila M, Kirchhoff M, Marle N, Hove HD, Chouchane M, Thauvin-Robinet C, et al. Delineation of a new chromosome 20q11.2 duplication syndrome including the ASXL1 gene. Am J Med Genet A. 2013;161A(7):1594–8.

40. Gimelli S, Capra V, Di Rocco M, Leoni M, Mirabelli-Badenier M, Schiaffino MC, et al. Interstitial 7q31.1 copy number variations disrupting IMMP2L gene are associated with a wide spectrum of neurodevelopmental disorders. Mol Cytogenet. 2014;7:54.

41. Lionel AC, Tammimies K, Vaags AK, Rosenfeld JA, Ahn JW, Merico D, et al. Disruption of the ASTN2/TRIM32 locus at 9q33.1 is a risk factor in males for autism spectrum disorders, ADHD and other neurodevelopmental phenotypes. Hum Mol Genet. 2014;23(10):2752–68.

42. Vergult S, Dheedene A, Meurs A, Faes F, Isidor B, Janssens S, et al. Genomic aberrations of the CACNA2D1 gene in three patients with epilepsy and intellectual disability. Eur J Hum Genet. 2015;23(5):628–32.

43. Jones RM, Cadby G, Blangero J, Abraham LJ, Whitehouse AJ, Moses EK. MACROD2 gene associated with autistic-like traits in a general population sample. Psychiatr Genet. 2014;24(6):241–8.

44. Matsunami N, Hadley D, Hensel CH, Christensen GB, Kim C, Frackelton E, et al. Identification of rare recurrent copy number variants in high-risk autism families and their prevalence in a large ASD population. PLoS One. 2013;8: e52239.

45. Rehm HL, Berg JS, Brooks LD, Bustamante CD, Evans JP, Landrum MJ, et al. ClinGen-the clinical genome resource. N Engl J Med. 2015;372:2235–42.

46. Lang B, Pu J, Hunter I, Liu M, Martin-Granados C, Reilly TJ, et al. Recurrent deletions of ULK4 in schizophrenia: a gene crucial for neuritogenesis and neuronal motility. J Cell Sci. 2014 Feb 1;127(Pt 3):630–40.

47. Neale BM, Kou Y, Liu L, Ma'ayan A, Samocha KE, Sabo A, et al. Patterns and rates of exonic de novo mutations in autism spectrum disorders. Nature. 2012 Apr 4;485(7397):242–5.

48. Bonnefond A, Raimondo A, Stutzmann F, Ghoussaini M, Ramachandrappa S, Bersten DC, et al. Loss-of-function mutations in SIM1 contribute to obesity and Prader-Willi-like features. J Clin Invest. 2013;123(7):3037–41.

49. Doche ME, Bochukova EG, Su HW, Pearce LR, Keogh JM, Henning E, et al. Human SH2B1 mutations are associated with maladaptive behaviors and obesity. J Clin Invest. 2012;122:4732–6.

50. Leroy C, Landais E, Briault S, David A, Tassy O, Gruchy N, et al. The 2q37-deletion syndrome: an update of the clinical spectrum including overweight, brachydactyly and behavioural features in 14 new patients. Eur J Hum Genet. 2013;21:602–12.

51. Willemsen MH, Vulto-van Silfhout AT, Nillesen WM, Wissink-Lindhout WM, van Bokhoven H, Philip N, et al. Update on Kleefstra Syndrome. Mol Syndromol. 2012;2(3–5):202–12.

52. De Rocker N, Vergult S, Koolen D, Jacobs E, Hoischen A, Zeesman S, et al. Refinement of the critical 2p25.3 deletion region: the role of MYT1L in intellectual disability and obesity. Genet Med. 2015;17:460–6.

53. Burns B, Schmidt K, Williams SR, Kim S, Girirajan S, Elsea SH. Rai1 haploinsufficiency causes reduced Bdnf expression resulting in hyperphagia, obesity and altered fat distribution in mice and humans with no evidence of metabolic syndrome. Hum Mol Genet. 2010;19:4026–42.

54. Kogelman LJA, Zhernakova DV, Westra H-J, Cirera S, Fredholm M, Franke L, Kadarmideen HN. An integrative systems genetics approach reveals potential causal genes and pathways related to obesity. Genome Med. 2015;7:105.

55. Bassett AS, Chow EW, Husted J, Weksberg R, Caluseriu O, Webb GD, Gatzoulis MA. Clinical features of 78 adults with 22q11 deletion syndrome. Am J Med Genet A. 2005;138(4):307–13.

56. Bassett AS, McDonald-McGinn DM, Devriendt K, Digilio MC, Goldenberg P, Habel A, et al. Practical guidelines for managing patients with 22q11.2 deletion syndrome. J Pediatr. 2011;159(2):332–9.

57. Voll SL, Boot E, Butcher NJ, Cooper S, Heung T, Chow EW, et al. Obesity in adults with 22q11.2 deletion syndrome. Genet Med. 2016; https://doi.org/10.1038/gim.2016.98.

58. D'Angelo CS, Jehee FS, Koiffmann CP. An inherited atypical 1 Mb 22q11.2 deletion within the DGS/VCFS 3 Mb region in a child with obesity and aggressive behavior. Am J Med Genet A. 2007;143A:1928–32.

59. Bassett JK, Chandler KE, Douzgou S. Two patients with chromosome 22q11.2 deletion presenting with childhood obesity and hyperphagia. Eur J Med Genet. 2016;59(8):401–3.

60. Mikhail FM, Descartes M, Piotrowski A, Andersson R, Diaz de Ståhl T, Komorowski J, et al. A previously unrecognized microdeletion syndrome on chromosome 22 band q11.2 encompassing the BCR gene. Am J Med Genet A. 2007;43A(18):2178–84.

61. Ben-Shachar S, Ou Z, Shaw CA, Belmont JW, Patel MS, Hummel M, et al. 22q11.2 distal deletion: a recurrent genomic disorder distinct from DiGeorge syndrome and velocardiofacial syndrome. Am J Hum Genet. 2008;82:214–21.

62. Fagerberg CR, Graakjaer J, Heinl UD, Ousager LB, Dreyer I, Kirchhoff M, et al. Heart defects and other features of the 22q11 distal deletion syndrome. Eur J Med Genet. 2013;56(2):98–107.

63. Mikhail FM, Burnside RD, Rush B, Ibrahim J, Godshalk R, Rutledge SL, et al. The recurrent distal 22q11.2 microdeletions are often de novo and do not represent a single clinical entity: a proposed categorization system. Genet Med. 2013;16(1):92–100.

64. Hauge X, Raca G, Cooper S, May K, Spiro R, Adam M, Martin L. Detailed characterization of and clinical correlations in ten patients with distal deletions of chromosome 9p. Genet Med. 2008;10(8):599–611.

65. Pober BR. Williams-Beuren syndrome. New Eng J Med. 2010;362:239–52.

66. Stagi S, Lapi E, Cecchi C, Chiarelli F, D'Avanzo MG, Seminara S, et al. Williams-Beuren syndrome is a genetic disorder associated with impaired glucose tolerance and diabetes in childhood and adolescence. New insights from a longitudinal study. Horm Res Pediatr. 2014;82:38–43.

67. Tropeano M, Ahn JW, Dobson RJB, Breen G, Rucker J, Dixit A, et al. Male-Biased Autosomal Effect of 16p13.11 Copy Number Variation in Neurodevelopmental Disorders. PLoS One. 2013;8(4):e61365.

68. Dolcetti A, Silversides CK, Marshall CR, Lionel AC, Stavropoulos DJ, Scherer SW, Bassett AS. 1q21.1 microduplication expression in adults. Genet Med. 2013;15:282–9.

69. Bartholdi D, Stray-Pedersen A, Azzarello-Burri S, Kibaek M, Kirchhoff M, Oneda B, et al. A newly recognized 13q12.3 microdeletion syndrome characterized by intellectual disability, microcephaly, and eczema/atopic dermatitis encompassing the HMGB1 and KATNAL1 genes. Am J Med Genet A. 2014;164A(5):1277–83.

70. Kaaman M, Ryden M, Axelsson T, Nordstrom E, Sicard A, Bouloumie A, et al. ALOX5AP expression, but not gene haplotypes, is associated with obesity and insulin resistance. Int J Obes. 2006;30:447–52.

71. Bonaglia MC, Marelli S, Novara F, Commodaro S, Borgatti R, Minardo G, et al. Genotype–phenotype relationship in three cases with overlapping 19p13.12 microdeletions. Eur J Hum Genet. 2010;18(12):1302–9.

72. Bi P, Kuang S. Notch signaling as a novel regulator of metabolism. Trends Endocrinol Metab. 2015;26(5):248–55.

73. Lehman AM, du Souich C, Chai D, Eydoux P, Huang JL, Fok AK, et al. 19p13.2 microduplication causes a Sotos syndrome-like phenotype and alters gene expression. Clin Genet. 2010;81:56–63.

74. McManaman JL, Bales ES, Orlicky DJ, Jackman M, MacLean PS, Cain S, et al. Perilipin-2-null mice are protected against diet-induced obesity, adipose inflammation, and fatty liver disease. J Lipid Res. 2013;54(5):1346–59.

75. Wang K, Li WD, Glessner JT, Grant SF, Hakonarson H, Price RA. Large copy-number variations are enriched in cases with moderate to extreme obesity. Diabetes. 2010;59(10):2690–4.

76. Saxena R, Saleheen D, Been LF, Garavito ML, Braun T, Bjonnes A, et al. Genome-wide association study identifies a novel locus contributing to type 2 diabetes susceptibility in Sikhs of Punjabi origin from India. Diabetes. 2013;62:1746–55.

77. Wu K-S, Hung Y-J, Lee C-H, Hsiao F-C, Hsieh P-S. The involvement of GAS6 signaling in the development of obesity and associated inflammation. Int J Endocrinol. 2015;2015:202513.

78. Tassano E, Alpigiani MG, Calcagno A, Salvati P, De Miglio L, Fiorio P, Gimelli G. Clinical and molecular delineation of a 16p13.2p13.13 microduplication. Eur J Med Genet. 2015;58(3):194–8.

2

Characterization of chromosome composition of sugarcane in nobilization by using genomic in situ hybridization

Fan Yu[1], Ping Wang[1], Xueting Li[1], Yongji Huang[1], Qinnan Wang[2], Ling Luo[1], Yanfen Jing[3], Xinlong Liu[3], Zuhu Deng[1,4*], Jiayun Wu[2], Yongqing Yang[1], Rukai Chen[1], Muqing Zhang[4] and Liangnian Xu[1*]

Abstract

Background: Interspecific hybridization is an effective strategy for germplasm innovation in sugarcane. Nobilization refers to the breeding theory of development and utilization of wild germplasm. *Saccharum spontaneum* is the main donor of resistance and adaptive genes in the nobilization breeding process. Chromosome transfer in sugarcane is complicated; thus, research of different inheritance patterns can provide guidance for optimal sugarcane breeding.

Results: Through chromosome counting and genomic in situ hybridization, we found that six clones with 80 chromosomes were typical *S. officinarum* and four other clones with more than 80 chromosomes were interspecific hybrids between *S. officinarum* and *S. spontaneum*. These data support the classical view that *S. officinarum* is characterized by 2n = 80. In addition, genomic in situ hybridization showed that five F$_1$ clones were products of a 2n + n transmission and one F$_1$ clone was the product of an n + n transmission in clear pedigree noble hybrids between *S. officinarum* and *S. spontaneum*. Interestingly, Yacheng 75–408 and Yacheng 75–409 were the sibling lines of the F$_1$ progeny from the same parents but with different genetic transmissions.

Conclusions: This is the first clear evidence of Loethers, Crystallina, Luohanzhe, Vietnam Niuzhe, and Nanjian Guozhe were typical *S. officinarum* by GISH. Furthermore, for the first time, we identified the chromosome transmission of six F$_1$ hybrids between *S. officinarum* and *S. spontaneum*. These findings may provide a theoretical basis for germplasm innovation in sugarcane breeding and guidance for further sugarcane nobilization.

Keywords: *Saccharum officinarum*, *Saccharum spontaneum*, Interspecific hybridization, Genomic in situ hybridization (GISH), Chromosome transmission

Background

Sugarcane, which belongs to the genus *Saccharum* in the family *Poaceae* and the tribe *Andropogoneae*, is related to *Miscanthus*, *Sclerostachya*, *Erianthus*, and *Narenga*, and constitutes the *Saccharum* complex. The genus *Saccharum* comprises six species, including *Saccharum officinarum*, *Saccharum robustum*, *Saccharum spontaneum*, *Saccharum sinense*, *Saccharum barberi*, and *Saccharum edule* [1]. Of these, *S. spontaneum* and *S. robustum* are considered to be wild species, as the

others have been cultivated [2]. Except for *S. edule*, five other native species, including *S. officinarum* (2n = 80) and *S. spontaneum* (2n = 40–128), have played an important role in sugarcane breeding [1]. *S. officinarum* (which is referred as "noble" cane) is essential for sugarcane breeding program, as it is the main source of alleles controlling high sugar content and almost all modern sugarcane cultivars contain its lineage [3]. Typically, *S. officinarum* have 2n = 80 chromosomes [4], with a basic chromosome number of x = 10 [5]. *S. spontaneum* is a wild species characterized by high stress-resistance, and then is the most valuable wild germplasm resources in the genus *Saccharum* [6]. It has a wide range of chromosome numbers, ranging from 2n = 40 to 128 [7, 8].

* Correspondence: xuliangnian@163.com; dengzuhu@163.com
[1]National Engineering Research Center for Sugarcane, Fujian Agriculture and Forestry University, Fuzhou, China
Full list of author information is available at the end of the article

Recently, research on *S. sinense* and *S. barberi* has shown that they are derived from natural interspecific hybridization between *S. officinarum* and *S. spontaneum* [9]. Furthermore, all modern sugarcane cultivars were hybrids between *S. officinarum* and *S. spontaneum* in the twentieth century [10]. The first artificial interspecific hybrids between these two species were created to overcome disease outbreaks and were followed by repeated backcrossing using *S. officinarum* as the recurrent female parent to restore high sucrose content. This procedure is referred as "nobilization".

Interspecific hybridization is an innovative and effective method for sugarcane breeding. This strategy allows for increasing stress-resistance from *S. spontaneum*, as well as maintaining high sugar genes from *S. officinarum*, which promote the genetic improvement process [3]. Through the process of sugarcane nobilization, utilization of diverse clones of *S. officinarum* and *S. spontaneum* has been proposed as a way to introduce genetic diversity [11, 12]. While a large number of germplasm resources are available for exploitation, a limited understanding of the quantitative aspects of nobilization makes the parent selection process for nobilization difficult. In 1922, Bremer discovered the classical cytological peculiarity of 2n chromosome transmission from *S. officinarum* in interspecific crosses with *S. spontaneum* [5]. Later studies verified his work and further demonstrated that the same process occurs in BC_1 when *S. officinarum* is used as the female parent [13]. Endoduplication, or fusion of two nuclei following the second meiosis, has been proposed by Bhat and Gill to explain this peculiar chromosome transmission [14]. However, Roach found that n + n transmission occurs in crosses between *S. officinarum* and *S. spontaneum* with 2n = 80, but seldom occurs in crosses between *S. officinarum* and *S. spontaneum* with 2n = 64 or 96 [15].

Modern sugarcane cultivars are derived from intercrossing between the first nobilized hybrids of a few parental clones with chromosome numbers ranging from 100 to 130, approximately 10% of which originating from *S. spontaneum* [5, 15]. The accurate number of *S. spontaneum* chromosomes in the different cultivars is not completely understood, as is their segregation during successive crosses. This problem impedes our understanding of the exact genetic contribution of *S. spontaneum* to sugarcane cultivars. To innovate germplasm in sugarcane breeding, study on chromosome composition of the progenies between *S. officinarum* and *S. spontaneum* in sufficient early generation is needed. Genomic in situ hybridization (GISH) is a highly efficient molecular cytogenetic tool that takes genomic DNA from one species as the labelled probe in hybridization experiments to chromosomal DNA in situ [16, 17]. The technique is mainly used to identify chromosome

recombination, genetic relationship of interspecific hybrids, and chromosome transmission [5, 18]. To date, many researches had verified the accuracy and high-efficiency of the GISH technology in studying the chromosome composition and chromosomal translocation in a wide range of natural allopolyploids or artificial polyploidy progenies [19–22]. D'Hont et al., for the first time, demonstrated that GISH can be used to differentiate parental chromosomes in interspecific hybrids between BNS 3066 (*S. officinarum*) and SES 14 (*S. spontaneum*) [5, 18]; in addition, they identified n + n transmission of parental chromosomes in the interspecific F_1 between *S. officinarum* and *S. spontaneum*. They also analyzed chromosomes of cultivar "R570" and found that approximately 10% originated from *S. spontaneum* and another approximately 10% were recombinant chromosomes, demonstrating that exchanges had occurred between chromosomes derived from *S. officinarum* and *S. spontaneum*. Recently, George Piperidis et al. used GISH to identify the occurrence of 2n + n transmission in crosses and the first backcrosses of *S. officinarum* and *S. spontaneum* [4]. GISH was also applied to identify parental genomes of an intergeneric hybrid between *S. officinarum* and a related wild species, *Erianthus arundinaceus*. These studies confirmed that the F_1 and BC_2 crosses resulted from an n + n chromosome transmission, while the BC_1 cross resulted from a 2n + n transmission [23].

To date, most modern sugarcane cultivars are derived from a few clones of *S. officinarum*. The limited number of parents have leaded to narrow genetic background of sugarcane, various *S. officinarum* should be identified for germplasm innovation. Additionally, clear chromosome composition of early progeny between *S. officinarum* and *S. spontaneum* will provide enough valid germplasm for further sugarcane nobilization. The aim of the present study was to verify the authenticity of ten clones classified as *S. officinarum* via chromosome counting and GISH. Six clear pedigree noble F_1 chromosome constitutions were analyzed using GISH. Our results will be applied to select the purest *S. officinarum* and valid germplasm for sugarcane breeding.

Results

Chromosome counting for identification of the authenticity of *S. officinarum*

We obtained chromosome preparations suitable for counting chromosomes in ten clones classified as *S. officinarum* (Table 2). The chromosomes were well spread with little cytoplasm background in all materials. Partial results are shown in Fig. 1, the rest results are shown in Additional file 1: Figure S1. The modal number of chromosomes for Muckche, Canablanca, 50uahapele, and Baimeizhe was 2n > 80, ranging from 86 to 114

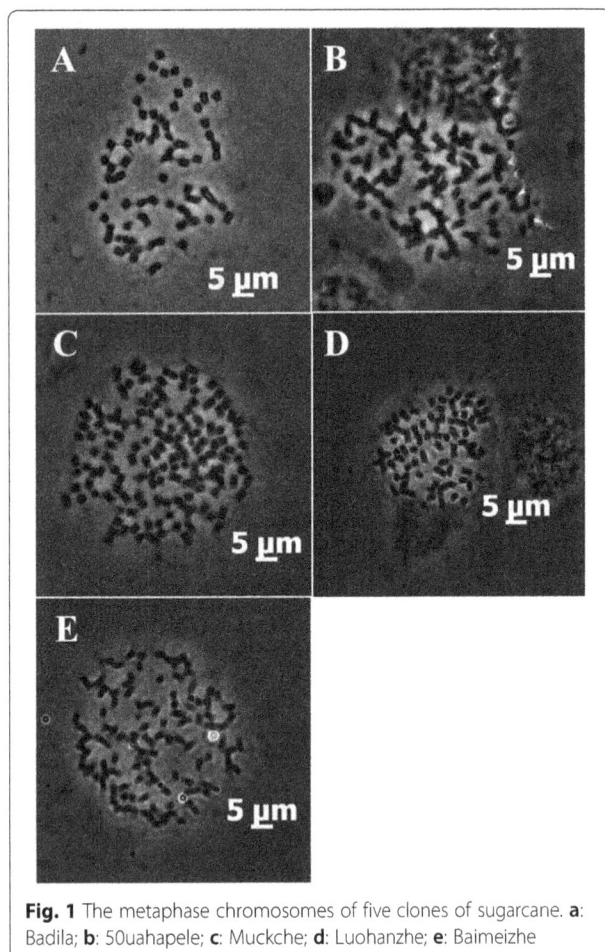

Fig. 1 The metaphase chromosomes of five clones of sugarcane. **a**: Badila; **b**: 50uahapele; **c**: Muckche; **d**: Luohanzhe; **e**: Baimeizhe

(Table 2); however, in others six clones the chromosome modal number was 2n = 80.

GISH for identification of the authenticity of *S. officinarum*
GISH was carried out on the metaphase chromosomes of ten clones classed as *S. officinarum*. In chromosomes, sequences homologous to *S. officinarum* total DNA fluoresced red and sequences homologous to *S. spontaneum* total DNA fluoresced green. However, due to the high homology of *S. officinarum* and *S. spontaneum* genomes, *S. officinarum*-derived and *S. spontaneum*-derived chromosomes were visualized in orange-yellow and green-yellow, respectively. The chromosomes of ten clones classed as *S. officinarum* were labeled in orange-yellow and green-yellow, respectively. The fluorescence of the two groups of chromosomes were differentially enhanced where their sequences were different, orange or green (Fig. 2d, e, f, and j).

In Badila, Loethers, Crystallina, Luohanzhe, Vietnam Niuzhe, and Nanjian Guozhe clones, all chromosomes fluoresced orange-yellow, indicating that the red signals were stronger than the green signals (Fig 2a, b, c, g, h, and i). These materials derived from only *S. officinarum* lineage.

However, according to the color, the chromosomes of Muckche, Canablanca, 50uahapele, and Baimeizhe can be identified as two groups, orange-yellow and green-yellow (Fig 2d, e, f, and j). These orange-yellow chromosomes were derived from *S. officinarum*. While, the rest chromosomes fluoresced green-yellow were derived from *S. spontaneum*. Thus, these materials were hybrids between *S. officinarum* and *S. spontaneum*.

GISH of F_1 hybrids between *S. officinarum* and *S. spontaneum*
In the six F_1 hybrids analyzed, five F_1 hybrids, including Yacheng 82–108, Yacheng 58–43, Yacheng 58–47, Yacheng 75–409, and Yacheng 75–419, had 2n = 112 or 120, of which 80 were derived from the *S. officinarum* female parent, and $n = 32$ or $n = 40$ derived from the male parents of *S. spontaneum*, being consistent with a typical 2n + n transmission of parental chromosomes (Table 3; Fig. 3a, b, c, d, f). However, Yacheng75–408, a sibling line of Yacheng 75–409 from the same parental combination, had 2n = 80, of which 40 were derived from the *S. officinarum* female parent and the other 40 were derived from the *S. spontaneum* male parent (Table 3; Fig. 3e). Therefore, Yacheng 75–408 is consistent with an n + n transmission of parental chromosomes.

Discussion
The authenticity of *S. officinarum*
Modern sugarcane cultivars have complex and unique genome structures and variable chromosome numbers. *S. officinarum*, which includes Badila, Black Cheribon, Crystallina, and Otaheite, has 2n = 80 chromosomes [24]; those with more than 80 chromosomes are likely to be hybrids [13, 24]. Badila is commonly used for sugarcane breeding and sugar production. Previous studies have indicated that of 31 clones in New Guinea, 29 were typical clones with chromosome number of 2n = 80 and two were atypical clones with chromosome number of 2n = 116 and 70 [25]. Piperidis et al. showed that six atypical clones (2n > 80) belong to hybrids from *S. officinarum* and *S. spontaneum*, indicating that more than 80 chromosome clones may not have originated from a pure *S. officinarum* [4]. In our study, the chromosome numbers of 50uahapele (2n ≈ 86), Muckche (2n ≈ 142), Baimeizhe (2n ≈ 104) and Canablanca (2n ≈ 114) were exceeded 80. Then, using GISH, we demonstrated that these cultivars were hybrids with a portion of chromosomes derived from *S. spontaneum*. Hence, these results were consistent with previous reports that *S. officinarum* may be characterized by 2n = 80 [26]. Furthermore, these differential typical *S. officinarum* will broaden the narrow genetic of sugarcane and provide larger pure *S. officinarum* for selecting cross parents in nobilization.

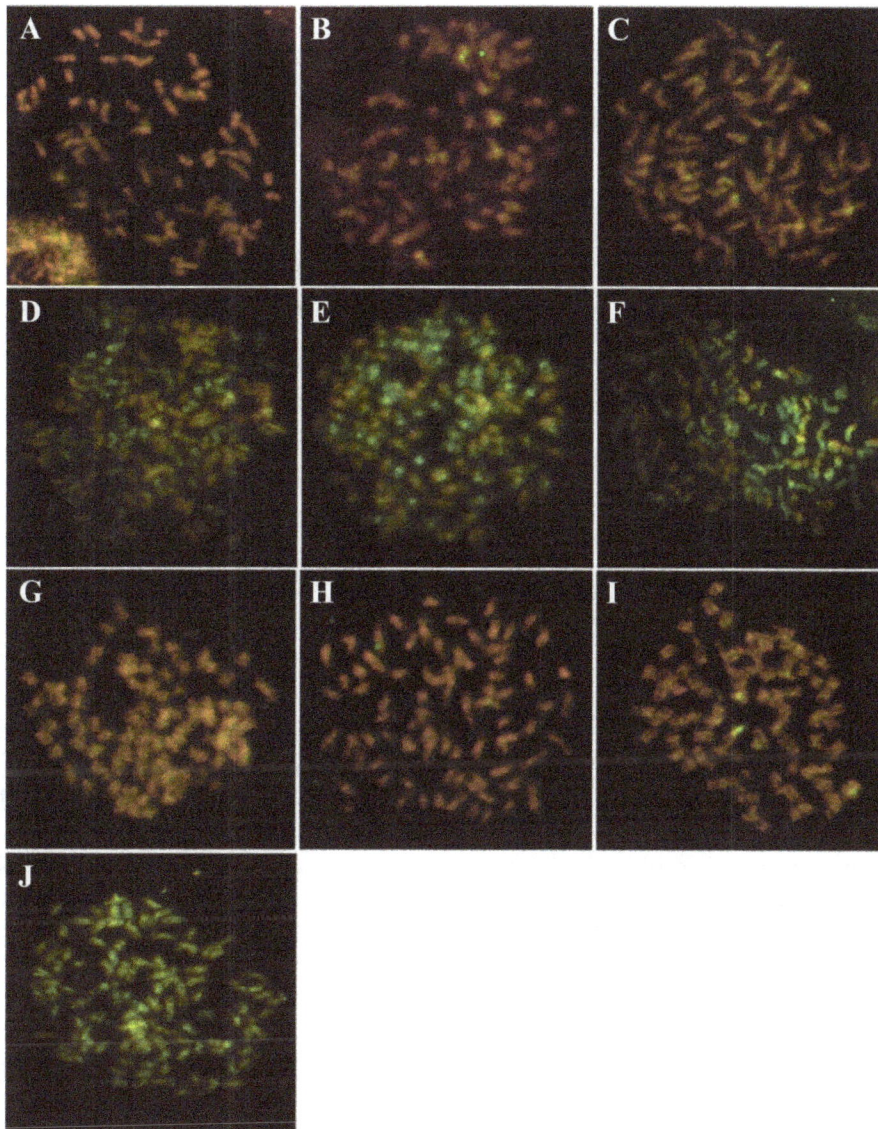

Fig. 2 GISH results of ten *S. officinarum* clones using biotin labelled *S. officinarum* genomic DNA and digoxigenin labelled *S. spontaneum* genomic DNA. **a**: Badila; **b**: Loethers; **c**: Crystallina; **d**: Muckche; **e**: Canablanca; **f**: 50uahapele; **g**: Luohanzhe; **h**: Vietnam Niuzhe; **i**: Nanjian Guozhe; **j**: Baimeizhe; The chromosomes of *S. officinarum* show orange-yellow fluorescent, while those of *S. spontaneum* show green-yellow fluorescent

Chromosome transmission in F$_1$ hybrids between *S. officinarum* and *S. spontaneum*

Interspecific hybridization had proved to be a major breakthrough for germplasm innovation in sugarcane breeding. POJ2878 is one of the most successful example in nobilization that has been widely applied [27]. However, the practical chromosome transmission is crucial for obtaining an ideal species with higher sugar, higher yield, and greater stress-resistance in nobilization. Diversity of chromosome transmission in F$_1$ hybrids had deeply affected the efficiency of sugarcane breeding. Different genetic inheritance would lead to diverse traits of the progeny. Cytogenetic studies have demonstrated that

2n + n chromosome transmission can occur in crosses between *S. officinarum* (female) and *S. spontaneum* (male); this was also confirmed by Piperidis [4]. The 2n + n transmission is key to the nobilization process since it accelerates return to the sugar-producing type. However, the results of chromosome counting showed that n + n transmission often occurs with crosses of *S. spontaneum* with 2n = 80 as a male parent and seldom in crosses of *S. spontaneum* with 2n = 64 and 96 [15]. D'Hont et al. revealed n + n transmission of parental chromosomes by using GISH to analyze an interspecific hybrid between *S. officinarum* (2n = 80) and *S. spontaneum* (2n = 64) [5]. Here, we confirmed that four F$_1$

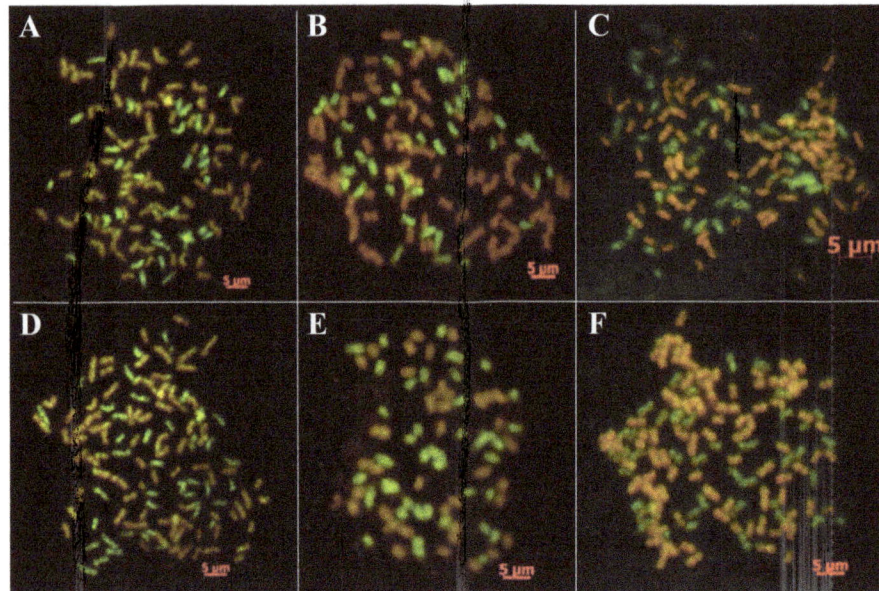

Fig. 3 GISH results of six F_1 hybrids between *S. officinarum* and *S. spontaneum* using biotin labelled *S. officinarum* genomic DNA and digoxigenin labelled *S. spontaneum* genomic DNA. **a**: Yacheng 82–108; **b**: Yacheng 58–43; **c**: Yacheng 58–47; **d**: Yacheng 75–419; **e**: Yacheng 75–408; **f**: Yacheng 75–409

clones of different series (*S. spontaneum* with 2n = 80 or 2n = 64 as male parents) were 2n + n. Furthermore, two different nobilization F_1 clones of the same series had two different transmissions simultaneously, 2n + n or n + n, with *S. spontaneum* (2n = 80) as the parent. Altogether, these results concluded that diverse transmissions, 2n + n or n + n, will occurs in two different ploidy *S. spontaneum* (2n = 80 or 2n = 64 as male parents). Therefore, different ploidy *S. spontaneum* have no influence on the type of chromosome transmission (2n + n versus n + n). Furthermore, nobilization may produce different frequencies of n + n, 2n + n, and aneuploid offspring in larger numbers of F_1 clones.

Many studies have shown that most F_1 crosses and BC_1 backcrosses result in chromosome doubling of the noble parent *S. officinarum* in transmission with the 2n chromosome [6–8, 28]. Although 2n + n is the main chromosome transmission in nobilization, there are also cases of n + n transmission [4, 5, 29]. Even more, in our study, we found that the differential transmissions in the

same parents using GISH. Indeed, chromosome transmission is complex in sugarcane and further studies should be performed to guide optimized sugarcane breeding. The 2n + n chromosome transmission in interspecific crosses is considered an important factor in the rapid breakthrough that interspecific hybridization has provided to sugarcane breeding, leading to a rapid reduction in the proportion of chromosomes from wild species of hybrids and subsequent backcrosses to rapidly recover clones with highest sugar content [3, 30].

Conclusions

Using GISH, this is the first direct evidence that Loethers, Crystallina, Luohanzhe, Vietnam Niuzhe, and Nanjian Guozhe with 80 chromosomes were typical *S. officinarum*; while 50uahapele, Muckche, Baimeizhe and Canablanca with more than 80 chromosomes were interspecific hybrids between *S. officinarum* and *S. spontaneum*. Additionally, GISH analysis demonstrated that five F_1 hybrids between *S. officinarum* and *S. spontaneum*,

Table 1 Crosses of A, B, C, and D

Cross	Clone	Female (♀)	Male (♂)
A	Yacheng 82–108	Badila (2n = 80; S.o)	Yunnan 75-2-11 (2n = 64; S.s)
B	Yacheng 58–43; Yacheng 58–47	Badila (2n = 80; S.o)	Yacheng (2n = 80; S.s)
C	Yacheng 75–419	Fiji (2n = 80; S.o)	Yacheng (2n = 80; S.s)
D	Yacheng 75–408; Yacheng 75–409	Vietnam Niuzhe (2n = 80; S.o)	Yacheng (2n = 80; S.s)

S.o S. officinarum, S.s S. spontaneum

Table 2 The chromosome numbers and ranges of ten clones in sugarcane

Clone	Total number of cells observed	Modal number of chromosomes	Range of total numbers of chromosomes
Badila	30	2n = 80	80
Loethers	30	2n = 80	80
Crystallina	30	2n = 80	80
Muckche	30	2n = 142	141–143
Canablanca	30	2n = 114	113–115
50uahapele	30	2n = 86	85–88
Luohanzhe	30	2n = 80	80
Vietnam Niuzhe	30	2n = 80	80
Nanjian Guozhe	30	2n = 80	80
Baimeizhe	30	2n = 104	104–106

Note: Since small variations in chromosome counts can occur due to the loss or the overlapping of a few chromosomes from the preparation, the modal number of chromosomes and range of total numbers of chromosomes in 2n cells are presented for the sugarcane clones analyzed

Yacheng 82–108, Yacheng 58–43, Yacheng 58–47, Yacheng 75–409, and Yacheng 75–419 were products of a 2n + n transmission; while, Yacheng 75–408 was the product of an n + n transmission. Although Yacheng 75–408 and Yacheng 75–409 are the sibling lines of the different F$_1$ progeny with the same parents, there was a large difference in chromosome numbers that led to different patterns of chromosome inheritance. The results of this study support previous reports that *S. officinarum* may be characterized by 2n = 80 and provide more useful molecular cytogenetic information for the larger germplasm resources of *S. officinarum*. Futhermore, clear chromosome composition of early progenies between *S. officinarum* and *S. spontaneum* will provide guidance for further sugarcane nobilization.

Methods

Plant materials and DNA extraction

In this study, ten experimental materials classified as *S. officinarum* were used, including Badila, Loethers, Crystallina, 50uahapele, Muckche, Canablanca, Luohanzhe,

Vietnam Niuzhe, Nanjian Guozhe, and Baimeizhe. Of these, 50uahapele, Canablanca, Baimeizhe were provided by the research Institute Ruili Station of Yunnan Agriculture Science Academy; the Sugarcane Research Institute of Yunnan Agriculture Science Academy provided the rest materials. The Hainan Sugarcane Breeding Station, Guangzhou Sugarcane Industry Research Institute provided six F$_1$ clones between *S. officinarum* and *S. spontaneum* for nobilization (Table 1). All plant materials used in this study were grown in the germplasm resources nursery at the Fujian Agriculture and Forestry University. Leaf tissues from the above materials were ground in liquid nitrogen and stored at − 80 °C. Total genomic DNA was extracted from young leaves following CTAB methodology [31].

Chromosome preparation

Root tips were obtained from ten clones classified as *S. officinarum* and six clones of F$_1$ between *S. officinarum* and *S. spontaneum*. Meristem of root-tips were treated with saturated p-dichlorobenzene solution for 1.5 h at

Table 3 Chromosome composition of six F$_1$ hybrids between *S. officinarum* and *S. spontaneum* in nobilization

Cross	Clone	No. of chromosomes	No. of S.o chromosomes	No. of S.s chromosomes	Chromosome composition	Chromosome transmission	No. of cells observed
A	Yacheng 82–108	112	80	32	80 S.o + 32 S.s	2n + n	30
B	Yacheng 58–43	120	80	40	80 S.o + 40 S.s	2n + n	35
	Yacheng 58–47	120	80	40	80 S.o + 40 S.s	2n + n	38
C	Yacheng 75–419	120	80	40	80 S.o + 40 S.s	2n + n	37
D	Yacheng 75–408	80	40	40	40 S.o + 40 S.s	n + n	32
	Yacheng 75–409	120	80	40	80 S.o + 40 S.s	2n + n	41

S.o *S. officinarum*, S.s *S. spontaneum*

25 °C. The root tips were then fixed in 3:1 (v/v) ethanol: acetic acid solution for 24 h and successive eluted in ethanol solution (75, 95 and 100% ethanol), finally kept at − 20 °C with 75% ethanol solution. The fixed roots were washed in water and digested in an enzyme solution (4% Onozuka R10 cellulose, 0.5% pectolyase Y-23 and 0.5% pectinase) for 4 h at 37 °C. The digestive meristematic cells were squashed on the clear slide in 20 μL of 3:1 (v/v) ethanol: acetic acid. Slides were stored at − 20 °C.

Probe labelling

Probes were labelled using a Nick-translation kit with biotin-dUTP (Roche, Germany) and digoxigenin (Roche, Germany). For in situ hybridization, 100 ng/μL of Badila (*S. officinarum*) genomic DNA, labeled with biotin-dUTP, and 100 ng/μL Yunnan 75–2-11 (*S. spontaneum*) genomic DNA, labeled with digoxigenin were used as probes.

Genomic in situ hybridization (GISH)

GISH technique were performed as described previously by D'Hont et al. [32] with moderate improvement. The denaturing solution included 70% formamide in 2× SSC. Slides were denatured in this solution for 3 min at 80 °C. Dehydration was performed in cold ethanol and slides were then air dried at room temperature. The probe mixture including hybridization buffer (50% formamide, 2× SSC, 10% dextransulfate) and 200 ng labeled probe after denaturation for 10 min at 97 °C was applied to each slide and incubated for 20 h at 37 °C in a humid dark box. The high stringency conditions of post-hybridization washes were carried out with 2 × SSC for 8 min at 42 °C, a second wash in 50% formamide, 2 × SSC, pH 7.0, for 3 × 8 min at 42 °C, followed by a rinse in 2 × SSC for 8 min at room temperature and a final wash in 0.1 × SSC for 3 × 8 min at 55 °C. The biotin-labelled probe was detected with avidin-conjugated Texas red and the digoxigenin-labelled probe was detected with FITC (fluorescein isothiocyanate)-conjugated anti-digoxigenin antibody. Slides then were counterstained with 4′, 6-diamidino-2-phenylindole (DAPI) in a Vectashield anti-fade solution (Vector Laboratories, Burlingame, CA). GISH signals were captured using the AxioVision measurement module of AxioScope A1 Imager fluorescent microscope (Zeiss, Germany).

Chromosome counting

The metaphase chromosomes of the above materials were captured using phase contrast microscope (Fig. 1) or fluorescence microscope (Additional file 1: Figure S1; Figs. 2 and 3). The number of chromosome was counted using the program Image-pro plus 6.0 (Media Cybernetics). Results were presented as the modal number (occurred the most times among different cells in each clone) and the number of cells observed at least 30 cells for each clone (Tables 2 and 3). Additionally, at least

three materials in one generation had been studied in six F_1 clones.

Abbreviations

DAPI: 4′, 6-diamidino-2-phenylindole; FISH: Fluorescence in situ hybridization; FITC: Fluorescein isothiocyanate; GISH: Genomic in situ hybridization

Acknowledgements

We thank the Sugarcane Research Institute of Yunnan Agriculture Science Academy, the Research Institute Ruili Station of Yunnan Agriculture Science Academy and the Hainan Sugarcane Breeding Station, Guangzhou Sugarcane Industry Research Institute for providing the plant materials used in this study. We greatly appreciate Bioscience Editing Solutions for critically reading this paper and providing helpful suggestions.

Funding

This work was funded by the Natural Science Foundation of Fujian Province of China (2016 J01094, http://yxmgl.fjkjt.gov.cn/) and supported by the earmarked fund for the Modern Agriculture Technology of China (CARS-20-1-5), the Natural Science Foundation of Guangdong Province of China (2015A030310286), and the science and technology major project of the Fujian Province of China (2015NZ0002–2, http://yxmgl.fjkjt.gov.cn/).

Authors' contributions

FY, PW, XL, ZD, and LX designed the study. FY, PW, and XL conducted the experiments. FY, PW, XL, YH, QW, LL, YJ, XL, ZD, JW, YY, RC, MZ, and LX analyzed the results. YH, PW, YH, ZD, and LX wrote the manuscript. All authors read and approved the final manuscript.

Competing interests

The authors declare that they have no competing interests.

Author details

[1]National Engineering Research Center for Sugarcane, Fujian Agriculture and Forestry University, Fuzhou, China. [2]Guangdong Provincial Bioengineering Institute, Guangzhou Sugarcane Industry Research Institute, Guangzhou, China. [3]Sugarcane Research Institute of Yunnan Agriculture Science Academy, Kaiyuan, China. [4]Guangxi Collaborative Innovation Center of Sugar Industries, Guangxi University, Nanning, China.

References

1. Irvine JE. *Saccharum* species as horticultural classes. Theor Appl Genet. 1999; 98:186–94.
2. Guimarães CT, Sobral BWS. The *Saccharum* Complex: relation to other *Andropogoneae*. In: Janick J, editor. Plant breeding reviews. New York: Wiley; 2010. p. 269–88.
3. Roach BT. Nobilisation of sugarcane. Proc Int Soc Sugar Cane Technol. 1972; 14:206–16.
4. Piperidis G, Piperidis N, D'Hont A. Molecular cytogenetic investigation of chromosome composition and transmission in sugarcane. Mol Gen Genomics. 2010;284:65–73.
5. D'Hont A, Grivet L, Feldmann P, Rao S, Berding N, Glaszmann JC. Characterisation of the double genome structure of modern sugarcane cultivars (*Saccharum* spp.) by molecular cytogenetics. Mol Gen Genomics. 1996;250:405–13.
6. Jianrong Z, Lianan T, Lihua D, Qingming Z, Huifen D, Lihe Y, Rudong A, Hongbo L, Yanfen J. Breeding potential of creation parents derived from China native *Saccharum spontaneum* in sugarcane. J Yunnan Agric Univ. 2011;26:12–9.
7. Jenkin MJ, Reader SM, Purdie KA, Miller TE. Detection of rDNA sites in sugarcane by FISH. Chromosom Res. 1995;3:444.

8. Panje RR, Babu CN. Studies in *Saccharum spontaneum* distribution and geographical association of chromosome numbers. Cytologia. 1960;25:152–72.
9. D'Hont A, Paulet F, Glaszmann JC. Oligoclonal interspecific origin of 'North Indian' and 'Chinese' sugarcanes. Chromosom Res. 2002;10:253–62.
10. Price S. Cytological studies in *Saccharum* and allied genera VII. Maternal chromosome transmission by *S. officinarum* in intra- and interspecific crosses. Int J Plant Sci. 1961;122:298–305.
11. Walker DIT. Utilization of noble and *Saccharum spontaneum* germplasm in the West Indies. Proc Int Sot Sug Cane Technol. 1971;14:224–32.
12. Daniels J. Improving sugarcane breeding methods to increase yields. Proc tnt Sot Sug Cane Technol. 1965;12:742–5.
13. Bremer G. Problems in breeding and cytology of sugar cane. Euphytica. 1961;10:59–78.
14. Bhat SR, Gill SS. The implication of 2n egg gametes in nobilisation and breeding of sugarcane. Euphytica. 1985;34:377–84.
15. Roach BT. Cytological studies in *Saccharum*. Chromosome transmission in interspecific and intergeneric crosses. Proc Int Soc Sugar Cane Technol. 1969;13:901–20.
16. Raina SN, Rani V. GISH technology in plant genome research. Methods Cell Sci. 2001;23:83–104.
17. Schwarzacher T, Leitch AR, Bennett MD, Heslop-Harrison JS. In situ localization of parental genomes in a wide hybrid. Ann Bot-London. 1989; 64:315–24.
18. Piperidis N. GISH: Resolving Interspecific and Intergeneric Hybrids. In: Besse P, editor. Molecular Plant Taxonomy: Methods and Protocols. Totowa, NJ: Humana Press; 2014. p. 325–36.
19. An D, Zheng Q, Zhou Y, Ma P, Lv Z, Li L, Li B, Luo Q, Xu H, Xu Y. Molecular cytogenetic characterization of a new wheat-rye 4R chromosome translocation line resistant to powdery mildew. Chromosom Res. 2013;21:419–32.
20. Harper J, Armstead I, Thomas A, James C, Gasior D, Bisaga M, Roberts L, King I, King J. Alien introgression in the grasses *Lolium perenne* (perennial ryegrass) and *Festuca pratensis* (meadow fescue): the development of seven monosomic substitution lines and their molecular and cytological characterization. Ann Bot. 2011;107:1313–21.
21. Mestiri I, Chague V, Tanguy AM, Huneau C, Huteau V, Belcram H, Coriton O, Chalhoub B, Jahier J. Newly synthesized wheat allohexaploids display progenitor-dependent meiotic stability and aneuploidy but structural genomic additivity. New Phytol. 2010;186:86–101.
22. Zhang P, Li WL, Friebe B, Gill BS. The origin of a "zebra" chromosome in wheat suggests nonhomologous recombination as a novel mechanism for new chromosome evolution and step changes in chromosome number. Genetics. 2008;179:1169–77.
23. Piperidis N, Chen JW, Deng HH, Wang LP, Jackson P, Piperidis G. GISH characterization of *Erianthus arundinaceus* chromosomes in three generations of sugarcane intergeneric hybrids. Genome. 2010;53:331–6.
24. Heinz DJ. Sugarcane improvement through breeding. In: Heinz DJ, editor. Plant Breeding Reviews. Amsterdam: Elsevier; 1987. p. 15–118.
25. Sobhakumari VP. New determinations of somatic chromosome number in cultivated and wild species of *Saccharum*. Caryologia. 2013;66:268–74.
26. Sreenivasan TV, Ahloowalia BS, Heinz DJ. Cytogenetics. In: Heinz DJ, editor. Sugarcane improvement through breeding. New York: Elsevier; 1987. p. 211–53.
27. Lam E, James Shine JR, Silva JD, Lawton M, Bonos S, Calvino M, Carrer H, Silva-Filho MC, Glynn N, Helsel Z. Improving sugarcane for biofuel: engineering for an even better feedstock. GCB Bioenergy. 2009;1:251–5.
28. Waclawovsky AJ, Sato PM, Lembke CG, Moore PH, Souza GM, Davies M, Campbell M, Henry R. Sugarcane for bioenergy production: an assessment of yield and regulation of sucrose content. Plant Biotechnol J. 2010;8:263–76.
29. Price S. Cytological studies in *Saccharum* and allied genera. III. Chromosome numbers in interspecific hybrids. Int J Plant Sci. 1957;118:146–59.
30. Roach BT. Evaluation and use of sugarcane germplasm. Proc Int Soc Sugar Cane Technol. 1986;1:492–503.
31. Jr SC, Via LE. A rapid CTAB DNA isolation technique useful for RAPD fingerprinting and other PCR applications. BioTechniques. 1993;14:748–50.
32. D'Hont A. Determination of basic chromosome numbers in the genus *Saccharum* by physical mapping of ribosomal RNA genes. Genome. 1998;41: 221–5.

3

Investigation of copy number variations on chromosome 21 detected by comparative genomic hybridization (CGH) microarray in patients with congenital anomalies

Wenfu Li, Xianfu Wang and Shibo Li[*]

Abstract

Background: The clinical features of Down syndrome vary among individuals, with those most common being congenital heart disease, intellectual disability, developmental abnormity and dysmorphic features. Complex combination of Down syndrome phenotype could be produced by partially copy number variations (CNVs) on chromosome 21 as well. By comparing individual with partial CNVs of chromosome 21 with other patients of known CNVs and clinical phenotypes, we hope to provide a better understanding of the genotype-phenotype correlation of chromosome 21.

Methods: A total of 2768 pediatric patients sample collected at the Genetics Laboratory at Oklahoma University Health Science Center were screened using CGH Microarray for CNVs on chromosome 21.

Results: We report comprehensive clinical and molecular descriptions of six patients with microduplication and seven patients with microdeletion on the long arm of chromosome 21. Patients with microduplication have varied clinical features including developmental delay, microcephaly, facial dysmorphic features, pulmonary stenosis, autism, preauricular skin tag, eye pterygium, speech delay and pain insensitivity. We found that patients with microdeletion presented with developmental delay, microcephaly, intrauterine fetal demise, epilepsia partialis continua, congenital coronary anomaly and seizures.

Conclusion: Three patients from our study combine with four patients in public database suggests an association between 21q21.1 microduplication of CXADR gene and patients with developmental delay. One patient with 21q22.13 microdeletion of DYRK1A shows association with microcephaly and scoliosis. Our findings helped pinpoint critical genes in the genotype-phenotype association with a high resolution of 0.1 Mb and expanded the clinical features observed in patients with CNVs on the long arm of chromosome 21.

Keywords: Chromosome 21, Microarray, CNV, Genotype-phenotype association, *CXADR, DYRK1A*

Background

Down Syndrome (DS) is the most prevalent genetic disorder resulting in intellectual disability, which is usually caused by an extra copy of chromosome 21. It is estimated that 1 in 700 newborn babies in United States are diagnosed with DS [1]. The phenotypes of DS frequently include congenital heart disease, intellectual disability, developmental abnormity and dysmorphic features [2].

Despite the fact that DS is mainly caused by trisomy 21, the genotype-phenotype association of typical DS features is yet to be determined.

Down Syndrome Critical Region (DSCR) hypothesis failed to provide solid evidence on the proposed theory of minimum gene responsible for all major DS phenotypes caused by a gene dosage effect [3–6]. Meanwhile, under limited circumstances partial monosomy 21 and partial trisomy 21 have been found to provide better understanding on the genotype-phenotype association of chromosome 21 [7–10]. Phenotypes with partial

* Correspondence: shibo-li@ouhsc.edu
Genetics Laboratory, University of Oklahoma Health Sciences Center, 1122 NE 13th Street, Suite 1400, Oklahoma City, OK 73104, USA

duplication or deletion of chromosome 21q are found to be highly variable among patients For instance, a child with Intellectual disability and dysmorphologic features of DS but without congenital heart disease was found to have a 2.78-Mb duplication on chromosome 21q22.11 [11]. Partial deletion of 21q21.1 are found to be associated with intellectual disability while deletion of 21q22.11 are considered associated with neurobehavioral disorder [8]. Despite the efforts to link DS clinical features with genes and regions, the association map resolution is low and details still remain incomplete.

Instead of trying to find a DSCR, our study focused on finding specific genotype-phenotype associations by investigating rare patients which involved a partial CNV on chromosome 21. Advancements in technology in comparative genomic hybridization (CGH) microarray enable laboratory to identify copy number variations (CNVs) on chromosome 21 as small as 10 k base pairs. From 2008 to 2018, 2768 samples were collected at the Genetics Laboratory at University of Oklahoma Health Sciences Center (OUHSC). During this period, we identified six patients with partial duplication and seven patients with partial deletion of chromosome 21. Among 13 patients with CNVs, two patients are related while others are independent. In this study, we report the molecular and clinical relationship of chromosomal imbalance on chromosome 21 and compare our results with current public data and literature to provide new way to naming patient with certain phenotypes.

Methods
Patients
The study was approved by the Institutional Review Board (IRB) of the University of Oklahoma. IRB number was 5938 and the reference number was 670,840. Retrospectively, 2768 pediatric patients sample were collected from 2008 to 2018 at the Genetics Laboratory at OUHSC. In-house software was developed to extract CNVs based on the following criteria:

1. CNVs only on chromosome 21, exclude whole chromosome 21 duplication/deletion and concurrent CNVs on other chromosomes.
2. CNV length larger than 100 kb.
3. CNV mean log2 ratio absolute value larger than 0.3.
4. CNV not overlap with common CNVs and segmental duplication regions.

After filtration, CNVs were manually curated to eliminate false positive cases based on background signal noise. A total of 13 samples were identified, six samples displayed partial duplication and seven samples showed partial deletion. The clinical information of the patients is summarized in Table 1.

CGH microarray
Fresh blood samples were collected for this study and genomic DNA was extracted from peripheral white blood cells according to our standard operating using Nucleic Acid Isolation System (QuickGene-610 L, FUJI-FILM Corporation, Tokyo, Japan). Patient D1's CGH microarray was performed on a 385-K oligonucleotide chip and all other samples were performed on a CGH 720 K Whole-Genome Tiling v3.0 array (Roche Nimble-Gen, Inc., Madison, WI) according to the manufacturer's protocol with minor modifications. As an internal hybridization control for each experiment, an opposite sex DNA came from normal population individuals pooled use as reference DNA (Promega Corporation, Madison, WI). Both the patients' DNA and reference DNA were labeled with either Cyanine 3 (Cy-3) or Cyanine 5 (Cy-5) by random priming (Trilink Biotechnologies, San Diego, CA) and then hybridized to the chip via incubation in the MAUI hybridization system (Biomicro Systems, Inc., Salt Lake City, UT). After 18 h of hybridization at 42 °C, slides were washed and scanned using an MS200 (Roche NimbleGen, Inc.). NimbleScan version 2.4 and the SignalMap version 1.9 were applied for data analysis (NimbleGen System Inc., Madison, WI). CGH microarray results were analyzed referring to University of California Santa Cruz (UCSC) Genome Browser (GRCh37/hg19) (http://genome.ucsc.edu/cgi-bin/hgGateway). Frequently affected regions that were recently identified as copy number polymorphisms were excluded from data analysis according to the Chromosome Number Variation (CNV) database in our lab and genomic variants in human genome (Build 37). Variants of interest were compared to disease-causing genes in DECIPHER v8.7 (Database of Chromosomal Imbalance and Phenotype in Humans using Ensembl Resources) (decipher.sanger.ac.uk/index), DGV (Database of Genomic Variants) (dgv.tcag.ca/dgv/app/home), ClinVar (www.ncbi.nlm.nih.gov/clinvar) and OMIM (www.omim.org). The patient's clinical phenotype and variants of interest were compared with available information from published reports.

Results
Duplications
Six patients (S1, S2, S3, S4, S5 and S6) were identified with duplication on chromosome 21. The size of chromosome 21 duplications ranged from 0.1 Mb to 1.2 Mb (Table 1, Fig. 1, and Additional file 1: Figure S1). Among the duplications, one CNV at 21q21.1 was maternally inherited by patient S3 from patient S4 and presented in another unrelated patient (S1) that includes the *CXADR* gene (Figs. 1 and 2). These three patients share the phenotype of developmental delay while patient S3 also demonstrated pulmonary stenosis and

Table 1 Molecular profile of patients

Patient #	Sex	Age at study	Chr21 location (hg19)	Gain/Loss	Size of CNVs (Mb)	Clinical features
DECIPHER280573	F	14y	18,582,895-18,983,265	Gain	0.4	DD, Intrauterine growth retardation, microcephaly, alopecia
S4	F	32 y	18,776,205-19,072,251	Gain	0.3	DD, Mother of S3
S1	M	2 y	18,781,100-18,885,813	Gain	0.1	DD, cleft palate, microcephaly, failure to thrive
S3	F	7 y	18,781,100-19,071,857	Gain	0.3	DD, pulmonary stenosis, autism, mild dysmorphic, daughter of S4
DECIPHER273421	M	4y	18,791,730-19,136,039	Gain	0.3	Intellectual disability
DECIPHER301183	F	2y	18,819,200-19,036,035	Gain	0.2	DD, microcephaly, seizures, hearing and visual abnormality
DECIPHER257242	F	7y	18,888,629-18,983,265	Gain	0.1	DD, Intrauterine growth retardation, intellectual disability
D6	F	2 y	21,427,690-24,133,154	Loss	2.7	DD
D4	F	33 y	22,271,313-23,399,894	Loss	1.1	Mother with Intrauterine fetal demise
D5	F	4 y	23,793,678-23,948,945	Loss	0.1	DD, epilepsia partialis continua
D3	M	2 m	23,840,342-23,941,319	Loss	0.1	Congenital coronary anomaly
D7	M	6 y	24,289,038-24,396,084	Loss	0.1	Seizures
S2	M	3 y	28,212,197-29,423,946	Gain	1.2	Preauricular skin tag, eye pterygium, speech delay
D2	F	1 y	31,005,158-31,236,003	Loss	0.2	Facial dysmorphic features
S6	F	9 d	35,902,679-36,149,583	Gain	0.2	Diaphragmatic hernia
S5	M	4 y	37,474,069-37,611,689	Gain	0.1	Pain insensitivity and minor dysmorphisms
D1	M	10 y	37,540,692-39,328,135	Loss	1.7	Microcephaly, levocurvature of thoracolumbar spine
Yamamoto, 2011	F	13y	38,528,931-39,009,341	Loss	0.4	DD, seizures, mild brain atrophy
Courcet, 2012	F	4y	38,722,631-38,791,771	Loss	0.1	Microcephaly, DD, ataxic gait, seizures
DECIPHER258106	F	N/A	38,865,151-38,885,792	Loss	0.1	Microcephaly, scoliosis, deeply set eye, Intrauterine growth retardation, short nose, sparse scalp hair, Hypoglycemia, DD, seizures
Van Bon, 2011	F	>20y	38,874,630-38,927,130	Loss	0.1	Microcephaly, DD, mild brain atrophy, anxious and autistic behaviour

Note: F female, M male, y year, m month, d day, DD developmental delay

autism. A 1.2-Mb duplication at 21q21.3 presented in patient S2 with preauricular skin tag, eye pterygium and speech delay (Fig. 2). Two genes, *ADAMTS1* and *ADAMTS5*, have been identified on this CNV. Diaphragmatic hernia presented in patient S6 with a 0.2-Mb duplication at 21q22.12 which includes the *RCAN1* and *CLIC6* genes (Fig. 2). Also with duplication at 21q22.12, another patient (S5) showed pain insensitivity along with minor dysmorphism. Two protein-coding genes, *CBR3* and *DOPEY2*, are located in this duplication region (Fig. 2).

Deletions
Seven patients (D1, D2, D3, D4, D5, D6 and D7) were identified with deletion on chromosome 21 ranged from 0.1 Mb to 2.7 Mb.Five patients (D3, D4, D5, D6 and D7) with various sizes of deletion at 21q21.1-q21.2 presented clinical features which included developmental delay, intrauterine fetal demise, epilepsia partialis

continua, congenital coronary anomaly and seizures (Table 1, Figs. 1 and 2 and Additional file 1: Figure S1). The *NCAM2* gene is located in this 21q21.1-q21.2 deletion region (Figs. 1 and 2). Patient D2 had a phenotype of facial dysmorphic features and a 0.2-Mb deletion on 21q21.3 that includes the *GRIK1* gene (Figs. 1 and 2). Patient D1 presented with a deletion of 1.7 Mb at 21q22.12-q22.13 that includes four OMIM genes: *CLDN14*, *HLCS*, *DYRK1A* and *KCNJ6* (Figs. 1 and 2). The phenotype associated with this patient was microcephaly and levocurvature of the thoracolumbar spine.

Discussion
Microduplication 21q21.1
The microduplication on 21q21.1 was found in three patients S1, S3 and S4. This CNV was inherited from S4 to S3. Published reports of this CNV are rare but four patients (DECIPHER 257242, 301,183, 273,421 and

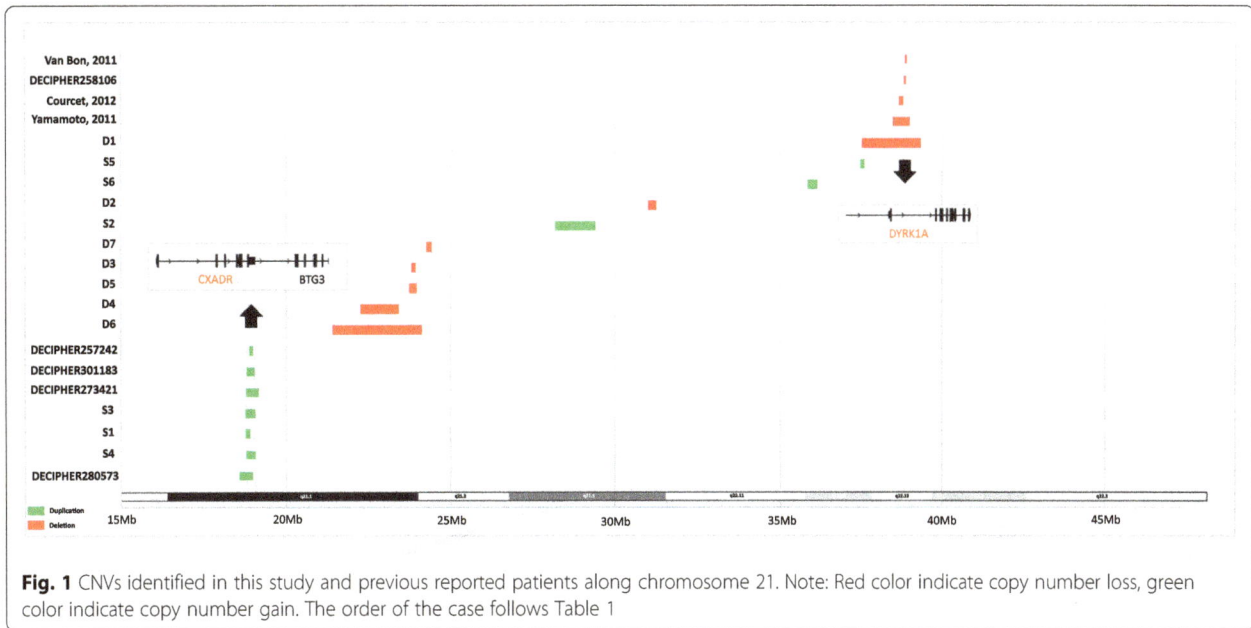

Fig. 1 CNVs identified in this study and previous reported patients along chromosome 21. Note: Red color indicate copy number loss, green color indicate copy number gain. The order of the case follows Table 1

280,573) were found to have similar duplication segments and shared phenotypes such as developmental delay and intellectual disability [12]. There are two protein-coding genes, *CXADR* and *BTG3*, in this region. The CNV identified with patient S1 is within the 0.3-Mb region but is smaller and only includes the *CXADR* gene. Patient S1 also displayed the same developmental delay features that patients S3 and S4 possessed.

The *CXADR* and *BTG3* genes were found to be expressed during early brain development and a balanced expression of *BTG3* is critical for neuron differentiation in the forebrain [13, 14]. *BTG3* is upregulated in trisomic fibroblasts compared to a control indicating a gene dosage effect on heart tissues [15]. Considering patient S3 displayed pulmonary stenosis while patient S1 did not, and the extra duplicated region of S3 includes *BTG3*, this gene could potentially contribute to this clinical distinction. *BTG3* has also been linked with autism because of its role in cellular apoptosis and responses to redox changes [16, 17]. The protein product of *BTG3* has also been found to have a critical impact on cell growth and differentiation of

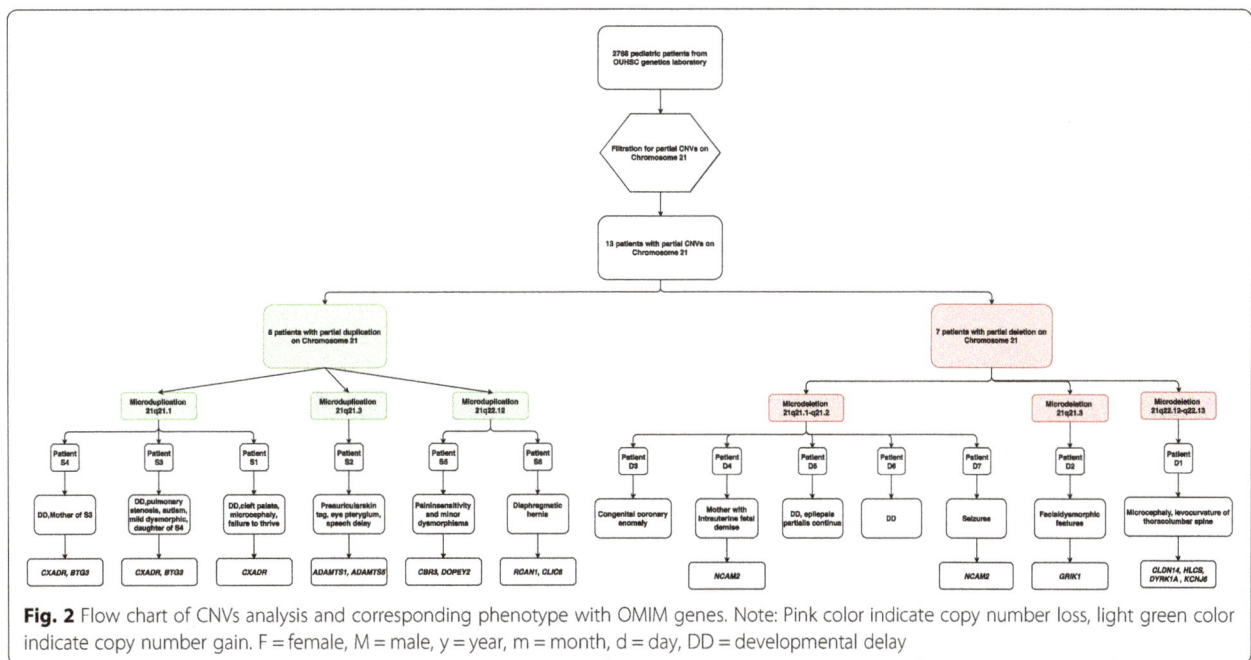

Fig. 2 Flow chart of CNVs analysis and corresponding phenotype with OMIM genes. Note: Pink color indicate copy number loss, light green color indicate copy number gain. F = female, M = male, y = year, m = month, d = day, DD = developmental delay

other cells like T lymphocytes, fibroblasts and epithelial cells [18].

CXADR has been associated with developmental delay in two patients with larger CNV deletions of 7.9 Mb and 8.5 Mb [19, 20]. Combined with our three cases and the four DECIPHER patients mentioned above, it shows a strong connection between the irregular expression levels of *CXADR* and developmental disorders [19]. Coxsackievirus and adenovirus receptor (CAR) is a protein encoded by the *CXADR* gene. CAR has dual function as a receptor in the immune response against virus and a signal transduction molecule during neurological system development [21]. CAR is highly expressed in tissues like brain and heart in the early development; it is mainly expressed in endothelial cells and cardiac cells postnatally [22, 23]. Excessive expression of CAR has been link to activation of mitogen-activated protein kinase (MAPK) pathway in heart which might contribute to the hyper M1 inflammatory response in DS [24]. Additional follow up with Cardiologist might provide better understanding on the clinical significance of *CXADR* gene for these three patients. Our study narrowed down the critical region of patients with microduplication 21q21.1 features from 0.4 Mb to 0.1 Mb and highlighted the clinical relevance of *CXADR* gene as a potential cause for developmental delay, abnormal development of cardio myocytes and intellectual disability [25, 26].

Microduplication 21q21.3

One patient S2 was found to have a 1.2-Mb microduplication at 21q21.3 with a preauricular skin tag, eye pterygium and speech delay. Our patient's CNV is the first ever reported on this region which includes *ADAMTS1* and *ADAMTS5*. The functions of these genes are not well understood but *ADAMTS1* was found to be associated with various inflammatory processes and cachexia and *ADAMTS5* may involve destruction of the aggrecan, a cartilage proteoglycan [20]. One case of an 8.8-Mb deletion which encompasses both *ADAMTS1* and *ADAMTS5* was reported before with a similar speech delay phenotype as patient S2 but without other clinical features [20]. Further study is needed to better understand the clinical significance of this CNV.

Microduplication 21q22.12

One patient S6, a 9-day-old female with a diaphragmatic hernia, was found to have a 0.2-Mb microduplication at 21q22.12. There are two genes in this region, *RCAN1* and *CLIC6*. Among them, *RCAN1* has been linked to contribute to the intellectual disability and neuronal degeneration in Alzheimer's disease [27]. Multiple studies using animal models and transcriptome analysis demonstrated the important function by *RCAN1* in regulation of the anxiogenic response and oxidative stress-induced

apoptosis [28–30]. Unfortunately, we were limited by the age of our patient (S6) so no other information is available other than the presence of the diaphragmatic hernia, which has not been found to be associated with either *RCAN1* or *CLIC6* before. The function of *CLIC6* is not exactly clear.

Another patient S5 was found to have a 0.1-Mb microduplication about 1.3 Mb downstream of S6's CNV. Literature research found several patients had this CNV and it mostly resulted in nervous system disorders or developmental delay (DECIPHER 276835,287,879, 317,546 etc.) [12]. Interestingly, one case reported a 6.5-Mb deletion on 21q22.12 and the patient also showed signs of pain insensitivity, however the genotype is deletion instead of duplication, the overlap region coordinate is chr21: 37,474,069-37,554,434 (hg19) and *CBR3* gene is in this region [31]. Two genes, *CBR3* and *DOPEY2*, are found in the duplicated region of patient S5. These genes were both found to be closely related with DS phenotypes and be subject to the gene dosage effect causing intellectual disability and early onset of Alzheimer's Disease [32–34]. However, no other pain insensitivity information was found to be associated with these genes.

Microdeletion 21q21.1-q21.2

Five patients (D3, D4, D5, D6 and D7) were found with various sizes of deletion at 21q21.1-q21.2. Patient D6 had a 2.7-Mb microdeletion on 21q21.1-q21.2. Three patients (D3, D4 and D5) also had microdeletions of 0.1 Mb, 1.1 Mb and 0.1 Mb, respectively, within the 2.7-Mb microdeletion region of patient D6. Patient D7 had a 0.1-Mb microdeletion on 21q21.2 with a clinical feature of seizures. A previous study showed one patient (DECIPHER 319386) had a similar, but slightly smaller, microdeletion compared to patient D6. DECIPHER 319386 had macrocephaly, autistic behavior and delayed speech and language development but no common phenotypic features were found between patient D6 and DECIPHER 319386. A common feature found in patients D5 and D6 was developmental delay. Patient D4 was a mother who experienced an intrauterine fetal demise. A congenital coronary anomaly was reported in D3.

On the molecular level, *NCAM2* overlaps with the microdeletion on patients D4 and D6. *NCAM2* is believed to be associated with certain DS phenotypes because, as the expression levels change, multiple folds related to the homotypic adhesion properties of cells will be altered [35]. *NCAM2* also has been suggested as a candidate gene for autism because it is highly expressed in the brain and nervous systems [20, 36–38]. There are no known protein-coding genes in the microdeletion region of patients D3, D5 and D7 which suggests an alternative explanation other than CNVs is responsible for their phenotype.

Microdeletion 21q21.3

One patient D2 had a microdeletion on 21q21.3 the size of 0.2 Mb and was found to be within the 0.4-Mb microdeletion region of DECIPHER 257308. Limited by the young age of patient D2 (one-year-old), only facial dysmorphic features were observed while DECIPHER 257308 displayed aggressive behavior, generalized tonic-clonic seizures and neurological speech impairment. *GRIK1*, a gene that encodes for a glutamatergic receptor subunit, is found in this microdeletion region. Glutamate is the most widely distributed excitatory neurotransmitter in the central nervous system acting on ionotropic and metabotropic receptors. Expression of *GRIK1* was found be to significantly lower in the hippocampus of DS patients and receptors were overexpressed in various areas of the brain [39, 40]. Also, trisomic animals were found to respond to glutamatergic stimuli differed from normal animals as well [41]. Based on the potential gene-dosage effect of *GRIK1* and the phenotypes displayed by DECIPHER 257308 which involved excitability, the *GRIK1* gene should be considered to be a strong candidate gene responsible for DS phenotypes.

Microdeletion 21q22.12-q22.13

One patient D1 had a 1.7-Mb deletion on 21q22.12-q22.13, which includes four OMIM genes: *CLDN14*, *HLCS*, *DYRK1A* and *KCNJ6*. Yamamoto et al. (2011) reported two cases with mosaic deletions on 21q22qter and one case with a 0.4-Mb deletion within the 21q22.12-q22.13 microdeletion region. One of the mosaic deletion cases displayed an identical phenotype to patient D1 which included microcephaly and scoliosis [42]. In addition, a DECIPHER case (258106) that had a 0.2-Mb microdeletion within the same region also had microcephaly and scoliosis. *DYRK1A* is the only gene affected in all three cases and is reported to play a role in neurogenesis and neural differentiation [43]. Previous studies showed an association between *DYRK1A* and microcephaly had been well established and around half of the patients also displayed scoliosis [44, 45]. Single Nucleotide Variances and small INDELs on this genes also demonstrate similar phenotype of microdeletion on 21q22.13 that reaffirms this strong association between *DYRK1A* gene and syndrome with microcephaly and scoliosis [44, 45].

Conclusions

In conclusion, our study expands the knowledge of the phenotypic consequences of CNVs on the long arm of chromosome 21. While the microduplications are associated with developmental delay, microcephaly, facial dysmorphic features, pulmonary stenosis, autism, preauricular skin tag, eye pterygium, speech delay and pain insensitivity, microdeletions are associated with developmental delay, microcephaly, intrauterine fetal demise, epilepsia partialis continua, congenital coronary anomaly and seizures. We suggest the *CXADR* gene is involved with developmental delay in patients with 21q21.1 microduplication and we provide additional evidence that *DYRK1A* is associated with microcephaly and scoliosis in patients with a 21q22 microdeletion. Both *CXADR* and *DYRK1A* are ranked high in the haploinsufficiency index of chromosome 21 gene list that indicates one allele with loss of function variant will result in a recognizable phenotype [46]. It also been found that haploinsufficient genes are more sensitive to dosage effect that might contribute to some of the DS phenotypes [47]. Our study demonstrates the clinical relevance of small CNVs as low as 0.1 Mb during CGH Microarray diagnostic testing and underlines the importance of prudent clinical interpretation of these CNVs. With the Next-generation sequencing (NGS) technology ability to detecting both single nucleotide variants and copy number variation in one test, Whole Genome Sequencing (WGS) could one day serve a more importance role in further establish the genotype-phenotype association. Large cohort studies with specific phenotypes subgroups will also be helpful to further our understanding of the genotype-phenotype association on chromosome 21.

Acknowledgements

The authors would like to thank the patients participating in this study and the technologists, including Hui Pang of OUHSC Genetics Laboratory, for their technical support.

Authors' contributions

WL gained the IRB approval, gathered clinical information, interpreted the array CGH data, and drafted the manuscript. XW performed the array CGH analysis and participated array CGH data interpretation. SL conceived this study and helped draft the manuscript. All authors read and approved the final manuscript.

Competing interests

The authors declare that they have no competing interests.

References

1. Parker SE, Mai CT, Canfield MA, Rickard R, Wang Y, Meyer RE, Anderson P, Mason CA, Collins JS, Kirby RS, et al. Updated National Birth Prevalence estimates for selected birth defects in the United States, 2004-2006. Birth Defects Res A Clin Mol Teratol. 2010;88(12):1008–16.
2. Scriver CR. The metabolic and molecular bases of inherited disease. 7th ed. New York: McGraw-Hill, Health Professions Division; 1995.
3. Delabar JM, Theophile D, Rahmani Z, Chettouh Z, Blouin JL, Prieur M, Noel B, Sinet PM. Molecular mapping of twenty-four features of Down syndrome on chromosome 21. Eur J Hum Genet. 1993;1(2):114–24.
4. Kahlem P, Sultan M, Herwig R, Steinfath M, Balzereit D, Eppens B, Saran NG, Pletcher MT, South ST, Stetten G, et al. Transcript level alterations reflect gene dosage effects across multiple tissues in a mouse model of Down syndrome. Genome Res. 2004;14(7):1258–67.
5. Amano K, Sago H, Uchikawa C, Suzuki T, Kotliarova SE, Nukina N, Epstein CJ, Yamakawa K. Dosage-dependent over-expression of genes in the trisomic region of Ts1Cje mouse model for Down syndrome. Hum Mol Genet. 2004; 13(13):1333–40.

6.   Crombez EA, Dipple KM, Schimmenti LA, Rao N. Duplication of the Down syndrome critical region does not predict facial phenotype in a baby with a ring chromosome 21. Clin Dysmorphol. 2005;14(4):183–7.

7.   Doran E, Keator D, Head E, Phelan MJ, Kim R, Totoiu M, Barrio JR, Small GW, Potkin SG, Lott IT. Down syndrome, partial trisomy 21, and absence of Alzheimer's disease: the role of APP. J Alzheimers Dis. 2017;56(2):459–70.

8.   Errichiello E, Novara F, Cremante A, Verri A, Galli J, Fazzi E, Bellotti D, Losa L, Cisternino M, Zuffardi O. Dissection of partial 21q monosomy in different phenotypes: clinical and molecular characterization of five cases and review of the literature. Mol Cytogenet. 2016;9(1):21.

9.   Pelleri MC, Cicchini E, Locatelli C, Vitale L, Caracausi M, Piovesan A, Rocca A, Poletti G, Seri M, Strippoli P, et al. Systematic reanalysis of partial trisomy 21 cases with or without Down syndrome suggests a small region on 21q22.13 as critical to the phenotype. Hum Mol Genet. 2016;25(12):2525–38.

10. Simioni M, Steiner CE, Gil-da-Silva-Lopes VL. De novo double reciprocal translocations in addition to partial monosomy at another chromosome: a very rare case. Gene. 2015;573(1):166–70.

11. Weisfeld-Adams JD, Tkachuk AK, Maclean KN, Meeks NL, Scott SA. A de novo 2.78-Mb duplication on chromosome 21q22.11 implicates candidate genes in the partial trisomy 21 phenotype. NPJ Genom Med. 2016;1

12. Firth HV, Richards SM, Bevan AP, Clayton S, Corpas M, Rajan D, Van Vooren S, Moreau Y, Pettett RM, Carter NP. DECIPHER: database of chromosomal imbalance and phenotype in humans using Ensembl resources. Am J Hum Genet. 2009;84(4):524–33.

13. Efron D. Autism: current theories and evidence (hbk). J Paediatr Child Health. 2010;46(1–2):70.

14. Rost I, Fiegler H, Fauth C, Carr P, Bettecken T, Kraus J, Meyer C, Enders A, Wirtz A, Meitinger T, et al. Tetrasomy 21pter-->q21.2 in a male infant without typical Down's syndrome dysmorphic features but moderate mental retardation. J Med Genet. 2004;41(3):e26.

15. Piccoli C, Izzo A, Scrima R, Bonfiglio F, Manco R, Negri R, Quarato G, Cela O, Ripoli M, Prisco M, et al. Chronic pro-oxidative state and mitochondrial dysfunctions are more pronounced in fibroblasts from Down syndrome foeti with congenital heart defects. Hum Mol Genet. 2013;22(6):1218–32.

16. Molloy CA, Keddache M, Martin LJ. Evidence for linkage on 21q and 7q in a subset of autism characterized by developmental regression. Mol Psychiatry. 2005;10(8):741–6.

17. Chauhan A, Chauhan V. Oxidative stress in autism. Pathophysiology. 2006; 13(3):171–81.

18. Matsuda S, Rouault J, Magaud J, Berthet C. In search of a function for the TIS21/PC3/BTG1/TOB family. FEBS Lett. 2001;497(2–3):67–72.

19. Petit F, Plessis G, Decamp M, Cuisset JM, Blyth M, Pendlebury M, Andrieux J. 21q21 deletion involving NCAM2: report of 3 cases with neurodevelopmental disorders. Eur J Med Genet. 2015;58(1):44–6.

20. Haldeman-Englert CR, Chapman KA, Kruger H, Geiger EA, McDonald-McGinn DM, Rappaport E, Zackai EH, Spinner NB, Shaikh TH. A de novo 8.8-Mb deletion of 21q21.1-q21.3 in an autistic male with a complex rearrangement involving chromosomes 6, 10, and 21. Am J Med Genet A. 2010;152A(1): 196–202.

21. Wilcock DM. Neuroinflammation in the aging Down syndrome brain; lessons from Alzheimer's disease. Curr Gerontol Geriatr Res. 2012;2012:170276.

22. Kashimura T, Kodama M, Hotta Y, Hosoya J, Yoshida K, Ozawa T, Watanabe R, Okura Y, Kato K, Hanawa H, et al. Spatiotemporal changes of coxsackievirus and adenovirus receptor in rat hearts during postnatal development and in cultured cardiomyocytes of neonatal rat. Virchows Arch. 2004;444(3):283–92.

23. Chen JW, Zhou B, Yu QC, Shin SJ, Jiao K, Schneider MD, Baldwin HS, Bergelson JM. Cardiomyocyte-specific deletion of the coxsackievirus and adenovirus receptor results in hyperplasia of the embryonic left ventricle and abnormalities of sinuatrial valves. Circ Res. 2006;98(7):923–30.

24. Yuen S, Smith J, Caruso L, Balan M, Opavsky MA. The coxsackie-adenovirus receptor induces an inflammatory cardiomyopathy independent of viral infection. J Mol Cell Cardiol. 2011;50(5):826–40.

25. Caceres M, Lachuer J, Zapala MA, Redmond JC, Kudo L, Geschwind DH, Lockhart DJ, Preuss TM, Barlow C. Elevated gene expression levels distinguish human from non-human primate brains. Proc Natl Acad Sci U S A. 2003;100(22):13030–5.

26. Iurov I, Vorsanova SG, Saprina EA, Iurov Iu B. Identification of candidate genes of autism on the basis of molecular cytogenetic and in silico studies of the genome organization of chromosomal regions involved in unbalanced rearrangements. Genetika. 2010;46(10):1348–51.

27. Hoeffer CA, Dey A, Sachan N, Wong H, Patterson RJ, Shelton JM, Richardson JA, Klann E, Rothermel BA. The Down syndrome critical region protein RCAN1 regulates long-term potentiation and memory via inhibition of phosphatase signaling. J Neurosci. 2007;27(48):13161–72.

28. Wong H, Levenga J, Cain P, Rothermel B, Klann E, Hoeffer C. RCAN1 overexpression promotes age-dependent mitochondrial dysregulation related to neurodegeneration in Alzheimer's disease. Acta Neuropathol. 2015;130(6):829–43.

29. Patel A, Yamashita N, Ascano M, Bodmer D, Boehm E, Bodkin-Clarke C, Ryu YK, Kuruvilla R. RCAN1 links impaired neurotrophin trafficking to aberrant development of the sympathetic nervous system in Down syndrome. Nat Commun. 2015;6:10119.

30. Wu Y, Song W. Regulation of RCAN1 translation and its role in oxidative stress-induced apoptosis. FASEB J. 2013;27(1):208–21.

31. Shirley MD, Frelin L, Lopez JS, Jedlicka A, Dziedzic A, Frank-Crawford MA, Silverman W, Hagopian L, Pevsner J. Copy number variants associated with 14 cases of self-injurious behavior. PLoS One. 2016;11(3):e0149646.

32. Fujita H, Torii C, Kosaki R, Yamaguchi S, Kudoh J, Hayashi K, Takahashi T, Kosaki K. Microdeletion of the Down syndrome critical region at 21q22. Am J Med Genet A. 2010;152A(4):950–3.

33. Cho CK, Drabovich AP, Karagiannis GS, Martinez-Morillo E, Dason S, Dimitromanolakis A, Diamandis EP. Quantitative proteomic analysis of amniocytes reveals potentially dysregulated molecular networks in Down syndrome. Clin Proteomics. 2013;10(1):2.

34. Swaminathan S, Huentelman MJ, Corneveaux JJ, Myers AJ, Faber KM, Foroud T, Mayeux R, Shen L, Kim S, Turk M, et al. Analysis of copy number variation in Alzheimer's disease in a cohort of clinically characterized and neuropathologically verified individuals. PLoS One. 2012;7(12):e50640.

35. Paoloni-Giacobino A, Chen H, Antonarakis SE. Cloning of a novel human neural cell adhesion molecule gene (NCAM2) that maps to chromosome region 21q21 and is potentially involved in Down syndrome. Genomics. 1997;43(1):43–51.

36. Nielsen J, Gotfryd K, Li S, Kulahin N, Soroka V, Rasmussen KK, Bock E, Berezin V. Role of glial cell line-derived neurotrophic factor (GDNF)-neural cell adhesion molecule (NCAM) interactions in induction of neurite outgrowth and identification of a binding site for NCAM in the heel region of GDNF. J Neurosci. 2009;29(36):11360–76.

37. Kulahin N, Walmod PS. The neural cell adhesion molecule NCAM2/OCAM/ RNCAM, a close relative to NCAM. Adv Exp Med Biol. 2010;663:403–20.

38. Chen CP, Lin YH, Chou SY, Su YN, Chern SR, Chen YT, Town DD, Chen WL, Wang W. Mosaic ring chromosome 21, monosomy 21, and isodicentric ring chromosome 21: prenatal diagnosis, molecular cytogenetic characterization, and association with 2-Mb deletion of 21q21.1-q21.2 and 5-Mb deletion of 21q22.3. Taiwan J Obstet Gynecol. 2012;51(1):71–6.

39. Reynolds GP, Warner CE. Amino acid neurotransmitter deficits in adult Down's syndrome brain tissue. Neurosci Lett. 1988;94(1–2):224–7.

40. Arai Y, Mizuguchi M, Takashima S. Excessive glutamate receptor 1 immunoreactivity in adult Down syndrome brains. Pediatr Neurol. 1996; 15(3):203–6.

41. Saud K, Arriagada C, Cardenas AM, Shimahara T, Allen DD, Caviedes R, Caviedes P. Neuronal dysfunction in Down syndrome: contribution of neuronal models in cell culture. J Physiol Paris. 2006;99(2–3):201–10.

42. Yamamoto T, Shimojima K, Nishizawa T, Matsuo M, Ito M, Imai K. Clinical manifestations of the deletion of Down syndrome critical region including DYRK1A and KCNJ6. Am J Med Genet A. 2011;155A(1):113–9.

43. Dowjat WK, Adayev T, Kuchna I, Nowicki K, Palminiello S, Hwang YW, Wegiel J. Trisomy-driven overexpression of DYRK1A kinase in the brain of subjects with Down syndrome. Neurosci Lett. 2007;413(1):77–81.

44. Courcet J-B, Faivre L, Malzac P, Masurel-Paulet A, Lopez E, Callier P, Lambert L, Lemesle M, Thevenon J, Gigot N, et al. The DYRK1A gene is a cause of syndromic intellectual disability with severe microcephaly and epilepsy. J Med Genet. 2012;49(12):731–6.

45. Ji J, Lee H, Argiropoulos B, Dorrani N, Mann J, Martinez-Agosto JA, Gomez-Ospina N, Gallant N, Bernstein JA, Hudgins L, et al. DYRK1A haploinsufficiency causes a new recognizable syndrome with microcephaly, intellectual disability, speech impairment, and distinct facies. Eur J Hum Genet. 2015;23(11):1473–81.

46. Antonarakis SE. Down syndrome and the complexity of genome dosage imbalance. Nat Rev Genet. 2017;18(3):147–63.

47. Conrad B, Antonarakis SE. Gene duplication: a drive for phenotypic diversity and cause of human disease. Annu Rev Genomics Hum Genet. 2007;8:17–35.

4

Human ring chromosome registry for cases in the Chinese population: re-emphasizing Cytogenomic and clinical heterogeneity and reviewing diagnostic and treatment strategies

Qiping Hu[1,2]*, Hongyan Chai[2], Wei Shu[1] and Peining Li[2]* (iD)

Abstract

Background: Constitutional ring chromosomes are rare orphan chromosomal disorders. Ring chromosome syndrome featuring growth retardation and mild to intermediate intellectual disability is likely caused by the dynamic behavior of ring chromosome through cell cycles. Chromosomal and regional specific phenotypes likely result from segmental losses and gains during the ring formation. Although recent applications of genomic copy number and sequencing analyses revealed various ring chromosome structures from an increasing number of case studies, there was no organized effort for compiling and curating cytogenomic and clinical finding for ring chromosomes.

Methods: A web-based interactive 'Human Ring Chromosome Registry' using Microsoft Access based relational database was developed to present genetic and phenotypic findings of ring chromosome cases. Chinese ring chromosome cases reported in the literature was reviewed and compiled as a testing data set to validate this registry.

Results: A total of 113 cases of ring chromosomes were retrieved in all chromosomes except for chromosomes 16, 17 and 19. The most frequently seen ring chromosomes by a decreasing order of relative frequencies were ring 13 (14%), X (12%), 22 (10%), 15 (9%), 14 (7%), and 18 (7%). Genomic imbalances were detected in 18 out of 19 cases analyzed by microarray or sequencing. Variable clinical manifestations of developmental delay, dysmorphic facial features, intellectual disability, microcephaly, and hypotonia were noted in most autosomal rings. Chromosomal specific syndromic phenotypes included Wolf-Hirschhorn syndrome in a ring chromosome 4, cri-du-chat syndrome in a ring chromosome 5, epilepsy in ring chromosomes 14 and 20, Turner syndrome in ring chromosome X, and infertility in ring chromosomes 13, 21, 22 and Y. Effective growth hormone supplemental treatment for growth retardation in a ring chromosome 18 was noted.

Conclusions: Based on findings from these Chinese ring chromosome cases, guidelines for cytogenomic diagnosis and criteria for case registration were proposed. Further research to define underlying mechanisms of ring chromosome formation and dynamic mosaicism, to delineate the genotype-phenotype correlations, and to develop chromosome therapy for ring chromosomes were discussed.

Keywords: Ring chromosome, Online registry, Ring chromosome instability, Dynamic mosaicism, Genomic imbalances, Syndromic phenotypes, Diagnostic guidelines, Chromosome therapy

* Correspondence: huqiping@gxmu.edu.cn; peining.li@yale.edu
[1]Department of Cell Biology and Genetics, School of Pre-Clinical Medicine,
Guangxi Medical University, Nanning, Guangxi 530021, China
[2]Laboratory of Clinical Cytogenetics and Genomics, Department of Genetics,
Yale School of Medicine, New Haven, CT 06520, USA

Background

Constitutional ring chromosomes are a rare type of intra-chromosome structural abnormality with an estimated occurrence of 1 in 50,000 newborns [1]. A ring chromosome is resulted from breakage and fusion at the telomeric or distal regions of both chromosome arms; this circular chromosome replaces one normal chromosome and presents unique mitotic behavior. Structurally, ring chromosomes are divided into two types: a complete ring chromosome without loss of genetic materials by telomere-telomere fusion or an incomplete ring with distal or interstitial deletions and duplications by one or multiple breakage-fusion events [2–4]. Through each cell cycle, ring chromosomes will experience mitotic disturbance induced by ring chromosome instability and result in three different fates of stable ring transmission, ring size changes by one sister chromatid exchange, or interlocked rings by two sister chromatid exchanges. This ring chromosome instability presents a 'dynamic mosaicism' with cells showing chromosomal or segmental aneuploidies and thus a portion of cell loss from mitotic arrest and apoptosis [5, 6]. Earlier reports of ring chromosome cases by karyotype analysis observed this dynamic mosaicism but failed to detect segmental or cryptic deletions and duplications due to the limited analytical resolution [7, 8]. The application of fluorescence in situ hybridization (FISH) enabled the differentiation of complete rings from incomplete ones and the monitoring of dynamic mosaicism using various probes targeted to the telomeric, subtelomeric, distal and centromeric regions of the involved chromosome [2, 3, 9]. Recently, genomic technologies such as array-comparative genomic hybridization (aCGH), single nucleotide polymorphism (SNP) chip, and whole-genome sequencing were applied to analyze copy number changes and complex rearrangements and revealed various genomic structures of human ring chromosomes [4, 10, 11].

Patients carrying an autosomal ring chromosome shared certain clinical manifestations including proportional growth retardation, developmental delay, mild to severe intellectual disability, microcephaly, and mild to intermediate dysmorphic facial features. These common manifestations were classified as 'ring chromosome syndrome' and were thought to be caused by ring chromosome instability from recognized cases of complete ring chromosome [8, 12]. However, ring chromosome cases with certain phenotypes associated with segmental deletions and duplications had been reported [3, 10]. In clinical practice, ring chromosomes were detected mostly from pediatric patients with growth retardation and occasionally from prenatal cases with intrauterine growth restriction [13, 14]. Ring chromosome X in females with premature ovarian failure and ring chromosome Y in males with azoospermia were noted in adult reproductive clinics [15, 16].

Despite an increase volume of case reports of ring chromosomes from prenatal to postnatal clinics and more detailed cytogenetic and genomic findings with the introduction of genomic technologies, it is still a challenge to interpret the compound effects and to predict the clinical consequences from the dynamic mosaicism and genomic imbalances of ring chromosomes. The rarity of ring chromosome cases demands organized efforts to compile and curate findings from ring chromosome cases for better diagnostic practice and disease classification. This report presented the design and implementation of an online interactive human ring chromosome registry and a comprehensive review of ring chromosome cases in the Chinese population. This initial effort could lead to future collaboration toward the construction of a human ring chromosome atlas as a clinical, research and educational resource for this rare type of chromosomal abnormality.

Design of an online human ring chromosome registry

A Microsoft Access based relational laboratory information management system had been developed and implemented for a clinical cytogenetics laboratory [17]. Following the design principles for a genetics home reference [18], a Microsoft Access based online interactive registry for human ring chromosomes was developed. This registry includes five modules of case information, figure, summary, reference, and glossary. The case module (ringchr_case) covers an assigned identification number, gender, age, cytogenetic and genomic results, and clinical findings. The figure module (fig_lib) stores illustrative images. The summary module (chr_summary) presents contents and statistics of major clinical features for a specific chromosome. The reference module collects case reports and articles of ring chromosome cases registered in the database. The glossary module contains genetic and clinical terms used in genetic diagnostic and clinical description. Relationships between these modules are determined using primary key (PK), unique key (UK) and foreign key (FK). Figure 1 shows the relationship model of the five modules and a view of the web page for this registry. This 'Human Ring Chromosome' registry is loaded online with a website of "http://web.gxmu.edu.cn/shengwu/HRC/home.asp". To validate the modular relations and functions of this human ring chromosome registry, ring chromosome cases in the Chinese population was collected as the initial testing data set.

Ring chromosome cases in the chinese population
Comprehensive review of ring chromosome cases

Case reports and original articles of constitutional ring chromosomes were searched from Chinese medical journals archived in the SinoMed (http://www.sinomed.ac.cn/), VIP (http://qikan.cqvip.com/), CNKI (China National

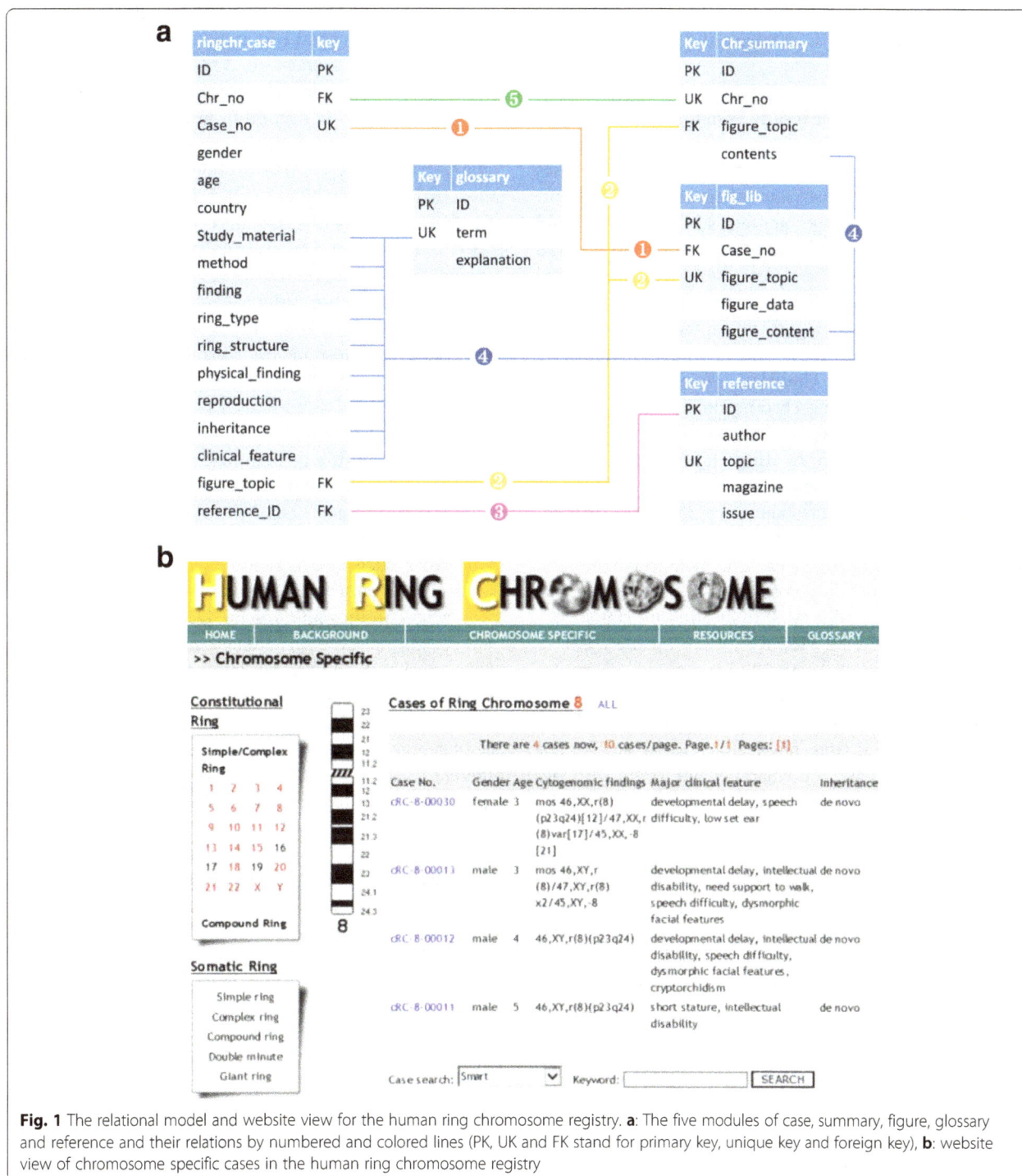

Fig. 1 The relational model and website view for the human ring chromosome registry. **a**: The five modules of case, summary, figure, glossary and reference and their relations by numbered and colored lines (PK, UK and FK stand for primary key, unique key and foreign key), **b**: website view of chromosome specific cases in the human ring chromosome registry

Knowledge Infrastructure, http://www.cnki.net) and WANFANG DATA (http://www.wanfangdata.com) as well as English journals archived in the PubMed (https://www.ncbi.nlm.nih.gov/pubmed/) for a period from 1979 to June 2017. For each case, the gender, age, cytogenetic and genomic results, clinical findings, and family history were retrieved, reviewed and registered into the ring chromosome registry. The relative

frequencies of ring chromosomes were calculated by the case number of a specific chromosome divided by the total number of cases. The presence and penetrance of clinical features was shown in a heat map by the observed frequency among cases of a chromosome or all autosomes. Cases with supernumerary small marker chromosomes (sSMC) in the form of a small ring chromosome were excluded because these cases and their cytogenomic and clinical findings were summarized in an online sSMC database (http://ssmc-tl.com/sSMC.html).

Cytogenetic and genomic results from ring chromosome cases

A systematic search of Chinese ring chromosome cases found a total of 113 cases from 94 case reports and four original articles. The age, gender, study materials and methods, cytogenetic and genomic results, major clinical findings, family history, and references are summarized in the Additional file 1: Table S1. Of these 113 cases, 95 cases were autosomal ring chromosomes except for no cases of chromosomes 16, 17 and 19 while 18 cases were sex chromosome rings. The relative frequencies by a decreasing order were ring chromosome 13 in 14%, ring chromosome X in 12%, ring chromosome 22 in 10%, ring chromosome 15 in 9%, ring chromosomes 14 and 18 each in 7%, ring chromosomes Y, 4, 5, 6, 8, 9 and 21 each in 4%, ring chromosome 2 in 3%, ring chromosomes 3, 7, 10 and 20 each in 2%, and ring chromosomes 1, 11 and 12 each in 1%. The male to female ratio for autosomal ring chromosome cases was 44 vs 51 (Chi-square test, P value 0.49), indicating no statistically significant gender bias. However, more female cases in ring chromosomes 13, 18 and 22 were noted. There is a need of more cases to evaluate the sex ratio for individual chromosome. Compound chromosomal abnormalities were noted in one physically normal adult male who was referred by a perinatal infant death and detected with a derivative chromosome 6 from a 6p/13q translocation and a ring chromosome 13 [19], and in an infant with XYY and a ring chromosome 13 [20].

Regional specific assays (RSA) such as FISH, multiple ligation probe amplification (MLPA), and short-tandem repeats (STR) were applied to 24 cases. Genome-wide aCGH and SNP-chip were used on 17 cases and genomic sequencing was used on two cases. Three out of 13 cases by RSA alone were noted with distal deletions while 18 out of 19 cases by genomic analysis were noted with distal deletions ranging from 160 Kb (kilo base-pair) to 34 Mb (mega base-pair). The latter result suggested that most cases of ring chromosome were incomplete rings although reporting bias of selected cases should be taken into consideration. The relative frequencies, the genomic imbalances, age and gender distribution of reported Chinese ring chromosome cases are shown in Fig. 2.

Dynamic mosaicism was detected in 63 cases by karyotype analysis of 20 to 250 metaphase cells. For cases with autosomal ring chromosomes, ring chromosome variants including ring size changes, interlocked rings, an extra copy of ring, or a derivative chromosome from ring breakage were noted in 2%–17% of cells with an average of 11%; monosomy due to the loss of the ring

chromosome was noted in 3%–31% of cells with an average of 13%, and normal karyotype was noted in 1%–84% of cells with an average of 32%. For cases with sex chromosome rings, ring chromosome variants were not seen but losses of ring chromosome X or Y were noted in 9%–93% of cells with an average of 62%. These results indicated that only a small portion of cells can tolerate autosomal ring instability but a relatively larger portion of cells can survive the loss of a sex chromosome ring. However, the lack of diagnostic guidelines specific for analyzing dynamic mosaicism has made it difficult for reliable case-by-case and chromosome-to-chromosome comparisons of ring chromosome instability. In a prenatal case with a ring chromosome 13, cytogenetic analysis showed similar dynamic mosaicism of ring chromosome 13, dicentric ring 13, and monosomy 13 in cultured amniocytes and cord blood leukocytes but a small marker chromosome 13 and monosomy 13 in placenta tissue; aCGH analysis revealed a 4.22 Mb deletion at 13q34 in the ring chromosome 13 and a 91.8 Mb deletion of 13q11-q34 in the marker chromosome. This fetoplacental chromosomal discrepancy suggested a tissue-specific karyotype evolution and the marker chromosome as a residual fragment from ring chromosome rescue [21]. The finding of a marker chromosome in prenatal analysis of chorionic villus specimen should be interpreted cautiously and followed by amniocentesis or cord blood study. Overall, cytogenomic heterogeneity was noted in the high percentage of genomic imbalances in ring chromosome structure, different levels of dynamic mosaicism, and variable karyotype evolution in different tissues.

Clinical findings in ring chromosome cases

Of the 113 cases with a ring chromosome, 89 cases (77 autosomal and 12 sex chromosomal rings) were assessed in perinatal or pediatric clinics, 14 cases (13 autosomal and one sex chromosome rings) were diagnosed prenatally, and 10 cases (six autosomal and four sex chromosome rings) were noted in infertility or reproductive clinics. Major clinical findings compiled from 82 postnatal cases with autosomal ring chromosomes are shown as a heat map in Fig. 3. Despite only one or two cases for several ring autosomes, the most common findings were developmental delay (52/82), dysmorphic facial features (41/82), intellectual disability (31/82), microcephaly (26/82), and hypotonia (18/82). These findings are considered as features of so-called 'ring chromosome syndrome' but variable clinical manifestations are obvious. Other frequently seen clinical presentations in different ring autosomes were speech difficulty, genitalia dysplasia in different forms, various types of congenital heart defects, and low birth weight.

Chromosome-specific syndromic phenotypes resulting from segmental imbalances were noted. Features

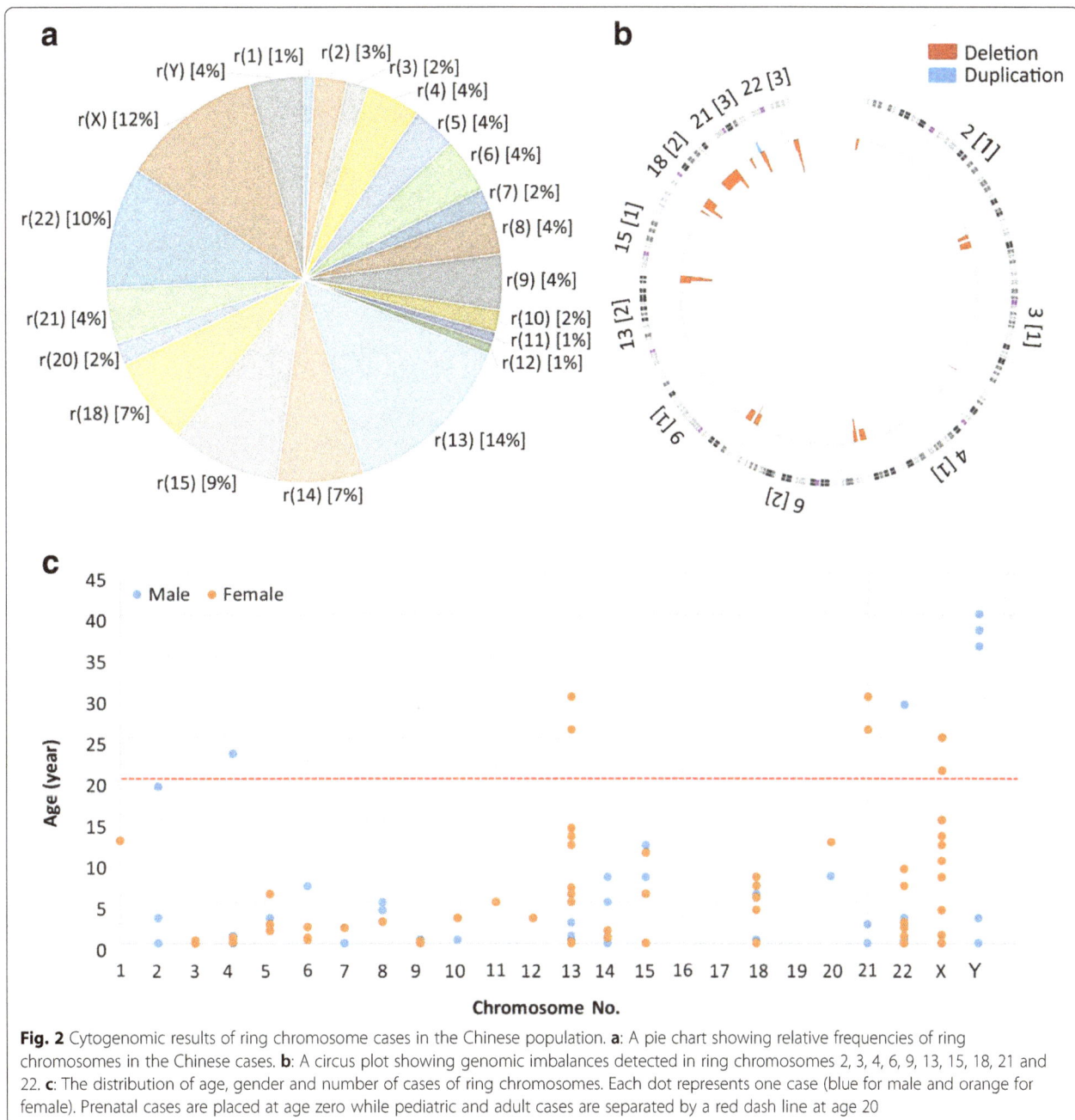

Fig. 2 Cytogenomic results of ring chromosome cases in the Chinese population. **a**: A pie chart showing relative frequencies of ring chromosomes in the Chinese cases. **b**: A circus plot showing genomic imbalances detected in ring chromosomes 2, 3, 4, 6, 9, 13, 15, 18, 21 and 22. **c**: The distribution of age, gender and number of cases of ring chromosomes. Each dot represents one case (blue for male and orange for female). Prenatal cases are placed at age zero while pediatric and adult cases are separated by a red dash line at age 20

of Wolf-Hirschhorn syndrome (OMIM#194190) known to 4p16.3 deletions was reported in a case with a ring chromosome 4. Cri-du-chat syndrome (OMIM#123450) related with 5p deletions was reported in one case with a ring chromosome 5 and another case with a ring chromosome 2. Wilms tumor caused by heterozygous mutations in the WT1 gene at 11p13 (OMIM#194070) was noted in one case with a ring chromosome 11. Retinal defect was noted in one case with a ring chromosome 13, inferring an increased risk for retinoblastoma (OMIM#180200) caused by deletions and mutations in the RB1 gene at 13q14.2. Epilepsy as a highly penetrant phenotype was noted in all seven cases with a ring chromosome 14 and two cases with a ring chromosome 20. Epilepsy and other symptoms in ring chromosome 14 are referred as ring chromosome 14 syndrome (OMIM#616606). Growth hormone deficiency was reported in one case with a ring chromosome 18; periodic growth hormone supplement treatment was effective [22]. Growth hormone deficiency was a key feature of distal 18q23 deletion with significant treatment implications [23]. For adult patients with infertility, aspermia was noted in two adult males with a ring chromosome 21 or 22, amenorrhea was noted in two adult females

Ring Chromosome	r(As)	r(1)	r(2)	r(3)	r(4)	r(5)	r(6)	r(7)	r(8)	r(9)	r(10)	r(11)	r(12)	r(13)	r(14)	r(15)	r(18)	r(20)	r(21)	r(22)
Case Number	82	1	2	2	5	4	4	1	4	5	2	1	1	14	7	7	7	2	4	9

Clinical Findings:
- Developmental delay
- Intellectual disability
- Dysmorphic facial features
- Microcephaly
- Hypotonia
- Low Birth weight
- Speech difficulty
- Congenital heart defect
- Cerebral palsy
- Epilepsy
- Hyperactivity
- Hypoactivity
- Hearing impairment
- Retinal defect
- Hypothiyroidism
- Genitalia dysplasia
- Aspermia/azoospemia
- Amenorrhea
- Infertility
- Cat-like cry
- Wolf-Hirschhorn syndrome
- Wilm's tumor
- Growth Hormone Deficiency

Legend: ■ 76-100% ■ 51-75% ■ 26-50% 1-25%   *r(As), autosomal chromosome rings

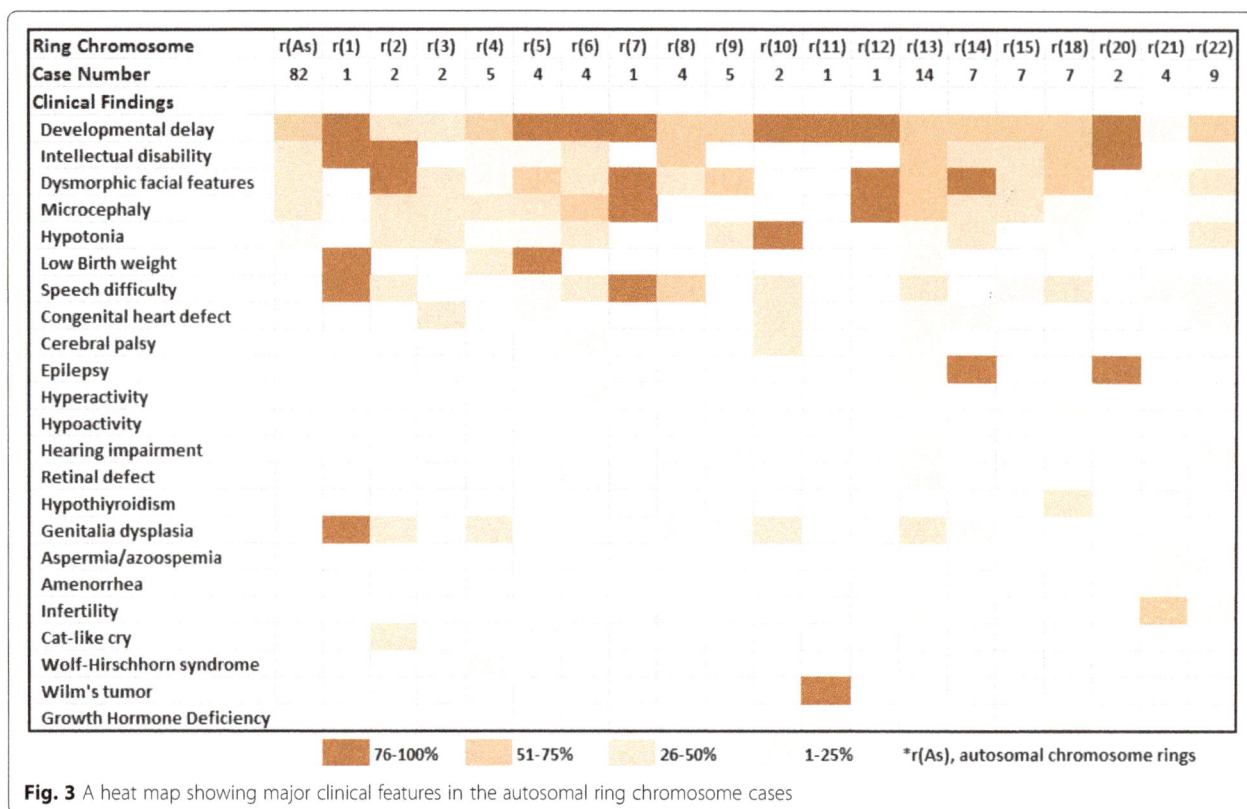

Fig. 3 A heat map showing major clinical features in the autosomal ring chromosome cases

with a ring chromosome 21, Tuner syndrome-like phenotype was noted in almost all cases with a ring chromosome X, and azoospermia, aspermia, small testes were seen in three cases with a ring chromosome Y. Overall, clinical heterogeneity for ring chromosomes was indicated by the incomplete penetrance, variable expressivity, and different age of onset of ring chromosome syndrome and the compound effects from chromosome-specific or region-specific phenotypes.

The clinical indications for prenatal diagnosis of ring chromosome cases included ultrasound findings of intrauterine growth restriction, oligohydramnios, microcephaly, lissencephaly, anencephaly, ventricular septal defect, and increased nuchal fold as well as abnormal prenatal screening results for increased risk of Down syndrome. Termination of pregnancy had been an option for fetus with severe anomalies and defined ring chromosome abnormalities. Excluding cases with parental denial or no follow up tests, parental studies performed in 60 families with a proband carrying a ring chromosome documented normal karyotypes for both parents. This result indicated that almost all ring chromosomes are de novo in origin. The clinical presentations from prenatal and postnatal cases with a ring chromosome and their family history could be helpful for genetic counseling.

Toward precise genetic diagnosis and clinical management

With annual births of 17.86 million in China for 2016 and the occurrence of 1/50,000 for a constitutional ring chromosome, there are an approximately 350 newborns with this group of rare orphan chromosomal disorders each year in the Chinese population. A comprehensive review of medical literature found only 113 reported Chinese cases with a ring chromosome which probably represented about 1% of total cases for the past four decades in the Chinese population. Even though only a small percentage of ring chromosome cases were published, this case series was by far the largest in an ethnic group. The findings from these cases provided insights into developing practice guidelines and research collaboration for genetic diagnosis, clinical management, and disease treatment.

Considerations of diagnostic guidelines for constitutional ring chromosomes

Integrated analyses by karyotype, FISH and SNP chip on a series of 14 cases of autosomal ring chromosomes detected the dynamic mosaicism of ring chromosome variants in 5%–16.3% of the 300 metaphase cells examined and distal deletions in the range of 364 Kb to 18 Mb in 12 cases [24]. The range of dynamic mosaicism and the portion of genomic imbalances in these 14 ring chromosome cases were consistent with findings from this Chinese case series. The analysis by aCGH and SNP chip can delineate the genomic imbalances in the ring chromosome, map critical regions containing candidate genes for certain phenotypes, and infer underlying gene dosage or position effects [10, 25]. A study of 27 patients with a ring chromosome 14 mapped the retinal abnormality and epilepsy within the proximal 14q11.2-q12 region containing the retinitis pigmentosa gene *RPGRIP1*, the neural retina leucine zipper gene *NRL*, and the *FOXG1* gene. It was speculated that the formation of the ring could induce the spreading of heterochromatinization and dysregulate the gene expression [26]. Dysregulation of *FOXG1* gene by an acentric ring chromosome 14 was noted in a patient with epilepsy [27]. Based on the clinical types per cytogenomic findings and reproductive patterns from male and female carriers per family history, recommendations for cytogenomic analysis specific for ring chromosome 21 was proposed [4]. Currently, except for the general cytogenetics guidelines and standards developed by American College of Medical Genetics and Genomics or other regional professional organizations, there were no diagnostic consensus and guidelines designated for analyzing the genomic structures and measuring the dynamic mosaicism from ring chromosomes. For all constitutional ring chromosomes, an integrated cytogenomic approach should be implemented for three purposes: 1) differentiating complete rings from incomplete ones, 2) delineating genomic imbalances in the ring chromosomes, and 3) defining levels of ring chromosome instability. The diagnostic guidelines for this approach should include the following:

- Routine chromosome analysis on a peripheral blood specimen should be performed on 100 metaphases for percentages of cells with typical ring chromosome, ring variants, and ring loss. FISH tests should be performed on 300 directly prepared interphase cells using chromosome-specific subtelomeric, centromeric, and targeted locus-specific probes to access distal deletions/duplications, ring variants and ring loss. This analysis of 100 to 300 cells will allow an accurate detection of dynamic mosaicism in 2%–3% of cells with a 95% confidence level [28]. If possible, the analysis of different tissues to further define the mosaic pattern should be considered.
- Genomic analysis by aCGH, SNP chip, or genomic sequencing should be performed to characterize the distal or interstitial copy number imbalances in the ring chromosomes. The result from this DNA-based genomic analysis should be correlated with findings from cell-based chromosome and FISH tests.

- Evidence-based interpretation should be provided regarding clinical significance for detected dynamic mosaicism and genomic imbalances of ring chromosomes. The implications on physical and mental development as well as risks for cancer and reproduction should be addressed [29]. Evidences for genomic imbalances could be collected from similar cases reported in the literature and databases of linear copy number variants. These databases include Database of Genomic Variants (DGV), ClinVar, and DatabasE of Chromosomal Imbalance and Phenotype in Humans using Ensembl Resources (DECIPHER). Tracks of these databases could be linked from the Human Genome Browser (http://genome.ucsc.edu/).
- Follow-up parental study should be considered to determine de novo or familial transmission of the ring chromosome. It was estimated that inherited ring chromosomes exist in approximately 1% of ring chromosome cases; familial cases usually presented relatively mild clinical manifestations but one third of the transmitted offspring were more severely affected [30].

There is an urgent need for consensus on defining level of ring chromosome instability by observed dynamic mosaicism. This report and a recent case series documented a range of 2%–17% for autosomal ring chromosome variants and ring loss [24]. A study of ring chromosome 20 cases found that the mosaic ratio of r(20) was directly correlated with the severity of cognitive impairment and inversely correlated with the onset age of epilepsy; this finding should be interpreted with caution since the level of mosaicism in blood may not reflect the level of mosaicism in other tissue, especially the brain [31]. A study of aneuploidy in the developing human brain determined an average aneuploidy frequency as 1.25–1.45% per chromosome and thus an estimated overall aneuploidy percentage of 30–35% for all chromosomes; these findings revealed confined chromosomal mosaicism in the brain and suggested a potential link between chromosome instability and human brain diseases [32]. These studies provided evidences on the importance of defining levels of ring chromosome instability. The low, intermediate and high levels of ring chromosome instability may be defined using an arbitrary measurement of less than 5%, 6–10% and more than 10% of metaphase/interphase dynamic mosaicism, respectively. For example, the analysis of 100 metaphase cells from a case (unpublished) revealed a primary pattern of a dicentric ring chromosome 18 in 91% of cells and secondary variant patterns of tri–/tetra-centric rings and monosomy 18 likely due to the loss of ring in 9% of cells. This could be considered as an intermediate level of ring chromosome instability. The cytogenetic results and the karyotypic evolution for this dicentric ring chromosome 18 are shown in Fig. 4. Recent progresses in the use of genomic analysis as the first-tier genetic testing and non-invasive prenatal screening of aneuploidies by sequencing of maternal serum cell-free DNA have improved the diagnostic efficacy for a wider spectrum of cytogenomic abnormalities [33–35]. However, for analyzing structural rearrangement like ring chromosomes, integrating cell-based karyotype and FISH analyses with DNA-based genomic analysis should be the gold standard.

General recommendations for clinical management of ring chromosome cases

Cases of ring chromosome presents a spectrum of clinical features caused by ring chromosome instability and additional features compounded by dosage effect from

genomic imbalances, position effect from structural rearrangement, or changes in epigenetic modification [5, 36]. Of the 113 cases in this report, approximately 12%, 79% and 9% of them were detected from prenatal, pediatric and reproductive clinics, respectively. Clinical features of ring chromosome syndrome and chromosome-specific syndromic phenotypes were presented. Variable clinical manifestations in ring chromosome cases were noted in one group with severe clinical symptoms and the other group with no obvious clinical problems apart from infertility [24]. Effective supplemental treatment of growth hormone deficiency in a ring chromosome 18 was noted [22]. The general principles for clinical management of ring chromosome cases should include: 1) thorough clinical assessment of developmental delay, intellectually disabilities, speech difficulties, facial features, ocular anomalies, epilepsy, genitalia dysplasia, and other related symptoms, 2) identifying medically actionable symptoms and providing targeted therapy

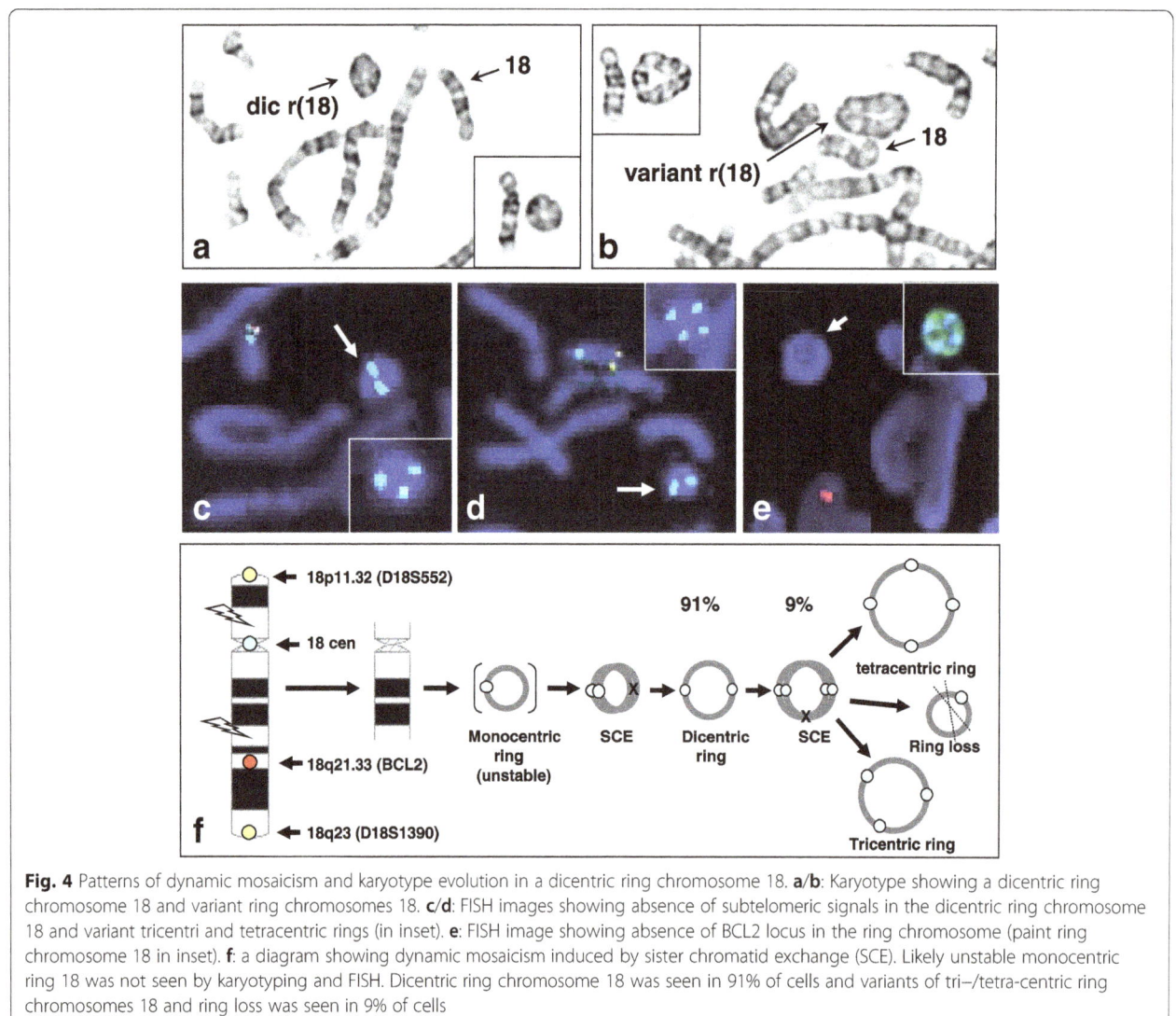

Fig. 4 Patterns of dynamic mosaicism and karyotype evolution in a dicentric ring chromosome 18. **a/b**: Karyotype showing a dicentric ring chromosome 18 and variant ring chromosomes 18. **c/d**: FISH images showing absence of subtelomeric signals in the dicentric ring chromosome 18 and variant tricentri and tetracentric rings (in inset). **e**: FISH image showing absence of BCL2 locus in the ring chromosome (paint ring chromosome 18 in inset). **f**: a diagram showing dynamic mosaicism induced by sister chromatid exchange (SCE). Likely unstable monocentric ring 18 was not seen by karyotyping and FISH. Dicentric ring chromosome 18 was seen in 91% of cells and variants of tri–/tetra-centric ring chromosomes 18 and ring loss was seen in 9% of cells

and follow up treatments, 3) delivering genetic counseling to parents of the affected with detailed information about the disease progression and related risks in cancer predisposition and reproduction failure.

An ad hoc task force proposed guideline recommendations for clinical diagnosis and management of ring chromosome 14 syndrome [37]. These guidelines were based on data from peer-review scientific literature and on a subsequent holistic summary by a heterogeneous panel of experts. For the major symptoms of epilepsy, hypotonia, recurrent infections, vision and hearing complications, respiratory complications, and communication and language disorders seen in patients with ring chromosome 14, recommendations for general management and specific treatments of each symptom were generated. For example, epilepsy should be treated from the onset with anticonvulsive therapy. Advices for taking care of a child with this rare and complex syndrome were offered to parents. This chromosome-specific symptom-oriented disease management and treatment set a model for cases involving other ring chromosomes.

For registering cases into the implemented human ring chromosome registry, a task force by clinical cytogeneticists and geneticists will be organized to review cytogenomic findings following the diagnostic guidelines and to curate clinical findings. Accumulation of more ring chromosome cases with defined genomic structures and dynamic mosaicism and detailed clinical manifestations will provide better genotype-phenotype correlation for predicting clinical consequences and planning treatments.

Understanding the biology of human ring chromosomes

It has been thought that human ring chromosomes are formed by a starting breakage-fusion event at the distal or telomeric ends of both arms [24] and then go through breakage-fusion-bridge (BFB) cycles for additional segmental imbalances in the ring or even chromothripsis to form a ring with randomly reassembly of multiple broken segments [38, 39]. The breakage-fusion point can be detected by aCGH or SNP chip analysis but the jointed sequences and underlying fusion mechanisms remain largely unknown. This ring chromosome replicates in the S phase with none, one, or two sister chromatid exchanges to generate intact ring, dicentric ring, or interlocked rings, respectively. During the mitotic phase, the dicentric or interlocked rings require breakage and thus show lagging at anaphase and nondisjunction into telophase. A dicentric chromosome can persist through mitosis and cytokinesis by forming a long chromatin bridge coated with nuclear membrane between daughter cells; this bridge resolves into single strand DNA by the cytoplasmic 3′ nuclease TREX1 and induces nuclear envelope rupture [40]. Mis-segregated or nondisjunction

chromosomes with various types of genomic rearrangements including chromothripsis are captured in a micronucleus [38]. DNA within micronuclei could go through replication in S-phase and repairing in G2 phase. High rate of cell deaths caused by mitotically unstable ring chromosome variants has been suggested for the evolution of cell lines with different ring chromosome components [41]. Somatic ring chromosomes have been seen in various types of cancers; chromothripsis in which multiple copy number gains or losses confined to one or a few chromosomes could contribute to the formation of somatic ring chromosomes [39]. Figure 5 shows the breakage-fusion-bridge cycle for a ring chromosome through a cell cycle. It was hypothesized that the anaphase lagging and resultant aneuploids could induce cell cycle arrest and cell death. Furthermore, it is hypothesized that there may be a selection process for karyotype evolution through a few early cell cycles to realize a ring structure sufficient for cell survive and tolerable for ring instability. To test these two hypotheses, methods for cell-based tracking and monitoring of ring chromosome behavior and cell fates and DNA-based targeted sequencing of various ring chromosomes should be developed.

It was suggested that larger ring chromosomes showed significantly more instability than small rings [8]. This correlation between ring instability and the size of the chromosome was partly reflected from the relative frequencies of ring chromosomes. The most frequently seen ring autosomes in the Chinese cases were chromosomes 13, 22, 15, 14, 18 and 21. Dynamic mosaicism from these ring chromosomes diverted a portion of cells with aneuploidy of the involved chromosome. As a comparison, the most frequently seen aneuploidy in products of conception were trisomies 13, 15, 16, 18, 21 and 22 [35]. There is an overlap in most of these small size autosomes. However, the absence of ring chromosomes 16, 17 and 19 in the reported Chinese cases suggested that, in addition to size, the content of a chromosome could affect the survive of cells or even the fetus. Cell lines from cases of ring chromosomes could be used as an in vitro cellular model for genetic mosaic analysis of chromosomal or segmental aneuploidy to understand the underlying mechanisms of chromosomal number control and the impact on human development and disease.

Reprograming human fibroblasts containing ring chromosomes 13 and 17 to induced pluripotent stem cells (iPSC) discovered the correction of ring chromosome through a compensatory uniparental disomy (UPD) mechanism [42]. This cell-autonomous correction involved first the loss of ring chromosome and then the duplication of the normal chromosome in five to ten cell culture passages; the correction ratio varied from different iPSC clones. A potential strategy for chromosome therapy to correct chromosome abnormalities using ring

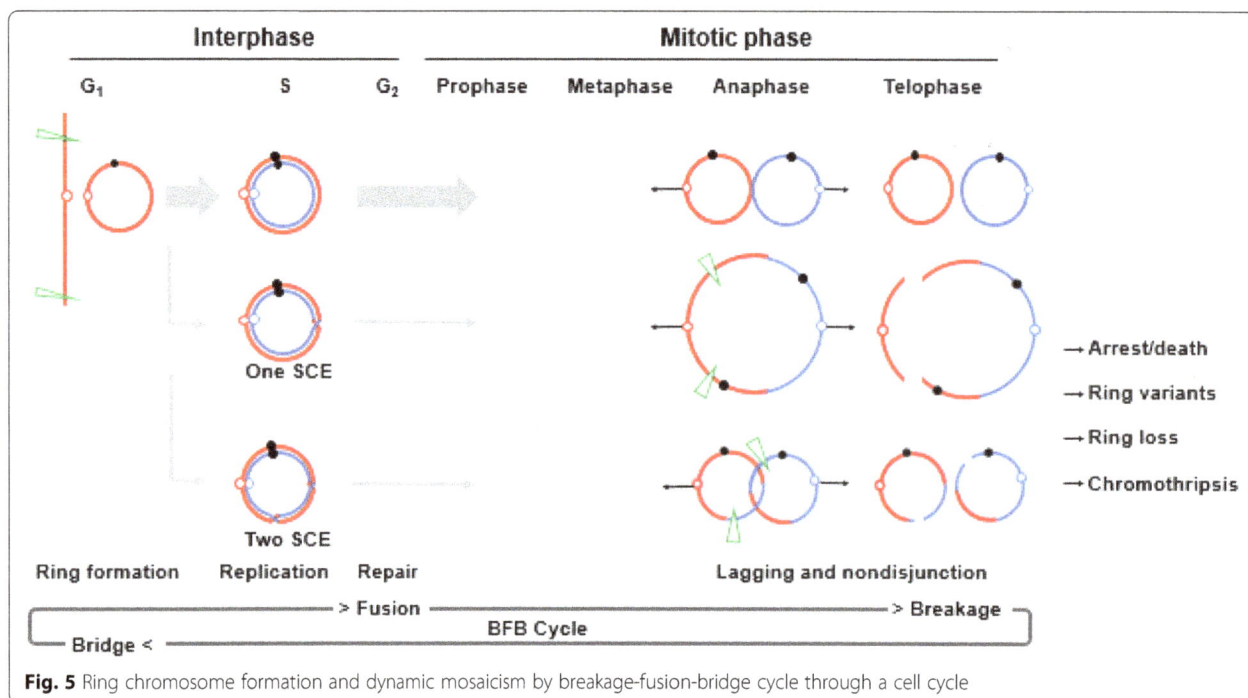

Fig. 5 Ring chromosome formation and dynamic mosaicism by breakage-fusion-bridge cycle through a cell cycle

chromosome was proposed [43]. Theoretically, loxP cassettes could be inserted into the p and q arm of an abnormal chromosome via CRISP-Cas9. Treatment with Cre-mediated recombinase will induce ring chromosome formation at the loxP loci. Cells containing the newly formed ring chromosome are grown for several passages to induce ring loss and then trigger compensatory UPD for monosomy rescue. This strategy could also be used to reduce trisomy to disomy by induced ring loss and to correct pathogenic CNVs or large aberration by compensatory UPD. Limitations in this chromosome therapy concept include validity and efficacy of the technical procedures, the risk of exposing recessive disease or imprinting disorders, and ethical considerations. Chromosome mosaicism is a relatively common finding in in vitro fertilization derived human embryos. Trisomy rescue and monosomy compensatory and resultant UPD have been documented in the prenatal findings of fetoplacental discrepancy and confined placenta mosaicism. Self-correction of chromosomal abnormalities in human preimplantation embryos and embryonic stem cells has been explained by increased death and decreased division of aneuploid cells or allocation of the aneuploidy in the trophectoderm [44, 45]. In a small case series, intrauterine transfer of mosaic aneuploid blastocysts developed into healthy euploid newborns [46]. However, if compensatory UPD is truly a cell-autonomous process, cases with ring chromosomes will showed self-corrected cells with normal disomic pattern for the involved chromosome. Of the 95 cases with an autosome ring in this report, only nine cases were noted with normal cells

and there was no study to determine a true mosaicism or a compensatory UPD. A study of 16 cases with ring chromosome 14 noted biparental inheritance and excluded UPD [26]. Therefore, the cytogenetic results did not observe a large-scale in vivo self-correction. Cellular reprogramming for iPSC may be a necessary step to trigger compensatory UPD. Further study to understand the mechanisms of ring chromosome loss and compensatory UPD is needed for practical chromosome therapy.

Future directions

The implemented human ring chromosome registry can play important roles in facilitating genetic diagnosis and developing translational research. With the formation of a task force by clinical cytogeneticists and geneticists, criteria and procedures for registering, compiling and curating cases into this human ring chromosome registry will be formulated; evidence-based diagnostic guidelines and management recommendations for ring chromosome patients will be proposed. Easy access to compiled and curated diagnostic and clinical data as well as properly preserved residual specimens are the key prerequisites for promoting collaborative research. Clinical cytogenetic laboratories should consider registering cases into the human ring chromosome registry and saving residual specimens. Standard operating procedures for proper biobanking of residual specimens should be developed and ethical and legal considerations for research applications should be resolved [47].

Conclusions

In summary, an online human ring chromosome registry was designed and implemented to review cytogenomic results and clinical manifestations from a set of ring chromosome cases reported in the Chinese population. Relative frequencies, age and gender distributions, and various phenotypes of all ring chromosomes except for chromosomes 16, 17 and 19 were revealed. Cytogenomic heterogeneity was noted in variable genomic imbalances in ring chromosomes, different levels of dynamic mosaicism, and possibly tissue-related karyotype evolution. Human ring chromosomes showed heterogeneous clinical findings ranging from intrauterine growth restriction, postnatal developmental delay and multiple congenital anomalies, adult reproduction failure, and risk for cancer. A framework of organized efforts for translational and basic research collaboration to define underlying mechanisms of ring chromosome formation and dynamic mosaicism, to delineate the genotype-phenotype correlations, and to develop chromosome therapy for ring chromosomes is under consideration.

Abbreviations
aCGH: Array comparative genomic hybridization; BFB: Breakage-fusion-bridge; CNKI: China National Knowledge Infrastructure; CNV: Copy Number Variants; DECIPHER: Database of Chromosomal Imbalance and Phenotype in Humans using Ensemble Resources; DGV: Database of Genomic Variants; FISH: Fluorescence in situ hybridization; FK: Foreign key; iPSC: Induced pluripotent stem cells; Kb: Kilo base-pair; Mb: Mega base-pair; MLPA: Multiple ligation probe amplification; OMIM: Online Mendelian Inheritance in Man; PK: Primary key; RSA: Regional specific assays; SNP: Single nucleotide polymorphism; sSMC: Supernumerary small marker chromosomes; STR: Short-tandem repeats; UK: Unique key; UPD: Uniparental disomy

Acknowledgements
We wish to thank Dr. Michael Baudis for the application of an online software Progenetix (www.progenetix.org) and Audrey Meusel for proofreading of this manuscript.

Web resources
China National Knowledge Infrastructure (CNKI): http://www.cnki.net
ClinVar: https://www.ncbi.nlm.nih.gov/clinvar/
Database of Genomic Variants (DGV): http://projects.tcag.ca/variation/
DatabasE of Chromosomal Imbalance and Phenotype in Humans using Ensembl Resources (DECIPHER): http://decipher.sanger.ac.uk/
Human Genome Browser: http://genome.ucsc.edu/
Online Mendelian Inheritance in Man (OMIM): http://www.ncbi.nlm.nih.gov/omim
PubMed: https://www.ncbi.nlm.nih.gov/pubmed/
SinoMed: http://www.sinomed.ac.cn/
Supernumerary small marker chromosomes (sSMC) database: http://ssmc-tl.com/sSMC.html
VIP: http://qikan.cqvip.com/
WANFANG DATA: http://www.wanfangdata.com

Funding
Not applicable.

Authors' contributions
HQ and LP designed and developed the web-based human ring chromosome registry; HQ, HC and SW performed the literature search and data analysis. HQ and LP wrote the manuscript. All authors read, review and approved this manuscript.

Competing interests
The authors declare that they have no competing interests.

References
1. Jacobs PA, Frackiewicz A, Law P, Hilditch CJ, Morton NE. The effect of structural aberrations of the chromosomes on reproductive fitness in man. II. Results. Clin Genet. 1975;8:169–78.
2. Pezzolo A, Gimelli G, Cohen A, Lavaggetto A, Romano C, Fogu G, Zuffardi O. Presence of telomeric and subtelomeric sequences at the fusion points of ring chromosomes indicates that the ring syndrome is caused by ring instability. Hum Genet. 1993;92:23–7.
3. Zhang HZ, Li P, Wang D, Huff S, Nimmakayalu M, Qumsiyeh M, Pober BR. FOXC1 gene deletion is associated with eye anomalies in ring chromosome 6. Am J Med Genet. 2004;124A:280–7.
4. Zhang HZ, Xu F, Seashore M, Li P. Unique genomic structure and distinct mitotic behavior of ring chromosome 21 in two unrelated cases. Cytogenet Genome Res. 2012;136:180–7.
5. Guilherme R, Klein E, Hamid A, Bhatt S, Volleth M, Polityko A, Kulpanovich A, Dufke A, Albrecht B, Morlot S, Brecevic L, Petersen M, Manolakos E, Kosyakova N, Liehr T. Human ring chromosomes - new insights for their clinical significance. Balkan J Med Genet. 2013;16:13–20.
6. Yip MY. Autosomal ring chromosomes in human genetic disorders. Transl Pediatr. 2015;4:164–74.
7. Cote GB, Katsantoni A, Deligeorgis D. The cytogenetic and clinical implication of a ring chromosome 2. Ann Genet. 1981;24:231–5.
8. Kosztolányi G. Does "ring syndrome" exist? An analysis of 207 case reports on patients with a ring autosome. Hum Genet. 1987;75:174–9.
9. Cui C, Shu W, Li P. Fluorescence in situ hybridization: cell-based genetic diagnostic and research applications. Front Cell Dev Biol. 2016;4:89.
10. Xu F, DiAdamo AJ, Grommisch B, Li P. Interstitial duplication and distal deletion in a ring chromosome 13 with pulmonary atresia and ventricular septal defect: a case report and review of the literature. N A J Med Sci. 2013;6:208–12.
11. Yao H, Yang C, Huang X, Yang L, Zhao W, Yin D, Qin Y, Mu F, Liu L, Tian P, Liu Z, Yang Y. Breakpoints and deleted genes identification of ring chromosome 18 in a Chinese girl by whole-genome low-coverage sequencing: a case report study. BMC Med Genet. 2016;17:49.
12. Burgemeister AL, Daumiller E, Dietze-Armana I, Klett C, Freiberg C, Stark W, Lingen M, Centonze I, Rettenberger G, Mehnert K, Zirn B. Continuing role for classical cytogenetics: case report of a boy with ring syndrome caused by complete ring chromosome 4 and review of literature. Am J Med Genet. 2017;173A:727–32.
13. Gu M, Su C, Chao S. 1272 cases cell karyotype analysis of peripheral blood chromosome. China Modern Doctor. 2015;53:81–3.
14. Guo CX, Xia JP, Shi JP, Tang Y, Zhao X, Wang JF. Analysis on prenatal diagnostic results of 181 cases with amniotic fluid chromosomal abnormalities and genetic counseling. Matern Child Health Care China. 2015;30:6275–80.
15. Lin YH, Lin YM, Lin YH, Chuang L, Wu SY, Kuo PL. Ring (Y) in two azoospermic men. Am J Med Genet. 2004;128A:209–13.
16. Jiao X, Qin C, Li J, Qin Y, Gao X, Zhang B, Zhen X, Feng Y, Simpson JL, Chen ZJ. Cytogenetic analysis of 531 Chinese women with premature ovarian failure. Hum Reprod. 2012;27(7):2201.
17. Xiang B, Hemingway S, Qumsiyeh M, CytoAccess LP. A relational laboratory information management system for a clinical cytogenetics laboratory. J Assoc Genet Technol. 2006;32:168–70.
18. Mitchell JA, Fun J, McCray AT. Design of genetics home reference: a new NLM consumer health resource. J Am Med Inform Assoc. 2004;11:439–47.
19. Tan YM, Tan YQ, Xu XQ, Song D, Wu FG, Qian WP. Identification of a ring chromosome 13 combined with terminal rearrangement of chromosome 6 and genetic counseling. Int J Genet. 2007;30:401–3.
20. Liao C, Fu F, Zhang L. Ring chromosome 13 syndrome characterized by high resolution array based comparative genomic hybridization in patient with 47, XYY syndrome: a case report. J Med Case Rep. 2011;5:99.

21. Chen CP, Tsai CH, Chern SR, Wu PS, Su JW, Lee CC, Chen YT, Chen WL, Chen LF, Wang W. Prenatal diagnosis and molecular cytogenetic characterization of mosaic ring chromosome 13. Gene. 2013;529:163–8.

22. Zhang YN, Yaheman P, Du HW WLJ. A case of ring chromosome 18 with growth hormone deficiency. Chin J Contemp Pediatr. 2014;16:947–8.

23. Margarit E, Morales C, Rodríguez-Revenga L, Monné R, Badenas C, Soler A, Clusellas N, Mademont I, Sánchez A. Familial 4.8 Mb deletion on 18q23 associated with growth hormone insufficiency and phenotypic variability. Am J Med Genet. 2012;158A:611–6.

24. Guilherme RS, Meloni VF, Kim CA, Pellegrino R, Takeno SS, Spinner NB, Conlin LK, Christofolini DM, Kulikowski LD, Melaragno MI. Mechanisms of ring chromosome formation, ring instability and clinical consequences. BMC Med Genet. 2011;12:171.

25. Su PH, Chen CP, Su YN, Chen SJ, Lin LL, Chen JY. Smallest critical region for microcephaly in a patient with mosaic ring chromosome 13. Genet Mol Res. 2013;12:1311–7.

26. Zollino M, Ponzi E, Gobbi G, Neri G. The ring 14 syndrome. Eur J Med Genet. 2012;55:374–80.

27. Alosi D, Klitten LL, Bak M, Hjalgrim H, Møller RS, Tommerup N. Dysregulation of FOXG1 by ring chromosome 14. Mol Cytogenet. 2015;8:24.

28. Hook EB. Exclusion of chromosomal mosaicism: Rables of 90%, 95% and 99% confidence limites and comments on use. Am J Hum Genet. 1977; 29:94–7.

29. Wei Y, Xu F, Li P. Technology-driven and evidence-based genomic analysis for integrated pediatric and prenatal genetic evaluation. J Genet Genomics. 2014;40:1–14.

30. Kosztolányi G, Mehes K, Hook EB. Inherited ring chromosomes: an analysis of published cases. Hum Genet. 1991;87:320–4.

31. Vignoli A, Bisulli F, Darra F, Mastrangelo M, Barba C, Giordano L, Turner K, Zambrelli E, Chiesa V, Bova S, Fiocchi I, Peron A, Naldi I, Milito G, Licchetta L, Tinuper P, Guerrini R, Dalla Bernardina B, Canevini MP. Epilepsy in ring chromosome 20 syndrome. Epilepsy Res. 2016;128:83–93.

32. Yurov YB, Iourov IY, Vorsanova SG, Liehr T, Kolotii AD, Kutsev SI, Pellestor F, Beresheva AK, Demidova IA, Kravets VS, Monakhov VV, Soloviev IV. Aneuploidy and confined chromosomal mosaicism in the developing human brain. PLoS One. 2007;2:e558.

33. Meng JL, Matarese C, Crivello J, Wilcox K, Wang DM, DiAdamo AJ, Xu F, Li P. Changes in and efficacies of indications for invasive prenatal diagnosis of cytogenomic abnormalities: 13 years of experience in a single center. Med Sci Monit. 2015;21:1942–8.

34. Li P, Xu F, Shu W. The spectrum of cytogenomic abnormalities in patients with developmental delay and intellectual disabilities. N a J Med Sci. 2015;8:166–72.

35. Zhou QH, Wu SY, Amato K, Diadamo A, Li P. spectrum Of cytogenomic abnormalities revealed by array comparative genomic hybridization in products of conception culture failure and normal karyotype samples. J Genet Genomics. 2016;43:121–31.

36. Guilherme RS, Moysés-Oliveira M, Dantas AG, Meloni VA, Colovati ME, Kulikowski LD, Melaragno MI. Position effect modifying gene expression in a patient with ring chromosome 14. J Appl Genet. 2016;57:183–7.

37. Rinaldi B, Vaisfeld A, Amarri S, Baldo C, Gobbi G, Magini P, Melli E, Neri G, Novara F, Pippucci T, Rizzi R, Soresina A, Zampini L, Zuffardi O, Crimi M. Guideline recommendations for diagnosis and clinical management of Ring14 syndrome-first report of an ad hoc task force. Orphanet J Rare Dis. 2017;12:69.

38. Zhang CZ, Spektor A, Cornils H, Francis JM, Jackson EK, Liu S, Meyerson M, Pellman D. Chromothripsis from DNA damage in micronuclei. Nature. 2015; 522:179–84.

39. Leibowitz ML, Chang CZ, Pellman D. Chromothripsis: a new mechanism for rapid karyotype evolution. Annu Rev Genet. 2015;49:183–211.

40. Maciejowski J, Li Y, Bosco N, Campbell PJ, de Lange T. Chromothripsis and kataegis induced by telomere crisis. Cell. 2015;163:1641–54.

41. Kaylor J, Alfaro M, Ishwar A, Sailey C, Sawyer J, Zarate YA. Molecular and cytogenetic evaluation of a patient with ring chromosome 13 and discordant results. Cytogenet Genome Res. 2014;144:104–8.

42. Bershteyn M, Hayashi Y, Desachy G, Hsiao EC, Sami S, Tsang KM, Weiss LA, Kriegstein AR, Yamanaka S, Wynshaw-Boris A. Cell-autonomous correction of ring chromosomes in human induced pluripotent stem cells. Nature. 2014; 507:99–103.

43. Plona K, Kim T, Halloran K, Wynshaw-Boris A. Chromosome therapy: potential strategies for the correction of severe chromosome aberrations. Am J Med Genet. 2016;172C:422–30.

44. Bazrgar M, Gourabi H, Valojerdi MR, Yazdi PE, Baharvand H. Self-correction of chromosomal abnormalities in human preimplantation embryos and embryonic stem cells. Stem Cells Dev. 2013;22:2449–56.

45. Taylor TH, Gitlin SA, Patrick JL, Crain JL, Wilson JM, Griffin DK. The origin, mechanisms, incidence and clinical consequences of chromosomal mosaicism in humans. Hum Reprod Update. 2014;20(4):571–81.

46. Greco E, Minasi MG, Fiorentino F. Healthy babies after intrauterine transfer of mosaic aneuploid blastocysts. N Engl J Med. 2015;373:2089–90.

47. Grommisch B, DiAdamo AJ, Xu ZY, Pan XH, Ma DQ, Xie JS, Qi Y, Li P. Biobanking of residual specimens from diagnostic genetics laboratories: standard operating procedures, ethical and legal considerations, and research applications. N a J Med Sci. 2013;6:200–7.

5

Importance and usage of chromosomal microarray analysis in diagnosing intellectual disability, global developmental delay, and autism; and discovering new loci for these disorders

Ahmet Cevdet Ceylan[1,2]* (iD), Senol Citli[1], Haktan Bagis Erdem[3], Ibrahim Sahin[3], Elif Acar Arslan[4] and Murat Erdogan[5]

Abstract

Background: Chromosomal microarray analysis is a first-stage test that is used for the diagnosis of intellectual disability and global developmental delay. Chromosomal microarray analysis can detect well-known microdeletion syndromes. It also contributes to the identification of genes that are responsible for the phenotypes in the new copy number variations.

Results: Chromosomal microarray analysis was conducted on 124 patients with intellectual disability and global developmental delay. Multiplex ligation-dependent probe amplification was used for the confirmation of chromosome 22q11.2 deletion/duplication. 26 pathogenic and likely pathogenic copy number variations were detected in 23 patients (18.55%) in a group of 124 Turkish patients with intellectual disability and global developmental delay. Chromosomal microarray analysis revealed pathogenic de novo Copy number variations, such as a novel 2.9-Mb de novo deletion at 18q22 region with intellectual disability and autism spectrum disorder, and a 22q11.2 region homozygote duplication with new clinical features.

Conclusion: Our data expand the spectrum of 22q11.2 region mutations, reveal new loci responsible from autism spectrum disorder and provide new insights into the genotype–phenotype correlations of intellectual disability and global developmental delay.

Keywords: Chromosomal microarray, Intellectual disability, Global developmental delay, Copy number variations, 22q11.2 homozygote duplication

Background

Advancements in molecular technology, such as chromosomal microarray analysis (CMA), has led to the discovery of new microdeletions and microduplications in patients with intellectual disability (ID), global developmental delay (GDD), epilepsy, and congenital anomalies (CA). ID and GDD are clinically heterogeneous neurodevelopmental disorders seen in 1–3% of children [1]. CMA is a first-tier test in the evaluation of individuals with ID and GDD with the diagnostic yield ranging from 5 to 20% varying based on population examined [2, 3]. The International Standard for the Consortium of Cytogenomic Array recommended CMA as a first-stage cytogenetic diagnostic test for patients with CA and ID / GDD.

CMA can detect well-known microdeletion syndromes. It also contributes to the identification of genes that are responsible for the phenotypes in the new copy number variations (CNVs). Chromosome 22q11.2 deletion syndrome and 22q11.2 duplication syndrome are good examples for microdeletion/microduplication syndromes.

* Correspondence: acceylan@yahoo.com
*This study has been presented at the ASHG 2017 annual meeting.
[1]Trabzon Kanuni Training and Research Hospital, Medical Genetics Unit, Trabzon, Turkey
[2]Ankara Yıldırım Beyazıt University, Ankara Atatürk Training and Research Hospital, Department of Medical Genetics, Ankara, Turkey
Full list of author information is available at the end of the article

Chromosome 22q11.2 duplication syndrome was first explained in 1999, but research continues to explore new phenotypes of this syndrome [4]. When there are three copies of the 22q11.2 region, it is called 22q11.2 duplication, whereas four copies of this region are referred to as the tetrasomy of 22q11.2 region. When there are two copies of 22q11.1 region in both alleles, this is referred to as 22q11.2 homozygote duplication. If there are three copies in one allele and one copy in the other, it is called 22q11.2 triplication.

Autism is a childhood disorder that expresses itself through core problems in communication and social interaction skills, along with the presence of stereotypical behaviors. Autism spectrum disorder (ASD) does not have a fixed pattern since a number of different genes have been reported as responsible for this disorder [5]. CMA studies have a high potential in revealing novel gene-phenotype associations in relation to this disorder. In this study, new loci for autism have been discovered which will help us better understand the cause of the disease.

Herein, we present the diagnostic rates for CNVs, and the aberrations, with major clinical findings detected by CMA in a group of 124 Turkish patients with ID and GDD. We also present a case with 22q11.2 homozygote duplication and new phenotypic findings as a result. Our study will help better explain the genotype-phenotype associations of the 22q11.2 region.

Methods

DNA extraction
Genomic DNA of family members was extracted according to the manufacturer's standard procedure using the MagNA Pure Compact Nucleic Acid Isolation Kit I (Roche Diagnostic GmbH, Mannheim, Germany).

Microarray analysis
Affymetrix CytoScan Optima® chips were used to perform CMA in 124 patients with ID and GDD at Trabzon Kanuni Training and Research Hospital. Data analysis was performed using Chromosome Analysis Suite 3.1 software. Data were presented as minimum coordinates (sequence positions of the first and last probes within the CNV) in the NCBI37/hg19 genome assembly. Variants were evaluated based on phenotype and using standard in silico tools [6]. The analysis and interpretation of the obtained results were performed by using public genomic databases, such as UCSC, OMIM, DGV, DECIPHER, CLINGEN.

MLPA (multiplex ligation-dependent probe Amplification) analysis
MLPA was performed as suggested by the manufacturer (MRC-Holland®, Amsterdam, The Netherlands). The SALSA® MLPA® probemix P250 DiGeorge was used for the confirmation of chromosome 22q11.2 deletion/duplication. The standard deviation of all probes in the reference samples were < 0.10 and the dosage quotient (DQ) of the reference probes in the patients' samples were between 0.80 and 1.20. DQ of the probes were between 0.40 and 0.65 for heterozygous deletion. DQ of the probes were between 1.30 and 1.65 for heterozygous duplication. DQ of the probes were between 1.75 and 2.15 for heterozygous triplication or homozygous duplication.

Results

Between May 2016 and April 2017, 124 patients were examined at the department of genetics for GDD/ID and CA. There were 73 males and 51 females. The age of the patients ranged from 15 days to 17 years. The Denver Developmental Test was used with patients up to 3 years of age, whereas the Standfort Benet Test was used for patients 4–6 years of age, and the WISC-R test for patients older than 6. This study was conducted with patients who were not diagnosed with any syndromes previously and CMA was performed as the first-tier test on the subjects. Table 1 shows the clinical features of these cases and the CMA results.

In 23 individuals (from 23 families), CMA analysis revealed CNVs including 6 microduplications (2p25p24, 22q11.2 [2 cases], 2p25, 14q32, and 15q11.2), 14 microdeletions (1p36.3, 1q21 [2 cases], 2q36, 6p25.1p23, 6q25q27, 14q32, 15q11.2, 16q24, 18p11.3, 18q22, 18q21q23, 19p23, and 22q11.2) and 1 homozygote duplication identified in same locus (22q11.2) in a patient (Fig. 1).

Twenty one of the 26 CNVs were interpreted as pathogenic, whereas 5 of the 26 CNVs were interpreted as having uncertain clinical significance (UCS); likely pathogenic in accordance with the clinical findings about the patients and literature [7]. 7 of 26 CNVs were associated with well-known microdeletion/ microduplication syndromes. Interestingly, multiple CNVs have been identified in two of the patients including 2 different deletions (6q13q14 and 8q21.3) in one and 1 deletion (6q25) and 2 duplications (6q24.1 and 6q26) in another (Table 1).

The length of 17 of the CNVs were below 5 Mb and they could not be detected with conventional karyotyping. The length of 7 of the CNVs were between 5 and 10-Mb. It is worth to note that siblings, whose parents were in consanguineous marriages and carried 22q11.2 duplication, were also diagnosed with 22q11.2 homozygote duplication. 23 of 26 CNVs were de novo. Eight out of 23 families had consanguineous marriages. Only two of the case studies are presented below in detail, however, the summary of all clinical features and mutations observed in patients can be found in Table 1.

Table 1 Clinical findings of 23 patients and CNV status

Case	Age	Region	OMIM Phenotype (number)	Comment	Type/Size	Inheritance	Genes involved	Likely pathogenic genes	Intellectual Disability	Developmental Delay	Dysmorphic features	Other findings
1	1,5 y	chr1:849466-3,152,968	1p36 deletion syndrome (607872)	Path	Del 2.3 Mb	De novo	76	DVL1, ATAD3A, GNB1, GABRD, SKI, PEX10, PRDM16	N/A	+	prominent forehead, pointed chin, deep-set eyes, straight eyebrows	dilated cardiomyopathy, epilepsy
2	4 m	chr1:145927661-148,588,367	1q21.1 deletion syndrome (612474)	Path	Del 2.6 Mb	Mother	31	NBPF10, HYDIN2, NBPF12, PRKAB2, FMO5, CHD1L, BCL9, ACP6, GJA5, GJA8, GPR89B, NBPF11, PPIAL4A, NBPF14, NBPF9	N/A	N/A	wide nasal bridge, bulbous nose and retrognathia.	pectoral muscle hypoplasis, radius and humerus hypoplasis, short and curved ribs
3	6 y	chr1:145607915-146,497,779		UCS/L-Path	Del 0.9 Mb	De novo	14	GPR89A, PDZK1, CD160, POLR3C, NBPF12	+	+	strabismus, hypertelorism	congenital hypothyroidism
4	2,5y	chr2:10266562-16,826,500		Path	Dup 6.5 Mb	De novo	20	ODC1, LPIN1, MYCN, NBAS,	N/A	+	prominent forehead, retrognathia, broad eyelashes, cupped ear, uplifted lobe	dysplastic aortic valve, hydrocephalus, cerebral atrophy
5	8 m	chr2:222686398-226,097,873		Path	Del 3.4 Mb	De novo	16	PAX3, AP1S3, MRPL44, CUL3	N/A	+	prominent forehead, hypoplastic alae nasi, epicanthal fold	
6	14,5 y	chr6:6806969-13,794,521		Path	Del 6.9 Mb	De novo	46	DSP, TFAP2A, GCNT2, MAK, GCM2, EDN1, TBC1D7	+	+	dolicocephaly, facial asymmetry, open mouth, depressed nasal tip, absent ear lobe,	atrial septal defect, bilateral cleft lip
7	8,5 y	chr6:70373236-79,654,154, chr8:7880 8754-81,835,864		Path Path	Del 9.2 Mb/Del 3 Mb	De novo	49	LMBRD1, COL9A1, RIMS1, KCNQ5, KHD3CL, MYO6,MTO1, SLC17A5, COL12A1,IMOG1	+	+	long face, wide mouth, high arched palate	potent ductus arteriosus, renal agenesis, pes equinovarus
8	4 m	chr6:151310706-170,919,482		Path	Del 19.6 Mb	De novo	115	SYNE1,ESR1, ARID1B, LPA, PDE10A,T, ERMARD,TBP,	N/A	+	sunset eye sign, low set ears, pointed chin	hydrocephalus, cerebral atrophy
9	1 m	chr6:163378290-16,709,184, chr6:160713926-16,287,570, chr6:141494387-144,877,906		Path UCS/L-Path Path Path	Dup 3.7 Mb Del 2.1 Mb Del 3.3 Mb	De novo	17 8 19	PACRG, QKI, PDE10A, T, MPC1, RPS6KA2, SLC22A3, LPAL2, LPA, PLG, MAP3K4, AGPAT4, PARK2, NMBR, VTA1, GPR126, HIVEP2, AIG1, PEX3, PLAGL1, HYMAI, STX11, UTRN	N/A	+	upslanting palpebral fissures, round face	neonatal diabetus, hypotonia, deafness
10	9 y	chr14:103255460-107,285,437		Path	Del 4 Mb	De novo	56	TRAF3, APOPT1, RCC3, INF2, AKT1, BRF1,IGHM	+	+	long face, pointed chin, anteverted ears, epicanthal fold	–
11	11,5 y	chr14:99528241-107,285,437		Path	Dup 7.7 Mb	De novo	183	YY1, DYNC1H1, TECPR2, APOPT1, XRCC, ADSSL1, AKT1, ZBTB42, BRF1, IGHG2,	+	+	facial asymmetry, downslanting palpebral fissures, prognathism, macrocephaly	strabismus, ptosis,
12	5 y	chr15:22770421-30, 295,864		Path	Dup 7.5 Mb	De novo	131	MKRN3, MAGEL2, NDN, SNRPN,UBE3A, GABRB3,OCA2, HER2	+	+	hypertelorism, depressed nasal bridge,	unilateral deafness, autism spectrum disorder

Table 1 Clinical findings of 23 patients and CNV status (*Continued*)

Case	Age	Region	OMIM Phenotype (number)	Comment	Type/Size	Inheritance	Genes involved	Likely pathogenic genes	Intellectual Disability	Developmental Delay	Dysmorphic features	Other findings
13	6 y	chr15:22770421–23,276,605		UCS/L-Path	Del 0.5 Mb	De novo	7	NIPA1, NIPA2, CYFIP1, TUBGCP5	+	+	hypertelorism, short palpebral fissures, blepharophimosis	corpus callosum agenesis, hypothyroidism
14	15 y	chr16:89342189–89,552,394	KBG Syndrome (148050)	Path	Del 0.2 Mb	De novo	2	ANKRD11	+	+	long and triangular face structure, large, protruding ears	degenerative myopia
15	13,5 y	chr18:136226–6,992,327		Path	Del 6.8 Mb	De novo	41	SMCHD1, LPIN2, TGIF1, LAMA1	+	+	hypertelorism, broad nasal bridge	obesity
16	10 y	chr18:59720983–78,014,123		Path	Del 18.2 Mb	De novo	72	PIGN,TNFRSF11A, BCL2, KDSR, SERPINB7, RTTN, CYB5A, TSHZ1, CTDP1, XNL4A	+	+	frontal bossing, deep set eyes, depressed nasal bridge	sensorineural deafness, strabismus
17	3 y	chr18:67847004–70,771,041		UCS/L-Path	Del 2.9 Mb	De novo	6	RTTN, SOCS6, CBLN2, NETO1	N/A	–	hypertelorism, broad nasal bridge	autism spectrum disorder
18	13 y	chr18:65852206–76,107,497		Path	Del 10 Mb	De novo	32	RTTN, SOCS6, CBLN2, NETO1, CYB5A, TSHXZ1, GALR1	+	+	frontal bossing, deep set eyes, protruding ears	feeding difficulties
19	9 m	chr19:11284538–13,555,660		UCS/L-Path	Del 2.2 Mb	De novo	78	KANK2, DOCK6, EPOR, PRKCSH, ACP5, MAN2B1, RNASEH2A, KLF1, CALR, NFIX, LYL1, NACC1, CACNA1A	N/A	+	deep set eyes, micrognatia	hypotonia
20	5 y	chr22:18917030–21,465,662	DiGeorge syndrome (188400)	Path	Del 2.5 Mb	De novo.	66	PRODH, SLC25A, CDC45, GP1BB, TBX1, COMT, TANGO2, RTN4R, CARF2, PI4KA, SERPIND1,	+	+	hypertelorism, blunted nose, high arched palate,	tetralogy of fallot
21	5 y	chr22:19004771–21,443,283	22q11.2 microduplication syndrome (608363)	Path	Dup 2.4 Mb	Father	63	SLC25A, CDC45, GP1BB, TBX1, COMT, TANGO2, RTN4R, CARF2, PI4KA, SERPIND1,	+	+	frontal bossing, synophrys, pytosis,	strabismus,
22	11,5 y	chr22:19077926–21,804,886	22q11.2 microduplication syndrome (608363)	Path	Dup 2.7 Mb	De novo	65	SLC25A, CDC45, GP1BB, TBX1, COMT, TANGO2, RTN4R, CARF2, PI4KA, SERPIND1,	–	–	no dysmorphic features	loss of cognitive functioning
23	11 y	chr22:18917030–21,421,425	22q11.2 microduplication syndrome (608363)	Path	Hom dup 2.5 Mb	Mother and father	66	PRODH, SLC25A, CDC45, GP1BB, TBX1, COMT, TANGO2, RTN4R, CARF2, PI4KA, SERPIND1,	+	+	Round face, broad nasal bridge, hypertelorism, downslanting palpebral fissures, long philtrum, overfolded helix	patent ductus arteriosus, hypoplasia of clivus

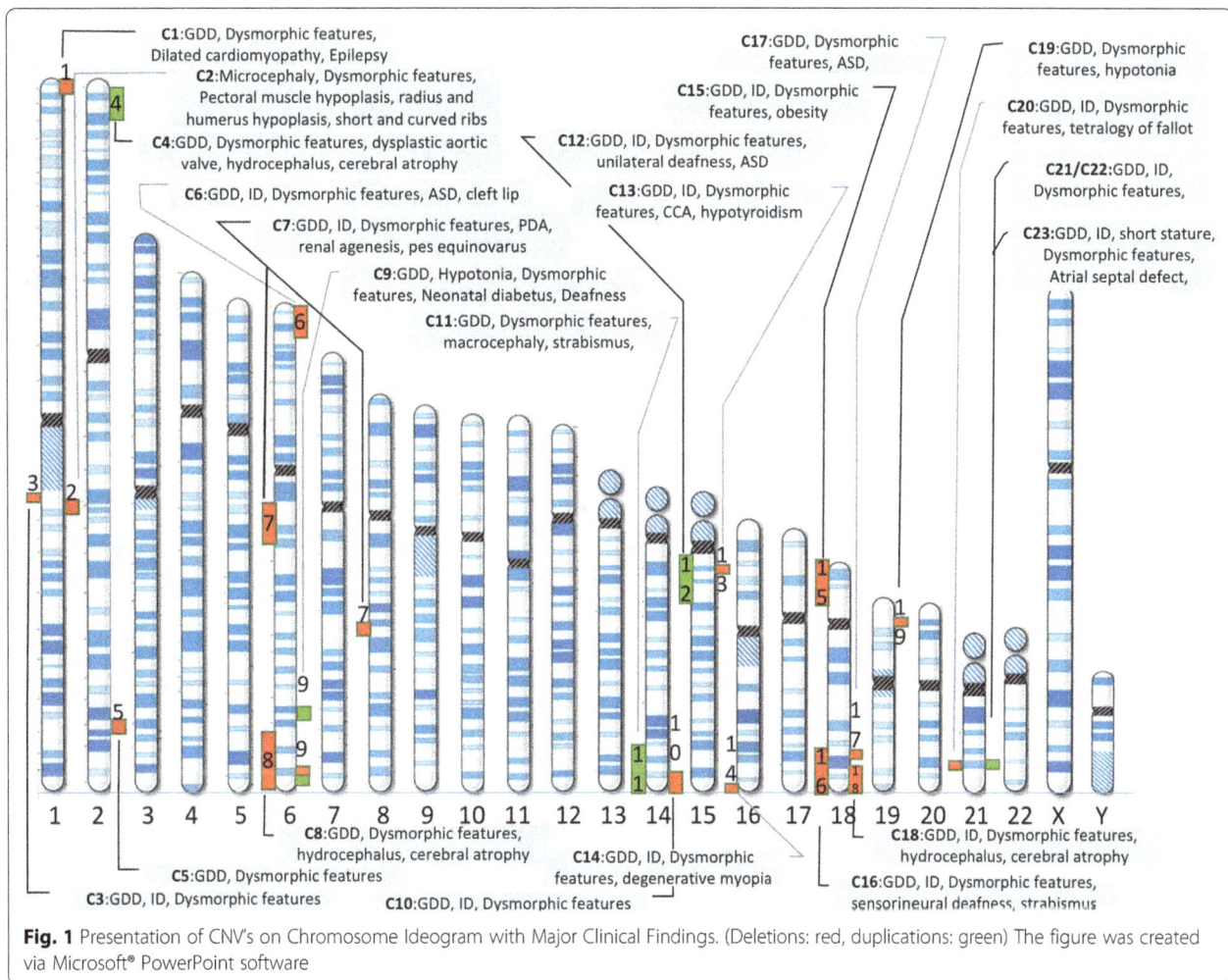

Fig. 1 Presentation of CNV's on Chromosome Ideogram with Major Clinical Findings. (Deletions: red, duplications: green) The figure was created via Microsoft® PowerPoint software

Region 22q11.2 duplication/ homozygote duplication family (cases 23 in Table 1)

An 11-year-old male patient (case 23) was diagnosed with learning disabilities. He started to walk in his first year and began speaking two-word sentences at the age of two. He was unable to learn how to read and write in his native language in the first year of elementary school, and was not able to keep up with his classmates. His history revealed that he had been hospitalized during the neonatal period due to high indirect bilirubinemia. His parents have a consanguineous marriage (Fig. 2a).

At his neurological examination, head circumference was 52 cm (25th–50th percentile), height was 121 cm (<3rd percentile), and weight was 25 kg (<3rd percentile). Round face, a broad nasal bridge, hypertelorism, downslanting palpebral fissures, long philtrum, and over-folded helix were observed (Fig. 2b). Hyperactivity and attention deficit disorder were not detected. No pyramidal system involvement was present, and reflexes were normoactive. Cerebellar system examinations were normal except for dysmetria and dysdiadochokinesia.

Tandem gait exhibited no abnormality. Echocardiography revealed small patent ductus arteriosus. T2 weighed MRI shows basillar impression and hypoplasia of clivus. Odontoid process was measured approximately 15 mm above the Chamberlain line (Fig. 2e). Serum electrolytes, electroencephalography, and abdominal ultrasonography were normal. Psychometric evaluation revealed borderline mental disability. 2.5 Mb triplication or homozygote duplication was detected at 22q11.2/ Di George Syndrome region with CMA. Both his mother and father had the duplication of same region. The results were in accordance with the MLPA analysis (Fig. 2d).

The patient's sister is 17 years old. She started to walk in her first year and began speaking two-word sentences at the age of 18 months. She was able to learn how to read and write in her native language in the first year of elementary school but she failed in mathematics. It was reported that she spoke less than her classmates and struggled building friendships. At her neurological examination, the circumference of her head was 54 cm

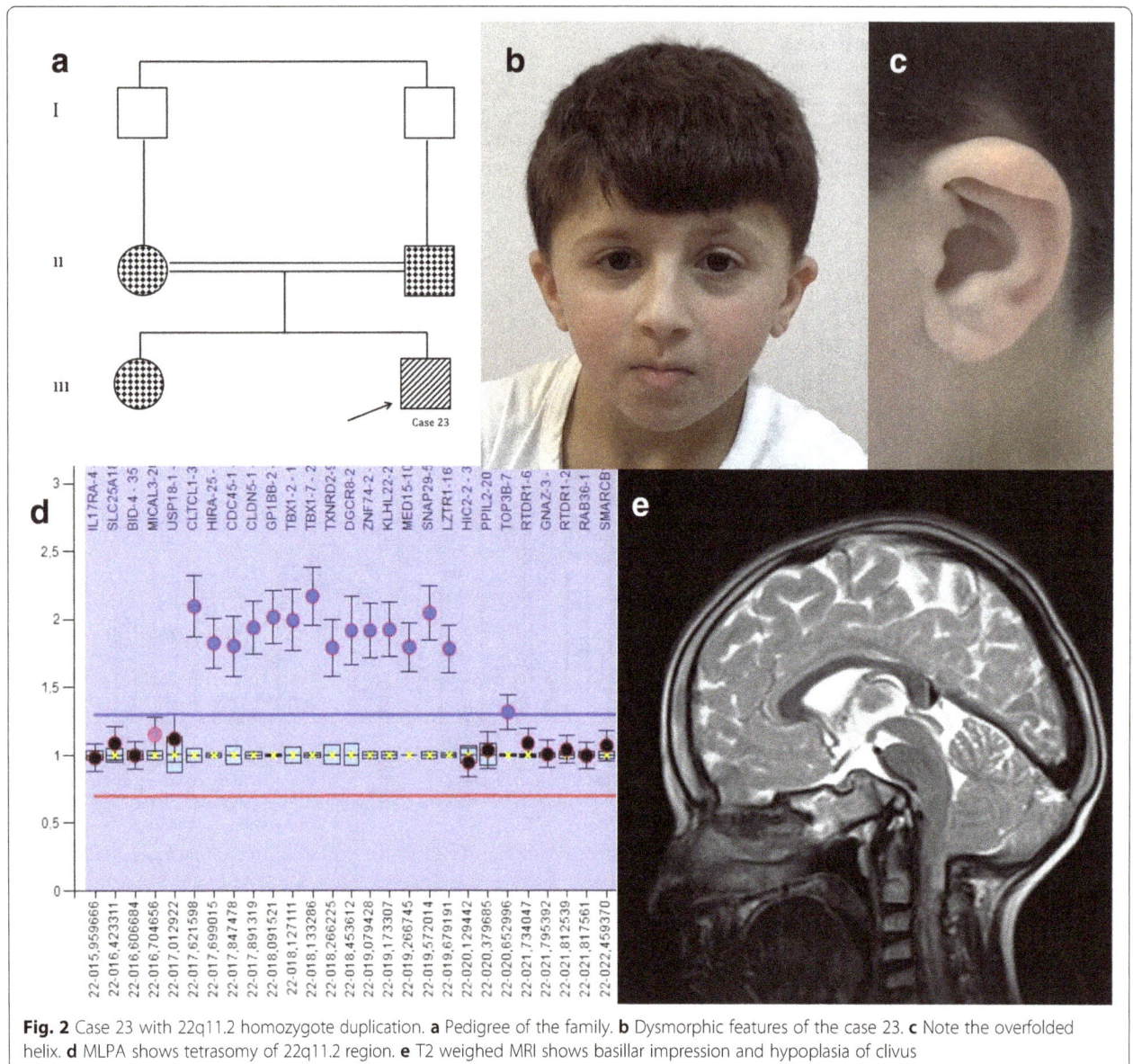

Fig. 2 Case 23 with 22q11.2 homozygote duplication. **a** Pedigree of the family. **b** Dysmorphic features of the case 23. **c** Note the overfolded helix. **d** MLPA shows tetrasomy of 22q11.2 region. **e** T2 weighed MRI shows basillar impression and hypoplasia of clivus

(25th–50th percentile), her height was 155 cm (25th–50th percentile), and weight was 45 kg (10th–25th percentile). Hypertelorism, broad nasal bridge, down-slanting palpebral fissures were observed. No pyramidal system involvement was present, and reflexes were normoactive. Echocardiography and brain MRI was normal. Psychometric evaluation revealed borderline mental disability. 2.5 Mb duplication was detected at 22q11.2/ Di George Syndrome region with CMA. The results were validated with MLPA analysis.

The patient's father is 48 years old. He is a primary school graduate and works in the transportation sector. There were no neuropsychiatric problems observed other than sudden irritation. The mother is 44 years old.

She is a primary school graduate. She is a housewife and is interested working in her own garden. She is capable of doing daily work, but has difficulty doing arithmetic calculations. Both the mother and the father had the duplication of the same 22q11.2/ Di George Syndrome region with CMA. The results were validated with MLPA analysis.

Case 17 with a new locus for ASD

A 3-year-old male patient (case 17) was diagnosed with speech delay. He started to walk in his first year and began speaking by using three words at two and half years of age. At neurological examination, head circumference was 48 cm (10th percentile), height was 93 cm

(10th–25th percentile), and weight was 13 kg (10th–25th percentile). Hypertelorism, broad nasal bridge, micrognathia were observed. Hyperactivity and poor eye contact were detected. No pyramidal system involvement was present, and reflexes were normoactive. Cerebellar system examinations were normal. Serum electrolytes, electroencephalography, and abdominal ultrasonography findings were within normal limits. He had stereotypical behaviors, deficits in communication, and autism spectrum disorder, which was diagnosed at 3 years of age. Denver developmental screening test showed one-year delay in speech and social skills. CMA revealed 2.9-Mb de novo deletion at 18q22 region. *RTTN, SOCS6, CBLN2, NETO1* genes were located at the deleted region.

Discussion

Global developmental delay is the term that is used to describe children (aged 5 years or younger) who have demonstrated several significant delays in the following areas: cognitive, speech, social/personal, fine/gross motor, and daily activities. Intellectual disability is a disorder with intellectual and adaptive deficits and can be diagnosed after the age of five [5]. CMA is a first-tier test in the evaluation of individuals with ID and GDD which provides opportunities to discover new ID/GDD associated syndromes, and helps uncover the genetic background of many syndromes by revealing genetic heterogeneity and by identifying new loci for novel candidate genes [3]. The widespread use of CMA allows patients to be diagnosed and provides families with guidance in genetic counseling.

This is the first study shows the diagnostic rate of chromosomal abnormalities in the northern part of Turkey, with yield of 18.55%, which is consistent with the results of previous studies (5–35%) [2, 3]. It is important to point out that our diagnostic rate is higher than the rate of other studies performed on a similar platform in Turkey (12–13.6%) [8, 9]. We found 26 CNV's in 23 patients, which indicates the importance of the CMA. Different diagnostic rates for different publications are related to the choice of patient group. If more patients were involved in the study, the rates could differ.

We also included parents in our study, and 23 of 26 CNVs were de novo. Although 8 out of 23 families had consanguineous marriages, our analyses revealed de novo variations in these families rather than homozygous mutations. In Turkish society, where the consanguineous marriage is common, it is necessary to investigate chromosomal abnormalities due to this phenomenon. We studied such a family, where mother and father were related and had a chromosome 22q11.2 duplication. The family had a girl with learning disability and was diagnosed with 22q11.2 duplication, and a boy (case 23) with milder intellectual disability, dysmorphic

features and short stature, who was diagnosed with tetrasomy of 22q11.2 region. In case 23, parents' diagnoses support the duplication of region 22q11.2 in both alleles, which can be described as homozygous duplication. Case 23 is the fifth patient diagnosed with 22q11.2 tetrasomy in the literature [4, 10, 11] and the third patient diagnosed with 22q11.2 homozygote duplication (Table 2). In other published 22q11.2 tetrasomy cases, three copies of an allele were reported. Bi et al. reported two cases with 22q11.2 homozygote duplication. However, there are other genomic changes, outside the 22q11.2 region, which could affect the phenotype of these patients [11]. As those two patients have region 22q11.2 homozygote duplication, case 23 can be added to this list as the third patient with a similar situation. Although our patient has cognitive deficiency and dysmorphic facial features in common with the other three cases, it is important to note that our patient does not suffer from hearing loss unlike the other three cases (Table 2). However, while other triplications may be three copies of a parental tract, it should be noted that our patient's mother and father have duplication of the region. Bi et al. reported that there was no phenotypic difference between duplication of 22q11.2 region and triplication of 22q11.2 [11]. While the T2 weighed MRI of the case 23 shows basillar impression and hypoplasia of clivus, hypoplasia of clivus has not been reported in the other region 22q11.2 triplication or duplication cases.

Case 17, who was diagnosed with autism spectrum disorder, had a 2.9 Mb deletion at 18q22 region. *RTTN, SOCS6, CBLN2, NETO1* genes are located at this region. *RTTN* homozygote mutations are associated with microcephaly, short stature, and polymicrogyria with seizures (OMIM 614833). [12]. Homozygote mutations of this gene also affect brain migration and volume [12]. Our patient had a deletion of 1-10th exons with milder phenotype. The MRI was normal and he had speech delay and autism spectrum disorder. These results show that the *RTTN* gene heterozygous mutations could be responsible for ASD.

SOCS6 gene, which encodes Suppressor of Cytokine Signaling 6 protein, was deleted in case 17. The SOCS6 gene has not yet been associated with a disease, however it may be related to syndromic obesity [13]. Although this gene is deleted in our patient, he is not yet obese. Even though *SOCS6* and *SOCS7* have been reported to be necessary for cortical neuron migration [14], there was no evidence of migration defect in the MRI of our patient. The other gene in the deletion region in case 17, which may be important for ASD/ID, is *CBLN2*. *CBLN2* gene encodes Precerebellin 2. Common variants of *CBLN2* are associated with increased risk of pulmonary arterial hypertension [15]. It is noteworthy that *CBLN2* expression is highest in cerebral cortex and hypothalamus of mouse reference [16].

Table 2 Clinical features of patients with tetrasomy of region 22q11.2

Features	Yobb et al. 2005	Bi et al. 2012	Vaz et al. 2015	This study (case 23)
22q11.2 region	4 copies (3/1)	4 copies (2/2)	4 copies (3/1)	4 copies (2/2)
Age at last evaluation	8 years	29 mounts	20 years	11 years
Gender	Female	Male	Female	Male
Heart defect	–	–	+	+
Velopharyngeal insufficiency	–	–	+	–
Hearing impairment	+	+	+	–
Failure to thrive	–	–	–	+
Sleep apnea	–	N/D	+	–
Urogenital abnormalities	–	N/D	+	–
Cognitive deficits	+	+	+	+
Psychiatric disorders	–	N/D	+	–
Behavioural problems	+	N/A	–	–
Headache	–	N/D	+	–
Recurrent infections	+	–	–	–
Hand/foot abnormality	+	+	–	–
Dysmorphic and other features	Epicanthal folds, Broad nasal bridge, Left ear pit, Secondary hearing impairment	Left preauricular pit, Plagiocephaly, Facial asymmetry, Teeth abnormality, Hypoplastic iris and corectopia	Long narrow face, Epicanthal folds, Hypertelorism, Downslanting palpebral fissures, Prominent nose, Long philtrum, Dental cavities, Retrognathia,	Round face, Hypertelorism, Downslanting palpebral fissures Broad nasal bridge, Long philtrum, Overfolded helix, Hypoplasia of clivus

Neuropilin and Tolloid-Like 1 (*NETO1*) gene was deleted in case 17. *NETO1* is a CUB domain-containing transmembrane protein, which have been reported to immuno-precipitate with assembled NMDA receptors via GluN2A or GluN2B subunits [17]. Ng D et al. have shown that *NETO1* plays a critical role in maintaining the delivery or stability of NR2A-containing NMDARs at CA1 synapses [18].

Cody et al. reported that genes located distal to 18q were associated with ASD, and *NETO1* was among these genes [19]. The only common point between the deletion in our patient and the region that Cody et al. have reported is the *NETO1*. O'Donnell et al. also reported that *NETO1* and *FBXO15* genes in region 18q22.3 may be risk factors for ASD [20]. When the synaptic plasticity is thought to be important in the development of ASD, heterozygous *NETO1* deletions may be considered as a risk factor for ASD. After doing a thorough evaluation of the literature, particularly the studies with mice, we conclude that *NETO1* should be added to the list of risky genes that should be investigated for ASD.

Conclusion

Our data expand the spectrum of 22q11.2 region mutations and provide insights for genotype–phenotype correlations of ID, GDD, and autism. It also underlines the importance of CMA and its use in understanding the pathophysiology of certain diseases. Based on our findings, we suggest that CMA should be used as a first-step test for the identification of new loci and the expansion of known phenotypes.

Abbreviations

ASD: Autism spectrum disorder; CA: Congenital anomalies; CMA: Chromosomal microarray analysis; CNVs: Copy number variations; DQ: Dosage quotient; GDD: Global developmental; ID: Intellectual disability; MLPA: Multiplex ligation-dependent probe amplification; UCS: Uncertain clinical significance;

Acknowledgements

We would like to thank the family of our patient for their assistance with the clinical evaluation.

Databases

Database of Chromosomal Imbalance and Phenotype in Humans Using Ensemble Resources [http://decipher.sanger.ac.uk].
Database of Genomic Variants [http://projects.tcag.ca/variation].
Online Mendelian Inheritance in Man [http://omim.org].
ClinGen Clinical Genome Resource [https://www.clinicalgenome.org].
University of California, Santa Cruz [https://genome.ucsc.edu].

Funding

This study was not supported by any foundation.

paper are however available from the corresponding author on reasonable request.

Authors' contributions

ACC designed the study. ACC and SC performed the experiments, analyzed the data and wrote the manuscript. ACC, SC, HBE, IS and, EAA are the main referring clinicians and performed the clinical assessment and physical examination of patients. ME performed the MLPA of the 22q11.2 chromosome region. All authors read and approved the final manuscript.

Competing interests

The authors declare that they have no competing interests.

Author details

[1]Trabzon Kanuni Training and Research Hospital, Medical Genetics Unit, Trabzon, Turkey. [2]Ankara Yıldırım Beyazıt University, Ankara Atatürk Training and Research Hospital, Department of Medical Genetics, Ankara, Turkey. [3]Ankara Diskapi Yildirim Beyazit Training and Research Hospital, Medical Genetics Unit, Ankara, Turkey. [4]Karadeniz Technical University, School of Medicine, Department of Child Neurology, Trabzon, Turkey. [5]Kayseri Training and Research Hospital, Department of Medical Genetics, Kayseri, Turkey.

References

1. Curry CJ, Stevenson RE, Aughton D, Byrne J, Carey JC, Cassidy S, et al. Evaluation of mental retardation: recommendations of a consensus conference. American College of Medical Genetics Am J Med Genet. 1997; 72:468–77.
2. Sagoo GS, Butterworth AS, Sanderson S, Shaw-Smith C, Higgins JP, Burton H. Array CGH in patients with learning disability (mental retardation) and congenital anomalies: updated systematic review and meta-analysis of 19 studies and 13,926 subjects. Genet Med. 2009;11:139–46.
3. Miller DT, Adam MP, Aradhya S, Biesecker LG, Brothman AR, Carter NP, et al. Consensus statement: chromosomal microarray is a first-tier clinical diagnostic test for individuals with developmental disabilities or congenital anomalies. Am J Hum Genet. 2010;86:749–64.
4. Yobb TM, Somerville MJ, Willatt L, Firth HV, Harrison K, MacKenzie J, et al. Microduplication and triplication of 22q11.2: a highly variable syndrome. Am J Hum Genet. 2005;76:865–76.
5. DSM-V. The 5th. Edition of the diagnostic and statistical manual of mental disorders from the American Psychiatric Association. In: American Psychiatric Association; 2013.
6. Wright CF, Fitzgerald TW, Jones WD, Clayton S, McRae JF, van Kogelenberg M, et al. Genetic diagnosis of developmental disorders in the DDD study: a scalable analysis of genome-wide research data. Lancet. 2015;385:1305–14.
7. Kearney HM, Thorland EC, Brown KK, Quintero-Rivera F, South ST, Working Group of the American College of medical genetics laboratory quality assurance C. American College of Medical Genetics standards and guidelines for interpretation and reporting of postnatal constitutional copy number variants. Genet Med. 2011;13:680–5.
8. Utine GE, Haliloglu G, Volkan-Salanci B, Cetinkaya A, Kiper PO, Alanay Y, et al. Etiological yield of SNP microarrays in idiopathic intellectual disability. Eur J Paediatr Neurol. 2014;18:327–37.
9. Ozyilmaz B, Kirbiyik O, Koc A, Ozdemir TR, Kaya OO, Guvenc MS, et al. Experiences in microarray-based evaluation of developmental disabilities and congenital anomalies. Clin Genet. 2017;92:372–9.
10. Vaz SO, Pires R, Pires LM, Carreira IM, Anjos R, Maciel P, et al. A unique phenotype in a patient with a rare triplication of the 22q11.2 region and new clinical insights of the 22q11.2 microduplication syndrome: a report of two cases. BMC Pediatr. 2015;15:95.
11. Bi W, Probst FJ, Wiszniewska J, Plunkett K, Roney EK, Carter BS, et al. Co-occurrence of recurrent duplications of the DiGeorge syndrome region on both chromosome 22 homologues due to inherited and de novo events. J Med Genet. 2012;49:681–8.
12. Kheradmand Kia S, Verbeek E, Engelen E, Schot R, Poot RA, de Coo IF, et al. RTTN mutations link primary cilia function to organization of the human cerebral cortex. Am J Hum Genet. 2012;91:533–40.
13. Vuillaume ML, Naudion S, Banneau G, Diene G, Cartault A, Cailley D, et al. New candidate loci identified by array-CGH in a cohort of 100 children presenting with syndromic obesity. Am J Med Genet A. 2014;164A:1965–75.
14. Lawrenson ID, Krebs DL, Linossi EM, Zhang JG, McLennan TJ, Collin C, et al. Cortical layer inversion and deregulation of Reelin signaling in the absence of SOCS6 and SOCS7. Cereb Cortex. 2017;27:576–88.
15. Ma L, Chung WK. The genetic basis of pulmonary arterial hypertension. Hum Genet. 2014;133:471–9.
16. Wei P, Pattarini R, Rong Y, Guo H, Bansal PK, Kusnoor SV, et al. The Cbln family of proteins interact with multiple signaling pathways. J Neurochem. 2012;121:717–29.
17. Cousins SL, Innocent N, Stephenson FA. Neto1 associates with the NMDA receptor/amyloid precursor protein complex. J Neurochem. 2013;126:554–64.
18. Ng D, Pitcher GM, Szilard RK, Sertie A, Kanisek M, Clapcote SJ, et al. Neto1 is a novel CUB-domain NMDA receptor-interacting protein required for synaptic plasticity and learning. PLoS Biol. 2009;e41:7.
19. Cody JD, Hasi M, Soileau B, Heard P, Carter E, Sebold C, et al. Establishing a reference group for distal 18q-: clinical description and molecular basis. Hum Genet. 2014;133:199–209.
20. O'Donnell L, Soileau B, Heard P, Carter E, Sebold C, Gelfond J, et al. Genetic determinants of autism in individuals with deletions of 18q. Hum Genet. 2010;128:155–64.

6

Understanding aneuploidy in cancer through the lens of system inheritance, fuzzy inheritance and emergence of new genome systems

Christine J. Ye[1], Sarah Regan[2], Guo Liu[2], Sarah Alemara[2] and Henry H. Heng[2,3]*

Abstract

Background: In the past 15 years, impressive progress has been made to understand the molecular mechanism behind aneuploidy, largely due to the effort of using various -omics approaches to study model systems (e.g. yeast and mouse models) and patient samples, as well as the new realization that chromosome alteration-mediated genome instability plays the key role in cancer. As the molecular characterization of the causes and effects of aneuploidy progresses, the search for the general mechanism of how aneuploidy contributes to cancer becomes increasingly challenging: since aneuploidy can be linked to diverse molecular pathways (in regards to both cause and effect), the chances of it being cancerous is highly context-dependent, making it more difficult to study than individual molecular mechanisms. When so many genomic and environmental factors can be linked to aneuploidy, and most of them not commonly shared among patients, the practical value of characterizing additional genetic/epigenetic factors contributing to aneuploidy decreases.

Results: Based on the fact that cancer typically represents a complex adaptive system, where there is no linear relationship between lower-level agents (such as each individual gene mutation) and emergent properties (such as cancer phenotypes), we call for a new strategy based on the evolutionary mechanism of aneuploidy in cancer, rather than continuous analysis of various individual molecular mechanisms. To illustrate our viewpoint, we have briefly reviewed both the progress and challenges in this field, suggesting the incorporation of an evolutionary-based mechanism to unify diverse molecular mechanisms. To further clarify this rationale, we will discuss some key concepts of the genome theory of cancer evolution, including system inheritance, fuzzy inheritance, and cancer as a newly emergent cellular system.

Conclusion: Illustrating how aneuploidy impacts system inheritance, fuzzy inheritance and the emergence of new systems is of great importance. Such synthesis encourages efforts to apply the principles/approaches of complex adaptive systems to ultimately understand aneuploidy in cancer.

Keywords: Adaptive system, Aneuploidy, Cancer evolution, Complexity, Emergence of new genome, Fuzzy inheritance, Genome theory, Non-clonal chromosome aberrations (NCCAs), Punctuated evolution, System inheritance

Background and progress

Why is aneuploidy commonly observed in various cancer types? How does aneuploidy directly or indirectly contribute to cancer? Is aneuploidy good or bad for cancer initiation and progression, and how does it affect treatment response? What is the relationship between aneuploidy and other genetic/epigenetic aberrations? How important is it to study each individual molecular mechanism that can be linked to aneuploidy? What are the general mechanisms (cause and effect) for generating aneuploidy? Why can aneuploidy be detected from other diseases? And what is the biological significance of aneuploidy in normal tissues for normal individuals? … These questions represent some long-debated issues in the field of cancer

* Correspondence: hheng@med.wayne.edu
[2]Center for Molecular Medicine and Genomics, Wayne State University School of Medicine, Detroit, MI 48201, USA
[3]Department of Pathology, Wayne State University School of Medicine, Detroit, MI 48201, USA
Full list of author information is available at the end of the article

research, ever since Theodor Boveri recognized the link between aneuploidy and cancer over a century ago [1–4].

Specific aneuploidy has been observed in various non-cancer diseases: Down syndrome with trisomy chromosome 21, Edwards syndrome with trisomy 18, Patau syndrome with trisomy 13, Klinefelter's syndrome with an extra X, and Turner's syndrome with the absence of one X. While clonal aneuploidy is also detected in some cancers, such as chronic lymphocytic leukemia (CLL) with trisomy 12 and acute myeloid leukemia (AML) with trisomy 8, the percentage of such cancer patients with the signature clonal aneuploidy is much lower (18% for CLL and 8.5% for AML) compared to those with Down syndrome (over 95% of all patients), suggesting that there are more diverse genomic factors contributing to cancer (even for the liquid cancer type) than those non-cancer genetic diseases.

Altogether, the complexity of aneuploidy makes studying its relationship with cancer extremely challenging (Table 1). Some known complications include: a) most cancer cases display non-clonal aneuploidy (impeding the fact that clonal aneuploidy has been much more commonly researched for decades) [5–9], b) aneuploidy often occurs in combination with other types of genetic/epigenetic and genomic aberrations (translocations and polyploidy) (Table 2) c) there is often a variable degree of somatic mosaicism [10–13], and d) there is a complex, dynamic relationship between aneuploidy and genome instability (Table 3). Interestingly, many common and complex diseases have been linked to non-clonal aneuploidy and somatic mosaicism as well [14, 15], which has led to efforts to search for commonly shared mechanisms among different diseases or illness conditions [16–19]. It is worth noting that aneuploidy can also be detected from the normal developmental process [20–22].

Such complexity did however discourage aneuploidy research, as cloning and characterizing individual cancer genes had promised much more certainty. During the peak era of oncogene- and tumor suppressor gene-focused research, for example, the importance of aneuploidy was largely ignored, due to high expectations from the gene mutation theory of cancer. As a result, efforts to systematically study aneuploidy in cancer, especially based on the belief that aneuploidy is much more important than gene mutations, are limited to a small number of research groups [23–26]. One of the popular viewpoints was that cancer gene mutations hold the key to understanding cancer, whereas chromosomes were just vehicles of genes; it was furthermore argued that most chromosomal changes are either incidental or the consequence of gene mutations.

While it was observed that some chromosomes display a tumor suppressor function following cell/chromosome fusion experiments [27], efforts were focused on cloning

Table 1 Explanations of key terminologies

Aneuploidy is a changed genomic state with an abnormal number of chromosomes in a cell. In cancer, most aneuploidy is not clonal or constitutional. Recently, a looser definition of aneuploidy has been used to analyze DNA sequence data, which includes partial chromosomal changes and somatic copy number aberration (SCNA). Such usage is not precise, as germline CNVs and SCNA represents the variable copy number of specific sequences, which is not the same as the entire abnormal chromosome(s). According to the genome theory, the chromosome represents a coding system, so the impact of aneuploidy is therefore much more significant than SCNA. The mechanisms causing somatic aneuploidy are many; examples can be found in Table 2.

CIN: Chromosome instability (CIN) refers the rate (cell-to-cell variability) of changed karyotypes of a given cell population. There are two types of CIN: numerical and structural. Numerical CIN is determined by the gain or loss of whole chromosomes or fractions of chromosomes (aneuploidy), as well as other forms. Structural CIN, on the other hand, is determined by structural NCCAs. Numerical and structural CIN often co-exist. CIN can be effectively measured by the frequency and type of NCCAs.

Type I and type II CIN: CIN can be classified into two types based on its involved molecular mechanisms. Type I CIN is directly linked to the maintenance of genome integrity within the chromosomal cycle, including the chromosomal machinery, checkpoints, and repair systems (see Table 3). Type I CIN is often detected in chromosome instability syndromes which provide good examples of direct "molecular causative relationship" between identified genes and CIN. However, mutations to type I genes are rare and they do not explain sporadic cancer. In contrast, the mechanisms of type II CIN are often associated with non-genetic factors such as the micro-environment and physiological processes, which do not have a direct molecular causative explanation. The diverse type II mechanisms all share one common feature: they are involved in the cellular system's response to stress, increasing heritable changes [50].

Fuzzy inheritance: In contrast to the gene theory, which states that a gene codes for a specific, fixed phenotype, the genome theory suggests that most genes code for a range of potential phenotypes. From this "fuzzy" range of phenotypes, the respective environment can then allow the best-suited status to be "chosen" [4, 37, 59]. For example, the gene for pea color codes for an entire potential spectrum of colors, from yellow to intense green (including blends of yellow and green, or green with yellow spots), not just two fixed, distinctive colors (yellow or intense green). In cancer, the emergence of "genomic context" adds yet another layer of complexity and instability that pushes fuzzy inheritance's dynamics to a maximal status.

Macro-and micro-cellular evolution: Macro-cellular evolution refers to karyotype change-mediated somatic cell evolution, which alters the genome context of a given cellular system. In contrast, micro-cellular evolution refers to gene/epigene change-mediated evolution, which modifies a given cellular system within the same karyotype. Macroevolution and microevolution respectively refer to organismal evolution at the above-species level and at the population level within a species.

System inheritance: Unlike the gene-defined "parts inheritance" (the instructions for making a given protein or RNA), a new three-dimensional genomic topologic coding, or the blueprint of the genome, is defined by the order of genes or other DNA sequences along and among the chromosomes of a given genome. This blueprint encodes how genes interact as an emergent property, which provides the instructions for how genomic networks work [4, 37, 66].

tumor suppressor genes [28]. The lack of easy-to-recognize patterns in aneuploidy has certainly reduced the enthusiasm of most funding agents about this topic, especially when gene mutation research has promised to identify the key common gene mutations for cancer.

One important publication has classified cancer into two major types based on observed molecular mechanisms: chromosome instability (CIN) and microsatellite

Table 2 Examples of different types of causative factors of aneuploidy

1. Gene mutations/epigenetic alterations	[111–113]
Mitotic checkpoint defects, e.g. *BUB1*, *MAD1* and *CENPE*	[114, 115]
Microtubule attachment defects, e.g. *aurora kinase B*, *Cydlin A*,	
Mitotic spindle and centrosome defects	[116]
Other CIN-related mutation, e.g. *p53*, *ATM*	[117]
2. Stress- (physiological, pathological and pharmaceutical) related responses	
Defective mitotic figures (condensation defects) (DMF, sticky chromosomes)	[50, 78, 106]
Chromosome fragmentations (C-Frags)	[115, 116]
Genome chaos	[5, 6, 37, 59, 67]
Chromosomal cycle variations (replication, condensation, segregation, de-condensation)	[104]
Non-specific stress (triggers type II CIN)	[50]
3. Genome system variability	
Fuzzy inheritance	[4, 37, 59]
Cellular adaptation	[37, 95]
Survival under high stress	[56, 67]

To illustrate the viewpoint that many genomic and environmental factors can contribute to aneuploidy, a few examples are presented, among a large number of publications. We focus more on the examples that feature a cytogenetic perspective, as these are currently less popular compared to gene mutation studies, despite their importance

Table 3 Examples of interesting observations in aneuploidy studies including some conflicting data. Some comments are also offered to explain them

1. The dynamic relationship between aneuploidy and CIN
Aneuploidy generates CIN, including increased chromosome loss, mutation rate and defective DNA damage repair [39, 119].
The relationship between aneuploidy and CIN can be envisioned as a "vicious cycle," wherein one potentiates the other [120].
The "stress–CIN–cancer evolution relationship" can also be used to discuss the relationship between aneuploidy and cancer [50].
Elevated transcriptome dynamics are linked to karyotype changes which impact multiple genetic/epigenetic interactions [121–123]
Aneuploidy is less influential compared to structure alterations [54].
CIN rates might be more predictive for tumor outcome than assessing aneuploidy rates alone [54, 124].
Many cancer cell lines with aneuploidy are relatively stable (an example of fuzzy inheritance of some relatively stable systems) [37].
Genome chaos, including karyoplast budding, giant cells and mitotic catastrophe, is often associated with aneuploidy [67, 125–127].
Chromosomal condensation defects (DMFs) and Chromosome fragmentation (C-Frags) can generate aneuploidy [37, 106, 118].
Aneuploidy (in the form of mosaicism) represents a common phenomenon. We may all have a touch of Down syndrome [128, 129].
Aneuploidy is a main feature among individual cancer cell lines. The rate of aneuploidy seems inherited [72].
Genomic *PTEN* deletion size influences the landscape of aneuploidy and outcome in prostate cancer [130].
ATM and p21 cooperate to suppress aneuploidy and tumor development [117]

2. The complex relationship between aneuploidy and immune response
When co-cultured with natural killer cells, aneuploidy cells with complex karyotype-induced senescent cells were selectively cleared [131].
High copy number alterations in melanoma patients are linked with less effective response to immune checkpoint blockade anti–CTLA-4 [52].

3. Biological impact of aneuploidy
Aneuploidy changes the genomic coding, which affects the transcriptome, proteome, network structure, incidence of CIN and phenotypes [4, 37, 132].
Chromosome mis-segregation per se can alter the genome in many ways in addition to chromosome gain or loss [133].
Aneuploidy puts pressure on the protein machinery and quality control, which generates a global stress response, reducing cell proliferation [133].
Both specific gene effects and the typical aneuploidy stress response contribute to new genomic coding or/and increased system stress, which can impact the emergent process of cancer evolution ([133], current paper)
Karyotype status (e.g. aneuploidy and polyploidy) can restore functions of specific genes (e.g. *MYO1*). Thus, genomic coding changes gene coding [83].
The chromosomal size involved in aneuploidy is inversely correlated to the resulting fitness [134].
The risk of cancers to metastasize is proportional to the degree of cancer-specific aneuploidy [48].
There is a dynamic relationship between epigenetic events and aneuploidy; epigenetic marks play a role in the control of chromosome segregation and integrity; aneuploidy impacts chromatin silencing [135–137].
New approaches are needed to study the complexity of systems, including that of aneuploidy-mediated karyotype evolution [138, 94, 110].

instability [29]. Remarkably, the majority of colon cancers display CIN. The fact that most cancers can be linked to chromosomal instability was a surprise to many who primarily study cancer genes.

If the majority of cancers are linked to CIN, and aneuploidy contributes to CIN, more attention needs to be paid to aneuploidy [30]. Based on this concept, increased efforts were focused on identifying genes that are responsible for aneuploidy. Many individual genes and molecular pathways involving chromosomal machinery/integrity have been linked to aneuploidy. For example, a list of identified genes that contribute to aneuploidy-mediated cancer includes germline BUBR1 mutation, which leads to aneuploidy and cancer predisposition [31]. Additional examples can be found in Table 2.

Another important factor that promotes aneuploidy research is the popularization of copy number variation studies of the human genome [32–34]. If various individual instances of CNV are of importance, large scale CNVs caused by aneuploidy should be too, despite the fact that the search for specific genes related to aneuploidy (such as chromosome 21) have traditionally been the main focus. The availability of various technologies that can detect CNV have now revolutionized molecular cytogenetics. It should be mentioned that the cytogenetically visible copy number variations (CG-CNVs) need more attention [35]. Regarding the framework of fuzzy inheritance, CNVs, CG-CNVs, small supernumerary marker chromosomes and aneuploidy represent different degrees of fuzziness, which are likely reflected by quantitative difference or combinational effect. It is important to integrate these with analyses of system emergence [4, 36, 37].

In recent years, due in part to the disappointment that has come from attempting to identify the common driver gene mutation, and more significantly, due to the realization that genome instability plays an important role in cancer, aneuploidy studies have gained momentum. In particular, the popularity of studying aneuploidy in cancer has been promoted by some yeast biologists. Taking advantage of yeast model systems, they have applied cutting-edge molecular and genomic technologies to illustrate the molecular mechanisms that link aneuploidy to biological functions [38–42]; by translating their discoveries into cancer research, they have brought the spotlight on aneuploidy research in cancer [43, 44] (Tables 2, 3). Interestingly, a complex relationship between aneuploidy and cancer has also been revealed, proposing that aneuploidy can either promote or inhibit cancer progression depending on the evolutionary context. This has led to the paradox of aneuploidy in cancer [45, 46].

There have been attitude changes towards the study of aneuploidy as well. When direct evidence simultaneously characterized gene mutation and chromosomal aberrations as drivers for the phenotypic implication of metastasis [47], the authors clearly emphasized CIN, and the potentially involved gene was not even mentioned in the title. This likely represents a new favored approach focusing on genome-level changes. There is also the realization that chromosomal aberrations contribute more significantly to metastasis than gene mutations do [48] which supports the hypothesis that chromosomal aberration-mediated genome evolution is responsible for all major transitions in cancer evolution, including metastasis and drug resistance [49, 50]. Furthermore, and surprisingly to many molecular researchers, chromosome aberration profiles have been demonstrated to have a much stronger prediction value in the clinic compared to DNA sequencing profiles [51]. This conclusion has gained strong support from various cancer genome sequencing projects [52, 53], which prompts an important question regarding the differential contribution of chromosome aberrations and gene mutations to the cancer genotype. All together, rapidly accumulated data has forcefully highlighted the importance of aneuploidy in current cancer research, and more detailed molecular information linking individual gene mutations or epigenetic events to aneuploidy will soon flourish.

Challenges for predicting cancer status based solely on the molecular mechanisms of aneuploidy

Like other hallmarks of cancer, aneuploidy has now become a hot topic. A predictable new trend is that more researchers will join the effort to link all possible genetic/epigenetic and environmental factors to aneuploidy and cancer. However, as we have extensively discussed, due to biocomplexity (i.e. that many individual factors can contribute to the same phenotype), it is possible that merely collecting more diverse molecular data linking gene mutation and environmental factors to aneuploidy is not the best way to advance this field. This is because there will be too many factors involved, most of them lacking the power to predict cancer status [54, 55].

This viewpoint has been articulated by the evolutionary mechanism of cancer and its relationship with individual molecular mechanisms [50, 56]. In brief, cancer evolution can be understood by the dynamic interaction among four key components: internal and external stress; elevated genetic and non-genetic variations (either necessary for cellular adaptation or resulting from cellular damages under stress); genome-based macro-cellular evolution (genome replacement, emergent as new systems); and multiple levels of system constraint which prevent/slow down cancer evolution (from tissue/organ organization to the immune system and mind-body interaction). Since the sources of stress are unlimited and unavoidable (as they are required by all living systems), there are large numbers of gene mutations/epigenetic events/chromosomal aberrations, such as aneuploidy, that can be linked to stress-mediated genomic variants; furthermore, as environmental constraints are constantly changing, even identical instances of aneuploidy will have completely different outcomes in the context of cancer evolution, as the results of each independent run of evolution will most likely differ. Solely knowing the mechanism of aneuploidy limits the predicting power for cancer. Furthermore, hundreds of gene mutations can contribute to aneuploidy, and the various contexts of cancer evolution are almost unlimited. Based on this rationale, we promote the idea of using the evolutionary mechanism of cancer to unify diverse individual molecular mechanisms of cancer (4).

Unfortunately, such ideas have received little attention within the cancer research community, due in part to the traditional molecular characterization of gene mutations, and possibly more so due to many cancer biologists' unfamiliarity with complexity science and a lack of understanding of the key principles of bio-emergence. It is thus necessary to discuss this issue of aneuploidy in cancer using the framework of the complex adaptive system [37].

A complex adaptive system is a system made up of many individual parts (agents) with nonlinear dynamical interaction. Due to the key emergent relationship between the lower level of heterogeneous agents and the behavior of the entire system, a detailed understanding of the individual parts does not automatically convey a determinist's understanding of the whole system's behavior. There are no fixed, dominant agents within the adaptive system, and when agents of the system are changed, the system adapts or reacts. Moreover, small changes in initial conditions can generate large changes in the system's outcome, and stochasticity is also frequently involved [57, 58]. As a result, the reductionist approaches which have triumphed in molecular biology may be fundamentally limiting when attempting to understand complex adaptive systems.

Cancer is typically a complex adaptive system involving multiple levels of agent interactions and genotype/phenotype emergence among different types of tissue/organ constraints. In such a system, aneuploidy represents only one type of agent, despite its importance. There is a complex interaction among different levels of genetic organization, which involves phase transitions among clonal and non-clonal cellular populations, and the final emergence of different genome-defined cellular systems under highly dynamic cellular environments and the process of cancer evolution. This reality of cancer evolution explains why it is so challenging to predict the final phenotype based on an understanding of one type of agent. The take-home message is that simply understanding the molecular mechanism (both cause and effect) of aneuploidy is far from enough. A better strategy is to monitor the evolutionary process by measuring evolutionary potential. For example, the overall degree of CIN is more predictive than individual gene mutation profile [54]; large-scale chromosomal structural aberrations can often have a more profound impact on cancer evolution (even though aneuploidy often leads to structural aberrations as well); and the landscape of chromosomal aberrations is more predictive than gene mutation landscapes. Furthermore, the initial factor and the evolutionary trajectory differ in complex systems. It is now accepted that treatment options can often drastically and rapidly change the genetic landscape of the cancer [59].

In addition to the challenge that cancer is a complex adaptive system, it should be understood that current molecular knowledge of aneuploidy is mainly derived from model systems, which can differ from cancer systems in patients. The following limitations are briefly mentioned to bring the reader's attention to them, and they are also useful for explaining some conflicting observations. First, the platform of the yeast model differs from human cellular populations within tissue. Different species display the feature of aneuploidy quite variably. In budding yeast *Saccharomyces cerevisiae*, aneuploidy is not uncommon and exists in natural populations; in plants, organisms can tolerate whole chromosome aneuploidy without triggering CIN; in mice, every single whole chromosome gain or loss is embryonic lethal [60]; in humans, the situation is similar to that of mice, with the exception of a few chromosome gains such as 13, 18 and 21. The pattern of evolution also differs when diverse types of cellular selection are involved, in addition to differing types of system constraints. For cancer evolution in reality, the overall complexity and the level of dynamics is much higher, which can often change the game completely. In the future, multiple cellular models might be helpful to certain degrees, especially when the

time variable (i.e. development and aging) is added in to the equation.

Second, the status of clonal and non-clonal aneuploidy differs between many model systems and the reality of cancer. So far, for many yeast and human cell models, aneuploidy stains are created with clonal populations in which most cells display the same extra chromosomes. In contrast, for many solid tumors, aneuploidy exists in non-clonal forms. Such differences may contribute to some misperceptions, thus requiring further studies. For example, the analysis of trisomic cells from human patients with congenital aneuploidy syndromes did not display any increased CIN, concluding that aneuploidy itself does not lead to cancer-like CIN [61]. We have mentioned the significant difference between constitutional aneuploidy and the acquired aneuploidy observed in cancers. Constitutional aneuploidy is a clonal-chromosome aberration (CCA), whereas many acquired somatic aneuploidies are nonclonal-chromosome aberrations (NCCAs). In the cellular environment of trisomy 21, trisomy 21 is the dominating "normal" genome, and any other genomes (including the "normal" 46 XY or XX karyotype) are relatively "abnormal;" the homeostasis of trisomy 21 could actually generate less cellular variation, which explains the resulting low levels of cell-to-cell variations. Based on this analysis, we suggested that although specific constitutional aneuploidy alone is not sufficient for generating numerical CIN, it is necessary to examine the impact of non-recurrent, stochastic aneuploidy on generating all types of CIN [62].

Third, many models feature simple types of aneuploidy (with one extra chromosome within an otherwise normal karyotype, for example), which is easier to analyze with repeatable results. In contrast, in the setting of cancer evolution, aneuploidy is often coupled with structural chromosomal changes and/or polyploidy. In addition, the rate of aneuploidy within the population is often lower than in clonal populations of model systems, while for each cell with aneuploidy, the heterogeneity is higher than cells from model systems (there are often multiple extra chromosomes, for example). Such differences between model systems (in which the majority of cells are isogenic) and cancer samples (which have high levels of chromosomal and gene mutation heterogeneity) are reflected by the display of mainly micro-evolutionary processes in model systems, and a mixture of macro-evolution plus micro-evolution in real cancer. In a sense, many model systems mimic a population of the same species, while real cancer systems mimic a population of the same species and different species [4, 63–65].

Fourth, when discussing the advantages/disadvantages of aneuploidy, the majority of studies are focused on growth status. It should be pointed out that while growth represents a key feature of cancer, during the earlier stages of cancer evolution, growth might not necessarily be the key precondition. The rationale of focusing on cell proliferation in cancer research was based on the concept of accumulating gene mutations during cancer initiation and progression; it was thus argued that the proliferated cell population could provide the basis for stepwise cancer evolution. Since the discovery that punctuated cancer evolution is achieved by genome reorganization events, such as genome chaos, the rationale of focusing on proliferation has been challenged [6–8, 50, 56, 66, 67]. Surely, the cancer genome sequencing project has failed to detect serial, stepwise gene mutation accumulation in the majority of cancer cases [4, 59, 68]. In contrast, system instability might not only be an important earlier event, but in fact the key event. According to the genome theory [4, 49, 50, 56], genome instability could be the key driver for all major transitions for cancer evolution, including transformation, metastasis, and drug resistance. It is likely that cellular proliferation contributed by the "oncogenes" often represents the later events which help cancer cells to become more dominant cell populations (for more, see reference [4, 37]). Similar patterns have been observed in metastasis and drug resistance. Therefore, system instability might be the most important aspect for the success of cancer: new systems' emergence from normal tissue [69, 70]. Recent single-cell sequencing of breast cancer cells supports this viewpoint. It was observed that copy number changes and rearrangements appeared early in tumorigenesis. In contrast, point mutations occurred gradually during tumor evolution (within the micro-evolutionary phase) [71].

Fifth, most current research efforts are focusing on molecular profiles based on an average population, and outliers are eliminated or ignored, either by the methods used or statistical tools. The traditional view of biological research is to identify patterns from "noise," without the realization that the so-called "noise" in fact is heterogeneity, which represents a key feature of cancer evolution by functioning as the evolutionary potential. Increased studies have demonstrated the importance of outliers in cancer evolution, as cancer is an evolutionary game of outliers [4, 72, 73].

Sixth, in the search for the molecular consequence of aneuploidy, the focus is still on the genes' function. Despite the fact that it is hard to make sense out of the data of altered profiles of a large numbers of genes, few have realized that aneuploidy, in fact, changes a new chromosomal-level coding system, which is namely the system inheritance [16, 37, 66].

Clearly, a new framework is needed to systematically study aneuploidy in cancer evolution. Since cancer is a complex adaptive system, and each run of successful evolution can be linked to different genome and gene mutation profiles, more attention needs to be paid to the gap between initial conditions and final emergence, the environmental and genome contexts, landscape dynamics, and system instability-mediated cancer evolutionary potential

[59]. Because cancer evolution requires inheritance, and involves the emergence of new systems, the following session will focus on these issues to redefine inheritance and the emergent bio-cellular system.

The genome theory of cancer evolution

Based on the ultimate importance of chromosomal aberrations in cancer evolution, especially within the punctuated phase of macro-cellular evolution, the genome theory of cancer evolution was introduced with the aim of departing from the gene mutation theory of cancer [4, 49, 66]. To illustrate how chromosomal changes play a key driving role in cancer evolution, we have redefined the genomic meaning of karyotype changes, and compared the evolutionary dynamics between clonal and non-clonal chromosomal aberrations [6–8, 64, 74]. Moreover, we have proposed the use of the genome-mediated evolutionary mechanism to unify the diverse molecular mechanisms of cancer [55, 75]. Since aneuploidy represents one important type of karyotype aberration [15, 74], the principles of genome theory can be easily applied to aneuploidy research in the context of somatic evolution, complexity, and how chromosomally-defined new genomic information plays a driving role for new system emergence.

System inheritance and aneuploidy

Genes encode proteins, and the sequence of ATGC within genes is the genetic coding. It has been challenging to study how aneuploidy affects genetic coding when there are over a thousand genes involved. Traditionally, attention has been paid to dosage effects. With the development of the technical platform for transcriptome profiling, it was surprisingly observed that the impact of aneuploidy is far beyond the dosage effect on genes located on gained or lost chromosomes [40, 76, 77]. Even more interestingly, different experimental systems differ in terms of the observed impact. The genomic basis for these unexpected findings is unknown.

During our watching-evolution-in-action experiments within an in vitro immortalization model, we constantly observed rapid and massive genome re-organization during the punctuated phase of cancer evolution [4, 6–8, 78]. Remarkably, during this phase, mother cells can generate daughter cells with similar DNA but drastically different karyotypes. To illustrate the biological meaning of this karyotype re-organization, we realized that the shattering of the genome and its subsequent reorganization represent a powerful means of creating new genomic information. Such a new mechanism functions above the coding of individual genes, and perhaps serves to organize gene interaction.

One of the biggest promises of the human genome sequencing project was to decipher the blueprint that makes us human. Unfortunately, we have failed to achieve this goal following the sequencing phase of the genome project. Despite that we know the sequence of nearly all genes, we have no idea what the genomic blueprint is. Systems biologists have suggested that the network structure defines the blueprint. But what defines the network structure in the first place?

Putting all of these questions together, we realized that the karyotype, in fact, represents a new genomic coding system, and the blueprint is encoded by the new genomic information which is defined by the order of genes along and among chromosomes [4, 37, 59]. More specifically, a gene only encodes a specific "part inheritance," while a set of the chromosomes of a given species encodes the "system inheritance" [16, 66]. Furthermore, we suggested that the karyotype defines the boundary of a network structure for a given species, which integrates the network into the genome-defined system [69, 70].

Further studies suggested that karyotype coding is maintained by the function of sex through the meiotic pairing mechanisms [79–82]. Nearly all significant karyotype aberrations will be eliminated by the "reproductive filter," which ensures the species identity. In this way, similar gene content can form different species by creating different karyotypes, which determine the physical platform for gene interactions in the 3-D nucleus [37]. Since different species display different karyotypes, a species is in fact preserved by its own chromosomal coding. Furthermore, it is likely that altered genomic information contributes to many common and complex diseases [4, 37].

Obviously, aneuploidy alters the karyotype and thus changes the genomic coding. Despite the fact that much work is needed to illustrate the details of how aneuploidy changes genomic coding, many experiments support this idea in principle. For example, aneuploidy not only changes the overall transcriptomes, but can specifically provide new functions to rescue cells lacking specific essential genes. When the only copy of the MYO 1 gene was knocked out, yeast should no longer have been able to survive, as MYO1 encodes the myosin II protein required for cytokinesis. Surprisingly, however, extensive polyploidy and aneuploidy (rather than reverse mutation) was demonstrated to rescue the dying populations, illustrating that genome-level changes can generate emergent new phenotypes without directly fixing the specific deleted gene [83]. In other words, re-organizing the karyotype coding can create functions encoded by specific genes in different systems. Ample evidence can be found in current literature [4, 37].

Fuzzy inheritance and aneuploidy
One key feature of cancer is its multiple levels of genetic/epigenetic/genomic heterogeneity. During time-course experiments designed to trace karyotype evolution in vitro, it was documented that the degree of karyotype heterogeneity can be drastically different depending on the phases of cellular evolution [6–8]. In addition, the different extents of karyotype heterogeneity are evolutionary phase-specific (extremely high within the punctuated phase and low within the stepwise phase), suggesting that karyotype heterogeneity is inheritable among different cell populations. A similar phenomenon has been observed from DNA mutation when discussing the mutant type [84]. Recently, the two phases of cancer evolution have been confirmed by gene mutation and copy number profiling [71, 85–88].

Following the characterization of various cancer cell lines, it became clear that each line displays a different degree of heterogeneity (reflected as the rate of NCCAs). To establish the baseline of karyotype heterogeneity in normal individuals, SKY karyotype analysis was used after short-term culture of lymphocytes, and the rate of structural NCCAs was found to be around 1–4%. Interestingly, drug treatment-induced frequencies of NCCAs are also different among cell lines or individuals with different levels of genome instability, and elevated frequencies of NCCAs from lymphocytes are detected from various diseases or illness conditions [17, 19, 89].

The above observations are highly significant in the context of missing inheritability [90, 91]. It is generally accepted that phenotype is the result of the interaction of genotype and environment, but its mechanism is not clearly understood. For example, for phenotype plasticity, the mechanism is unknown. It is also unclear how different genotypes display different extents of phenotypic plasticity, and why environment can win over the power of genetics or vice versa.

The link between the frequency of NCCAs and phenotype heterogeneity has promoted the concept that the previously regarded "noise," in fact, represents karyotype heterogeneity. Further research/synthesis has led to the realization that it is likely that the coded message at the karyotype level is heterogeneous in nature, which results in high phenotypic plasticity.

Important questions were then asked. Is it possible that inheritance itself is not precise but fuzzy, even for the coding of a single gene-determined phenotype? Do genetic elements code a spectrum of potential information rather than a fixed one? What if these highly penetrant relationships between genotype and phenotype only represent exceptions in which environmental factors are well-controlled? Does the major role of environmental factors select a specific possibility encoded by the genetic coding? Do stress conditions increase the heterogeneity of phenotype by increasing the fuzziness of the genetic coding? To address these questions, fuzzy inheritance has been introduced by us as the mechanism of various levels of genetic and epigenetic heterogeneity [4, 37, 70].

Since non-clonal aneuploidy belongs within the category of NCCAs and represents karyotype heterogeneity, it is important to integrate aneuploidy into fuzzy inheritance. Despite the fact that the frequencies of aneuploidy in various normal tissues are low, when combined with other NCCAs, the level of altered karyotypes is rather high, especially under stress conditions [50, 92, 93, 94]. In addition, the drastic difference between the spontaneous rate of aneuploidy in cells from normal tissue and in those from cancers supports the idea that specific cell populations display different degrees of fuzzy inheritance which are related to aneuploidy. For example, the mis-segregation rate in a stable, diploid cell line is one chromosome per 100–1000 cell divisions. In contrast, the mis-segregation rate in cultured cancer cells with CIN is approximately once every 1–5 divisions [95–97]. More remarkably, during the genome chaos phase, almost all cells display a high rate of mis-segregation with large number of aneuploidies, plus all sorts of karyotype variants [6, 50, 67]. The high degree of fuzzy inheritance in cancer, in fact, can also explain why non-clonal aneuploidy is a common feature of even later stages of cancer. All tumors are under high stress from surrounding tissues or higher systems, so fuzzy inheritance-mediated karyotype heterogeneity is essential for tumor survival and further progression. Clearly, how aneuploidy quantitatively contributes to fuzzy inheritance-mediated genomic heterogeneity needs further study.

The relationship between cellular adaptation and trade-off

Traditionally, aneuploidy has long been blamed as the result of bio-errors. Most of the molecular evidence supports this viewpoint, as when specific genes are dysfunctional as a result of experimental manipulation, a phenotype of increased aneuploidy can be observed. Many gene mutations involving cell cycle/chromosomal integrity can achieve the same phenotype. While the baseline of aneuploidy in normal individual tissues is low in many cases, in some tissue types, the spontaneous aneuploidy is high. Moreover, the overall rate of NCCAs is not low at all in most normal tissues.

Obviously, the higher than expected frequency of karyotype changes, including aneuploidy, cannot simply be explained as bio-error. In recent years, the biological significance of these seemingly random genetic "backgrounds" were studied, which has led to the appreciation of genomic heterogeneity in cancer evolution. Further synthesis suggests a relationship between stress-induced NCCAs and the advantages offered by their presence for cellular adaptation, as well as the trade-offs caused by their presence in cancer evolution and possibly in other disease conditions [4, 92]. Moreover, many diseases are the results of genomic variants which do not fit the current environments. Due to the dynamics of environments and the nature of fuzzy inheritance, it is impossible to eliminate all of these variants. Paradoxically, these genomic variants might be necessary for the species' long-term survival, and they should be considered as a life insurance policy despite their

high costs. Such a concept of trade-off not only addresses the key evolutionary mechanism of many diseases including cancer, but may also provide some answers to patients who ask the "why me" question. In a sense, cancer as an evolutionary trade-off can be illustrated by different perspectives: at the mechanistic level, cancers are the by-products of evolution (that is, the same mechanisms which make us human also make cancer successful); at the species level, as population heterogeneity is important for species survival, an individual with high genome instability can be considered as paying the price for our species; and at the individual level, most bio-features, including lifestyle, could be beneficial in some aspects and yet harmful in other aspects. Even for non-clonal aneuploidy-mediated cellular heterogeneity, while this phenomenon can provide a potential advantage for cellular adaptation, it can also, paradoxically, generate non-specific system stress, which can further produce more genetic and non-genetic variants which favor the disease condition [4]. Based on this rationale, we have attempted to use type I and type II CIN to unify diverse gene mutations under the principle of CIN-mediated cancer evolution, as many gene mutations and molecular pathways which are not directly involved in maintaining genome integrity can still be linked to CIN [50].

Emergence and luck

The unpredictability of emergence represents a common challenge for using parts characterization to predict phenotype at higher levels in a complex adaptive system. How aneuploidy triggers the successful evolution of cancer, especially during the phase transitions, is almost unknown. The situation worsens when the type of aneuploidy is non-clonal, and when both the context of other types of genetic changes and cellular environments keeps changing. For example, different tissues can tolerate different degrees of aneuploidy; aneuploidy can be detected at the early development stage with high frequencies, but the developmental process can overcome them, whereas the impact of aneuploidy can become serious during cancer evolution later in life; even in tissues that are sensitive to aneuploidy, most instances of aneuploidy will not lead to cancer. It seems that in different tissue types, different stages of development and aging, and different physiological and pathological processes, there are different "roles" for the cellular society which favor different types of emergence [19, 37]. For example, in a normal physiological cellular society, the average profile can overrule outliers, while in the setting of cancer evolution and under high stress, the outliers may triumph.

To understand how non-clonal karyotype aberrations can contribute to the emergence of cancer evolution, we proposed that instances of non-clonal aneuploidy, like other types of non-clonal karyotype aberrations, serve as heterogeneous agents that can impact the emergent properties of the cellular evolution. While the details of how aneuploidy affects emergence are not yet known, this model illustrates the importance of how even a portion of non-clonal aneuploidy can change the emergence process (Fig. 1). A similar general model of how the heterogeneity of genetic agents impacts diseases has been proposed to explain how NCCAs can contribute to different diseases [18, 98].

Due to the complex combinations of aneuploidy and the genetic and environmental contexts, a vast majority of these combinations will not directly lead to cancer's success, as they are either not powerful enough to contribute to the phase transition which leads to cancer, or they are eliminated by system constraint. For example, it was recently demonstrated that the complex karyotypes derived from aneuploidy can trigger the immune system to eliminate them (Table 3). Another example is drug therapy in which a high dosage of drugs is used. The majority of the cancer cells will be eliminated by the initial drug treatment, and only a tiny portion of the cancer cells can survive (through the formation of genome chaos). It is extremely challenging to predict which aberrations will be successful, even though drug-resistant clones often arise.

As a consequence of the highly heterogeneous nature of karyotypes featuring aneuploidy, as well as the diverse genomic/environmental contexts involved, most genomic aberrations will not lead to the success of cancer, despite their potential. A "perfect storm" is needed for any cancer

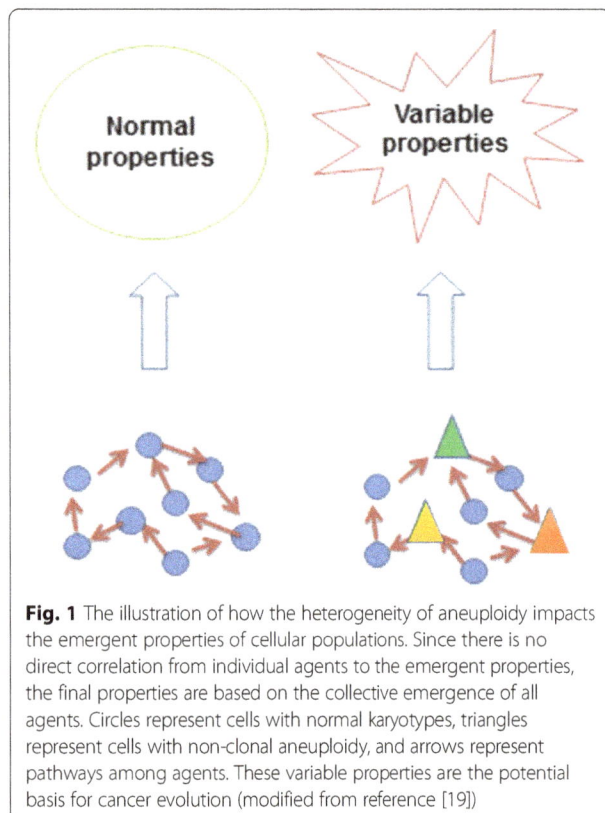

Fig. 1 The illustration of how the heterogeneity of aneuploidy impacts the emergent properties of cellular populations. Since there is no direct correlation from individual agents to the emergent properties, the final properties are based on the collective emergence of all agents. Circles represent cells with normal karyotypes, triangles represent cells with non-clonal aneuploidy, and arrows represent pathways among agents. These variable properties are the potential basis for cancer evolution (modified from reference [19])

to be successful. Under such conditions, luckiness or unluckiness can be considered agents which impact the emergent properties.

Such interplay during cancer evolution is ultimately responsible for the emergence of a new genome system from normal tissue, and aneuploidy-mediated genome re-organization plays a key role for creating these new systems [4, 37, 66]. For altered cells to become cancer cells, they have to complete many key transitions, including immortalization, transformation and metastasis, all of which require the emergence of different genome systems; gene mutation alone is not sufficient for creating a new system. The alteration of system inheritance and the increased degree of fuzzy inheritance mainly contribute to the macro-cellular evolution which leads to new systems. In contrast, genes that promote cell proliferation can expand cancer cell populations following the formation and selection of cancer cells with unique karyotype-defined systems (Fig. 2).

Conclusion and future research

Within the framework that represents cancer as a complex adaptive system, the following elements become highly important for understanding both the key feature and common mechanism of cancer: internal and external stress-mediated adaptation and its trade-off (trigger factors); the multiple levels of genetic/environmental heterogeneity (essential conditions for cancer evolution); the involvement of system inheritance and fuzzy inheritance (how genomics works during cancer evolution); the two phases of cancer evolution (the mechanism of cellular evolution and the relationship between gene/epigene and genome changes); the emergence of new, karyotype-defined systems (the formation of a cancer seed and the importance of NCCAs and outliers); and the population of cancer cells that become clinically significant (the dominance of cancer). It is necessary to integrate these elements during studies of aneuploidy.

Despite the recent exciting progress of aneuploidy research, some great challenges remain. Simply focusing on the molecular characterization of agents at lower levels is neither sufficient for understanding the emergent properties of a complex adaptive system nor for predicting the contribution of aneuploidy to cellular evolution.

To change the status quo, the crucial first step is to acknowledge the fundamental limitation of the reductionist approach in aneuploidy research, as there is no precise, predictable relationship between an understanding of the individual mechanism of aneuploidy and clinical certainty, nor between many diverse individual agents and the emergent properties of cancer evolution. It is thus equally difficult to search for patterns based on diverse molecular pathways. In addition, the dynamic interaction of average cells and outliers further complicates this prediction. To

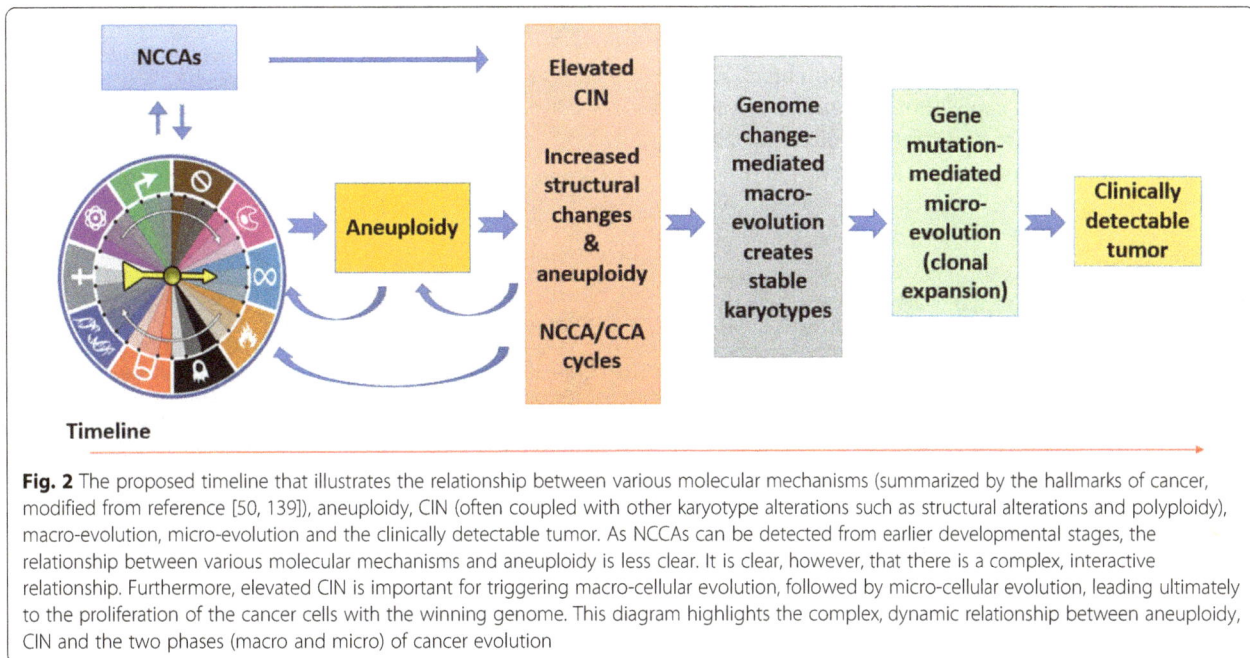

Fig. 2 The proposed timeline that illustrates the relationship between various molecular mechanisms (summarized by the hallmarks of cancer, modified from reference [50, 139]), aneuploidy, CIN (often coupled with other karyotype alterations such as structural alterations and polyploidy), macro-evolution, micro-evolution and the clinically detectable tumor. As NCCAs can be detected from earlier developmental stages, the relationship between various molecular mechanisms and aneuploidy is less clear. It is clear, however, that there is a complex, interactive relationship. Furthermore, elevated CIN is important for triggering macro-cellular evolution, followed by micro-cellular evolution, leading ultimately to the proliferation of the cancer cells with the winning genome. This diagram highlights the complex, dynamic relationship between aneuploidy, CIN and the two phases (macro and micro) of cancer evolution

make sense of this complexity and to increase predictability, a better strategy is to consider aneuploidy as an agent and cancer as a complex adaptive system. Expectations regarding the predictive power of aneuploidy must also change, as the success of cancer evolution depends on both evolutionary potential (which can be measured) as well as on chance or accidents (which are hard to predict) [99, 100]. The importance of special "circumstances" or "accidents" in evolutionary success is receiving our increased attention [4, 37, 66].

An innovative type of biomarkers is needed to integrate aneuploidy with other karyotype alterations, and these should be used to measure evolutionary potential (based on the degree of heterogeneity and karyotype complexity) rather than specific pathways. This approach will likely bridge the gap between basic research and clinical implications. There are some examples of applying aneuploidy in clinical analysis [101]. High somatic copy number alterations in melanoma patients have recently been linked with less effective response to immune checkpoint blockade anti–CTLA-4 (cytotoxic T lymphocyte–associated protein 4) therapy [52]. Clearly, aneuploidy status is associated with response to precise immunotherapy. We have engaged in the effort of using NCCAs (mainly structural NCCAs) to monitor clinical outcomes. One approach is to measure an individual's overall genome instability and its linkage to cancer status. We have observed a strong correlation between the frequencies of structural NCCAs from short term lymphocytes culture and prostate cancer [37]. This work has expanded into other health conditions [17]. A similar concept of monitoring overall genome instability to detect cancer can be found in literature

involving telomere length and the overall chromosomal aberration rate [102–107]. More aneuploidy data should be integrated into this effort. In particular, since chromosome data (CIN statuses, for example) have much more clinical predictive power than sequenced gene mutation data [4, 50–53, 74], bioinformaticians should be encouraged to search for new platforms for mining sequences in the context of evolutionary potential, through the use of AI (artificial intelligence) approaches. For example, this strategy could be used to search for the principle of how aneuploidy changes the blueprint, its overall impact on the gene network, and the quantitative contribution of elements for the higher level of emergence.

Further research is also needed to compare emergence based on average profiles and outliers with various degrees of system stress. Such analysis needs to be done within the context of the cellular society concept [4, 108]. As for the technical platforms, new monitoring methods should be developed to study single cells, especially to profile non-dividing cell populations. Recently, the CRISPR/Cas9 system has been used to eliminate targeted chromosomes. This new approach offers an effective way to develop animal models with aneuploidy, which can be used as a potential therapeutic strategy for human aneuploidy diseases [109]. Certainly, among these advances, one immediate priority is to illustrate how aneuploidy triggers structural alterations of the karyotype and provides the maximal diversity and plasticity needed for new system emergence and domination. For example, can aneuploidy lead to genome chaos [110]? How does the heterogeneity of aneuploidy impact the newly emergent karyotype?

Finally, and perhaps most importantly, the ultimate goal of establishing better concepts and platforms for cancer research is to apply them in the clinic. Further studies are needed to apply this new understanding of aneuploidy for patient stratification, directing therapy schedules, and predicting drug resistance.

Abbreviations

CCA: clonal chromosome aberrations; C-Frags: chromosome fragmentations; CIN: chromosomal instability; CNV: copy number variations; DMFs: defective mitotic figures; NCCA: non clonal chromosome aberrations

Acknowledgements

This manuscript is part of our series of publications on the subject of "the mechanisms of cancer and organismal evolution." This work was also partially supported by the start-up fund for Christine J. Ye from the University of Michigan's Department of Internal Medicine, Hematology/Oncology Division. We thank Dr. Emanuela Volpi, the special issue editor, for her kind invitation. We also thank two anonymous reviewers for their valuable suggestions, and Julie Heng for partial editing.

Funding

This work was partially supported by the start-up fund for CJY from the department of internal medicine, division of hematology/oncology, University of Michigan.

Authors' contributions

CY and HH drafted the manuscript. SR, GL and SA contributed to discussion and editing. All authors read and approved the final manuscript.

Competing interests

The authors declare that they have no competing interests.

Author details

[1]The Division of Hematology/Oncology, Department of Internal Medicine, University of Michigan, Ann Arbor, MI 48109, USA. [2]Center for Molecular Medicine and Genomics, Wayne State University School of Medicine, Detroit, MI 48201, USA. [3]Department of Pathology, Wayne State University School of Medicine, Detroit, MI 48201, USA.

References

1. Boveri T. Concerning the origin of malignant tumors. J Cell Sci. 2008; 121: Suppl1, 1–84.
2. Holland AJ, Cleveland DW. Boveri revisited: chromosomal instability, aneuploidy and tumorigenesis. Nature Rev Mol Cell Biol. 2009;10:478–87.
3. Rasnick D. The chromosomal imbalance theory of cancer: the autocatalyzed progression of aneuploidy is carcinogenesis: CRC Press; 2011.
4. Heng HH. Debating Cancer. The paradox in Cancer research. New Jersey: World Scientific Publishing Company; 2015.
5. Mitelman F. Recurrent chromosome aberrations in cancer. Mutat Res. 2000; 462:247–53.
6. Heng HH, Stevens JB, Liu G, Bremer SW, Ye KJ, Reddy PV, et al. Stochastic cancer progression driven by nonclonal chromosome aberrations. J Cell Physiol. 2006;208:461–72.
7. Heng HH, et al. Cancer progression by non-clonal chromosome aberrations. J Cell Biochem. 2006;98(6):1424–35.
8. Heng HH, et al. Clonal and non-clonal chromosome aberrations and genome variation and aberration. Genome. 2006;49(3):195–204.
9. Vargas-Rondón N, Villegas VE, Rondón-Lagos M. The Role of Chromosomal Instability in Cancer and Therapeutic Responses. Cancers (Basel). 2017;10(1): pii: E4.
10. Hall JG. Somatic mosaicism: observations related to clinical genetics. Am J Hum Genet. 1988;43:355–63.
11. Yurov YB, et al. Aneuploidy and confined chromosomal mosaicism in the developing human brain. PLoS One. 2007;2:e558.
12. Astolfi PA, Salamini F, Sgaramella V. Are we genomic mosaics? Variations of the genome of somatic cells can contribute to diversify our phenotypes. Curr Genomics. 2010;11(6):379–86.
13. Sgaramella V. The hypergenome in inheritance and development. Cytogenet Genome Res. 2013;139(3):215–22.
14. Heng HH. The contribution of genomic heterogeneity. Preface. Cytogenet Genome Res. 2013;139(3):141–3.
15. Heng HH, Liu G, Stevens JB, Abdallah BY, Horne SD, Ye KJ, et al. Karyotype heterogeneity and unclassified chromosomal abnormalities. Cytogenet Genome Res. 2013;139(3):144–57.
16. Heng HH, Liu G, Stevens JB, Bremer SW, Ye KJ, Abdallah BY, et al. Decoding the genome beyond sequencing: the next phase of genomic research. Genomics. 2011;98(4):242–52.
17. Heng HH. Challenges and new strategies for gulf war illness research. Environ Dis. 2016;1:118–25.
18. Heng HH, Regan S, Ye CJ. Genotype, environment and evolutionary mechanism of diseases. Environ Dis. 2016;1:14–23.
19. Heng HH, Liu G, Regan S, Ye CJ. Chapter 7, Linking Gulf War Illness to genome instability, somatic evolution and complex adaptive systems. In Putting systems and complexity sciences into practice, J. P. Sturmberg (ed). Switzerland: Springer, Cham ; 2018. p. 83–95.
20. Ambartsumyan G, Clark AT. Aneuploidy and early human embryo development. Hum Mol Genet. 2008;17(R1):R10–5.
21. Rehen SK, et al. Chromosomal variation in neurons of the developing and adult mammalian nervous system. Proc Natl Acad Sci U S A. 2001;98:13361–6.
22. Lee A, Kiessling AA. Early human embryos are naturally aneuploid—can that be corrected. J Assist Reprod Genet. 2017;34:15–21.
23. Li R, Yerganian G, Duesberg P, Kraemer A, Willer A, Rausch C, Hehlmann R. Aneuploidy correlated 100% with chemical transformation of Chinese hamster cells. Proc Natl Acad Sci U S A. 1997;94(26):14506–11.
24. Duesberg P, Rausch C, Rasnick D, Hehlmann R. Genetic instability of cancer cells is proportional to their degree of aneuploidy. Proc Natl Acad Sci U S A. 1998;95(23):13692–7.
25. Duesberg P, Rasnick D, Li R, Winters L, Rausch C, Hehlmann R. How aneuploidy may cause cancer and genetic instability. Anticancer Res. 1999; 19(6A):4887–906.
26. Duesberg P, Li R, Fabarius A, Hehlmann R. Aneuploidy and cancer: from correlation to causation. Contrib Microbiol. 2006;13:16–44.
27. Wiener F, Klein G, Harris H. The analysis of malignancy by cell fusion. VI. Hybrids between different tumour cells. J Cell Sci. 1974;16(1):189–98.
28. Guan XY, Zhang HE, Zhou H, Sham JS, Fung JM, Trent JM. Characterization of a complex chromosome rearrangement involving 6q in a melanoma cell line by chromosome microdissection. Cancer Genet Cytogenet. 2002;134(1):65–70.
29. Lengauer C, Kinzler KW, Vogelstein B. Genetic instabilities in human cancers. Nature. 1998;396(6712):643–9.
30. Gibbs WW. Untangling the roots of cancer. Sci Am. 2003;289(1):56–65.
31. Hanks S, Coleman K, Reid S, Plaja A, Firth H, Fitzpatrick D, et al. Constitutional aneuploidy and cancer predisposition caused by biallelic mutations in BUB1B. Nat Genet. 2004;36(11):1159–61.
32. Iafrate AJ, Feuk L, Rivera MN, Listewnik ML, Donahoe PK, Qi Y, et al. Detection of large-scale variation in the human genome. Nat Genet. 2004; 36:949–51.
33. Sebat J, Lakshmi B, Troge J, Alexander J, Young J, Lundin P, et al. Large-scale copy number polymorphism in the human genome. Science. 2004; 305:525–8.
34. Feuk L, Carson AR, Scherer SW. Structural variation in the human genome. Nat Rev Genet. 2006;7(2):85–97.
35. Liehr T. Cytogenetically visible copy number variations (CG-CNVs) in banding and molecular cytogenetics of human; about heteromorphisms and euchromatic variants. Mol Cytogenet. 2016;22:9–5.
36. Liehr T, Cirkovic S, Lalic T, Guc-Scekic M, de Almeida C, Weimer J, et al. Complex small supernumerary marker chromosomes - an update. Mol Cytogenet. 2013;6:46.

37. Heng HH. Genome chaos: rethinking genetics, evolution and molecular medicine (in press). Academic Press.

38. Torres EM, et al. Effects of aneuploidy on cellular physiology and cell division in haploid yeast. Science. 2007;317:916–24.

39. Sheltzer JM, et al. Aneuploidy drives genomic instability in yeast. Science. 2011;333:1026–30.

40. Siegel JJ, Amon A. New insights into the troubles of aneuploidy. Annu Rev Cell Dev Biol. 2012;28:189–214.

41. Zhu J, Pavelka N, Bradford WD, Rancati G, Li R. Karyotypic determinants of chromosome instability in aneuploid budding yeast. PLoS Genet. 2012;8: e1002719.

42. Bonney ME, Moriya H, Amon A. Aneuploid proliferation defects in yeast are not driven by copy number changes of a few dosage-sensitive genes. Genes Dev. 2015;29(9):898–903.

43. Pavelka N, Rancati G, Li R. Dr Jekyll and Mr Hyde: role of aneuploidy in cellular adaptation and cancer. Curr Opin Cell Biol. 2010;22:809–15.

44. Gordon DJ, Resio B, Pellman D. Causes and consequences of aneuploidy in cancer. Nat Rev Genet. 2012;13:189–203.

45. Weaver BA, Silk AD, Montagna C, Verdier-Pinard P, Cleveland DW. Aneuploidy acts both oncogenically and as a tumor suppressor. Cancer Cell. 2007;11:25–36.

46. Weaver BA, Cleveland DW. The aneuploidy paradox in cell growth and tumorigenesis. Cancer Cell. 2008;14:431–3.

47. Gao C, Su Y, Koeman J, Haak E, Dykema K, Essenberg C, et al. Chromosome instability drives phenotypic switching to metastasis. Proc Natl Acad Sci U S A. 2016;113(51):14793–8.

48. Bloomfield M, Duesberg P. Inherent variability of cancer-specific aneuploidy generates metastases. Mol Cytogenet. 2016;9:90.

49. Heng HH. Cancer genome sequencing: the challenges ahead. BioEssays. 2007;29(8):783–94.

50. Heng HH, Bremer SW, Stevens JB, Horne SD, Liu G, Abdallah BY, et al. Chromosomal instability (CIN): what it is and why it is crucial to cancer evolution. Cancer Metastasis Rev. 2013;32(3–4):325–40.

51. Jamal-Hanjani M, Wilson GA, McGranahan N, Birkbak NJ, Watkins TBK, et al. Tracking the evolution of non-small-cell lung Cancer. N Engl J Med. 2017; 376(22):2109–21.

52. Davoli T, Uno H, Wooten EC, Elledge SJ. Tumor aneuploidy correlates with markers of immune evasion and with reduced response to immunotherapy. Science. 2017;355(6322). pii: eaaf8399.

53. Zanetti M. Chromosomal chaos silences immune surveillance. Science. 2017; 355(6322):249–50.

54. Ye CJ, Stevens JB, Liu G, Bremer SW, Jaiswal AS, Ye KJ, et al. Genome based cell population heterogeneity promotes tumorigenicity: the evolutionary mechanism of cancer. J Cell Physiol. 2009;219:288–300.

55. Horne SD, Pollick SA, Heng HH. Evolutionary mechanism unifies the hallmarks of cancer. Int J Cancer. 2015;136(9):2012–21.

56. Heng HH, Stevens JB, Bremer SW, Liu G, Abdallah BY, Ye CJ. Evolutionary mechanisms and diversity in cancer. Adv Cancer Res. 2011;112:217–53.

57. Heng HH. The conflict between complex systems and reductionism. JAMA. 2008;300(13):1580–1.

58. Coffey DS. Self-organization, complexity and chaos: the new biology for medicine. Nat Med. 1998;4(8):882–5.

59. Heng HH. The genomic landscape of cancers (chapter 5) in ecology and evolution of Cancer, eds Ujvari, Roche, Thomas (eds). Acadmic Press, 2017. Pp69–86.

60. Hernandez D, Fisher EM. Mouse autosomal trisomy: two's company, three's a crowd. Trends Genet. 1999;15(6):241–7.

61. Valind A, Jin Y, Baldetorp B, Gisselsson D. Whole chromosome gain does not in itself confer cancer-like chromosomal instability. Proc Natl Acad Sci U S A. 2013;110(52):21119–23.

62. Heng HH. Distinguishing constitutional and acquired nonclonal aneuploidy. Proc Natl Acad Sci U S A. 2014;111(11):E972.

63. Duesberg P, Rasnick D. Aneuploidy, the somatic mutation that makes cancer a species of its own. Cell Motil Cytoskeleton. 2000;47(2):81–107.

64. Ye CJ, Liu G, Bremer SW, Heng HH. The dynamics of cancer chromosomes and genomes. Cytogenet Genome Res. 2007;18:237–46.

65. Vincent MD. The animal within: carcinogenesis and the clonal evolution of cancer cells are speciation events sensu stricto. Evolution. 2010;64(4):1173–83.

66. Heng HH. The genome-centric concept: resynthesis of evolutionary theory. BioEssays. 2009;31(5):512–25.

67. Liu G, Stevens JB, Horne SD, Abdallah BY, Ye KJ, Bremer SW, et al. Genome chaos: survival strategy during crisis. Cell Cycle. 2014;13(4):528–37.

68. Horne SD, Ye CJ, Abdallah BY, Liu G, Heng HH. Cancer genome evolution. Transl Cancer Res. 2015;4(3):303–13.

69. Heng HH, Regan S. A systems biology perspective on molecular cytogenetics. Cur bioinformatics. 2017;12:4–10.

70. Heng HH, Horne SD, Chaudhry S, Regan SM, Liu G, Abdallah BY, Ye CJ. A Postgenomic Perspective on Molecular Cytogenetics. Cur Genomics. 2018; 19(3):227–39.

71. Wang Y, Waters J, Leung ML, Unruh A, Roh W, Shi X, et al. Clonal evolution in breast cancer revealed by single nucleus genome sequencing. Nature. 2014;512:155–60.

72. Abdallah BY, Horne SD, Stevens JB, Liu G, Ying AY, Vanderhyden B, et al. Single cell heterogeneity: why unstable genomes are incompatible with average profiles. Cell Cycle. 2013;12(23):3640–9.

73. Abdallah BY, Horne SD, Kurkinen M, Stevens JB, Liu G, Ye CJ, et al. Ovarian cancer evolution through stochastic genome alterations: defining the genomic role in ovarian cancer. Syst Biol Reprod Med. 2014;60(1):2–13.

74. Heng HH, Regan SM, Liu G, Ye CJ. Why it is crucial to analyze non clonal chromosome aberrations or NCCAs? Mol Cytogenet. 2016;9:15.

75. Heng HH, Stevens JB, Bremer SW, Ye KJ, Liu G, Ye CJ. The evolutionary mechanism of cancer. J Cell Biochem. 2010;109(6):1072–84.

76. Sheltzer JM, Torres EM, Dunham MJ, Amon A. Transcriptional consequences of aneuploidy. Proc Natl Acad Sci U S A. 2012;109(31):12644–9.

77. Zhang H, Yang X, Feng X, Xu H, Yang Q, et al. Chromosome-wide gene dosage rebalance may benefit tumor progression. Mol Genet Genomics. 2018; https://doi.org/10.1007/s00438-018-1429-2. [Epub ahead of print].

78. Heng HH, Stevens JB, Liu G, Bremer SW, Ye CJ. Imaging genome abnormalities in cancer research. Cell Chromosome. 2004;3(1):1.

79. Heng HH. Elimination of altered karyotypes by sexual reproduction preserves species identity. Genome. 2007;50(5):517–24.

80. Wilkins AS, Holliday R. The evolution of meiosis from mitosis. Genetics. 2009; 181(1):3–12.

81. Gorelick R, Heng HH. Sex reduces genetic variation: a multidisciplinary review. Evolution. 2011;65(4):1088–98.

82. Horne SD, Abdallah BY, Stevens JB, Liu G, Ye KJ, Bremer SW, Heng HH. Genome constraint through sexual reproduction: application of 4D-Genomics in reproductive biology. Syst Biol Reprod Med. 2013;59(3):124–30.

83. Rancati G, Pavelka N, Fleharty B, Noll A, Trimble R, Walton K, et al. Aneuploidy underlies rapid adaptive evolution of yeast cells deprived of a conserved cytokinesis motor. Cell. 2008;135(5):879–93.

84. Loeb LA. Human Cancers Express a Mutator Phenotype: Hypothesis, Origin, and Consequences. Cancer Res. 2016;76(8):2057–9.

85. Baca SC, Prandi D, Lawrence MS, Mosquera JM, Romanel A, Drier Y, et al. Punctuated evolution of prostate cancer genomes. Cell. 2013;153(3): 666–77.

86. Notta F, Chan-Seng-Yue M, Lemire M, Li Y, Wilson GW, Connor AA, et al. A renewed model of pancreatic cancer evolution based on genomic rearrangement patterns. Nature. 2016;538(7625):378–82.

87. Sun R, Hu Z, Curtis C. Big Bang Tumor Growth and Clonal Evolution. Cold Spring Harb Perspect Med. 2017; pii: a028381.

88. Markowetz F. A saltationist theory of cancer evolution. Nat Genet. 2016; 48(10):1102–3. https://doi.org/10.1038/ng.3687.

89. Chandrakasan S, Ye CJ, Chitlur M, Mohamed AN, Rabah R, Konski A, et al. Malignant fibrous histiocytoma two years after autologous stem cell transplant for Hodgkin lymphoma: evidence for genomic instability. Pediatr Blood Cancer. 2011;56(7):1143–5.

90. Eichler EE, Flint J, Gibson G, Kong A, Leal SM, Moore JH, et al. Missing heritability and strategies for finding the underlying causes of complex disease. Nat Rev Genet. 2010;11(6):446–50.

91. Heng HH. Missing heritability and stochastic genome alterations. Nat Rev Genet. 2010;11:813.

92. Horne SD, Chowdhury SK, Heng HH. Stress, genomic adaptation, and the evolutionary trade-off. Front Genet. 2014;5:92.

93. Stevens JB, Abdallah BY, Liu G, Ye CJ, Horne SD, Wang G, et al. Diverse system stresses: common mechanisms of chromosome fragmentation. Cell Death Dis. 2011;2:e178.

94. Heng HH, Horne SD, Stevens JB, Abdallah BY, Liu G, Chowdhury SK, Et. al. chapter 9, heterogeneity mediated system complexity: the ultimate challenge for studying common and complex diseases. The value of systems and complexity sciences for healthcare. Joachin P Sturmberg (eds). New York: Springer, 2016. p101–115.

95. Cimini D, Tanzarella C, Degrassi F. Differences in malsegregation rates obtained by scoring ana-telophases or binucleate cells. Mutagenesis. 1999;14(6):563–8.

96. Thompson SL, Compton DA. Examining the link between chromosomal instability and aneuploidy in human cells. J Cell Biol. 2008;180(4):665–72.

97. Milena Dürrbaum and Zuzana Storchová Effects of aneuploidy on gene expression: implications for cancer. The FEBS Journal. 2016; 283: 791–802.

98. Heng HH. Heterogeneity-mediated cellular adaptation and its trade-off: searching for the general principles of diseases. J Eval Clin Pract. 2017 Feb; 23(1):233–7.

99. Tomasetti C, Vogelstein B. Cancer etiology. Variation in cancer risk among tissues can be explained by the number of stem cell divisions. Science. 2015;347:78–81.

100. Tomasetti C, Li L, Vogelstein B. Stem cell divisions, somatic mutations, cancer etiology, and cancer prevention. Science. 2017;355(6331):1330–4.

101. Park SY, Gönen M, Kim HJ, Michor F, Polyak K. Cellular and genetic diversity in the progression of in situ human breast carcinomas to an invasive phenotype. J Clin Invest. 2010 Feb;120(2):636–44.

102. Barrios L, Caballin MR, Miro R, Fuster C, Guedea F, Subias A, et al. Chromosomal instability in breast cancer patients. Hum Genet. 1991;88:39–41.

103. Bonassi S, Hagmar L, Stromberg U, Montagud AH, Tinnerberg H, Forni A, et al. Chromosomal aberrations in lymphocytes predict human cancer independently of exposure to carcinogens. European study group on cytogenetic biomarkers and health. Cancer Res. 2000;60:1619–25.

104. El-Zein R, Gu Y, Sierra MS, Spitz MR, Strom SS. Chromosomal instability in peripheral blood lymphocytes and risk of prostate cancer. Cancer Epidemiol Biomark Prev. 2005;14:748–52.

105. Hagmar L, Bonassi S, Stromberg U, Mikoczy Z, Lando C, Hansteen IL, et al. Cancer predictive value of cytogenetic markers used in occupational health surveillance programs. Recent Results Cancer Res. 1998;154:177–84.

106. Heng HQ, Chen WY, Wang YC. Effects of pingyanymycin on chromosomes: a possible structural basis for chromosome aberration. Mutat Res. 1988;199(1):199–205.

107. Hsu TC. Genetic instability in the human population: a working hypothesis. Hereditas. 1983;98:1–9.

108. Heppner GH. Cancer cell societies and tumor progression. Stem Cells. 1993; 11(3):199–203.

109. Zuo E, Huo X, Yao X, Hu X, Sun Y, Yin J, et al. CRISPR/Cas9-mediated targeted chromosome elimination. Genome Biol. 2017 Nov 24;18(1):224. https://doi.org/10.1186/s13059-017-1354.

110. Ye CJ, Liu G, Heng HH. Chapter 21: experimental induction of genome chaos. Chromothripsis: methods and protocols, 2018 springer, Ed frank Pellestor. Methods Mol Biol. 2018;1769:337–52.

111. Solomon et al. Mutational inactivation of STAG2 causes aneuploidy in human cancer. Science. 2011;333:1039–43.

112. Sansregret L, Swanton C. The Role of Aneuploidy in Cancer Evolution. Cold Spring Harb Perspect Med. 2017;7(1). pii: a028373.

113. Roussel-Gervais A, Naciri I, Kirsh O, Kasprzyk L, Velasco G, Grillo G, et al. Loss of the methyl-CpG-binding protein ZBTB4 alters mitotic checkpoint, increases aneuploidy, and promotes tumorigenesis. Cancer Res. 2017;77(1):62–73.

114. Giam M, Rancati G. Aneuploidy and chromosomal instability in cancer: a jackpot to chaos. Cell Div. 2015;10:3.

115. Schvartzman JM, Duijf PH, Sotillo R, Coker C, Benezra R. Mad2 is a critical mediator of the chromosome instability observed upon Rb and p53 pathway inhibition. Cancer Cell. 2011;19:701–14.

116. Ganem NJ, Godinho SA, Pellman D. A mechanism linking extra centrosomes to chromosomal instability. Nature. 2009;460:278–82.

117. Shen KC, Heng H, Y Wang SL, Liu G, Deng CX, Brooks SC, Wang YA. ATM and p21 cooperate to suppress aneuploidy and subsequent tumor development. Cancer Res. 2005;65(19):8747–53.

118. Stevens JB, Liu G, Bremer SW, Ye KJ, Xu W, Xu J, et al. Mitotic cell death by chromosome fragmentation. Cancer Res. 2007;67(16):7686–94.

119. Ohashi A, Ohori M, Iwai K, Nakayama Y, Nambu T, et al. Aneuploidy generates proteotoxic stress and DNA damage concurrently with p53-mediated post-mitotic apoptosis in SAC-impaired cells. Nat. Commun. 2015; 6:7668.

120. Potopova TA, Zhu J, Li R. Aneuploidy and chromosomal instability: a vicious cycle driving cellular evolution and cancer genome chaos. Cancer Metastasis Rev. 2013;32(3–4):377–89.

121. Heng HH, Bremer WS, Stevens JB, Ye KJ, Liu G, Ye CJ, et al. Genetic and epigenetic heterogeneity in Cancer: a genome centric perspective. J Cell Physiol. 2009;220(3):538–47.

122. Stevens JB, Liu G, Abdallah BY, Horne SD, Ye KJ, Bremer SW, et al. Unstable genomes elevate transcriptome dynamics. Int J Cancer. 2014;134(9):2074–87.

123. Stevens JB, Horne SD, Abdallah BY, Ye CJ, Heng HH. Chromosomal instability and transcriptome dynamics in cancer. Cancer Metastasis Rev. 2013 Dec;32(3–4):391–402.

124. Schukken KM, Foijer F. CIN and aneuploidy: different concepts, different consequences. BioEssays. 2018;40(1)

125. Walen KH. Budded karyoplasts from multinucleated fibroblast cells contain centrosomes and change their morphology to mitotic cells. Cell Biol Int. 2005;29(12):1057–65.

126. Erenpreisa J, Cragg MS. MOS, aneuploidy, and the ploidy cycle of cancer cells. Oncogene. 2010;29(40):5447–51.

127. Zhang S, Mercado-Uribe I, Sun B, Kuang J, Liu J. Generation of cancer-stem-like cells through the formation of polyploid giant cancer cells. Oncogene. 2014;33(1):116–28.

128. Hultén MA, Jonasson J, Iwarsson E, Uppal P, Vorsanova SG, Yurov YB, et al. Trisomy 21 mosaicism: we may all have a touch of Down syndrome. Cytogenet Genome Res. 2013;139(3):189–92.

129. Iourov IY, Vorsanova SG, Yurov YB. Chromsomal mosaicism goes global. Mol Cytogenet. 2008;1:26.

130. Vidotto T, Tiezzi DG, Squire JA. Distinct subtypes of genomic PTEN deletion size influence the landscape of aneuploidy and outcome in prostate cancer. Mol Cytogenet. 2018;11(1)

131. Santaguida S, Richardson A, Iyer DR, M'Saad O, Zasadil L, Knouse KA, et al. Chromosome Mis-segregation Generates Cell-Cycle-Arrested Cells with Complex Karyotypes that Are Eliminated by the Immune System. Dev Cell. 2017;41(6):638–651.e5.

132. Rutledge SD, Cimini D. Consequences of aneuploidy in sickness and in health. Curr Opin Cell Biol. 2016;40:41–6.

133. Santaguida S, Amon A. Short- and long-term effects of chromosome mis-segregation and aneuploidy. Nat Rev Mol Cell Biol. 2015;16(8):473–85.

134. Sheltzer JM, Ko JH, Replogle JM, Habibe Burgos NC, Chung ES, et al. Single-chromosome Gains Commonly Function as Tumor Suppressors. Cancer Cell. 2017;31(2):240–55.

135. Herrera LA, Prada D, Andonegui MA, Dueñas-González A. The epigenetic origin of aneuploidy. Curr Genomics. 2008;9(1):43–50.

136. Davidsson J. The epigenetic landscape of aneuploidy: constitutional mosaicism leading the way. Epigenomics. 2014;6(1):45–58.

137. Mulla WA, Seidel CW, Zhu J, Tsai HJ, Smith SE, Singh P et al., Aneuploidy as a cause of impaired chromatin silencing and mating-type specification in budding yeast. Elife. 2017;6. pii: e27991.

138. Heng HH. Bio-complexity: Challenging reductionism. In: Sturmberg JP, Martin CM, editors. Handbook on systems and complexity in health. New York: Springer; 2013. p. 193–208.

139. Hanahan D, Weinberg RA. Hallmarks of cancer: the next generation. Cell. 2011;144(5):646–74.

7

Monoallelic and biallelic deletions of 13q14 in a group of CLL/SLL patients investigated by CGH Haematological Cancer and SNP array (8x60K)

Beata Grygalewicz[1,4*], Renata Woroniecka[1], Jolanta Rygier[1], Klaudia Borkowska[1], Iwona Rzepecka[1], Martyna Łukasik[1], Agnieszka Budziłowska[1], Grzegorz Rymkiewicz[2], Katarzyna Błachnio[2], Beata Nowakowska[3], Magdalena Bartnik[3], Monika Gos[3] and Barbara Pieńkowska-Grela[1]

Abstract

Background: Deletion of 13q14 is the most common cytogenetic change in chronic lymphocytic leukemia/small lymphocytic lymphoma (CLL/SLL) and is detected in about 50 % of patients by fluorescence in situ hybridization (FISH), which can reveal presence of del(13)(q14) and mono- or biallelic deletion status without information about the size of the lost region. Array-comparative genomic hybridization (aCGH) and single nucleotide polymorphism (SNP) can detect submicroscopic copy number changes, loss of heterozygosity (LOH) and uniparental disomy (UPD) regions. The purpose of this study was detection of the size of del(13)(q14) deletion in our group of patients, comparing the size of the monoallelic and biallelic deletions, detection of LOH and UPD regions.

Results: We have investigated 40 CLL/SLL patients by karyotype, FISH and CGH and SNP array. Mutational status was of immunoglobulin heavy-chain variable-region (IGVH) was also examined. The size of deletion ranged from 348,12 Kb to 38.97 Mb. Detected minimal deleted region comprised genes: TRIM13, miR-3613, KCNRG, DLEU2, miR-16-1, miR-15a, DLEU1. The RB1 deletions were detected in 41 % of cases. The average size in monoallelic 13q14 deletion group was 7,2 Mb while in biallelic group was 4,8 Mb. In two cases 13q14 deletions were located in the bigger UPD regions.

Conclusions: Our results indicate that bigger deletion including RB1 or presence of biallelic 13q14 deletion is not sufficient to be considered as adverse prognostic factor in CLL/SLL. CytoSure Haematological Cancer and SNP array (8x60k) can precisely detect recurrent copy number changes with known prognostic significance in CLL/SLL as well as other chromosomal imbalances. The big advantage of this array is simultaneous detection of LOH and UPD regions during the same test.

Keywords: CLL/SLL, 13q14 deletion, CGH and SNP array, UPD

* Correspondence: beata.grygalewicz@coi.pl
[1]Cancer Genetic Laboratory, Pathology and Laboratory Diagnostics Department, Centre of Oncology, M. Skłodowska-Curie Memorial Institute, Warsaw, Poland
[4]Department of Pathology and Laboratory Diagnostics, Maria Skłodowska-Curie Memorial Cancer Center and Institute of Oncology, 15B Wawelska Str, 02-034, Warsaw, Poland
Full list of author information is available at the end of the article

Background

CLL/SLL is the most common leukemia in adults in Western countries [1]. The clinical course of this disease is very variable from indolent disease which is stable for many years to very rapid progression toward advanced stages, intensive treatment and short patients survival [2, 3]. Clinical staging systems developed by Rai and Binet can recognize advanced stage of disease, but they cannot predict disease course of the earlier stages [4]. Several prognostic markers have been described. Among genetic factors, prognostic significance have mutational status of *IGVH* and recurrent cytogenetic abnormalities [5, 6]. Somatic hypermutation of the *IGVH* gene is observed in approximately 50 % of patients, and its presence is associated with a more benign clinical course. Chromosomal changes of prognostic value as del(13)(q14), tris12, del(11)(q22.3) and del(17)(p13) can be detected in up to 50 % of patients by conventional cytogenetic analysis and up to 80 % by routine FISH analysis [7].

Deletion of 13q14 is the most common cytogenetic change in CLL/SLL and is detected in about 50 % of patients by FISH [5, 8]. This is a good prognostic factor if is detected as a sole aberration in FISH analysis. In karyotype del(13)(q14) is visible only in 8-10 % of patients, because in most of cases deletion size is submicroscopic [9]. Deletions vary considerably in size. The breakpoints are heterogeneous ranging from only 300 Kb up to more than 70 Mb [10–12]. The minimal deleted region (MDR) is described as located distal to *RB1* and comprises leukemia 2 (*DLEU2*) gene, which includes microRNA miR-15a/16-1 cluster [13–15]. In recent studies two main types of 13q14 deletions are proposed: del(13)(q14) type I (short), which breaks close to the miR16/15a locus and does not involve *RB1*; and del(13q)(q14) type II (larger), which includes *RB1* and has been suggested to be associated with greater genomic complexity and a more aggressive course [11, 16, 17]. Additionally 13q14 deletions may be heterozygous (monoallelic) or homozygous (biallelic). Studies of serial samples suggest that heterozygous deletion is an early event, whereas deletion of the second copy of this region occurs at a later stage [18, 19]. Biallelic del(13)(q14) are present in 30 % of 13q-deleted patients [20]. They are described as smaller and not involving *RB1* [11]. The large 13q deletions are most often monoallelic, whereas a minor proportion carries biallelic deletions. The 13q14 MDR includes miR-15a and miR-16-1, which are described as negative regulators of the *BCL2* expression [21]. One of the documented biological functions of miR-15a and 16–1 is down-regulation of the anti-apoptotic *BCL2* through post-translational mRNA repression, which may lead to an increased anti-apoptotic resistance [22]. This deletion allows the CLL/SLL cells to survive. Mouse models have formally proven the pathogenetic role of del(13q)(14) in

CLL/SLL development. Three different lines of transgenic mice designed to mimic del(13q)(14) developed CLL/SLL and other del(13)(q14)-associated lymphoproliferative disorders [21, 23].

Array-based genomic technologies allow a genome wide screening for genetic lesions. An aCGH array enables the detection of acquired genomic copy number variations (CNV), excluding balanced chromosomal translocations. SNP array allows to detect the presence of deletions which are visible as a LOH regions and regions of copy-neutral LOH, which are also called uniparental disomies. The resolution of array is much higher than cytogenetic classical methods and enables detection of submicroscopic chromosomal changes. In the current study, we performed molecular analysis of 39 CLL/SLL patients using CytoSure Haematological Cancer and SNP array containing 60.000 probes. This array combines on one slide long oligo aCGH probes for copy number detection with SNP content for accurate identification of LOH also without concurrent changes in gene copy number. The aims of the current study were detection of the size of del(13)(q14) deletion in our group of CLL/SLL patients, comparing the size of the monoallelic and biallelic deletions, detection of LOH and UPD regions.

Results

Patients

Detailed genetic examination was conducted on a group of 40 patients, who had a loss of 13q14 region in the tumor cells in FISH analysis. At that time of analysis 25 % of patients were treated and 75 % of patients remain without treatment. Characteristics of patients are given in Table 1. The median age at the time of diagnosis was 62 years (range 24–78). The 55 % of the patients were male.

Conventional G-banding analysis

Among the 40 examined patients the karyotype analysis was successful in 35 of cases (Table 2). In 12 of patients the karyotype was normal and 23 of patients showed non-random karyotype aberrations. Deletion of 13q14 was karyotypically visible in two patients (cases 3,12), monosomy 13 in one case (case 39) while translocations with 13q14 break point were noticed twice, as t(9;13)(q34;q14) and t(2;13)(q37;q14) (case 30 and 33). Six patients showed deletion of 11q, three presented trisomy 12, one patient displayed deletion of 17p as t(17;18)(p11.2;q11.2) translocation. Other changes had random occurrence.

FISH analysis

In 40 CLL/SLL cases with the presence of 13q14 deletion detailed analysis showed 21 of patients with

Table 1 Clinical characteristics of 40 CLL/SLL patients

Case No.	Sex	Age at diagnosis (y)	Diagnosis	Binet stage at enrollment	Time to treatment (mo)	Overall survival (mo)	CD38 > 30 % (1) CD38 ≤ 30 % (0)
1.	M	55	CLL	C	13	70+	1
2.	M	59	CLL	C	2	54	1
3.	M	73	CLL	C	18	43+	0
4.	M	58	SLL	C	1	27	1
5.	F	75	CLL	B	nd	73	1
6.	F	69	CLL	A	84	95+	0
7.	F	61	CLL	A	7	141+	1
8.	M	47	CLL	A	36	80+	0
9.	M	63	CLL	C	36	70+	1
10.	M	47	CLL	B	30	76+	0
11.	M	47	CLL	A	36	72+	0
12.	M	51	CLL	A	36+	36+	0
13.	M	34	CLL	A	20	139	0
14.	M	57	SLL	A	3	71+	1
15.	K	54	CLL	A	nt	138+	0
16.	M	67	CLL	C	1	17+	1
17.	M	24	CLL	C	64	148	1
18.	M	52	CLL	B	28	83	0
19.	F	63	SLL	A	76	96+	0
20.	M	64	CLL	C	4	42	1
21.	M	41	CLL	C	3	31+	1
22.	F	74	CLL	A	78	111	1
23.	F	63	CLL	B	53	62+	1
24.	M	78	CLL	C	7	32+	0
25.	M	64	CLL	C	0	66+	0
26.	F	51	CLL	A	nt	59+	0
27.	F	60	CLL	A	nt	175+	0
28.	F	66	CLL	A	nt	16+	0
29.	F	76	CLL	A	nt	8+	0
30.	M	76	CLL	C	30	48	1
31.	F	67	CLL	B	21	187+	0
32.	F	51	SLL	B	60	144+	0
33.	F	64	CLL	B	23	40+	1
34.	M	75	CLL	A	nt	39+	0
35.	F	64	CLL	B	89	107+	0
36.	M	76	CLL	C	0	5	0
37.	F	66	CLL	A	nt	59+	nd
38.	F	56	CLL	C	nt	131+	0
39.	M	53	CLL	C	1	8+	0
40.	F	60	CLL	C	0	39	nd

y years, *mo* months, *nd* no data, *nt* not treated

Table 2 Results of karyotype analysis, FISH and *IGVH* mutation status of 40 CLL patients

Case no.	Karyotype	FISH analysis				Mutational status *IGVH*
		del 13q14	tris 12	del *ATM*	del *TP53*	
Cases with monoallelic deletion 13q14						
1.	46,XY[10]	97 %	N	N	N	UM
2.	-	97 %	N	88 %	N	UM
3.	46,XY,del(13)(q14q32)[2]/46,XY[17]	96 %	N	N	N	UM
4.	45,XY,-6,-13,+mar [6]/ 46,XY [1]	95 %	N	N	N	UM
5.	46,XX,del(11)(q21)[10]	95 %	N	99 %	N	UM
6.	46,XX[15]	94 %	N	N	N	UM
7.	46,XX,t(?;14)(?;q32),?add(18)(q23)[3]/46,XX[7]	93 %	N	N	N	M
8.	46,XY[12]	90 %	N	92 %	N	UM
9.	46,XY[20]/45 ~ 46,XY,-10[2], +1 ~ 3mar[cp3]	90 %	N	92 %	N	UM
10.	-	86 %	N	N	N	M
11.	47,XY,+?2,-8,+mar[3]/46,XY[37]	84 %	N	N	N	UM
12.	46,XY,del(13)(q14q14)[9]/46,XY[11]	80 %	N	N	N	UM
13.	-	71 %	N	N	N	M
14.	46,XY,del(11)(q21q24)[3]/46,XY[4]	71 %	N	81 %	N	UM
15.	46,XX[38]	69 %	N	N	N	M
16.	46,XY,del(11)(q23)[7]/46,XY,-13,+mar[7]/ 46,XY[4]	63 %	N	20 %	N	UM
17.	46,XY,add(1)(q?44),del(11)(q?14) [2]/46,XY [18]	58 %	N	38 %	N	UM
18.	47,XY,+12[1]/46,XY[10]	57 %	N	N	N	UM
19.	46,XX[20]	55 %	N	N	N	UM
20.	46,XY[19]	50 %	N	N	N	UM
21.	46,XY[19]	43 %	N	N	N	UM
Cases with biallelic deletion 13q14						
22.	-	**98 %**	N	N	39 %	UM
23.	46,XX,del(11)(q14)[10]	**90 %**	N	90 %	N	UM
24.	47,XY,-6,del(12)(p11.2),+del(12)(p11.2), +der(?) (?- > ?cen- > ?::6p25- > 6q21:6q14- > 6qter)[10] /46,XY[2]	**89 %**	76 %	N	N	M
25.	-	**89 %**	N	N	94 %	UM
26.	46,XX[20]	**87 %**	N	N	N	M
27.	46,XX,t(2;7)(p11;q22)[6]/46,XX[7]	**86 %**	N	N	N	M
28.	45,X,-X[6]/46,XX[14]	**80 %**	N	N	N	M
29.	47,XX,+12[9]/46,XX[1]	**56 %**	41 %	N	N	M
30.	46,XY,t(9;13)(q34;q14)[17]/46,XY[1]	**90 %**10 %	N	N	N	UM
31.	46,XX[20]	**67 %**19 %	N	N	N	M
32.	46,XX,+12,[6]/46,XX[5]	**44 %**32 %	80 %	N	N	M
33.	46,XX,t(2;13)(q37;q14)[6]/46,XX[3]	**40 %**53 %	N	N	N	UM
34.	46,XY[13]	**40 %**40 %	N	N	N	M
35.	44 ~ 47,XX,+12[7]/46,XX[5]	**35 %**7 %	74 %	N	N	M
36.	45,XY,der(17)t(17;18)(p11.2;q11.2),-18[2]/ 45,idem,-11,+mar[6]	**26 %**70 %	N	27 %	93 %	UM
37.	46,XX[20]	**23 %**21 %	N	N	N	M
38.	46,XX,del(5)(p11.2)[2]/46,XX[14]	**20 %**62 %	N	N	N	M
39.	46,XY,del(11)(q21)[7]/45,idem,-13 [4]/46,XY[4]	**19 %**76 %	N	85 %	N	UM
40.	46,XX[5]	**11 %**86 %	N	95 %	N	UM

„-'' no katryotype, *del* deletion, *tris* trisomy, *N* 100 % cells with two normal copies, *M* mutated *IGVH*, *UM* unmutated *IGVH*, bold type 13q14 biallelic deletion clone monoallielic and 19 of patients with biallelic deletion. FISH results are shown in Table 2. Monoallelic deletion was present in the range of 43–97 % of cells (average 77.8 %) in individual cases. Biallelic deletion accounted 56–98 % (average 84.4 %) of cells population in separate cases. Pure biallelic deletion was observed in 8 patients (42 %) and accounted 56–98 % (average 84,4 %) of cells. The next 11 patients (58 %) had separate clones with combined monoallelic and biallelic 13q14 deletions (cases 30–40). Biallelic deletion clones were detected in 19–90 % of interphase nuclei (average 37.7 %) and monoallelic deletion clones were present in the range of 7–85 % of cells (average 43.3 %) in distinct cases. Other FISH changes were visible in 18/40 cases. The deletion of ATM was shown in 7 out of 21 monoallelic cases and in 4 out of 19 biallelic cases. Trisomy 12 (4 cases) as well as TP53 deletion (3 cases) were seen only in biallelic group.

IGVH mutational status

Analysis of the mutational status of IGVH in all 40 patients indicated 62 % of patients with unmutated (UM) and 38 % of patients with mutated (M) IGVH (Table 2). In monoallelic 13q14 deletion group UM status showed 81 % of patients while mutation of IGVH was detected in 19 % of patients. All 7 patients with ATM deletion in this group had UM IGVH. In biallelic 13q14 deletion group 58 % of patients revealed mutated IGVH status and 42 % unmutated status. All three patients with TP53 deletion and four patients with ATM deletion showed UM IGVH, on the contrary all four patients with trisomy 12 had mutated IGVH.

aCGH analysis

CGH array analysis was performed on 39 available from 40 studied cases. Analysis confirmed 13q14 deletion in all patients (Table 3, Fig. 1). The size of deletion ranged from 348,12 Kb to 38.97 Mb. In all cases except one (case 14) deleted region contained miR-16-1 (position 50,623,109–50,623,197) and miR-15a (position 50,623,255–50,623,337) genes (Fig. 1a). The deletions including RB1 were detected in 41 % of cases. In all 21 monoallelic cases the loss of 13q14 was detected as a single region. The average size in monoallelic 13q14 deletion group was 7,2 Mb. The smallest monoallelic MDR of 13q14 was 348,12 Kb and comprised genes: TRIM13, miR-3613, KCNRG, DLEU2, miR-16-1, miR-15a, DLEU1. The size of the biggest monoallelic deletion was 34,82 Mb. In case 14 monoallelic deletion of 13q14 not included miR-16-1 and miR-15a and contained fragment of DLEU2, DLEU1, DLEU7. The deletion proximal breakpoint was located 25,1 Kb telomeric direction from miR-16-1 and 24,9 Kb from miR-15a. The deletions including RB1 were detected in 9/21 (43 %) of monoalelic cases. Among 18 biallelic cases the same region

of deletion on the both copies of chromosome 13 was identified in 11 (61 %) cases, while in next 7 patients (39 %) two different deleted regions were detected. The median size of 13q14 deletion in biallelic group was 4,8 Mb. The size of the MDR was 505,17 Kb. The biggest lost region was 38,97 Mb. All cases showed deletion of miR-16-1 and miR-15a. Deletion RB1 was identified in 7/18 (39 %) of biallelic cases. Part of cytogenetic changes, detected by array CGH, confirmed presence of typical chromosomal aberrations identified by FISH (Table 4). Deletion of 11q was identified in 8 of 11 patients with ATM deletion detected by FISH. The smallest deletion del(11)(q22.1q23.3) was 16,96 Mb and the biggest del(11)(q14.1q25) covered 50,41 Mb. In six patients 11q deletion was interstitial whereas in other two cases (17,39) deletion was terminal. Trisomy 12 was identified in 4 patients (cases 24,29,32,35). In three out of these cases array analysis showed typical trisomy 12, while one patient (case 24) showed partial trisomy covering whole long arm of chromosome 12. Deletion of 17p was detected in all three patients with one copy of TP53 in FISH (cases 22,25,36). The smallest 17p deletion del(17)(p13.3p13.1) was 7,64 Mb and in the biggest del(17)(p13.3p11.2) comprising almost whole short arm of chromosome 17 was 21,08 Mb. Additional changes, with respect to those detected by FISH, were similar in both groups with monoallelic and biallelic deletion of 13q14. The most common aberrations included losses and gains of different regions of 1q (4 cases), gains of 2p (3 cases) and 19q13 (3 cases) as well as changes of Xq (3 cases). The minimal gained region on 2p16.1-p15 (case 21) was 3,23 Mb and covered genes: FANCL, EIF3FP3, BCL11A, PAPOLG, REL, NONOP2, PUS10, PEX13, KIAA1841, AHSA2, USP34. Rest of copy number alternations had random occurrence. Additional copy number aberrations, in relation to the already described, were detected in 12 patients with monoallelic group and in 10 patients in biallelic group, with total number of alternation equal 20 in each group.

SNP analysis

SNP analysis was performed on 25/39 cases of which 13/25 showed aberrant SNP pattern (Table 4). Chromosome 13 changes were detected in 7/25 patients. In five cases (2,7,12,13,39) SNP distribution confirmed big 13q14 deletions as LOH regions. In six cases (2,5,8,9,14,39) SNP analysis showed LOH in 11q deletion regions. In two patients (25,39) LOH regions matched deletions of 8p, 17p and 12p, respectively. Regions of no changes in copy number but with aberrant pattern in SNP analysis were considered as UPD. In two cases (25,29) 13q14 deletions were located in the bigger (at least 10 Mb larger than deletion regions) copy neutral LOH regions (Fig. 2). In case 25 this UPD covered whole chromosome 13. Remaining UPD regions included: 2p25.3-p14, 3p26.1-p24.3, 7q21.11-q22.1, 17q21.2-

Table 3 Results of chromosome 13 array CGH analysis of 39 CLL patients

Case No.	Position of 13q14 deletion		Size of deletion	miR 15a/16-1 deletion	*RB1* deletion
	Monoallelic				
5.	arr 13q14.2q14.3	(50,561,374-50,909,490)x1	348,12 Kb	+	-
18.	arr 13q14.2q14.3	(50,575,469-51,213,898)x1	638,43 Kb	+	-
14.	arr 13q14.2q14.3	(50,648,212-51,296,645)x1	648.43Kb	-	-
10.	arr 13q14.2q14.3	(50,532,206-51,502,524)x1	970,32 Kb	+	-
11.	arr 13q14.2q14.3	(50,506,929-51,502,525)x1	995,60 Kb	+	-
17.	arr 13q14.2q14.3	(49,975,238-51,581,258)x1	1,61 Mb	+	-
6.	arr 13q14.2q14.3	(50,547,426-52,293,661)x1	1.75 Mb	+	-
19.	arr 13q14.2q14.3	(49,667,023-51,766,748)x1	2,10 Mb	+	-
21.	arr 13q14.2q14.3	(49,466,784-51,789,968)x1	2,32 Mb	+	-
1.	arr 13q14.2q14.3	(48,796,715-51,126,898)x1	2,33 Mb	+	-
4.	arr 13q14.2q14.3	(49,643,767-52,415,185)x1	2,77 Mb	+	-
20.	arr 13q14.2q14.3	(48,852,953-52,024,641)x1	3,17 Mb	+	-
9.	arr 13q14.2q14.3	(48,476,853-51,937,417)x1	3,46 Mb	+	+
3.	arr 13q14.2q14.3	(48,229,933-51,827,408)x1	3,60 Mb	+	+
8.	arr 13q14.2q14.3	(48,875,709-52,722,490)x1	3,85 Mb	+	+
16.	arr 13q14.13q14.3	(47,067,473-52,293,661)x1	5,23 Mb	+	+
7.	arr 13q14.11q14.3	(44,820,708-51,472,821)x1	6.65 Mb	+	+
12.	arr 13q14.12q21.31	(45,230,434-65,085,253)x1	19,85 Mb	+	+
15.	arr 13q13.3q21.2	(37,178,772-60,025,895)x1	22,85 Mb	+	+
2.	arr 13q13.3q21.33	(39,377,596-71,248,873)x1	31,87 Mb	+	+
13.	arr 13q13.3q21.33	(36,430,114-71,248,873)x1	34,82 Mb	+	+
	Biallelic				
33.	arr13q14.2q14.3	(50,659,348-51,164,513)x0	505,17Kb	-	-
	arr 13q14.2q14.3	(50,337,728-51,897,968)x0	1,56 Mb	+	-
38.	arr 13q14.2q14.3	(50,575,469-51,360,705)x0	785,24 Kb	+	-
25.	arr 13q14.2q14.3	(50,597,418-51,454,330)x0	856.91Kb	+	-
27.	arr 13q14.2q14.3	(50,575,469-51,441,414)x1	865,95 Kb	+	-
24.	arr 13q14.2q14.3	(50,561,374-51,441,414)x0	880,04 Kb	+	-
26.	arr 13q14.2q14.3	(50,575,469-51,472,821)x0	897,35 Kb	+	-
35.	arr 13q14.2q14.3	(50,575,469-51,502,524)x1	927,06 Kb	+	-
	arr 13q14.2q14.3	(48,754,460-52,536,626)x1	3,78 Mb	+	+
29.	arr 13q14.2q14.3	(50,575,469-51,523,591)x1	948,12 Kb	+	-
37.	arr 13q14.2q14.3	(50,532,206-51,502,524)x1	970,32 Kb	+	-
28.	arr 13q14.2q14.3	(50,484,540-51,524,424)x1	1,04 Mb	+	-
	arr 13q14.2q14.3	(50,241,416-51,524,424)x1	1,28 Mb	+	-
34.	arr 13q14.2q14.3	(50,484,540-51,572,737)x1	1.09 Mb	+	-
32.	arr 13q14.2q14.3	(50,408,714-51,572,737)x0	1,16 Mb	+	-
	arr 13q13.3q14.3	(39,596,989-51,624,965)x1	12,03 Mb	+	+
31.	arr 13q14.2q14.3	(50,305,714-51,469,354)x1	1,16 Mb	+	-
	arr 13q12.3q21.31	(31,346,665-64,680,548)x1	33,33 Mb	+	+
36.	arr 13q14.2q14.3	(49,579,386-51,404,793)x1	1,83 Mb	+	-
40.	arr 13q14.2q14.3	(49,667,023-51,641,879)x1	1,97 Mb	+	-
	arr 13q14.2q14.3	(48,783,721-52,722,490)x1	3,94 Mb	+	+

Table 3 Results of chromosome 13 array CGH analysis of 39 CLL patients *(Continued)*

22.	arr 13q14.2q14.3	(48,841,955-50,976,908)x0	2,13 Mb	+	+
	arr 13q14.13q14.3	(46,934,009-52,663,754)x0	5,73 Mb	+	+
30.	arr13q14.2q14.3	(48,801,028-51,680,357)x0	2,88 Mb	+	+
39.	arr 13q14.11q31.1	(41,246,428-80,220,989)x1	38.97 Mb	+	+

In biallelic 13q14 deletion group digit x1 suggests monoallelic change, but this value is associated with lower percentage of cells with biallelic deletion in whole cell population

q21.33, 7q32.2-q36.6, 7q35-q36.3, 12q23.1-q24.13. In case 25 big UPD region (65 Mb) on 2p covered smaller deletion (7,27 Mb).

Survival and time to treatment

Clinical follow-up of 40 CLL patients ranged from 8 to 187 months, with a median follow-up of 71 months. At the time of last follow-up 5 of 21 patients in monoallelic group and 4 of 19 patients in biallelic group had died. Time to treatment (TTT) for all patients ranged from 8 to 175 months, with a median TTT of 59 months. We investigated the relationship of 13q14 deletion status

(monoallelic vs. biallelic; monoallelic vs. biallelic excluding cases with *TP53* and *ATM* deletion), size of 13q14 deletion (13q14 with *RB1* deletion vs.13q14 without *RB1* deletion) and *IGVH* mutation status with TTT and overall survival (OS) (Table 5). This analysis showed that only mutational status has statistically significant relation (Fig. 3). Median TTT was shorter in the unmutated group (18 months vs. 89 months, $P = 0.003$, 95 % CI: 0–45 and 16–162). Median OS was also shorter in *IGVH* unmutated group (110 months, $P = 0.003$; 95 % CI: 62–160) compared to the mutated group (median has not been reached).

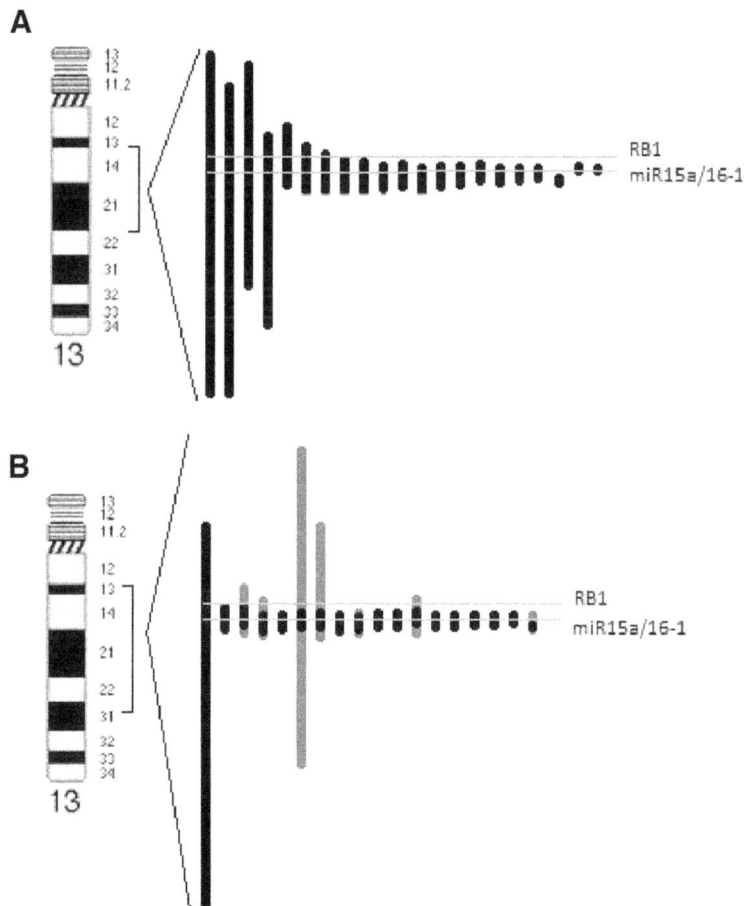

Fig. 1 Pattern of chromosome 13q deletions of 39 CLL/SLL patients detected by CGH array. **a** monoallelic deletions (black lines); **b** biallelic deletion (grey lines indicate deletion size on the second chromosome 13 copy, if was different than on the first copy identified in array analysis)

Table 4 Results of aCGH analysis of copy number variations, and SNP results revealing loss of heterozygosity, and uniparental disomy status of 39 CLL patients

Case no.	CNV	LOH	UPD
Cases with monoallelic deletion			
1.	arr 13q14.2q14.3(48,796,715-51,126,898)x1 (2,33 Mb)	n.t.	n.t.
2.	arr 11q13.4-q23.3(70,503,170-116,961,197)x1 (46,46 Mb)	11q14q22.3(81,735,918-104,024,380) (22,29 Mb)	No changes
	arr 13q13.3q21.33(39,377,596-71,248,873)x1 (31,87 Mb)	13q13.2 q22.1(33,900,810-74,999,739) (41,09 Mb)	
3.	arr 13q14.2q14.3(48,229,933-51,827,408)x1 (3,60 Mb)	No changes	No changes
	arr 19q13.41(52,273,095-52,540,512)x3 (267,42 Kb)		
4.	arr 13q14.2q14.3 (49,643,767-52,415,185)x1 (2,77 Mb)	No changes	No changes
5.	arr 4p15.2(25,475,860-26,940,881)x1 (1,47 Mb)		7q35q36.3(147,741,217-157,731,561)x2 (9,99 Mb)
	arr 11q14.3(89,656,697-91,983,518)x1 (2,33 Mb)		
	arr 11q21-q24.3(94,371,784-128,262,880)x1 (33,89 Mb)	11q22.1q24.3(99,501,357-129,280,824) (29,78 Mb)	
	arr 13q14.2q14.3(50,561,374-50,909,490)x1 (348,12Kb)		
	arr 17q21.31(44,204,228-44,418,272)x1 (214,04Kb)		
	arr Xp22.31(6,493,087-8,034,106)x3 (1,54 Mb)		
	arr Xq28(155,169,566-155,234,551)x3 (64,98 Mb)		
6.	arr 13q14.2q14.3(50,547,426-52,293,661)x1 (1.75 Mb)	No changes	No changes
7.	arr 13q14.11q14.3(44,820,708-51,472,821)x1 (6.65 Mb)	13q14.11q14.3(44,820,708-51,472,821)x1 (6.65 Mb)	No changes
8.	arr 11q22.1-q23.3(98,280,345-115,237,704)x1 (16,96 Mb)	11q22.1q23.3(97,723,221-115,807,318) (18,08 Mb)	No changes
	arr 13q14.2q14.3(48,875,709-52,722,490)x1 (3,85 Mb)		
9.	arr 2p25.3-p11.2(28,080,-84,775,088)x3 (84,75 Mb)		No changes
	arr 11q21-q23.3(93,076,720-116,285,664)x1 (23.21 Mb)	11q21q23.3(92,940,850-119,863,407) (26,92 Mb)	
	arr 13q14.2q14.3(48,476,853-51,937,417)x1 (3,46 Mb)		
	arr 17p13.3(10,152-1,130,849)x1 (1,12 Mb)		
10.	arr 13q14.2q14.3(50,532,206-51,502,524)x1 (970,32 Kb)	n.t.	n.t.
11.	arr 8q21.3-q24.3(89,582,111-143,980,245)x3 (54,4 Mb)	No changes	No changes
	arr 13q14.2q14.3(50,506,929-51,502,525)x1 (995,60Kb)		
12.	arr 13q14.12q21.31(45,230,434-65,085,253)x1 (19,85 Mb)	13q14.11q21.31(41,189,113-64,888,985) (23,70 Mb)	7q21.11q22.1(86,118,243-99,637,271) (13,52 Mb)
	arr 16q23.2 (79,630,721-79,634,651)x3 (3,93Kb)		
13.	arr 1q21.3-q22(154,947,320-155,300,504)x3 (353,18Kb)		No changes

Table 4 Results of aCGH analysis of copy number variations, and SNP results revealing loss of heterozygosity, and uniparental disomy status of 39 CLL patients *(Continued)*

	arr 13q13.3q21.33(36,430,114-71,248,873)x1 (34,82 Mb)	13q13.3q21.33(36,430,114-71,248,873) (34,82 Mb)	
14.	arr 11q14.1-q23.3(77,433,358-119,173,987)x1 (41,74 Mb)	11q13.1q23.3(64,336,971-115,680,986) (51,34 Mb)	No changes
	arr 13q14.2q14.3(50,648,212-51,296,645)x1 (648.43Kb)		
15.	arr 13q13.3q21.2 (37,178,772-60,025,895)x1 (22,85 Mb)	n.t.	n.t
16.	arr 13q14.11(41,500,387-42,681,278)x1 (1,18 Mb)	No changes	3p26.1p24.3 (6,131,168-18,306,025) (12,17 Mb)
	arr 13q14.13q14.3(47,067,473-52,293,661)x1 (5,23 Mb)		
17.	arr 8q24.23-q24.3(139,637,331-146,147,478)x3 (6,51 Mb)	n.t.	n.t
	arr 9p24.1(5,073,751-5,093,784)x3 (20,03Kb)		
	arr 11q14.1-q25(84,360,979-134,772,193)x1 (50,41 Mb)		
	arr 13q14.2q14.3(49,975,238-51,581,258)x1 (1,61 Mb)		
	arr Xq27.2(140,354,604-140,762,836)x0 (408,23Kb)		
18.	arr 6q15-q22.31(92,567,028-122,238,549)x1 (29,67 Mb)	n.t.	n.t.
	arr 13q14.2q14.3 (50,575,469-51,213,898)x1 (638,43Kb)		
19.	arr 3q23(140,617,291-142,215,033)x1 (1,6 Mb)	No changes	No changes
	arr 10q25.1(110,247,081-111,224,354)x3 (977,27Kb)		
	arr 13q14.2q14.3(49,667,023-51,766,748)x1 (2,10 Mb)		
20.	arr 13q14.2q14.3(48,852,953-52,024,641)x1 (3,17 Mb)	n.t.	n.t.
	arr 19q13.41(53,209,131-53,472,835)x3 (263,7Kb)		
21.	arr 2p16.1-p15(58,413,294-61,643,329)x3 (3,23 Mb)	No changes	No changes
	arr 13q14.2q14.3(49,466,784-51,789,968)x1 (2,32 Mb)		
Cases with biallelic deletion			
22.	arr 3p12.3-p11.1(77,467,782-90,191,784)x3 (12,72 Mb)	n.t.	n.t.
	arr 13q14.2q14.3(48,841,955-50,976,908)x0 (2,13 Mb)		
	arr 13q14.13q14.3(46,934,009-52,663,754)x0 (5,73 Mb)		
	arr 15q14-q15.1(40,067,479-42,229,801)x1 (2,16 Mb)		
	arr 17p13.3-p13.1(111,956-9,547,885)x1 (9,44 Mb)		
24.	arr 6p25.3(209,906-1,318,308)x3 (1,11 Mb)	n.t.	n.t
	arr 6p21.1-q13(45,388,754-72,422,581)x1 (27,03 Mb)		

Table 4 Results of aCGH analysis of copy number variations, and SNP results revealing loss of heterozygosity, and uniparental disomy status of 39 CLL patients *(Continued)*

	arr 12q11-q24.33(37,896,066-133,773,393)x3 (95,88 Mb)		
	arr 13q14.2q14.3(50,561,374-51,441,414)x0 (880,04Kb)		
25.[a]	arr 1q42.12q42.3(225,534,669-234,720,224)x1 (9.19 Mb)		
	arr 1q44(247,898,601-249,228,445)x3 (1.33 Mb)		
	arr 2p16.1p14(59,068,992-66,342,421)x3 (7.27 Mb)	2p16.1p14(59,068,992-66,342,421)x3 (7.27 Mb)	2p25.3p14(852,240-65,905,900) (65.05 Mb)
	arr 5q21.3 (108,305,821-108,763,974)x1 (458.5Kb)		
	arr 8p23.3p11.21(1,775,777-42,326,846)x1 (40.55 Mb)	8p23.3p11.1(591,022-43,149,647) (42.56 Mb)	
	arr 13q14.2q14.3(50,597,418-51,454,330)x0 (856.91Kb)	13q14.2q14.3(50,597,418-51,454,330)x0 (856.91Kb)	13q12.11q34(19,813,548-114,888,975) (95.08 Mb)
	arr 17p13.3p13.1(10,152-7,654,148)x1 (7.64 Mb)	17p13.3p13.1 (1,135,130-8,800,337) (7.67 Mb)	
	arr 17p12p11.2(11,403,886-21,438,821)x1 (10.03 Mb)	17p12p11.2 (11,724,886-21,047,102) (9.32 Mb)	
	arr 19q13.43(56,465,808-59,057,705)x3 (2.59 Mb)		
	arr Xq28(154,844,440-155,234,551)x2 (390.11Kb)		
26.	arr 7q34(142,034,557-142,424,354)x3 (389,8Kb)	No changes	No changes
	arr 13q14.2q14.3(50,575,469-51,472,821)x0 (897,35Kb)		
27.	arr 13q14.2q14.3(50,575,469-51,441,414)x1 (865,95Kb)		
	arr 17q21.31(44,204,228-44,342,442)x0 (138,21Kb)	17q21.31(44,204,228-44,342,442)x0 (138,21Kb)	17q21.2q21.33 (38,973,99-48,047,566) (9,07 Mb)
28.	arr 13q14.2q14.3(50,484,540-51,524,424)x1 (1,04 Mb)	No changes	No changes
	arr 13q14.2q14.3(50,241,416-51,524,424)x1 (1,28 Mb)		
29.			7q32.2q36.1(129,639,751-148,168,183) (18,53 Mb)
	arr 12p13.33-q24.33(207,344-133,773,393)x3 (133,57 Mb)		12q23.1q24.13(100,260,227-113,728,620) (13,49 Mb)
	arr 13q14.2q14.3(50,575,469-51,523,591)x1 (948,12Kb)	13q14.2q14.3(50,575,469-51,523,591)x1 (948,12Kb)	13q14.11q21.32(40,405,019-66,081,272) (25,68 Mb)
30.	arr13q14.2q14.3(48,801,028-51,680,357)x0 (2,88 Mb)	n.t.	n.t.
31.	arr 13q14.2q14.3(50,305,714-51,469,354)x1 (1,16 Mb)	n.t.	n.t
	arr 13q12.3q21.31(31,346,665-64,680,548)x1 (33,33 Mb)		
32.	arr 7q33-q34(134,286,767-143,042,219)x1 (8,76 Mb)	n.t.	n.t.
	arr 12p13.3-q24.33(207,344-133,773,393)x3 (133,57 Mb)		
	arr 13q14.2q14.3(50,408,714-51,572,737)x0 (1,16 Mb)		
	arr 13q13.3q14.3(39,596,989-51,624,965)x1 (12,03 Mb)		

Table 4 Results of aCGH analysis of copy number variations, and SNP results revealing loss of heterozygosity, and uniparental disomy status of 39 CLL patients (Continued)

33.	arr 2q37.3(238,903,162-242,335,337)x1 (3,43 Mb)	No changes	No changes
	arr 13q14.2q14.3(50,659,348-51,164,513)x0 (505,17Kb)		
	arr 13q14.2q14.3(50,337,728-51,897,968)x0 (1,56 Mb)		
34.	arr 13q14.2q14.3(50,484,540-51,572,737)x1 (1.09 Mb)	No changes	No changes
35.	arr 1q23.3(161,493,499-161,619,000)x3 (125,5Kb)	No changes	No changes
	arr 12p13.33-q24.33(151,196-133,773,393)x3 (133,62 Mb)		
	arr 13q14.2q14.3(50,575,469-51,502,524)x1 (927,06Kb)		
	arr 13q14.2q14.3(48,754,460-52,536,626)x1 (3,78 Mb)		
36.	arr 13q14.2q14.3(49,579,386-51,404,793)x1 (1,83 Mb)	n.t.	n.t.
	arr 17p13.3-p11.2(10,152,21-21,088,538)x1 (21,08 Mb)		
	arr 18p11.32-p11.21(2,857,465-14,096,343)x1 (11,24 Mb)		
37.	arr 13q14.2q14.3(50,532,206-51,502,524)x1 (970,32Kb)	n.t.	n.t.
38.	arr 13q14.2q14.3(50,575,469-51,360,705)x0 (785,24Kb)	No changes	No changes
39.	arr 1q43q44(240,340,273-249,228,445)x3 (8.89 Mb)		No changes
	arr 11q21q25(93,214,146-134,931,948)x1 (41.72 Mb)	11q21q25(92,940,850-133,599,968) (40.66 Mb)	
	arr 12p13.31p12.3(8,514,368-15,095,031)x1 (6.58 Mb)	12p13.32p12.3(3,782,056-18,007,840) (14.23 Mb)	
	arr 13q14.11q31.1(41,246,428-80,220,989)x1 (38.97 Mb)	13q14.11q22.1(41,189,113-73,649,362) (32.46 Mb)	
40.	arr 11q14.1-q24.2(83,780,266-127,200,577)x1 (43,42 Mb)	n.t.	n.t.
	arr 13q14.2q14.3(49,667,023-51,641,879)x1 (1,97 Mb)		
	arr 13q14.2q14.3(48,783,721-52,722,490)x1 (3,94 Mb)		

Changes are described in a cytogenetic region, molecular position and size in base pairs

CNV copy number variations, LOH loss of heterozygosity, UPD uniparental disomy, n.t not tested,[a]UPD of whole chromosome 13 with deletion 13q14

Discussion

Only 8–10 % of 13q14 deletion can be detected in karyotype analysis in CLL/SLL patients because of its submicroscopic size [9]. By FISH method deletion of 13q14 is revealed in 50 % of patients. This technique can show the presence or absence of the deletion without information about the size of the lost region. Here we present detailed size analysis of 39 CLL/SLL patients performed by CytoSure Haematological Cancer and SNP array. The smallest identified 13q14 deleted region was 348,12 Kb. This observation is concordant with other studies, were MDRs were similar sizes and also comprised

DLEU1, DLEU2 and DLEU7 genes [12, 24, 25]. In the most CLL/SLL cases 13q14 deletion leads to loss of two microRNA genes miR-15a and miR-16-1, which are considered to be a key genes of this deletion. Studies on the structure of genes in 13q14 deleted region revealed that in MDR is located DLEU2 gene which encodes part of first exon of DLEU1 as well as two microRNA miR-15a and miR-16-1 which are located between exons 2 and 5 of the DLEU2 [26]. Previous data reported downregulation of miR-15a and miR-16-1 in about 65 % of CLL cases with 13q14 deletion [15]. However recent reports describe much smaller proportion of patients with downregulation

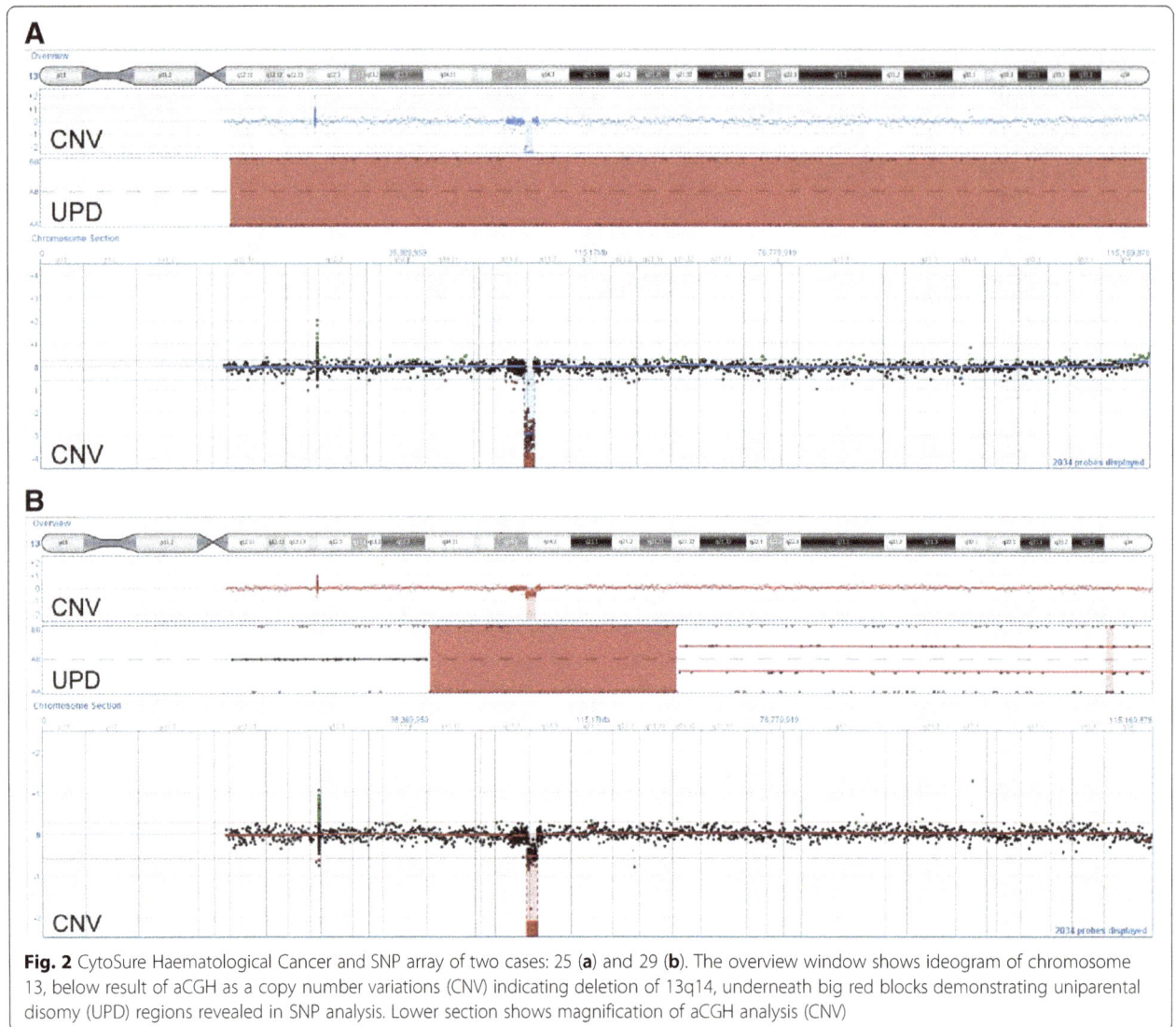

Fig. 2 CytoSure Haematological Cancer and SNP array of two cases: 25 (**a**) and 29 (**b**). The overview window shows ideogram of chromosome 13, below result of aCGH as a copy number variations (CNV) indicating deletion of 13q14, underneath big red blocks demonstrating uniparental disomy (UPD) regions revealed in SNP analysis. Lower section shows magnification of aCGH analysis (CNV)

of both micoRNAs which accounts near 10 % of CLL and mostly in patients with biallelic 13q14 deletion [11, 27, 28]. MiR-15a and miR-16-1 expression was inversely correlated to *BCL2* expression in CLL [22]. *BCL2* is an oncogene promoting survival by inhibiting cell death. In light of recent research that do not indicate a reduced expression of miR-15a and miR-16-1 in the majority of patients with 13q14 deletion but in the same time shows elevated level of *BCL2* protein in patients with monoallelic and biallelic 13q14 deletion, this point out that the regulation of BCL2 protein levels is more complex and do not mainly determined by miR-15a and miR-16-1 levels [28]. In our study one patient with 13q14 deletion detected by FISH retained both copies of miR-15a and miR-16-1. The proximal deletion breakpoint was situated telomeric direction relative to both microRNA genes. Similar phenomenon of 13q14 deletions without loss

of miR-15a and miR-16-1 were described by Mosca et al. and Edelmann et al. [12, 24].

Deletion of the second copy of D13S319 locus in CLL/SLL is well documented. Biallelic 13q14 deletion can have the same or different sizes [16, 17, 24, 29]. Generally, biallelic deletions of 13q14 are reported as smaller in comparison with monoallelic deletions [10, 12, 24]. Our results indicate that biallelic 13q14 deletion regions can be the same or different sizes on both copies of chromosome 13. Concurrently the median size of deletion in biallelic group was much smaller than in monoallelic group what is consistent with the literature data. Some authors define biallelic 13q14 deletion presence as well as bigger deletion region covering *RB1* (called type II deletions) as adverse prognostic factors connected with faster lymphocyte growth and associated with inferior prognosis [11, 30, 31]. The statistical analysis of our data regarding to TTT and OS do not confirm this observations. Our data

Table 5 Statistical analysis of 40 CLL/SLL patients

Genetic feature		Number of patients		Median TTT (months)	Median OS (months)
		TTT	OS		
IGHV status	unmutated	24	25	18	110
	mutated	15	15	89	Not reached
	P-value			p = 0,003	p = 0,003
13q14 deletion	monoallelic	20	21	19	140
	biallelic	19	19	53	148
	P-value			p = 0,203	p = 0,511
13q14 deletion without delTP53	monoallelic	20	21	19	140
	biallelic	16	16	60	Not reached
	P-value			p = 0,099	p = 0,237
13q14 deletion without del TP53 and del ATM	monoallelic	14	14	19	140
	biallelic	14	14	60	Not reached
	P- value			p = 0,141	p = 0,444
13q14 deletion	with Rb deletion	16	16	21	140
	without Rb deletion	23	24	30	148
	P- value			p = 0,426	p = 0,942

TTT time to treatment, OS overall survival

are in line with results of other groups, which showed that loss of second copy of 13q14 is not enough to cause a worst prognosis in CLL and there is not any significant difference in the baseline characteristic and TTT between patients with shorter (biallelic) and wider (monoallelic) 13q14 deletions [12, 25, 32, 33].

The presence of all cytogenetic aberrations identified by FISH was confirmed by aCGH. Only in three cases deletion 11q was not recognized in aCGH study. In two patients percentage of cells with ATM deletion was less than 30 % what was below the sensitivity of the method

and one patient with del 11q was not analysed by aCGH. Among the most frequent additional changes revealed by aCGH the most significant was gain of 2p detected in three patients. This aberration is described as recurrent genetic change in CLL associated disease progression. Some studies defined in common 2p gained region presence of REL, MYCN and ALK oncogenes [34, 35]. The results of other research by Pfeifer and Edelmann delineated much smaller minimal 2p gained regions, which included 2p16 (size 3,5 Mb) and 2p16.1-p15 (size 1,9 Mb), respectively. Both regions contained two

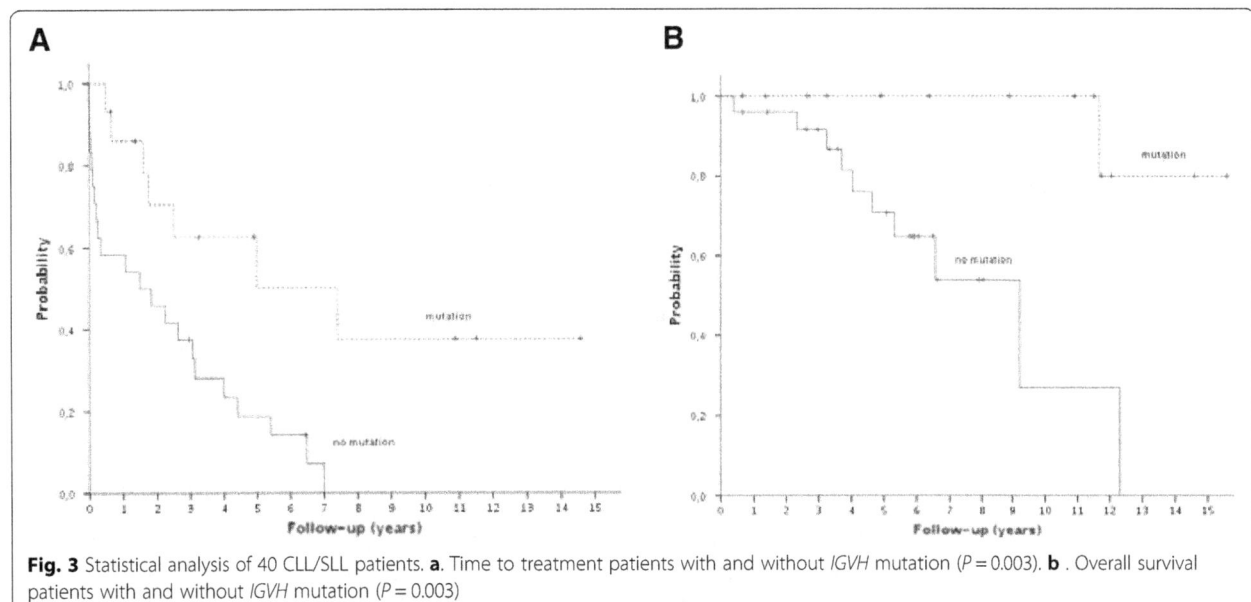

Fig. 3 Statistical analysis of 40 CLL/SLL patients. **a**. Time to treatment patients with and without IGVH mutation (P = 0.003). **b** . Overall survival patients with and without IGVH mutation (P = 0.003)

oncogenes *REL* and *BCL11A* [24, 30]. Our results are consistent with these observations. The size of minimal detected 2p16.1-p15 gained region was 3.23 Mb and included *REL* and *BCL11A* oncogenes. In second patient duplicated 2p16.1-p14 region was bigger and covered 7.27 Mb, consisting *REL* and *BCL11A*, but not *MYCN* and *ALK*. Third patient revealed duplication of the whole 2p. Additional copies of 2p in CLL are associated with unmutated *IGVH*, frequent occurrence of deletion 11q and 17p and advanced stage of disease [30, 34, 35]. In our studied group all three patients revealed unmutated *IGVH* and Binet stage C. One patients had deletion of *ATM* and other deletion of *TP53*. The presence of 2p gain often is accompanied by adverse genetic changes and more advanced stage of disease what confirms the poor prognosis of this change.

There is an association between prognosis and the somatic hypermutation status of the *IGHV* genes in CLL [5, 6]. Patients with unmutated *IGHV* display a more aggressive disease, high-risk cytogenetics and a poor outcome, while mutated *IGHV* are associated with a more favourable clinical course with long OS. In our analysed group all CLL/SLL patients with unfavourable cytogenetic prognostic factors as deletions of *TP53* and *ATM* had unmutated *IGVH* status, what confirms poor prognosis. On the contrary all patients with trisomy 12, which is associated with an intermediate prognosis and a good response to treatment, had mutated *IGVH*. Mutational status of *IGVH* was the only factor in our study with statistical significance in relation to TTT and OS. In both analysis patients with unmutated *IGVH* had shorter TTT and OS.

SNP array can identify LOH regions as well as copy neutral LOH, which are also called UPD in cancer genome. These chromosomal regions are characterized by loss of heterozygosity and normal copy number of DNA segments which are not homozygous in the germ-line or normal somatic genome [36]. Due to a lack of change in the copy number, UPD remains undetected by karyotyping, FISH and aCGH. The CytoSure Haematological Cancer and SNP array (8x60k) can identify on one slide during the same experiment both copy number variations and SNP, which enables detection of corresponding LOH and UPD regions. A significant advantage of this method is also no need to use the corresponding control DNA from the same patient. In our analysis big LOH regions matched to deletion regions confirming presence of these changes by using another method. In most cases LOH corresponded to deletions with prognostic significance in CLL as 11q, 13q and 17p, what is in accordance with previous SNP array studies in CLL [24, 29]. UPD regions, showing changes in SNP distribution but not in copy number, were included in our analysis when covered regions bigger than 10 Mb [29]. In two patients

with biallelic 13q14 deletion we have detected UPD regions. In one patient this neutral copy number LOH covered whole chromosome 13. In the second case small biallelic deletion was located in much bigger UPD region. Similar observation regarding the coexistence of UPD and biallelic 13q14 deletions was reported by other authors [16, 24, 29, 30]. The same size of deletion in both cases with UPD on chromosome 13 confirms duplication of deleted region, which is different from biallelic deletions with different sizes which probably arisen by two events. Biallelic 13q14 deletions of the same size but without copy neural LOH can be created by other genetic mechanism or the second deletion is invisible in array analysis because of to low percentage of clone with the second loss. UPD containing deletions may implicate the elimination of tumor suppressor genes. In one patient big UPD segment covered small gain region on 2p. In this case UPD is connected with gain of two oncogenes *REL* and *BCL11A* and hypothetically can concern unmutated gene copies or gene mutations increasing the activity of oncogenes. The significance of a common occurrence of UPD and copy number changes is not exactly defined, but can be related with clonal evolution favouring alleles with greater growth potential.

In the summary, the CytoSure Haematological Cancer and SNP array (8x60k) can precisely detect recurrent copy number changes with known prognostic significance in CLL/SLL as well as other chromosomal imbalances. The big advantage of this array is simultaneous detection of LOH and UPD regions during the same test. Resolution of this technique can accurately define size of 13q14 deletion with detection of miR-15a and miR-16-1 involvement. The average size of monoallelic 13q14 deletions was larger than in biallelic group. Our results show that bigger deletion including *RB1* or presence of biallelic 13q14 deletion is not sufficient to be considered as adverse prognostic factor. Uniparental disomies especially on chromosome 13 are quite frequent phenomenon in CLL patients, especially with biallelic 13q14 deletion and its impact on the disease course has to be determined.

Methods

Patients

The study group included 40 patients with diagnosis of CLL/SLL. All patients were evaluated in MSCM Institute and Cancer Center, Warsaw from February 2005 to November 2014. All samples had approval of the Bioethics Committee of the Oncology Centre - Institute Maria Sklodowska-Curie. The diagnosis of CLL/SLL was established between September 1999 and June 2014, according to the current WHO classification [29, 37]. For the present study patients were selected on the basis of the presence of 13q14 deletion detected by routine FISH analysis and the availability of specimens.

Cell culture and cytogenetics

Fresh blood (CLL) or biopsy samples (SLL) were fixed directly or cultured in a 5 % CO2 atmosphere at 37 °C. The growth medium was DMEM (Lonza, Verviers, Belgium), enriched with 15 % fetal calf serum (GIBCO, Invitrogen GmbH, Karlsruhe, Germany) and antibiotics. Blood was cultured for 72 h and stimulated in two variants: with TPA (phorbol 12- myristate 13-acetate)(Sigma-Aldrich, Steinheim, Germany) or with DSP-30 (2 µM; TIBMolBiol, Berlin, Germany) together with IL-2 (200 U/ml; R&D Systems, Minneapolis, MN, USA). For biopsy material following cell cultures were performed: direct, 24 h without mitogens and 72 h with TPA or with DSP-30 plus IL-2. Cells for cytogenetic and FISH analysis were harvested according to standard procedures, cultures were treated with colcemid, afterwards cells were exposed to hypotonic solution and fixed in Cornoy's solution. Chromosomes were Wright stained for G,C-banding. At least 7 metaphases were analyzed. Karyotypes were classified according to the International System for Human Cytogenetic Nomenclature (2013)[38].

Fluorescence in situ hybridization (FISH)

FISH analysis was performed on tumor cells obtained directly from a biopsy or after unstimulated or stimulated in vitro culture. FISH was performed to establish the status of TP53, ATM, centromere12 and D13S319 region. Following commercially available probes were used: LSI TP53, LSI ATM, CEP12, LSI D13S319 and LSI 13q34 (Vysis Abbott Molecular, Downers, Grove, IL, USA). Loss of one D13S319 signal was equal with monoallelic 13q14 deletion and loss of both D13S319 signals was equivalent biallelic 13q14 deletion. The procedures for all commercial probes were applied according to the manufacturer's protocol. At least 100 interphase cells were analysed. Slides were analyzed using an epifluorescence microscope Axioskop2 (Carl Zeiss, Jena, Germany) and documented by ISIS Imaging System (Metasysytems, Altlussheim, Germany).

Array comparative genomic hybridization (aCGH)

DNA was extracted from fresh biopsy material or cytogenetic fixed cell suspension by QIAmp DNA Blood Mini Kit (Qiagen, Valencia, CA) according to the manufacturer's recommendation. For aCGH analysis CytoSureTM Haematological Cancer and SNP Array (8x60k) (Oxford Gene Technology (OGT), Yarnton, Oxford OX5 1PF UK) was used. On this array average gene resolution was 68 Kb and SNP resolution was equal 30 Mb. The procedure of aCGH was performed following the manufacturer's protocol. The reference DNA was from two pools of normal individuals (male and female), run as a same-sex control. Each patient and reference DNA was labeled with Cy3 and Cy5, respectively. Purification of labeled products, hybridization, and post-wash of the array was carried out according to OGT's recommendation and with their proprietary solutions. Array slides were scanned with Agilent's DNA Microarray Scanner and extraction software (Agilent, Santa Clara, USA).

aCGH analysis

CytoSure Interpret software 020022 (OGT) was used for analysis of array data. The program uses the Circular Binary Segmentation (CBS) algorithm to generate segments along the chromosomes that have similar copy number relative to reference chromosome [39]. Averaging of the segments is with median value of all segments on a chromosome as the baseline. Deletion or duplication calls are made using the log2 ratio of each segment that has a minimum of four probes. Threshold factor for deletions was set as a log2 ratio of −0.6 that is less stringent than the theoretical log2 score of −1 (heterozygous deletion $\log2(1/2) = -1$; No change in allele number $\log2(2/2) = 0$; heterozygous duplication $\log2(3/2) = 0.59$). The software uses the Derivative Log Ratio (DLR) Spread, which is used as a quality control check. This metric calculates probe-to-probe log ratio noise of an array and hence of the minimum log ratio difference required to make reliable amplification or deletion calls. A DLR of 0.08–0.19 is accepted, 0.20- 0.29 is borderline, and ≥0.30 is rejected. The DLR for all arrays was scored by this scale. Genes positions were identified according to human genome build hg19. The software calculated the total percentage homozygosity of each sample containing SNP data based on the method described by Sund et al.[40].

PCR amplification of immunoglobulin rearrangements and sequence analysis

Genomic DNA was isolated from cell culture using the QIAamp DNA Extraction Kit (Qiagen, Hilden, Germany) according to the kit's instructions. Immunoglobulin heavy chain variable gene (IGHV) rearrangements were amplified by the Multiplex polymerase chain reaction (PCR), following the BIOMED–2 protocol [41]. In this instance, each reaction contained a mixture of six family-specific framework region (FR) primers (VH1-VH6) and an antisense primer (JH). However, for cases, where mutations weren't detected, *IGHV* rearrangement were determined by amplifying DNA using the appropriate leader primers. The cycling conditions were: an initial denaturation step at 95o C for 7 min, followed by 35 cycles at 94o C for 30 s, 60o C for 30 s and 72o C for 30 s, with a final extension step at 72o C for 7 min and ended at 4o C. The PCR products were determined by 2 % agarose gel electrophoresis.

DNA bands were observed on the UV transilluminator and documented using the Bio-RAD software. PCR products were then purified using a mixture of two enzymes: alkaline phosphatase and exonuclease I (in the ratio 1:1). The purified amplicons were sequenced using the Big Dye Terminator and analysed with an automatic ABI PRISM 3100 Sequencer (Life Technology, Foster City, SA). Nucleotide sequences were analysed using the ImMunoGeneTics database (IMGT) [42]. Mutational status was identified by comparing the sequence of the IGHV of the patient with the most homologous germline V sequence. IGHV sequences with <98 % homology to a germline were defined as mutated, while sequences with of homology of 98 % or higher were considered as unmutated.

Statistical methods

TTT was measured from the date of diagnosis until first treatment or, for untreated patients, to last follow-up (censored observation). OS was estimated from the date of diagnosis to the death (whatever the cause) or the last follow up. The cumulative probability of OS and TTT were plotted as curves according to the Kaplan-Meier method. A log-rank (Mantel-Cox) test was performed for all categorical variables. A P–value of <0.05 was considered as statistically significant.

Abbreviations
CLL/SLL: Chronic lymphocytic leukemia/small lymphocytic lymphoma; FISH: Fluorescence in situ hybridization; aCGH: Array-comparative genomic hybridization; SNP: Single nucleotide polymorphism; LOH: Loss of heterozygosity; UPD: Uniparental disomy; IGVH: Immunoglobulin heavy-chain variable-region; MDR: Minimal deleted region; CNV: Copy number variations; M: Mutated IGVH status; UM: Unmutated IGVH status; TTT: Time to treatment; OS: Overall survival; TPA: Phorbol 12- myristate 13-acetate; DSP-30: CpG-oligonucleotide; IL-2: Interleukin 2; PCR: Polymerase chain reaction; IMGT: ImMunoGeneTics database.

Competing interests
The authors declare that they have no competing interests.

Authors' contributions
BG planed, organized the study, did all aCGH study and analysis, part of FISH and karyotype analysis, wrote the paper; RW performed all aCGH study and analysis, part of FISH and karyotype analysis, statistical analysis, collected patients data, paper revision; JR, KB performed part of FISH and karyotype analysis; IRz,MŁ,AB,MG carried out IGVH mutational status analysis; GR,KB prepared patients data; BN,MB helped with aCGH experiments and analysis; BPG did final drafting of the paper. All authors read and approved the paper.

Acknowledgements
This work was supported by grant 4/GNB/K001/2013 of Polish Oncological Society.

Author details
[1]Cancer Genetic Laboratory, Pathology and Laboratory Diagnostics Department, Centre of Oncology, M. Skłodowska-Curie Memorial Institute, Warsaw, Poland. [2]Flow Cytometry Laboratory, Pathology and Laboratory Diagnostics Department, Centre of Oncology, M. Skłodowska-Curie Memorial Institute, Warsaw, Poland. [3]Department of Medical Genetics, Mother and Child Institute, Warsaw, Poland. [4]Department of Pathology and Laboratory Diagnostics, Maria Skłodowska-Curie Memorial Cancer Center and Institute of Oncology, 15B Wawelska Str, 02-034, Warsaw, Poland.

References
1. Zwiebel JA, Cheson BD. Chronic lymphocytic leukemia: staging and prognostic factors. Semin Oncol. 1998;25:42–59.
2. Seiler T, Dohner H, Stilgenbauer S. Risk stratification in chronic lymphocytic leukemia. Semin Oncol. 2006;33:186–94.
3. Chiorazzi N, Rai KR, Ferrarini M. Chronic lymphocytic leukemia. N Engl J Med. 2005;352:804–15.
4. Rai KR, Sawitsky A, Cronkite EP, Chanana AD, Levy RN, Pasternack BS. Clinical staging of chronic lymphocytic leukemia. Blood. 1975;46:219–34.
5. Dohner H, Stilgenbauer S, Benner A, Leupolt E, Kröber A, Bullinger L, et al. Genomic aberrations and survival in chronic lymphocytic leukemia. N Engl J Med. 2000;343:1910–6.
6. Shanafelt TD, Geyer SM, Kay NE. Prognosis at diagnosis: integrating molecular biologic insights into clinical practice for patients with CLL. Blood. 2004;103:1202–10.
7. Dohner H, Stilgenbauer S, Dohner K, Bentz M, Lichter P. Chromosome aberrations in B-cell chronic lymphocytic leukemia: reassessment based on molecular cytogenetic analysis. J Mol Med. 1999;77:266–81.
8. Mehes G. Chromosome abnormalities with prognostic impact in B-cell chronic lymphocytic leukemia. Pathol Oncol Res. 2005;11:205–10.
9. Atlas of Genetics and Cytogenetics in Oncology and Haematology. Available at: http://AtlasGeneticsOncology.org
10. Gunnarsson R, Mansouri L, Isaksson A, Göransson H, Cahill N, Jansson M, et al. Array-based genomic screening at diagnosis and during follow-up in chronic lymphocytic leukemia. Haematologica. 2011;96:1161–9.
11. Ouillette P, Erba H, Kujawski L, Kaminski M, Shedden K, Malek SN. Integrated genomic profiling of chronic lymphocytic leukemia identifies subtypes of deletion 13q14. Cancer Res. 2008;68:1012–21.
12. Mosca L, Fabris S, Lionetti M, Todoerti K, Agnelli L, Morabito F, et al. Integrative genomics analyses reveal molecularly distinct subgroups of B-cell chronic lymphocytic leukemia patients with 13q14 deletion. Clin Cancer Res. 2010;16:5641–53.
13. Liu Y, Corcoran M, Rasool O, Ivanova G, Ibbotson R, Grandér D, et al. Cloning of two candidate tumor suppressor genes within a 10 kb region on chromosome 13q14, frequently deleted in chronic lymphocytic leukemia. Oncogene. 1997;15:2463–73.
14. Migliazza A, Bosch F, Komatsu H, Cayanis E, Martinotti S, Toniato E, et al. Nucleotide sequence, transcription map, and mutation analysis of the 13q14 chromosomal region deleted in B-cell chronic lymphocytic leukemia. Blood. 2001;97:2098–104.
15. Calin GA, Dumitru CD, Shimizu M, Bichi R, Zupo S, Noch E, et al. Frequent deletions and down-regulation of micro-RNA genes miR15 and miR16 at 13q14 in chronic lymphocytic leukemia. Proc Natl Acad Sci U S A. 2002;99: 15524–9.
16. Parker H, Rose-Zerilli MJ, Parker A, Chaplin T, Wade R, Gardiner A, et al. 13q deletion anatomy and disease progression in patients with chronic lymphocytic leukemia. Leukemia. 2011;25:489–97.
17. Hanlon K, Ellard S, Rudin CE, Thorne S, Davies T, Harries LW. Evaluation of 13q14 status in patients with chronic lymphocytic leukemia using single nucleotide polymorphism-based techniques. J Mol Diagn. 2009; 11:298–305.
18. Stilgenbauer S, Sander S, Bullinger L, Benner A, Leupolt E, Winkler D, et al. Clonal evolution in chronic lymphocytic leukemia: acquisition of high-risk genomic aberrations associated with unmutated VH, resistance to therapy, and short survival. Haematologica. 2007;92:1242–5.
19. Shanafelt TD, Witzig TE, Fink SR, Jenkins RB, Paternoster SF, Smoley SA, et al. Prospective evaluation of clonal evolution during long-term follow-up of patients with untreated early-stage chronic lymphocytic leukemia. J Clin Oncol. 2006;24:4634–41.
20. Reddy KS. Chronic lymphocytic leukaemia profiled for prognosis using a fluorescence in situ hybridisation panel. Br J Haematol. 2006;132:705–22.
21. Klein U, Lia M, Crespo M, Siegel R, Shen Q, Mo T, et al. The DLEU2/miR-15a/16-1 cluster controls B cell proliferation and its deletion leads to chronic lymphocytic leukemia. Cancer Cell. 2010;17:28–40.
22. Cimmino A, Calin GA, Fabbri M, Iorio MV, Ferracin M, Shimizu M, et al. miR-15 and miR-16 induce apoptosis by targeting BCL2. Proc Natl Acad Sci U S A. 2005;102:13944–9.

23. Lia M, Carette A, Tang H, Shen Q, Mo T, Bhagat G, et al. Functional dissection of the chromosome 13q14 tumor-suppressor locus using transgenic mouse lines. Blood. 2012;119:2981–90.

24. Edelmann J, Holzmann K, Miller F, Winkler D, Bühler A, Zenz T, et al. High-resolution genomic profiling of chronic lymphocytic leukemia reveals new recurrent genomic alterations. Blood. 2012;120:4783–94.

25. Lehmann S, Ogawa S, Raynaud SD, Sanada M, Nannya Y, Ticchioni M, et al. Molecular allelokaryotyping of early-stage, untreated chronic lymphocytic leukemia. Cancer. 2008;112:1296–305.

26. Pekarsky Y, Croce CM. Role of miR-15/16 in CLL. Cell Death Differ. 2015;22:6–11.

27. Fulci V, Chiaretti S, Goldoni M, Azzalin G, Carucci N, Tavolaro S, et al. Quantitative technologies establish a novel microRNA profile of chronic lymphocytic leukemia. Blood. 2007;109:4944–51.

28. Sellmann L, Scholtysik R, Kreuz M, Cyrull S, Tiacci E, Stanelle J, et al. Gene dosage effects in chronic lymphocytic leukemia. Cancer Genet Cytogenet. 2010;203:149–60.

29. Müller-Hermelink HK A, Montserrat E, Catovsky D, Campo E, Harris NL, Stein H. Chronic lymphocytic leukaemia/small lymphocytic lymphoma. In: Swerdlow SH, Campo E, Harris NL, editors. WHO classification of tumours of haematopoietic and lymphoid tissues. 4th ed. Lyon: IARC; 2008. p. 180–2.

30. Pfeifer D, Pantic M, Skatulla I, Rawluk J, Kreutz C, Martens UM, et al. Genome-wide analysis of DNA copy number changes and LOH in CLL using high-density SNP arrays. Blood. 2007;109:1202–10.

31. Ouillette P, Collins R, Shakhan S, Li J, Li C, Shedden K, et al. The prognostic significance of various 13q14 deletions in chronic lymphocytic leukemia. Clin Cancer Res. 2011;17:6778–90.

32. Garg R, Wierda W, Ferrajoli A, Abruzzo L, Pierce S, Lerner S, et al. The prognostic difference of monoallelic versus biallelic deletion of 13q in chronic lymphocytic leukemia. Cancer. 2012;118:3531–7.

33. Puiggros A, Delgado J, Rodriguez-Vicente A, Collado R, Aventín A, Luño E, et al. Biallelic losses of 13q do not confer a poorer outcome in chronic lymphocytic leukaemia: analysis of 627 patients with isolated 13q deletion. Br J Haematol. 2013;163:47–54.

34. Jarosova M, Urbankova H, Plachy R, Papajik T, Holzerova M, Balcarkova J, et al. Gain of chromosome 2p in chronic lymphocytic leukemia: significant heterogeneity and a new recurrent dicentric rearrangement. Leuk Lymphoma. 2010;51:304–13.

35. Chapiro E, Leporrier N, Radford-Weiss I, Bastard C, Mossafa H, Leroux D, et al. Gain of the short arm of chromosome 2 (2p) is a frequent recurring chromosome aberration in untreated chronic lymphocytic leukemia (CLL) at advanced stages. Leuk Res. 2010;34:63–8.

36. Bacolod MD, Schemmann GS, Giardina SF, Paty P, Notterman DA, Barany F. Emerging paradigms in cancer genetics: some important findings from high-density single nucleotide polymorphism array studies. Cancer Res. 2009;69:723–7.

37. Craig FE B, Foon KA. Flow cytometric immunophenotyping for haematology neoplasms. Blood. 2008;111:3941–67.

38. ISCN. An International System for Human Cytogenetic Nomenclature (2013). Shaffer LG, McGowan-Jordan J, Schmid M: S Karger 2013.

39. Olshen AB, Venkatraman ES, Lucito R, Wigler M. Circular binary segmentation for the analysis of array-based DNA copy number data. Biostatistics. 2004;5:557–72.

40. Sund KL, Zimmerman SL, Thomas C, Mitchell AL, Prada CE, Grote L, et al. Regions of homozygosity identified by SNP microarray analysis aid in the diagnosis of autosomal recessive disease and incidentally detect parental blood relationships. Genet Med. 2013;15:70–8.

41. van Dongen JJ, Langerak AW, Brüggemann M, Evans PA, Hummel M, Lavender FL, et al. Design and standardization of PCR primers and protocols for detection of clonal immunoglobulin and T-cell receptor gene recombinations in suspect lymphoproliferations: report of the BIOMED-2 Concerted Action BMH4-CT98-3936. Leukemia. 2003;17:2257–317.

42. The International ImMunoGeneTics information system. Available at: http://www.imgt.org/

8

Cytogenetically visible copy number variations (CG-CNVs) in banding and molecular cytogenetics of human; about heteromorphisms and euchromatic variants

Thomas Liehr

Abstract

Background: Copy number variations (CNVs) having no (obvious) clinical effects were rediscovered as major part of human genome in 2004. However, for every cytogeneticist microscopically visible harmless CNVs (CG-CNVs) are well known since decades. Harmless CG-CNVs can be present as heterochromatic or even as euchromatic variants in clinically healthy persons.

Results: Here I provide a review on what is known today on the still too little studied harmless human CG-CNVs, point out which can be mixed up with clinically relevant pathological CG-CNVs and shortly discuss that the artificial separation of euchromatic submicroscopic CNVs (MG-CNVs) and euchromatic CG-CNVs is no longer timely.

Conclusion: Overall, neither so-called harmless heterochromatic nor so-called harmless euchromatic CG-CNVs are considered enough in evaluation of routine cytogenetic analysis and reporting. This holds especially true when bearing in mind the so-called two-hit model suggesting that combination of per se harmless CNVs may lead to clinical aberrations if they are present together in one patient.

Keywords: Heteromorphism, Copy number variations (CNVs), Banding cytogenetics, Molecular cytogenetics, Euchromatic variants (EVs)

Background

In 2004 it was a kind of big surprise for geneticists that within the human genome there are hundreds or more regions prone to so-called submicroscopic copy number variations (CNVs) [1–3]. As this kind of CNVs is detectable primarily by molecular genetics, they are abbreviated as MG-CNVs in the following. These MG-CNVs are located in euchromatic regions of, and dispersed over the entire human genome. They are detected by microarray-analyses in each healthy as well as in each (due to other reasons) diseased person [1–4]. Even though still it is not clear if such repeatedly found MG-CNVs have any kind of long term effects on e.g. health, cancer susceptibility, intelligence or life expectance [5–7],

at present they are considered as harmless and as not worth to be reported [8].

Before detection of MG-CNVs in 2004 [1–3] it was suggested that no two clinically healthy individuals in human, apart from monozygote twins, are alike due to different gene/allele combinations and point mutations leading to new alleles along the human genome [9]. This is emphasized e.g. by the possibility to perform paternity tests based on single nucleotide polymorphisms [10]. However, studying thousands of patients and normal controls by microarray revealed, that each person distinguishes from another in euchromatic MG-CNVs by the size of up to 1.5 megabasepairs (Mb); also several 0.1 Mb of MG-CNVs are lost or amplified during meiosis from generation to generation [11].

Still, considering what was known and common sense among cytogeneticists on harmless cytogenetically visible CNVs (= CG-CNVs) since decades, the excitement from

Correspondence: Thomas.Liehr@med.uni-jena.de
Jena University Hospital, Friedrich Schiller University, Institute of Human Genetics, Kollegiengasse 10, D-07743 Jena, Germany

2004 is somehow unknowable. Harmless CG-CNVs were first found as heterochromatic variants in the 1960s [12, 13] and later-on in the 1990s even as euchromatic variants (EVs) in clinically healthy persons (for review see [14, 15]). An already early finding of cytogenetics was that on chromosomal level the numbers and kinds of CG-CNVs detected during routine cytogenetics is high; this led to the statement that there are no individuals which are really the same on a chromosomal level, especially concerning the pericentric regions, the acrocentric short arms and - in male - cytoband Yq12 [12, 13, 15]. Thus, the gender-specific interindividual differences in genome size are for sure not only in an average range of only 0.5 Mb as previously suggested [11]; based on variety of heterochromatic CG-CNVs at least 2-4 Mb have to be added.

In the following a review on the overall too little studied, so-called harmless human CG-CNVs is provided, including what is nowadays known on their standard sizes and their anchorage within the human reference genome. As, according to the literature, the major importance of these harmless CG-CNVs is to know the available tools to distinguish them from clinically relevant pathological CG-CNVs, this is also a point covered here. Finally, the question of reporting CG-CNVs and MG-CNVs is discussed in light of the so-called two-hit model, suggesting that combination of at least two per se harmless CNVs may lead to clinical aberrations if they are present together in one individual [11].

What are harmless human CG-CNVs and where are they localized?

Harmless human CG-CNVs can include heterochromatic and even euchromatic regions. Euchromatic regions are here designated as such which contain genes and are sequence- and alignable. The constitutive heterochromatin, was already earlier defined as "regions that are generally late replicating, rich in repetitive DNA sequences, and genetically inert" [16], and as "that portion of the genome that remains condensed and intensely stained with DNA intercalating dyes throughout the cell cycle. It represents a significant fraction of most eukaryotic genomes and is generally associated with pericentric regions of chromosomes. Contrary to euchromatin, heterochromatic regions consist predominantly of repetitive DNA, including satellite sequences and middle repetitive sequences related to transposable elements and retroviruses. Although not devoid of genes, these regions are typically gene-poor. Establishment of heterochromatin depends on two basic elements: the histonemodification code and the interaction of nonhistone chromosomal proteins" [17].

CG-CNVs can be found mostly at specific spots of the human genome as shown in Fig. 1. Heterochromatic CG-CNVs seem to be restricted to pericentric regions of all human chromosomes, all acrocentric short arms and the regions 1q12, 9q12, 16q11.2 and Yq12. Euchromatic CG-CNVs can be divided in such which are repeatedly found and such which are rarely reported. Repeatedly

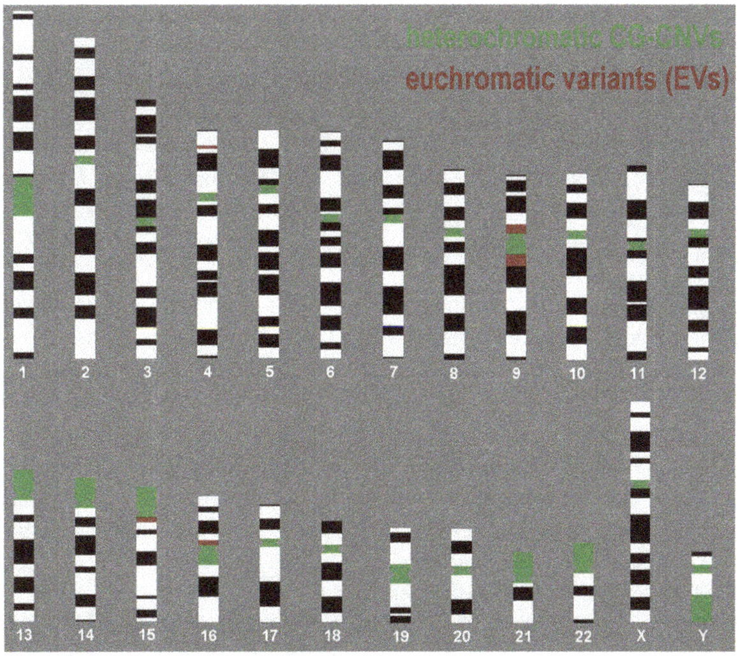

Fig. 1 Heterochromatic regions (CG-CNVs) and euchromatic variants (EVs). CG-CNVs and EVs of the human genome are highlighted in a schematically depicted haploid set of human chromosomes

found ones are called "euchromatic variants" (EVs) and are located in 4p16, 8p23.1, 9p12, 9q13-q21.12, 15q11.2 and 16p11.2 (Fig. 1) [14, 15]. Less frequently found euchromatic CG-CNVs, which are not treated here in more detail, include the majority of all pericentric regions and are most often gains of copy numbers due to presence of small supernumerary marker chromosomes (for review see [18]). Finally, CG-CNVs can be present in single cases / families at various regions of the human genome as deletions or duplications (for review see [15]). In the later only occasionally observed cases large euchromatic deletions or duplications (in the range of 5 or more Mb) do not lead to any clinical problems in the corresponding carriers; those are called carriers of unbalanced chromosome abnormalities without phenotypic consequences (UBCA) [14]. It remains to be determined if this is, as in case of EVs due to absence of dosage dependent genes in the affected copy number altered regions of the genome, or due to other reasons, as recently discussed by Crabtree [19, 20] and Mitchell [21]. The text below refers only to harmless euchromatic CG-CNVs which were mentioned before as EVs.

While due to technical reasons heterochromatic CG-CNVs cannot be detected by microarray-technologies, euchromatic CG-CNVs can be found there together with other MG-CNVs. In rare cases MG-CNVs can even have such a size that they become visible on the banding cytogenetic level and are detectable also by molecular cytogenetics [22]. Thus, it has been postulated that MG-CNVs and euchromatic CG-CNVs are biologically the same [15]. The latter may also partly explain the event of rare UBCAs, which, similar to MG-CNVs can be dispersed throughout all the genome (for localization of most frequent MG-CNVs see [23] Fig. 3).

Standard sizes of harmless human CG-CNVs

Yet there are, due to lack of data, no standard sizes defined for MG-CNVs and for euchromatic CG-CNVs. In other words, it is not known what is to be considered as 'the normal size' of those regions [14, 15]. For euchromatic CG-CNVs it can be at least stated that as long as the corresponding regions show a GTG-banding pattern according to the actual international system for human cytogenetic nomenclature [24] they seem to have a size in the normal range. Still, as the resolution of banding cytogenetics is below 5-10 Mb this still leaves space for a wide range of variability. Also, euchromatic CG-CNVs and MG-CNVs, the latter being per definition euchromatic, are anchored in the human reference sequence, i.e. in genome browsers [15], given there as copy number variant, but no standard size is available from there, as well.

For heterochromatic CG-CNVs the story is much more complicated. First of all these regions are not depicted in the human reference sequence. It is argued that this is due to the facts that, (i) nothing is known about the DNA-sequences present there, and (ii) that these regions cannot be sequenced and aligned properly, as they are repetitive. However, both arguments are only partly true. There are studies from 1980, where researchers managed to clone and sequence multiple so-called satellite DNAs derived from the centromeres, the heterochromatic regions on chromosomes 1, 9, 16 and Y and the acrocentric short arms (for review see [15]). Sequences of all centromeric probes used nowadays in molecular cytogenetic diagnostics are known on their base pair level. Besides, many other satellite-DNA-sequences have been reported back in these years, however, later neither studied any more nor included in the genome browsers [15].

Furthermore, even though the international system for human cytogenetic nomenclature [24] was established to achieve a worldwide uniform nomenclature for description of chromosomal alterations, no universal agreement has been included there yet, how to define the standard sizes of (i) centromeres, (ii) heterochromatic regions of chromosomes 1, 9, 16 and Y or (iii) acrocentric short arms. As recently shown it is even worse, and e.g. the sizes of acrocentric short arms vary between different versions of the international system for human cytogenetic nomenclature [15].

Thus, the following norms were suggested:

– Considered as normal could be for short arm sizes of the acrocentric chromosomes if they are about the same size of the short arm of a chromosome 18 of the same metaphase spread; in other words if it is between half of a chromosome 18p and up to 2/3 of the length of a 17p, the short arm has a normal size. If smaller than half 18p it is a "p-" variant and if it is larger than 2/3 of a 17p it is a 'p+' variant [15] (Fig. 2a);

– for the regions 1q12, 9q12, 16q11.2 and Yq12 normal could be if they have about the same size as the short arm of chromosome 16 of the same metaphase spread. As long as the size is in between half of 16p and complete 16p it is a normal sized region; if smaller than half 16p it is a "qh-" variant and if larger than 16p it is "qh+" variant [15] (Fig. 2b);

– for centromeric regions visualized by molecular cytogenetics a norm may be that those are about the size of a chromatid (Fig. 2c).

Frequencies of harmless human CG-CNVs

Incidences of euchromatic CG-CNVs in human population are not available from the literature yet. For MG-CNVs, at least some of them are known to be more

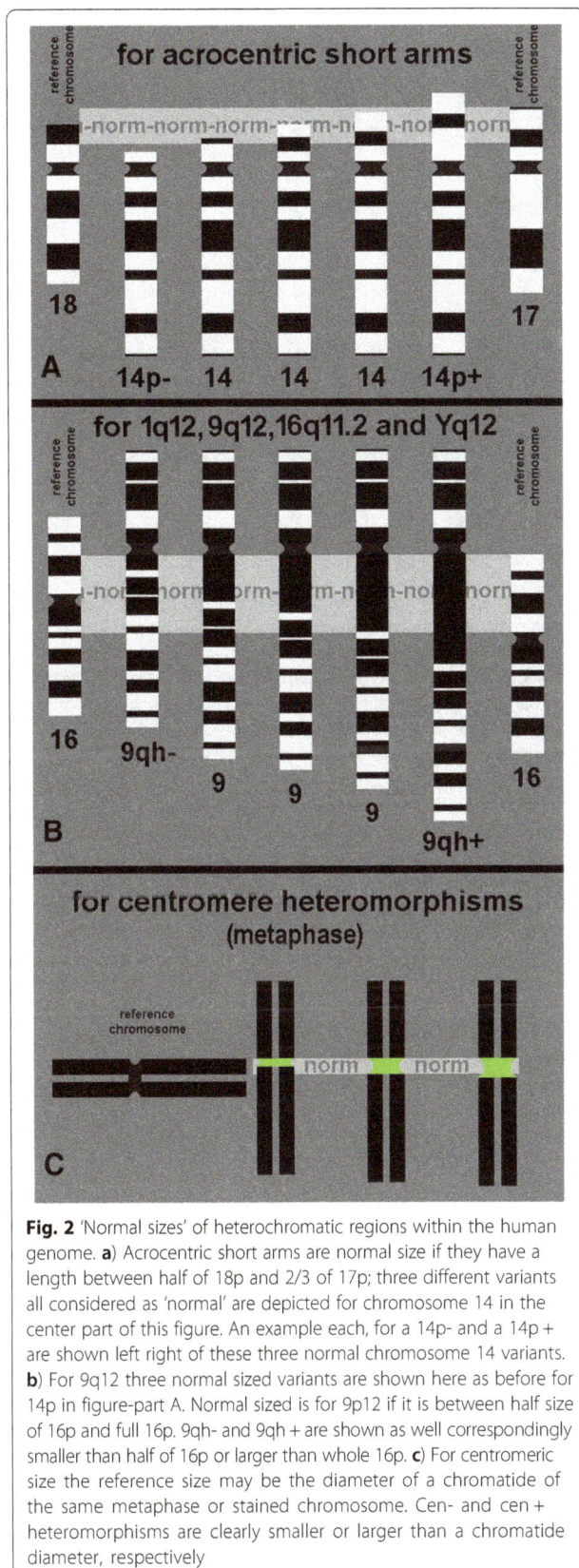

Fig. 2 'Normal sizes' of heterochromatic regions within the human genome. **a)** Acrocentric short arms are normal size if they have a length between half of 18p and 2/3 of 17p; three different variants all considered as 'normal' are depicted for chromosome 14 in the center part of this figure. An example each, for a 14p- and a 14p + are shown left right of these three normal chromosome 14 variants. **b)** For 9q12 three normal sized variants are shown here as before for 14p in figure-part A. Normal sized is for 9p12 if it is between half size of 16p and full 16p. 9qh- and 9qh + are shown as well correspondingly smaller than half of 16p or larger than whole 16p. **c)** For centromeric size the reference size may be the diameter of a chromatide of the same metaphase or stained chromosome. Cen- and cen + heteromorphisms are clearly smaller or larger than a chromatide diameter, respectively

frequent than others; still, one has to consider that most available data for MG-CNVs was obtained from Caucasian people, while highest variance is to be expected for Africans [25]. Undoubtedly the MG-CNV present in 15q11.2, also being an EV, is a really common variant seen in many samples in diagnostics; for sure depending on the used reference, it is expresses as gain or loss of copy numbers [26].

As especially heterochromatic CG-CNVs seem to have no direct impact on the phenotype [15], these genomic regions do not underlie the same evolutionary rules as other ones. Thus, these regions may be enlarged or smaller, duplicated, inverted or otherwise rearranged, and these changes may be stabilized within a population [27]. Especially, the short arms of the acrocentric chromosomes being in major parts identical and present in overall 10 copies per cell show nicely this effect. The aforementioned fact that there are practically no single individuals (maybe apart from monozygotic twins), which are really alike on chromosomal level, is mainly due to the variations of acrocentric short arms.

Even though not based on uniform assessments (see part for standard sizes of CG-CNVs) there is data available on approximate frequencies of harmless heterochromatic CG-CNVs as summarized in Table 1. The most frequently observed chromosomal heteromorphism is an inversion polymorphism of chromosome 9, for which my group previously showed that this includes at least 37 different variants in parts combined with CG-CNVs of this chromosomal region and resolvable by molecular cytogenetics [28]. Given the statement on acrocentric short arms before, it is not surprising that length variations of those are present in ~2.5 % of the general population. Due to technical reasons the acrocentric p- and p + variants could not be further distinguished as cases with inversions, loss of nucleolus organizing regions (NOR), translocations or other rearrangements, even though they exist (see Figs. 3a-d and

Table 1 Frequency of CG-CNVs in general human population

Kind of aberration	Frequency [%]
inv(9)(p11q13)	2.86
acrocentric p+	2.38
Yqh+	0.78
16qh+	0.37
9qh+	0.33
1qh+	0.25
acrocentric p-	0.11
inv(2)(p11.2q13)	0.11
Yqh-	0.09

The data was adapted from [15]

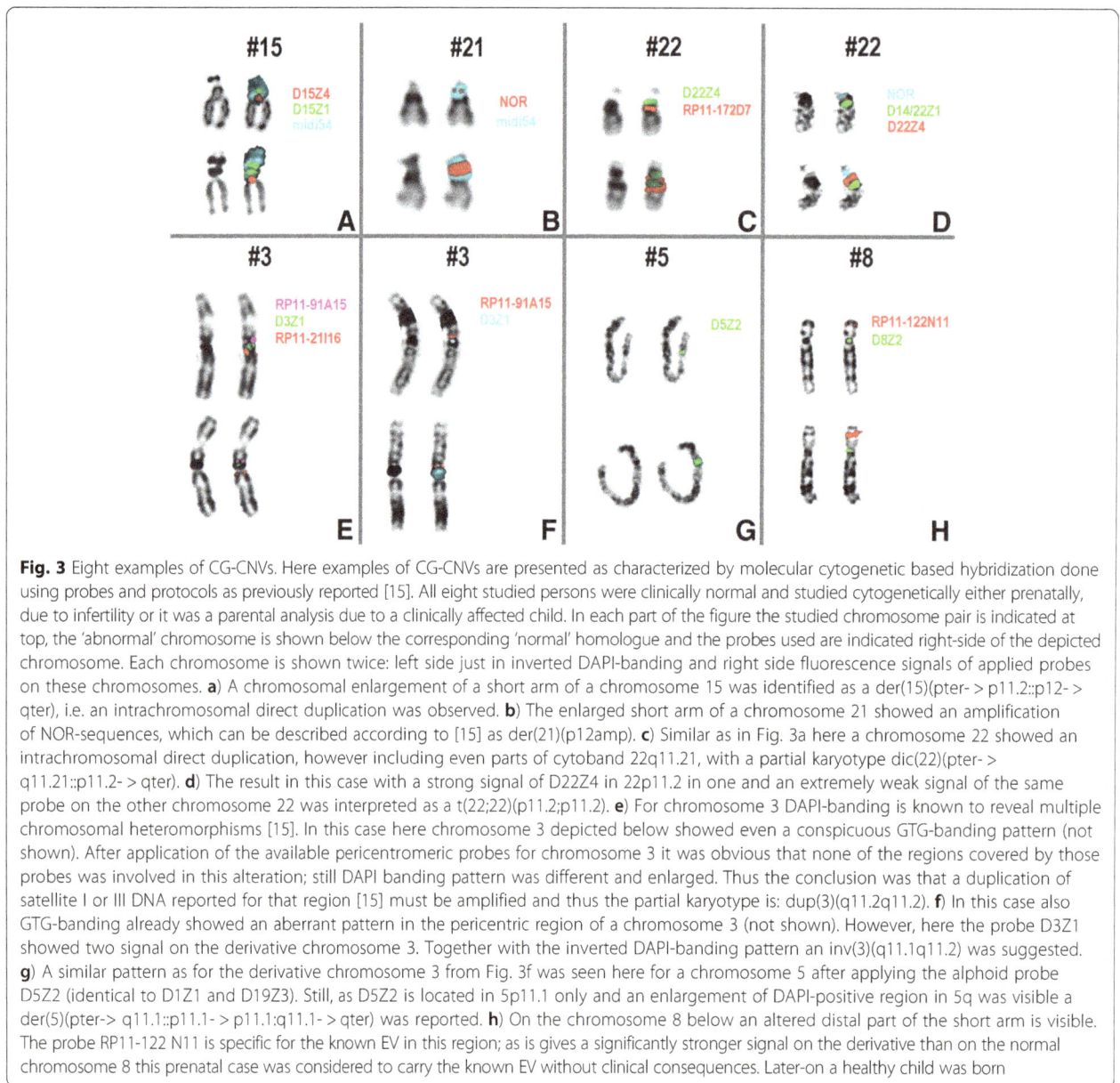

Fig. 3 Eight examples of CG-CNVs. Here examples of CG-CNVs are presented as characterized by molecular cytogenetic based hybridization done using probes and protocols as previously reported [15]. All eight studied persons were clinically normal and studied cytogenetically either prenatally, due to infertility or it was a parental analysis due to a clinically affected child. In each part of the figure the studied chromosome pair is indicated at top, the 'abnormal' chromosome is shown below the corresponding 'normal' homologue and the probes used are indicated right-side of the depicted chromosome. Each chromosome is shown twice: left side just in inverted DAPI-banding and right side fluorescence signals of applied probes on these chromosomes. **a**) A chromosomal enlargement of a short arm of a chromosome 15 was identified as a der(15)(pter- > p11.2::p12- > qter), i.e. an intrachromosomal direct duplication was observed. **b**) The enlarged short arm of a chromosome 21 showed an amplification of NOR-sequences, which can be described according to [15] as der(21)(p12amp). **c**) Similar as in Fig. 3a here a chromosome 22 showed an intrachromosomal direct duplication, however including even parts of cytoband 22q11.21, with a partial karyotype dic(22)(pter- > q11.21::p11.2- > qter). **d**) The result in this case with a strong signal of D22Z4 in 22p11.2 in one and an extremely weak signal of the same probe on the other chromosome 22 was interpreted as a t(22;22)(p11.2;p11.2). **e**) For chromosome 3 DAPI-banding is known to reveal multiple chromosomal heteromorphisms [15]. In this case here chromosome 3 depicted below showed even a conspicuous GTG-banding pattern (not shown). After application of the available pericentromeric probes for chromosome 3 it was obvious that none of the regions covered by those probes was involved in this alteration; still DAPI banding pattern was different and enlarged. Thus the conclusion was that a duplication of satellite I or III DNA reported for that region [15] must be amplified and thus the partial karyotype is: dup(3)(q11.2q11.2). **f**) In this case also GTG-banding already showed an aberrant pattern in the pericentric region of a chromosome 3 (not shown). However, here the probe D3Z1 showed two signal on the derivative chromosome 3. Together with the inverted DAPI-banding pattern an inv(3)(q11.1q11.2) was suggested. **g**) A similar pattern as for the derivative chromosome 3 from Fig. 3f was seen here for a chromosome 5 after applying the alphoid probe D5Z2 (identical to D1Z1 and D19Z3). Still, as D5Z2 is located in 5p11.1 only and an enlargement of DAPI-positive region in 5q was visible a der(5)(pter-> q11.1::p11.1- > p11.1:q11.1- > qter) was reported. **h**) On the chromosome 8 below an altered distal part of the short arm is visible. The probe RP11-122 N11 is specific for the known EV in this region; as is gives a significantly stronger signal on the derivative than on the normal chromosome 8 this prenatal case was considered to carry the known EV without clinical consequences. Later-on a healthy child was born

elsewhere [15]); their frequencies were never studied and/or reported.

CG-CNVs in diagnostics

From the above mentioned data it may be obvious already, that CG-CNVs may be a more than suited target of future research. Still CG-CNVs play also a role in diagnostics and are matter of discussion concerning the attention which is necessary to be given to them in terms of detailed evaluation and reporting [15, 29].

Heterochromatic CG-CNVs in metaphase-diagnostics

Examples how heterochromatic CG-CNVs may look like can be found in Fig. 2a-g; more examples can be found elsewhere [15]. Some of them can really make you

worried and suggest that there is not only heterochromatin involved but maybe something like balanced or unbalanced translocations behind. Thus molecular cytogenetic studies are necessary to resolve the findings; suited probes may be directed against centromeric regions, 15p11.2 (D15Z1), 22p11.2 (D22Z4), NOR, short arms of all acrocentrics, and Yq12 [15, 30]. Based on such studies one may learn more about how these CG-CNVs may be formed, e.g. by unequal crossing-over events, translocations or amplifications/deletions. Still systematic studies therefore lack [15].

The necessity for thorough characterization, description and reporting of heterochromatic CG-CNVs in diagnostics is highlighted by the following examples:

– Most important is for sure to distinguish between heterochromatic CG-CNVs and semicryptic imbalanced or balanced translocation. An example was previously reported by our group [30] where an enlarged p-arm of a chromosome 13 was indicative for a der(13)t(6;13)(p22.2;p12). Similar cases with semicryptic translocations can also be found elsewhere [15, 31].

– In case of enlargement and/or strange banding pattern of an acrocentric short arm (e.g. Fig. 2a-d) detected in case of a leukemia sample may suggest clinically relevant acquired translocations or oncogene-amplification. In case this was already found earlier and correctly reported as heteromorphism in a previous peripheral blood based chromosomal analyses of the same patient for other reasons, this possibility can be excluded immediately and save important diagnostic time and resources.

– The same holds true for centromeric changes like shown in Figs. 2e-2g, including centromeric enlargement, loss or inversions; misinterpretation in tumor samples can be omitted and additional clarifying studies are not necessary, if the CG-CNV was correctly reported previously.

Still many guidelines recommend not to report such alterations [29, 32], a statement which is only rarely questioned [15].

Heterochromatic CG-CNVs in interphase-diagnostics

Application of centromeric probes in interphase cells is a major field of molecular cytogenetics [33]. However, without having metaphases in parallel one can never be really sure if the obtained results are interpreted correctly. There are pitfalls reported when applying centromeric probes for chromosomes X, Y and 18 in uncultured amniocytes [34] as well as for a corresponding centromeric probe for chromosome 7 in leukemia [35]. CG-CNVs being relevant here can mimic chromosome loss or gain. Apparent loss can be due to coincidental reduction of alpha-satellite sequences at one tested centromere; apparent gain can be due to by chance amplification of the tested sequences at another, non-homologous chromosome [15, 34, 36]. Thus, in case of interphase-diagnostics without the possibility to study metaphases of the patient, locus-specific probes should always be preferred against heterochromatin-oriented probes.

Euchromatic CG-CNVs in metaphase-diagnostics

For euchromatic CG-CNVs/EVs two aspects are diagnostically relevant. On the one hand there are such EVs which may be mixed up with adverse copy number changes of the same regions as reported e.g. for the EVs in chromosomes 8 (see Fig. 2h) and 16 [14, 15]. Second, EVs may be a problem in leukemia cases, as EVs may be misinterpreted as translocations, insertions, deletions or oncogene-amplifications.

CG-CNVs and MG-CNVs in light of the so-called two-hit model

As recently stated, "MG-CNVs are determined as variable copy numbers when compared to a reference genome and may include deletions and duplications of genomic loci. They may encompass as much as 12 % of the human genome. Most of them are considered as benign MG-CNVs and are usually inherited from a parent. When determined as de novo, genomic imbalances are considered more likely pathological. It is also known that each human being carries about thousand MG-CNVs ranging from only a few hundred basepairs to over 1 Mb. The major determinant for the clinical impact of a CNV seems to be, if dosage sensitive genes are present in the corresponding DNA-stretch" [23]. Besides, it was recently found that more than one MG-CNV (larger than 500 kb) can contribute to phenotypic variability associated with genomic disorders and may be the reason for developmental impairment; this phenomenon is called "two-hit"-model [11]. To the best of my knowledge there is no study aligning, or even considering the possibility that euchromatic, and/or (even though being less likely) heterochromatic CG-CNV may contribute to phenotypes or age-related conditions. This is, from my point of view, something to be tested urgently in future! As it is known nowadays that regions of heterochromatic DNA are expressed in early embryogenesis [15, 17] copy number alterations of these regions should have some effect.

Conclusion

Besides a unique DNA-primary sequence, each human has also an individual combination of CG-CNVs and MG-CNVs; this includes even monozygote twins as differences in MG-CNVs were already found there [37, 38]. If a genetic analyses is performed in a person one has to consider that depending on the chosen test one will always be blind for a part of his genome. If (molecular) cytogenetics is done a genome wide view with low resolution is obtained - including the detection of heterochromatic CG-CNVs. In case of microarray or sequencing based studies a high-resolution of the analyzed genome is the result, but heterochromatic CG-CNVs are missed as well as the information if a copy number change is due to an insertion, translocation or an extra derivative chromosome. Overall, a study in which MG-CNVs and CG-CNVs are evaluated together is still waiting to be done. Combining (molecular) cytogenetics with molecular genetics could help to avoid being blind for possible solutions of yet not understood phenomena in human health.

Abbreviations
CG-CNVs: Cytogenetically visible CNVs; CNVs: Copy number variations; EVs: Euchromatic variants; Mb: Megabasepairs; MG-CNVs: Submicroscopic CNVs detectable by molecular genetics; UBCA: Unbalanced chromosome abnormalities without phenotypic consequences.

Competing interests
The author declare that he has no competing interests.

Authors' contributions
The article was drafted and worked out by TL.

Acknowledgements
For providing clinical cases shown in Fig. 1 many thanks to Dr. B. Belitz, Berlin, Germany; Dr. U. Jung, Rostock, Germany; Dr. A. Louis, Heidelberg, Germany; Dipl. Biol. W. Trawicki, Essen, Germany; and Dr. A. Ujfalusi, Debrecen, Hungary.

References
1. Iafrate AJ, Feuk L, Rivera MN, Listewnik ML, Donahoe PK, Qi Y, et al. Detection of large-scale variation in the human genome. Nat Genet. 2004; 36:949–51.
2. Sebat J, Lakshmi B, Troge J, Alexander J, Young J, Lundin P, et al. Large-scale copy number polymorphism in the human genome. Science. 2004; 305:525–8.
3. Buckley PG, Mantripragada KK. Piotrowski A, Diaz de Ståhl T, Dumanski JP. Copy-number polymorphisms: mining the tip of an iceberg. Trends Genet. 2005;21:315–7.
4. Database of Genomic Variants - A curated catalogue of human genomic structural variation. 2015. http://dgv.tcag.ca/dgv/app/home. Accessed on 11 December 2015.
5. Grant SF, Hakonarson H. Recent development in pharmacogenomics: from candidate genes to genome-wide association studies. Expert Rev Mol Diagn. 2007;7:371–93.
6. Hong S, Kim Y, Park T. Practical issues in screening and variable selection in genome-wide association analysis. Cancer Inform. 2015;13 Suppl 7:55–65.
7. Ku CS, Loy EY, Pawitan Y, Chia KS. The pursuit of genome-wide association studies: where are we now? J Hum Genet. 2010;55:195–206.
8. South ST, Lee C, Lamb AN, Higgins AW, Kearney HM, Working Group for the American College of Medical Genetics and Genomics Laboratory Quality Assurance Committee. ACMG Standards and Guidelines for constitutional cytogenomic microarray analysis, including postnatal and prenatal applications: revision 2013. Genet Med. 2013;15:901–9.
9. Cinader B. Aging, evolution and individual health span: introduction. Genome. 1989;31:361–7.
10. Sobrino B, Brión M, Carracedo A. SNPs in forensic genetics: a review on SNP typing methodologies. Forensic Sci Int. 2005;154(2-3):181–94.
11. Girirajan S, Rosenfeld JA, Cooper GM, Antonacci F, Siswara P, Itsara A, et al. A recurrent 16p12.1 microdeletion supports a two-hit model for severe developmental delay. Nat Genet. 2010;42:203–9.
12. Ferguson-Smith MA, Ferguson-Smith ME, Ellis PM, Dickson M. The sites and relative frequencies of secondary constrictions in human somatic chromosomes. Cytogenetics. 1962;1:325–43.
13. Makino S, Muramoto JI, Tabata S. A survey of a familial transmission of an anomalous autosome in group 13-15. Chromosoma. 1966;18:371–9.
14. Barber JC. Directly transmitted unbalanced chromosome abnormalities and euchromatic variants. J Med Genet. 2005;42:609–29.
15. Liehr T. Benign & Pathological Chromosomal Imbalances. 1st ed. Oxford: Academic; 2014.
16. Jalal SM, Ketterling RP. Euchromatic variants. In: Wyandt HE, Tonk VS, editors. Atlas of Human Chromosome Heteromorphisms. Dordrecht: Kluwer Academic Publishers; 2004. p. 75–86.
17. Rizzi N, Denegri M, Chiodi I, Corioni M, Valgardsdottir R, Cobianchi F, et al. Transcriptional activation of a constitutive heterochromatic domain of the human genome in response to heat shock. Mol Biol Cell. 2004;15:543–51.
18. Liehr T. Small Supernumerary Marker Chromosomes (sSMC) A Guide for Human Geneticists and Clinicians; With contributions by UNIQUE (The Rare Chromosome Disorder Support Group). 1st ed. Berlin, New York: Springer; 2012.
19. Crabtree GR. Our fragile intellect. Parts I and II. Trends Genet. 2013;29:1–5.
20. Mitchell KJ. Genetic entropy and the human intellect. Trends Genet. 2013; 29:59–60.
21. Crabtree G. Our fragile intellect: response to Dr Mitchell. Trends Genet. 2013; 29:60–2.
22. Manvelyan M, Cremer FW, Lancé J, Kläs R, Kelbova C, Ramel C, et al. New cytogenetically visible copy number variant in region 8q21.2. Mol Cytogenet. 2011;4:1.
23. Liehr T. Copy number variations - is there a biological difference between submicroscopic and microscopically visible ones? OA Genetics. 2013;1:2.
24. ISCN. In: Shaffer LG, McGowan-Jordan J, Schmid M, editors. An International System for Human Cytogenetic Nomenclature. 1st ed. Basel: S. Karger; 2013.
25. Henn BM, Cavalli-Sforza LL, Feldman MW. The great human expansion. Proc Natl Acad Sci U S A. 2012;109:17758–64.
26. Buiting K, Dittrich B, Dworniczak B, Lerer I, Abeliovich D, Cottrell S, et al. A 28-kb deletion spanning D15S63 (PW71) in five families: a rare neutral variant? Am J Hum Genet. 1999;65:1588–94.
27. Genest P. An eleven-generation satellited Y chromosome. Lancet. 1972;1: 1073.
28. Kosyakova N, Grigorian A, Liehr T, Manvelyan M, Simonyan I, Mkrtchyan H, et al. Heteromorphic variants of chromosome 9. Mol Cytogenet. 2013;6:14.
29. Brothman AR, Schneider NR, Saikevych I, Cooley LD, Butler MG, Patil S, et al. Cytogenetic heteromorphisms: survey results and reporting practices of giemsa-band regions that we have pondered for years. Arch Pathol Lab Med. 2006;130:947–9.
30. Trifonov V, Seidel J, Starke H, Martina P, Beensen V, Ziegler M, et al. Enlarged chromosome 13 p-arm hiding a cryptic partial trisomy 6p22.2-pter. Prenat Diagn. 2003;23:427–30.
31. Cockwell AE, Jacobs PA, Beal SJ, Crolla JA. A study of cryptic terminal chromosome rearrangements in recurrent miscarriage couples detects unsuspected acrocentric pericentromeric abnormalities. Hum Genet. 2003; 112:298–302.
32. Gardner RJM, Sutherland GR, Shaffer LG. Chromosome abnormalities and genetic counseling. Oxford Monographs on Medical Genetcis. Oxford: Oxford University Press; 2012.
33. Vorsanova SG, Yurov YB, Iourov IY. Human interphase chromosomes: a review of available molecular cytogenetic technologies. Mol Cytogenet. 2010;3:1.
34. Liehr T, Ziegler M. Rapid prenatal diagnostics in the interphase nucleus: procedure and cut-off rates. J Histochem Cytochem. 2005;53:289–91.
35. Duval A, Feneux D, Sutton L, Tchernia G, Léonard C. Spurious monosomy 7 in leukemia due to centromeric heteromorphism. Cancer Genet Cytogenet. 2000;119:67–9.
36. Cockwell AE, Jacobs PA, Crolla JA. Distribution of the D15Z1 copy number polymorphism. Eur J Hum Genet. 2007;15:441–5.
37. Bruder CE, Piotrowski A, Gijsbers AA, Andersson R, Erickson S, Diaz de Ståhl T, et al. Phenotypically concordant and discordant monozygotic twins display different DNA copy-number-variation profiles. Am J Hum Genet. 2008;82:763–71.
38. Mkrtchyan H, Gross M, Hinreiner S, Polytiko A, Manvelyan M, Mrasek K, et al. The human genome puzzle - the role of copy number variation in somatic mosaicism. Curr Genomics. 2010;11:426–31.

9

Evaluation of three read-depth based CNV detection tools using whole-exome sequencing data

Ruen Yao[1], Cheng Zhang[2], Tingting Yu[1], Niu Li[1], Xuyun Hu[1,2], Xiumin Wang[3], Jian Wang[1] and Yiping Shen[1,2]*

Abstract

Background: Whole exome sequencing (WES) has been widely accepted as a robust and cost-effective approach for clinical genetic testing of small sequence variants. Detection of copy number variants (CNV) within WES data have become possible through the development of various algorithms and software programs that utilize read-depth as the main information. The aim of this study was to evaluate three commonly used, WES read-depth based CNV detection programs using high-resolution chromosomal microarray analysis (CMA) as a standard.

Methods: Paired CMA and WES data were acquired for 45 samples. A total of 219 CNVs (size ranged from 2.3 kb – 35 mb) identified on three CMA platforms (Affymetrix, Agilent and Illumina) were used as standards. CNVs were called from WES data using XHMM, CoNIFER, and CNVnator with modified settings.

Results: All three software packages detected an elevated proportion of small variants (< 20 kb) compared to CMA. XHMM and CoNIFER had poor detection sensitivity (22.2 and 14.6%), which correlated with the number of capturing probes involved. CNVnator detected most variants and had better sensitivity (87.7%); however, suffered from an overwhelming detection of small CNVs below 20 kb, which required further confirmation. Size estimation of variants was exaggerated by CNVnator and understated by XHMM and CoNIFER.

Conclusion: Low concordances of CNV, detected by three different read-depth based programs, indicate the immature status of WES-based CNV detection. Low sensitivity and uncertain specificity of WES-based CNV detection in comparison with CMA based CNV detection suggests that CMA will continue to play an important role in detecting clinical grade CNV in the NGS era, which is largely based on WES.

Keywords: Clinical sequencing, Copy number variants, Whole exome sequencing, Structural variation

Background

Copy number variants are important human genomic variants known to be responsible for Mendelian disorders as well as for common genetic conditions such as autism, intellectual disability, and schizophrenia [1–3]. Chromosomal microarray analysis (CMA) has demonstrated its technical validity and has remained the method of choice for the detection of genome-wide copy number variants (CNVs) in clinical settings. It has also demonstrated its clinical validity for both pre- and postnatal diagnostic testing [4, 5]. CMA is currently regarded as the gold standard for detection of CNVs that range from several kilobases to several megabases in size [6, 7].

The advent of next-generation sequencing (NGS) technology has dramatically improved our capability for examining small-scale sequence variants; it has also provided new options for the evaluation of large scale structural variants such as CNVs [8]. Whole-exome sequencing (WES) has been accepted as the most comprehensive test currently implemented in the clinical setting for small sequence variants [9, 10]. Much effort has been focused to generate CNV information from WES data [11]; however, low sensitivity and high false positive rates have been reported in previous studies using

* Correspondence: yiping.shen@childrens.harvard.edu
[1]Department of Medical Genetics and Molecular Diagnostic Laboratory, Shanghai Children's Medical Center, Shanghai Jiaotong University School of Medicine, Shanghai 200127, China
[2]Boston Children's Hospital, Boston, MA 02115, USA
Full list of author information is available at the end of the article

cancer cell lines [12], publicly available exome data [13], or comparing with whole genome sequencing data based CNV calling [14–16]. Thus, its technical validity has yet to be thoroughly evaluated.

Here, we evaluated three representative and popular read-depth based CNV detection programs: the eXome-Hidden Markov Model (XHMM), the Copy Number Inference From Exome Reads (CoNIFER), and CNVnator using clinical grade WES data. XHMM and CoNIFER detect rare CNVs based on a batched-comparison principle, while CNVnator detects CNVs based on a mean-shift approach within single samples. CNVs detected from the CMA platform were used as reference standard.

Methods
Samples and ethics statement
A total of 45 clinical diagnostic samples were enrolled from the Shanghai Children's Medical Centre and the Maternal and Child Health Hospital of the Guangxi Zhuang autonomous region with the approval of respective institutional ethics review committees. Genomic DNA was extracted using the QIAamp Blood DNA Mini kit® (Qiagen GMBH, Hilden, Germany).

WES and WES-based CNV detection
Exome targets were captured using the Agilent SureSelect Human All Exon V4 or V5 kit (Agilent Technologies, Santa Clara, CA). Raw sequencing data (FASTQ format) were generated via the Illumina HiSeq 2000 platform (Illumina, Inc., San Diego, CA). The Burrows Wheeler Alignment tool (BWA) v0.2.10 [17] was employed for sequencing data alignment to the Human Reference Genome (NCBI build 37, hg 19). All data were assessed using FastQC (version 0.11.2) (http://www.bioinformatics.babraham.ac.uk/projects/fastqc/) for quality.

CNVs were generated using the following three CNV detection programs: (1) XHMM v1.0 [18], (2) CoNIFER v0.2.2 [19], and (3) CNVnator v0.2.7 [20]. XHMM includes several analytic steps and involves a number of parameters. In our study, we set all parameters to default (minTargetSize: 10; maxTargetSize: 10,000; minMeanTargetRD: 10; maxMeanTargetRD: 500; minMeanSampleRD: 25; maxMeanSampleRD: 20; maxSdSampleRD: 150) for filtering samples and targets, and prepared the data for normalization via XHMM. The only parameter that could be adjusted on Conifer was SVD, which was set to 1. For CNVnator, we set the bin size to 50–60 according to the average coverage depth of our sequencing data (45–70 X). XHMM and CoNIFER used a pooled sample calling approach as input, and CNVnator called CNVs sample by sample after individually generating a baseline.

CMA and CMA-based CNV detection
CMA were performed using three different array platforms including the SurePrint G3 customized array (Agilent Technologies, Santa Clara, CA), CytoScan HD (Affymetrix, Santa Clara, CA), and Infinium iSelect HD and HTS Custom Genotyping BeadChips (Illumina, San Diego, CA). Prior validated settings for each platform were consistently utilized for CNV detection and filtering. CNVs in the size range of 2 kb – 400 kb were detected via CMA and were further confirmed by manual inspection.

Results
Quality control of WES data
Fourteen samples were prepared using the Agilent SureSelect Human All Exon V4 kit and the remaining samples were prepared using the V5 kit. The mean read depth of all samples ranged around 50 X and the average read quality was well above the standard of 20 X. Details of sequence data are available in the supplemental data (Additional file 1: Table S1).

Size distribution of CNV detected via CMA and WES
A total of 219 CNVs were detected via CMA from all samples. Forty-eight CNVs were located in regions that had no exome capture probes; consequently, they were removed from being used as true CNVs when comparing data between CMA and NGS. The remaining 171 CNVs were in regions involving at least one exon. The CNVs were examined and compared for size distribution, detection sensitivity, boundaries, and overlap among three programs and between two platforms.

   1. CNV size

We arbitrarily constructed six size bins as shown in Fig. 1. The largest portion (37.9%) of CNV detected by CMA ranged within 100–500 kb whereas CNV detected by NGS data were of much smaller size; 35.3, 44.5 and 79.5% of CNVs were detected by XHMM, CoNIFER, and CNVnator, respectively and belong to the 0–20 kb bin. CNVnator in particular detected many smaller CNVs (42.2% below 10 kb, 27.3% below 5 kb).

   2. Detection sensitivity

We defined the detection of any particular CNV when there was a 50% overlap with a CNV detected via CMA. Using this definition for the presence/absence of CNV, 25, 38, and 150 CNVs were found to be detected by CoNIFER, XHMM, and CNVnator respectively; thus, the detection sensitivities of three programs were 14.6, 22.2 and 87.7%, respectively. CoNIFER and XHMM have an even poorer detection sensitivity for smaller CNVs involving fewer capturing probes, whereas CNVnator had

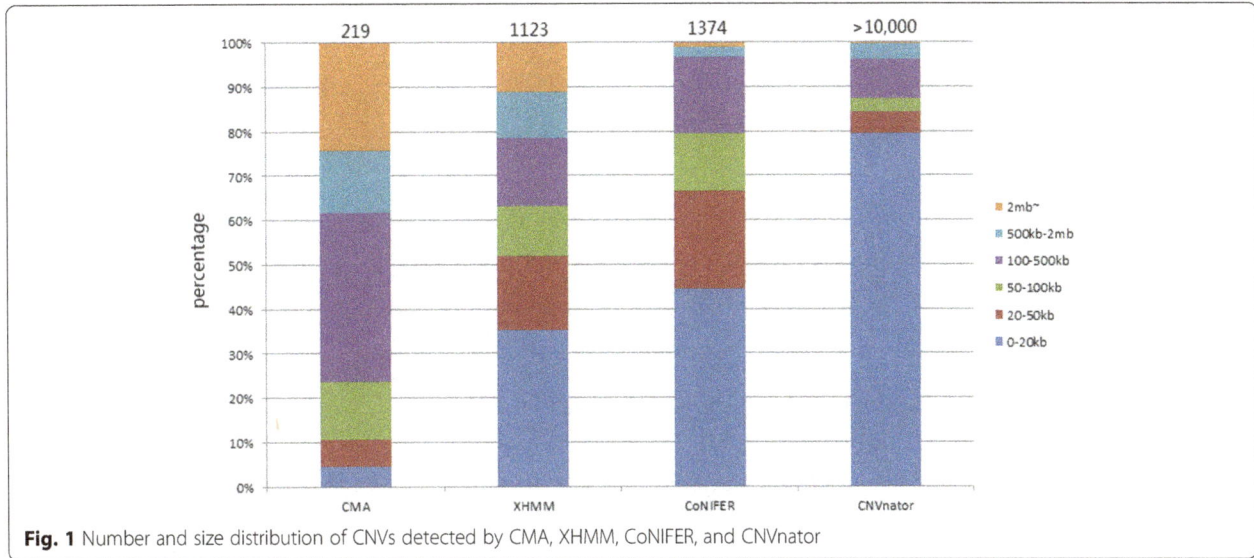

Fig. 1 Number and size distribution of CNVs detected by CMA, XHMM, CoNIFER, and CNVnator

a rather consistent detection sensitivity for all size CNVs (> 3 kb) (Fig. 2).

3. Precision of CNV detection

Among the 171 variants detected by CMA, 152 variants were detected by at least one WES program. Forty-six variants were detected by XHMM and CoNIFER, which are shown in Fig. 3(A). We plotted the size ratio of those detected from three programs, using CMA as reference. XHMM and CoNIFER detected more accurate size of variants, while CNVnator reported a significantly larger CNV size (Fig. 3(B)).

4. Characteristics of CNV missed by exome data (Fig. 3 (C))

A large number of CNVs (125) were missed by CoNIFER and XHMM combined detection and were further investigated. The WES read coverage and capture probes distribution were insufficient for both CoNIFER and XHMM detection of 42 CNVs. XHMM and CoNIFER automatically filtered capturing probes located in the region within recurrent CNV detected in the same batch; thus, 43 variants were missed and had to be confirmed with involving probes. Details of all 171 variants are available in the supplemental data (Additional file 2: Table S2).

5. Poor concordance among three programs (Fig. 3 (D))

Although CoNIFER and XHMM used a similar batched input approach, poor CNV detection concordance was

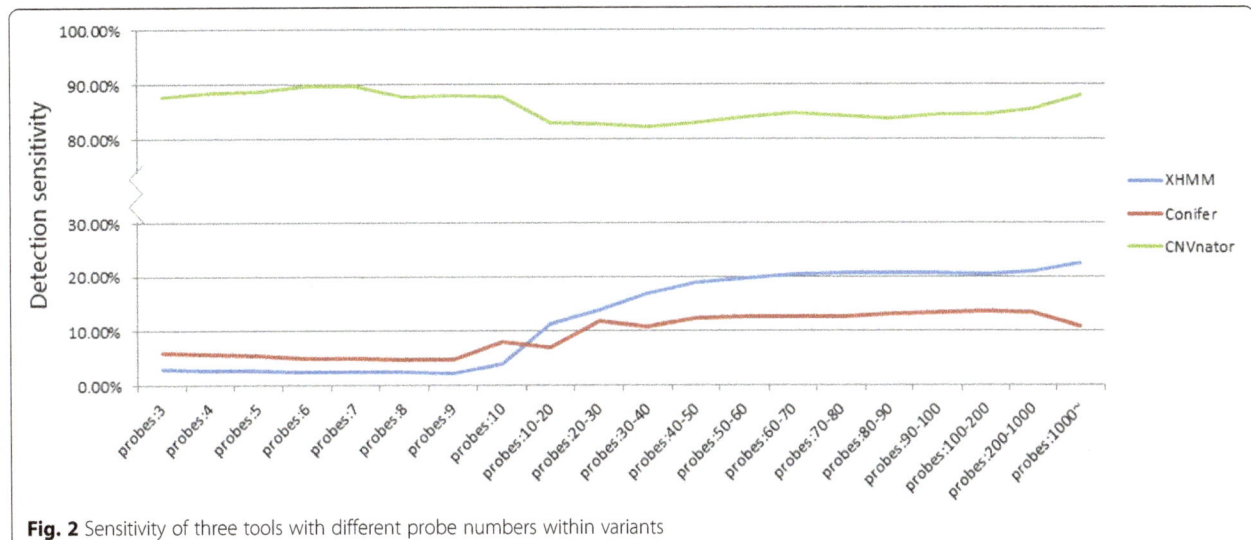

Fig. 2 Sensitivity of three tools with different probe numbers within variants

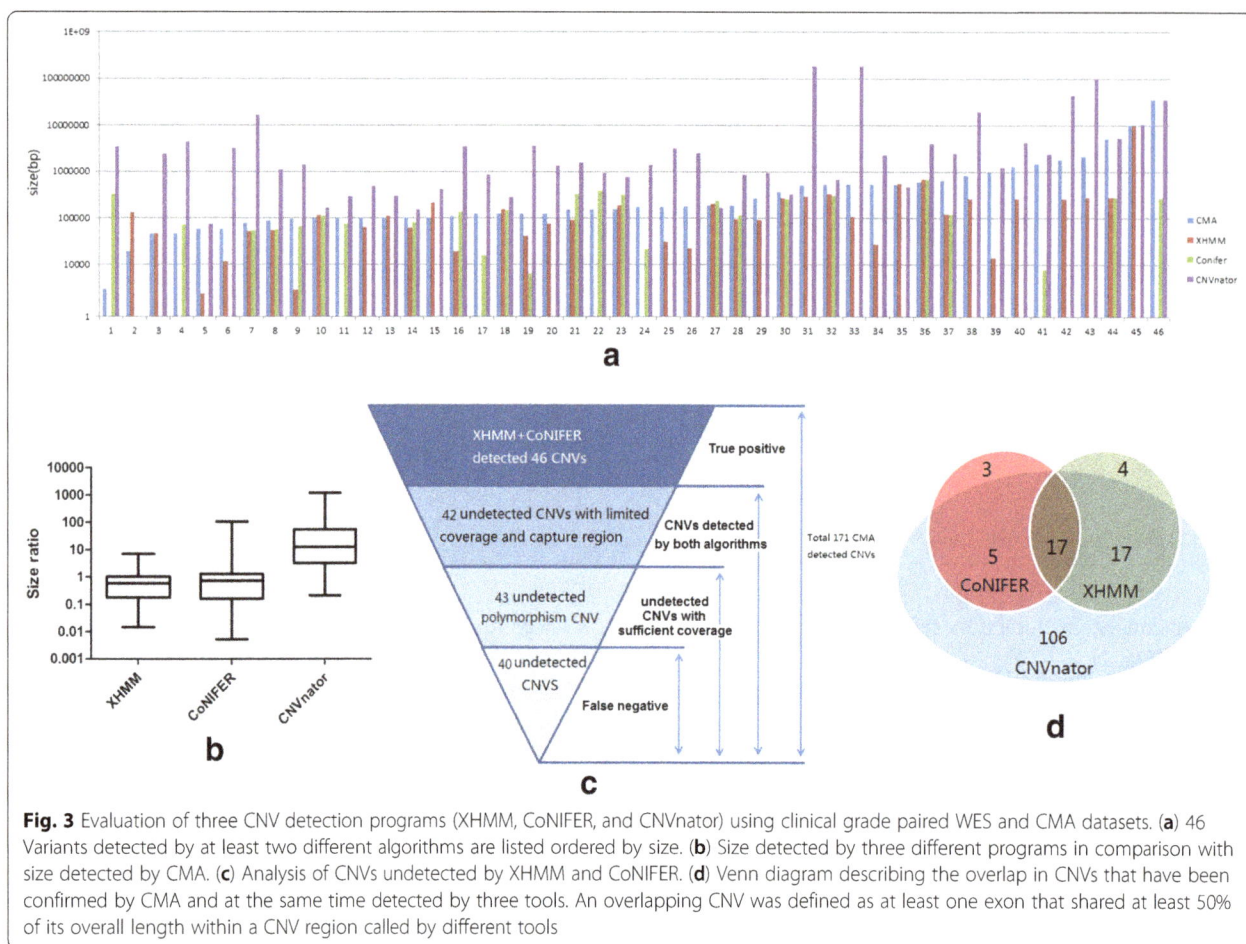

Fig. 3 Evaluation of three CNV detection programs (XHMM, CoNIFER, and CNVnator) using clinical grade paired WES and CMA datasets. (**a**) 46 Variants detected by at least two different algorithms are listed ordered by size. (**b**) Size detected by three different programs in comparison with size detected by CMA. (**c**) Analysis of CNVs undetected by XHMM and CoNIFER. (**d**) Venn diagram describing the overlap in CNVs that have been confirmed by CMA and at the same time detected by three tools. An overlapping CNV was defined as at least one exon that shared at least 50% of its overall length within a CNV region called by different tools

still identified in our study. CNVnator discovered most variants and covered most variants that could be detected through WES data. Only 17 CNVs were detected by all three programs.

6. Detection of clinical relevant variants

All variants were evaluated with our in-house standard for clinical relevant variants and eight CNVs were categorized as pathogenic or likely pathogenic variants ranging from 306 kb – 35 mb. Six of these variants were detected by WES programs. A 306 kb variant on chromosome 3 remained undetected due to particularly low capture probe coverage within the variant region. Another 11 mb variant on chromosome 2 remained undetected despite sufficient capture probes and depth coverage (Additional file 3: Table S3).

Discussion

Copy number variants (CNVs) are a very important target in the clinical diagnosis of genetic diseases. CMA has been proven as the most stable and accurate platform for CNV detection and has been implemented as a

clinical test for more than a decade. NGS now provided a new approach for detecting CNV, which can potentially replace CMA. Before implementing NGS-based CNV detection, extensive validation is required to evaluate the validity of the new method.

Numerous WES based CNV detection programs have been developed, including the 15 read-depth based CNV detection tools currently available [21]. We selected three representative and well-known methods for this study. XHMM is the most commonly accepted software, which employs the classical hidden Markov model (HMM) for CNV identification and achieves a sensitivity of 8–14% via XHMM, reported against CNV detection based on WGS data [13]. The XHMM framework starts with aligned BAM files to calculate the depth of coverage; then, utilizing normalized read depths via principal component analysis (PCA). Finally, XHMM uses the normalized data to train and run a Hidden Markov Model (HMM) for CNV detection. CoNIFER was the first developed tool to deal with rare CNVs from multiple samples and has been chosen as representative software, which can be used as reference in evaluating other new softwares [22]. CoNIFER calculates the RPKM (reads per kilobase per million mapped reads) values for each sample, and utilizes the singular value decomposition (SVD) method (originating from linear algebra) to reduce data dimensions for detecting obvious CNV signals. Evaluation against the array CGH platform in breast cancer samples characterized CoNIFER as leading to high false positives, low sensitivity, and obvious duplication bias [11]. Another study showed that CoNIFER achieves higher precision, but at a cost of reduced sensitivity below 5% [13]. XHMM and CoNIFER have been evaluated in parallel in patients with nonsyndromic hearing loss showing poor concordance on size of detected CNV [23]. However, both tools are noted for advantages of identification of rare CNV from a population of WES samples [24]. CNVnator was previously used in whole genome data for CNVs identification based on read depth, and was accessed to achieve better resolution of CNV borders than the other WGS data-based tools [25]. The main methodology for CNVnator is a mean-shift. The software first divides the whole genome into equal sized, non-overlapping bins, and treats the mapped reads of each bin as a read depth signal. To estimate copy number change in each genome segment, it then calculates the *P*-value for a one-sample t-test, testing whether the mean RD signal of a segment would be close to the genome average. In a comprehensive comparison study, CNVnator was accessed to be outstanding in break point position and copy number estimation; however, disconcordance of variants was also discovered among all tools evaluated in the study [26].

In our study, large differences were observed in number and size distribution of CNVs detected from CMA and three WES based tools. Microarray platforms have a smaller capacity to detect small variants that are not covered by a sufficient number of probes. Several studies have tried to understand the roles of these small variants. The detection of small, non-recurrent pathogenic or likely pathogenic CNVs could help to increase the diagnostic yield of CMA clinical testing by ~3% [27, 28]. WES-based tools, such as XHMM and CoNIFER, are capable of detecting small variants as long as a sufficient number of capturing probes (> 10) are covered in the region and enable a sensitivity of 14.6 and 22.2%, respectively, indicating the importance of probe number for CNVs detection. The overwhelming number of variants CNVnator detected from samples was due to the extreme resolution of the algorithm [19]. This extreme resolution is affected by sequencing depth and high resolution could result in splitting large CNVs into small pieces, which are more sensitive in detecting smaller variants. Larger bin size setting in CNVnator could help to merge consecutive small CNVs as integrated variants; however, this parameter was limited by the average sequencing depth of our clinical WES data.

125 CMA confirmed CNVs that were not detected by XHMM and CoNIFER were further investigated for possible explanations. Low sequencing depth (< 10 X) and limited capture probes (< 10) were detected in 42 variants and these regions were automatically excluded during the normalization step of both tools. The detection for these CNV may be improved if sequence depth increased. The programs filter out capture probes located in recurrent variants that detected the same batch during data processing; thus, 43 polymorphism CNVs were neglected during the detection, which was also confirmed by our in-house array database [http://database.gdg-fudan.org/DB_HTML/DataSub.html]. Thus, only 40 (23.4%) CNVs remained theoretically undetected. Limitation of sample number and sequencing depth of XHMM and CoNIFER could be a possible explanation of these undetected variants. CoNIFER requires at least 50 million mapped reads and a minimum of eight exome samples to run at a time, while XHMM recommends ~50 exome samples with at least 60–100 X coverage [18, 29]. Characteristics of samples in each batch also contribute to the effectiveness of CNV detection in XHMM and CoNIFER. Recurrent pathogenic or likely pathogenic variants may be filtered out erroneously, if they existed in multiple samples; therefore, including non-abnormal reference samples as part of the batch could help to detect these CNVs. Conservative predefined thresholds in default settings of the CoNIFER might be a further reason for missing variants. Read-depth based tools are fairly limited to repeated regions of the reference genome [30]; thus, the sequence nature of specific locations also hinders detection of variants. CNVnator was designed for CNV discovery and genotyping from read-depth analysis based on a mean-shift approach. The number of nucleotides covered in each shift is called bin size (50–60 in our study), which can be determined by the average coverage of sequencing data (45–70 for our samples). CNVnator had the highest sensitivity of 87.7% since 150 of 171 CMA confirmed variants were detected by CNVnator. A Venn diagram was used to show the poor disconcordance among WES based tools, which was attributed to unsatisfying sequencing depth and inadequate number of batched samples. Therefore, CNV detection from WES based tools was affected by the following factors (ranked in the order of importance): probe number, reading depth, sample constituent in the batch, software parameters, and sequence nature of variants.

Using CMA detected variants as standard, the three tested WES based CNV detecting tools were not able to detect the accurate size of variants from WES data. XHMM and CoNIFER have lower sensitivity, but more accurate size of CNVs compared to CNVnator. CNVnator reached higher sensitivity at the cost of high false positive rates and exaggerated readout of the variant size. Poor concordance of CNV detection was observed in the study. Increasing the number of batch samples and valid sequencing depth were the most realizable approaches to improve performance of these WES based tools. At this stage, CMA still remains the first-choice and gold standard for CNV detection for clinical diagnostic purpose. CNV detection tools using WES data could be used as a screening tool.

Conclusion

Low concordances of CNV detection were observed via three different read-depth based programs indicating that WES-based CNV detection still remains immature and unstable compared to CMA. Since WES based CNV detection was evaluated to have low sensitivity and uncertain specificity in comparison with CMA based CNV detection, CMA will continue to play an important role in detecting clinical grade CNV in the NGS era, which is largely based on WES. CNV detection tools using WES data could be considered as a complementary way with only computational effort, but where further validation has been suggested for the purpose of clinical diagnosis.

Acknowledgements
The authors would like to thank all members of family for their participation in this study.

Funding
This research was supported by the National Natural Science Foundation of China (Grant No. 81371903 and 81,472,051), the Project of Shanghai Municipal Science and Technology Commission (Grant No. 15410722800), and the Project of Shanghai Municipal Education Commission- Gaofeng Clinical Medicine (Grant No. 20152529).

Authors' contributions
RY was the major contributor in writing the manuscript and analyzing the data; CZ, TY, and XH contributed to the computational analysis of CMA data and WES data; NL and XW helped in summarizing data and interpretation; JW and YS performed a critical review of the manuscript. All authors read and approved the final manuscript.

Competing interests
The authors declare that they have no competing interest.

Author details
[1]Department of Medical Genetics and Molecular Diagnostic Laboratory, Shanghai Children's Medical Center, Shanghai Jiaotong University School of Medicine, Shanghai 200127, China. [2]Boston Children's Hospital, Boston, MA 02115, USA. [3]Department of Endocrinology and Metabolism, Shanghai Children's Medical Center, Shanghai Jiaotong University School of Medicine, Shanghai 200127, China.

References
1. Feuk L, Carson AR, Scherer SW. Structural variation in the human genome. Nat Rev Genet. 2006;7(2):85–97.
2. Sharp AJ, Cheng Z, Eichler EE. Structural variation of the human genome. Annu Rev Genomics Hum Genet. 2006;7:407–42.
3. Martin CL, Kirkpatrick BE, Ledbetter DH. Copy number variants, aneuploidies, and human disease. Clin Perinatol. 2015;42(2):227–42. vii
4. Fiorentino F, Napoletano S, Caiazzo F, Sessa M, Bono S, Spizzichino L, Gordon A, Nuccitelli A, Rizzo G, Baldi M. Chromosomal microarray analysis as a first-line test in pregnancies with a priori low risk for the detection of submicroscopic chromosomal abnormalities. Eur J Hum Genet. 2013;21(7): 725–30.
5. Manning M. Hudgins L; professional practice and guidelines committee. Array-based technology and recommendations for utilization in medical genetics practice for detection of chromosomal abnormalities. Genet Med. 2010;12(11):742–5.
6. Liang D, Peng Y, Lv W, Deng L, Zhang Y, Li H, Yang P, Zhang J, Song Z, Xu G, Cram DS, Wu L. Copy number variation sequencing for comprehensive diagnosis of chromosome disease syndromes. J Mol Diagn. 2014;16(5):519–26.
7. Boone PM, Bacino CA, Shaw CA, Eng PA, Hixson PM, Pursley AN, Kang SH, Yang Y, Wiszniewska J, Nowakowska BA, del Gaudio D, Xia Z, Simpson-Patel G, Immken LL, Gibson JB, Tsai AC, Bowers JA, Reimschisel TE, Schaaf CP, Potocki L, Scaglia F, Gambin T, Sykulski M, Bartnik M, Derwinska K, Wisniowiecka-Kowalnik B, Lalani SR, Probst FJ, Bi W, Beaudet AL, Patel A, Lupski JR, Cheung SW, Stankiewicz P. Detection of clinically relevant exonic copy-number changes by array CGH. Hum Mutat. 2010;31(12):1326–42.
8. Mills RE, Walter K, Stewart C, Handsaker RE, Chen K, Alkan C, Abyzov A, Yoon SC, Ye K, Cheetham RK, Chinwalla A, Conrad DF, Fu Y, Grubert F, Hajirasouliha I, Hormozdiari F, Iakoucheva LM, Iqbal Z, Kang S, Kidd JM, Konkel MK, Korn J, Khurana E, Kural D, Lam HY, Leng J, Li R, Li Y, Lin CY, Luo R, Mu XJ, Nemesh J, Peckham HE, Rausch T, Scally A, Shi X, Stromberg MP, Stütz AM, Urban AE, Walker JA, Wu J, Zhang Y, Zhang ZD, Batzer MA, Ding L, Marth GT, McVean G, Sebat J, Snyder M, Wang J, Ye K, Eichler EE, Gerstein MB, Hurles ME, Lee C, SA MC, Korbel JO, 1000 Genomes Project. Mapping copy number variation by population-scale genome sequencing. Nature. 2011;470(7332):59–65.
9. Ng SB, Turner EH, Robertson PD, Flygare SD, Bigham AW, Lee C, Shaffer T, Wong M, Bhattacharjee A, Eichler EE, Bamshad M, Nickerson DA, Shendure J. Targeted capture and massively parallel sequencing of 12 human exomes. Nature. 2009;461(7261):272–6.
10. Rabbani B, Tekin M, Mahdieh N. The promise of whole-exome sequencing in medical genetics. J Hum Genet. 2014;59(1):5–15.
11. Miyatake S, Koshimizu E, Fujita A, Fukai R, Imagawa E, Ohba C, Kuki I, Nukui M, Araki A, Makita Y, Ogata T, Nakashima M, Tsurusaki Y, Miyake N, Saitsu H, Matsumoto N. Detecting copy-number variations in whole-exome sequencing data using the eXome hidden Markov model: an 'exome-first' approach. J Hum Genet. 2015;60(4):175–82.
12. Guo Y, Sheng Q, Samuels DC, Lehmann B, Bauer JA, Pietenpol J, Shyr Y. Comparative study of exome copy number variation estimation tools using array comparative genomic hybridization as control. Biomed Res Int. 2013; 2013:915636.
13. Samarakoon PS, Sorte HS, Kristiansen BE, Skodje T, Sheng Y, Tjønnfjord GE, Stadheim B, Stray-Pedersen A, Rødningen OK, Lyle R. Identification of copy number variants from exome sequence data. BMC Genomics. 2014;15:661.
14. Tan R, Wang Y, Kleinstein SE, Liu Y, Zhu X, Guo H, Jiang Q, Allen AS, Zhu M. An evaluation of copy number variation detection tools from whole-exome sequencing data. Hum Mutat. 2014;35(7):899–907.
15. Belkadi A, Bolze A, Itan Y, Cobat A, Vincent QB, Antipenko A, Shang L, Boisson B, Casanova JL, Abel L. Whole-genome sequencing is more powerful than whole-exome sequencing for detecting exome variants. Proc Natl Acad Sci U S A. 2015;112(17):5473–8.
16. Hehir-Kwa JY, Pfundt R, Veltman JA. Exome sequencing and whole genome sequencing for the detection of copy number variation. Expert Rev Mol Diagn. 2015;15(8):1023–32.
17. Li H, Durbin R. Fast and accurate short read alignment with burrows-wheeler transform. Bioinformatics. 2009;25(14):1754–60.
18. Fromer M, Moran JL, Chambert K, Banks E, Bergen SE, Ruderfer DM, Handsaker RE, McCarroll SA, O'Donovan MC, Owen MJ, Kirov G, Sullivan PF, Hultman CM, Sklar P, Purcell SM. Discovery and statistical genotyping of copy-number variation from whole-exome sequencing depth. Am J Hum Genet. 2012;91(4):597–607.
19. Krumm N, Sudmant PH, Ko A, O'Roak BJ, Malig M, Coe BP; NHLBI Exome Sequencing Project., Quinlan AR, Nickerson DA, Eichler EE. Copy number variation detection and genotyping from exome sequence data. Genome Res 2012;22(8):1525-1532.

20. Abyzov A, Urban AE, Snyder M, Gerstein M. CNVnator: an approach to discover, genotype, and characterize typical and atypical CNVs from family and population genome sequencing. Genome Res. 2011;21:974–84.

21. Kadalayil L, Rafiq S, Rose-Zerilli MJ, Pengelly RJ, Parker H, Oscier D, Strefford JC, Tapper WJ, Gibson J, Ennis S, Collins A. Exome sequence read depth methods for identifying copy number changes. Brief Bioinform. 2015;16(3):380–92.

22. Bansal V, Dorn C, Grunert M, Klaassen S, Hetzer R, Berger F, Sperling SR. Outlier-based identification of copy number variations using targeted resequencing in a small cohort of patients with Tetralogy of Fallot. PLoS One. 2014;9(1):e85375.

23. Bademci G, Diaz-Horta O, Guo S, Duman D, Van Booven D, Foster J 2nd, Cengiz FB, Blanton S, Tekin M. Identification of copy number variants through whole-exome sequencing in autosomal recessive nonsyndromic hearing loss. Genet Test Mol Biomarkers. 2014;18(9):658–61.

24. Zhao M, Wang Q, Wang Q, Jia P, Zhao Z. Computational tools for copy number variation (CNV) detection using next-generation sequencing data: features and perspectives. BMC Bioinformatics. 2013;14(Suppl 11):S1.

25. Legault MA, Girard S, Lemieux Perreault LP, Rouleau GA, Dubé MP. Comparison of sequencing based CNV discovery methods using monozygotic twin quartets. PLoS One. 2015;10(3):e0122287.

26. Duan J, Zhang JG, Deng HW, Wang YP. Comparative studies of copy number variation detection methods for next-generation sequencing technologies. PLoS One. 2013;8(3):e59128.

27. Hollenbeck D, Williams CL, Drazba K, Descartes M, Korf BR, Rutledge SL, Lose EJ, Robin NH, Carroll AJ, Mikhail FM. Clinical relevance of small copy-number variants in chromosomal microarray clinical testing. Genet Med. 2017;19(4):377–85.

28. Poultney CS, Goldberg AP, Drapeau E, Kou Y, Harony-Nicolas H, Kajiwara Y, De Rubeis S, Durand S, Stevens C, Rehnström K, Palotie A, Daly MJ, Ma'ayan A, Fromer M, Buxbaum JD. Identification of small exonic CNV from whole-exome sequence data and application to autism spectrum disorder. Am J Hum Genet. 2013;93(4):607–19.

29. Fromer M, Purcell SM. Using XHMM Software to detect copy number variation in whole-exome sequencing data. Curr Protoc Hum Genet. 2014; 81:7.23.1–21.

30. Alkan C, Kidd JM, Marques-Bonet T, Aksay G, Antonacci F, Hormozdiari F, Kitzman JO, Baker C, Malig M, Mutlu O, Sahinalp SC, Gibbs RA, Eichler EE. Personalized copy number and segmental duplication maps using next-generation sequencing. Nat Genet. 2009;41(10):1061–7.

10

Molecular cytogenetic identification of three rust-resistant wheat-*Thinopyrum ponticum* partial amphiploids

Yanru Pei[1], Yu Cui[1], Yanping Zhang[2], Honggang Wang[1,2], Yinguang Bao[2] and Xingfeng Li[1,2]*

Abstract

Background: *Thinopyrum ponticum* (2n = 10x = 70, $J^S J^S J^S J^S JJJJJJ$) is an important wild perennial *Triticeae* species that has a unique gene pool with many desirable traits for common wheat. The partial amphiploids derived from wheat-*Th. ponticum* set up a bridge for transferring valuable genes from *Th. ponticum* into common wheat.

Results: In this study, genomic in situ hybridization (GISH), multicolor GISH (mcGISH) and fluorescence in situ hybridization (FISH) were used to analyze the genomic constitution of SN0389, SN0398 and SN0406, three octoploid accessions with good resistance to rust. The results demonstrated that the three octoploids possessed 42 wheat chromosomes, while SN0389 contained 12 *Th. ponticum* chromosomes and SN0398 and SN0406 contained 14 *Th. ponticum* chromosomes. The genomic constitution of SN0389 was 42 W + 12J^S, and for SN0398 and SN0406 it was 42 W + 12J^S + 2 J. Chromosomal variation was found in chromosomes 1A, 3A, 6A, 2B, 5B, 6B, 7B, 1D and 5D of SN0389, SN0398 and SN0406 based on the FISH and McGISH pattern. A resistance evaluation showed that SN0389, SN0398 and SN0406 possessed good resistance to stripe and leaf rust at the seedling stage and adult-plant stage.

Conclusions: The results indicated that these wheat-*Th. ponticum* partial amphiploids are new resistant germplasms for wheat improvement.

Keywords: *Thinopyrum ponticum*, Common wheat, Partial amphiploids, In situ hybridization, Stripe rust, Leaf rust

Background

Thinopyrum ponticum (Podp.) Barkworth & D.R. Dewey [syn. *Agropyron elongatum* (Host) P. Beauv., *Lophopyrum ponticum* (Popd.) A. Löve, *Elytrigia pontica* (Popd.) Holub] (2n = 10x = 70), a perennial Triticeae species that is closely related to wheat, has been used for more than half a century to enrich the wheat germplasm with desirable traits [3]. Many important genes have been successfully transferred to common wheat from *Th. ponticum*, including resistance to powdery mildew [18], stripe rust [12, 30], leaf rust [24], stem rust [7, 23], Fusarium head blight [9, 14, 26, 27] and wheat streak mosaic virus [17], as well as abiotic stress tolerance [4, 28], and even yield-related traits [16, 21]. Although it is widely used in wheat improvement, the genomic composition of *Th. ponticum* has been long debated. Past research suggests that *Th. ponticum* is a decaploid with the genome formula JJJJJJJJJJ [22]. Using St genomic DNA from the diploid *Pseudoroegneria strigosa* as a probe and the E genomic DNA from *Th. elongatum* for blocking, Chen et al. [3] revealed that the genomic composition of *Th. ponticum* was $J^S J^S J^S J^S JJJJJJ$. The J genome of *Th. ponticum* is homologous to the J genome of the diploid *Thinopyrum bessarabicum*, while the J^S genome is a modified J genome of unknown origin [3].

Stripe rust and leaf rust are both severe foliar diseases in wheat (*Triticum aestivum* L.) all over the world. Stripe rust is caused by the fungus *Puccinia striiformis* f. sp. *Tritici.*, and it can cause severe yield loss in common wheat [25]. Leaf rust is caused by *Puccinia recondita f. sp. Tritici.*, which is the most widespread and regularly occurring rust on wheat and can also cause yield losses up to 50% in extremely susceptible cultivars [6]. Breeding resistant cultivars is the most effective and economical means to control the disease [13]. At the present

---

* Correspondence: lixf@sdau.edu.cn
[1]State Key Laboratory of Crop Biology, Shandong Agriculture University, Tai'an 271018, Shandong, China
[2]College of Agronomy, Shandong Agriculture University, Tai'an 271018, Shandong, China

time, many of the existing resistance genes have been overcome by newly emerged virulent isolates. Thus, it is necessary and pressing to exploit new resistant genes for wheat breeding.

Genomic in situ hybridization (GISH) is widely used and is an effective means for detecting alien chromosomes and chromosome segments in wheat-alien species amphiploids, addition lines, and translocation lines. Multicolor GISH (mcGISH) is used to discriminate the A, B, D and E genomes of wheat - *Th. ponticum* addition, substitution and translocation lines [9, 10]. Fluorescence in situ hybridization (FISH), which uses repetitive DNA clones or oligonucleotides as a probe, is an extremely useful method for identifying chromosomes within a species or detecting intergenomic chromosome rearrangements in a polyploid species [5, 15, 19].

In this study, three novel wheat-*Th. ponticum* partial amphiploids were developed from derivatives of common wheat and *Th. ponticum*, and FISH, GISH and mcGISH analyses were used to identify their genomic constitution. Furthermore, the resistance to stripe and leaf rust of the three partial amphiploids was also identified.

Methods
Plant materials
The plant materials used in this study included *Th. ponticum*, *Pseudoroegneria spicata* (StSt, 2n = 14), *Aegilops speltoides* (SS, 2n = 14), *Aegilops tauschii* (DD, 2n = 14), the common wheat cultivar Yannong15 (YN15) and three wheat-*Thinopyrum ponticum* partial amphiploids (SN0389, SN0398 and SN0406). Among them, *Th. ponticum* was provided by Prof. Zhensheng Li (formerly of the Northwest Institute of Botany at the Chinese Academy of Sciences, Yangling, China). *Ps. spicate, Triticum urartu, A. speltoides* and *A. tauschii* were provided by Prof. Lihui Li from the Institute of Crop Science, Chinese Academy of Agricultural Sciences, Beijing, China. The partial amphiploids SN0389, SN0398 and SN0406 were selected from BC_1F_7 of common wheat Yannong15 crossed with *Th. ponticum*, based on the stability and good phenotypic characteristics, such as long spikes, advanced fluorescence, and so on. The amphiploids were maintained by selfing in our laboratory.

Mitotic and meiotic studies
The seeds were germinated at 25 °C on moistened filter paper in petri dishes for 24 h, were maintained at 4 °C for approximately 1 day, and were then transferred to 25 °C for approximately 12 h. Roots, of a length of 1–2 cm, were collected and immediately placed in ice water. After 24–32 h, these roots were fixed in Carnoy's solution for 24 h and were then stored in 70% (v/v) ethanol. The root tips were squashed in acetic acid and were observed under a phase contrast microscope. When the

flag leaf of the wheat was spread, the young spikes were sampled, and the anthers, at metaphase I (MI) of meiosis, were fixed in Carnoy's solution, dissociated in 1 M HCl at 60 °C for 6–8 min, and homogenized in 1% acetocarmine.

Genomic in situ hybridization (GISH)
Genomic DNA from *Ps. spicata* was labeled with Texas red-5-dCTP by the nick translation method and was used as a probe. Sheared genomic DNA from Yannong15 was used as the blocking DNA. The slides were counterstained with DAPI in Vectashield mounting medium (Vector Laboratories, USA). The detailed procedures of the chromosome spread preparation and hybridization are described by Bao et al. [1, 2]. The J^S-genomic and J-genomic chromosomes were distinguished by the GISH signals [3, 29], and those with centromeres labeled by the red signals were the J^S-genome and those with two arm ends of chromosomes labeled by signals were the J-genome.

Multicolor genomic in situ hybridization (mcGISH)
Total genomic DNA from *T. urartu*, *A. speltoides* and *A. tauschii* was isolated from the young leaves via a modified CTAB method. The total genomic DNA from *T. urartu* was labeled with fluorescein-12-dUTP, and the genomic DNA from *A. tauschii* was labeled with Texas-red-5-dUCP by the nick translation method. Total genomic DNA from *A. speltoides* was used a blocker (at a ratio of 1:160). After hybridization, the slides were washed in 2× saline sodium citrate (SSC) and mounted in Vectashield mounting medium.

Fluorescence in situ hybridization (FISH)
Two probes were used in the multicolor FISH. pAs1 was labeled with fluorescein-12-dUTP, and the repeated DNA sequence, $(GAA)_8$, was labeled with Texas-red-5-dUCP. Before hybridization, the two probes were mixed at a ratio of 4:1. The detailed procedures for the hybridization were previously described by He et al. [11]. Images were captured with an Olympus BX-60 fluorescence microscope equipped with a CCD (charge-coupled device) camera.

Stripe rust and leaf rust resistance evaluation
The stripe rust resistance of the three partial amphiploids, at the seedling stage, was evaluated with stripe rust race CYR32 in a greenhouse that had a favorable environment for stripe rust development at the Shandong Academy of Agricultural Sciences, Jinan, China. At the adult-plant stage, stripe rust and leaf rust resistance were evaluated under natural conditions. YN15 (the susceptible cultivar for stripe rust and leaf rust) and *Th. ponticum* were planted as contrasts at the

same time. When the control variety YN15 was all fully infected, the evaluation results were scored according to the standard classification system with 6 scales from 0 to 4 as follows: 0 for no visible symptoms; 0, for necrotic flecks without sporulation; and 1, 2, 3, and 4 for strongly resistant, resistant, susceptible and strongly susceptible, respectively.

Results

Chromosomal constitution of three partial amphiploids

An analysis of the mitotic chromosomes showed that SN0389 contained a chromosome number of 2n = 54, and both SN0398 and SN0406 had a mitotic chromosome number of 2n = 56 (Fig. 1). The meiotic observations of the three partial amphiploids indicated that most of the chromosomes in the observed pollen mother cells of SN0389 formed 27 bivalents at meiotic MI, and SN0398 and SN0406 both formed into 28 bivalents,

which proved that these three partial amphiploids exhibited high cytological stability.

GISH, mcGISH and FISH were used to analyze the genomic constitution of SN0389, SN0398 and SN0406. The results of the GISH (Fig. 1-A1) and FISH (Fig. 1-A3) analyses revealed that SN0389 had 42 wheat chromosomes and 12 *Th. ponticum* chromosomes, including six pairs of J^S-genome chromosomes (Fig. 2). SN0398 contained 42 wheat chromosomes and 14 *Th. ponticum* chromosomes (Fig. 1-B1, B2, B3), including six pairs of J^S-genome chromosomes and one pair of J-genome chromosomes (Fig. 2). The genomic constitution of SN0406 (Fig. 1-C1, C2, C3 and Fig. 2) was similar to SN0398. According to the configuration and signal of the alien chromosomes, the alien chromosomes of SN0389 were different compared to SN0398 and SN0406, while some of the alien chromosomes in SN0398 were probably identical to that in SN0406. For example, the J^S-4*, J^S-6* and J-1*

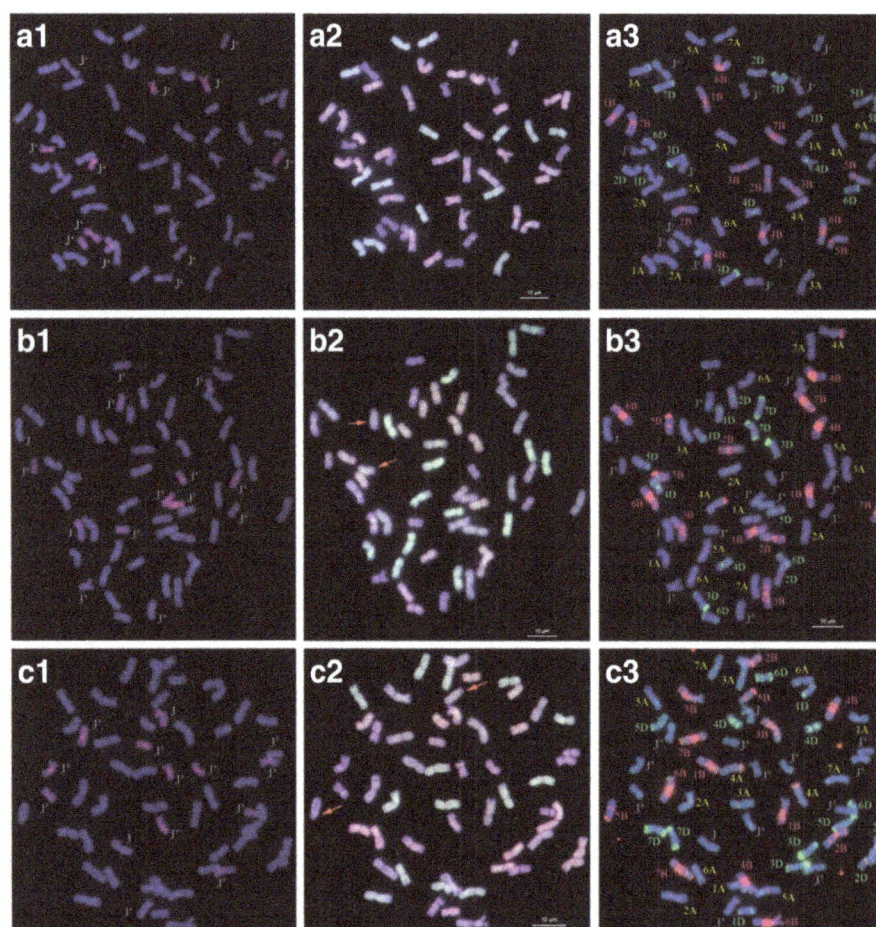

Fig. 1 GISH, McGISH and FISH patterns of SN0389, SN0398 and SN0406. GISH patterns of SN0389 (**a1**), SN0398 (**b1**) and SN0406 (**c1**): *Ps. spicata* (St) genomic DNA labeled with Texas-Red-5-dCTP was used as the probe, and YN15 genome DNA was used to block. McGISH patterns of SN0389 (**a2**), SN0398 (**b2**) and SN0406 (**c2**): A-genomic DNA was labeled with green fluorescence, D-genomic DNA was labeled with red fluorescence and B-genomic DNA (gray) was used to block. As a result, *Th. ponticum* chromosomes showed purple signals. The FISH patterns of SN0389 (**a3**), SN0398 (**b3**) and SN0406 (**c3**): red signals were (GAA)$_8$ and green signals were pAs1

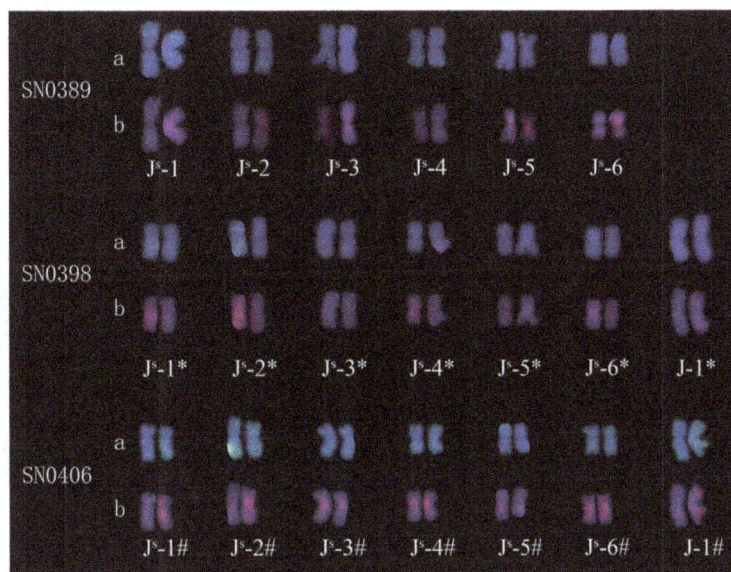

Fig. 2 FISH and GISH patterns of the alien chromosomes of SN0389, SN0398 and SN0406. a. FISH patterns of the alien chromosomes; b. GISH patterns of the alien chromosome. * behind the chromosome numbers indicate the J^S and J chromosomes in SN0398. # behind the chromosome numbers indicate the J^S and J chromosomes in SN0406. The alien chromosomes in SN0389, SN0398 and SN0406 with the same number did not mean the same chromosomes

chromosomes in SN0398 were similar with the J^S-$4^\#$, J^S-$6^\#$ and J-$1^\#$ chromosomes in SN0406 (Fig. 2). But as *Th. ponticum* contained 14 pairs of J^S and 21 pairs of J chromosomes, and there were lack of specific in situ hybridization signals and specific molecular markers of each pairs of chromosomes in *Th. ponticum*, so it's difficult to identify the alien chromosomes in these three amphiploids.

Wheat chromosome variation of three partial amphiploids

The wheat chromosome variation in the three partial amphiploids was analyzed using FISH and McGISH signals, and the results of the common wheat parent YN15 were used as a comparison (Fig. 3). For the A-genome chromosomes, the results showed that the additional red $(GAA)_8$ signals were detected at the terminal of 1AL in SN0389 (Fig. 3-E). Additional, apparently green, signals of the pAs1 probe were also found on 3AS of SN0389. Moreover, the green signal present in the terminal of 6AS in YN15 disappeared in the three partial amphiploids, and a pair of $(GAA)_8$ signals of 6AL in SN0398 and SN0406 was absent (Fig. 3-E).

The red signals of $(GAA)_8$ in the B-genome chromosomes of SN0389, SN0398 and SN0406 were also changed a lot. For example, the $(GAA)_8$ signals at the long arm of 2B were absent in SN0398 and SN0406, while the red signal still remained in SN0389, and the absence was also observed on the satellite of 6B in SN0389. Additional red signals were observed on 7BL

of the three partial amphiploids. Furthermore, the $(GAA)_8$ signal on the terminal of 6BL in SN0389 was different from the other three materials and approached the end of 6BL in SN0389. Moreover, part of the 5B short arm in SN0398 and SN0406 was absent, compared with that of YN15 and SN0389. A few green signals of pAs1 were present on the 6BL chromosomes in YN15, while they were not observed in the three germplasms (Fig. 3-E).

For the D-genome chromosomes in SN0389, SN0398 and SN0406, variations occurred in the 1D, 2D and 5D chromosomes. First, the red signals of $(GAA)_8$ on 1DS were absent in SN0389, while they were preserved in YN15, SN0398 and SN0406. Additionally, the green signals of pAs1, near the terminal of 2DL, were also absent in SN0398 and SN0406. Moreover, the pAs1 signal near the centromere of the 5D chromosomes in SN0389 and SN0398 was absent (Fig. 3-E).

Phenotypic evaluation of three partial amphiploids

The stripe rust resistance of SN0389, SN0398 and SN0406 at the seedling stage was evaluated in a greenhouse, while stripe and leaf rust resistance was evaluated under natural conditions (Table 1, Additional file 1: Figure S1). The results showed that SN0389, SN0398 and SN0406 showed good resistance to stripe rust race CYR32 in the seedling stage. At the adult-plant stage, these three partial amphiploids were immune to stripe rust and showed good resistance to leaf rust

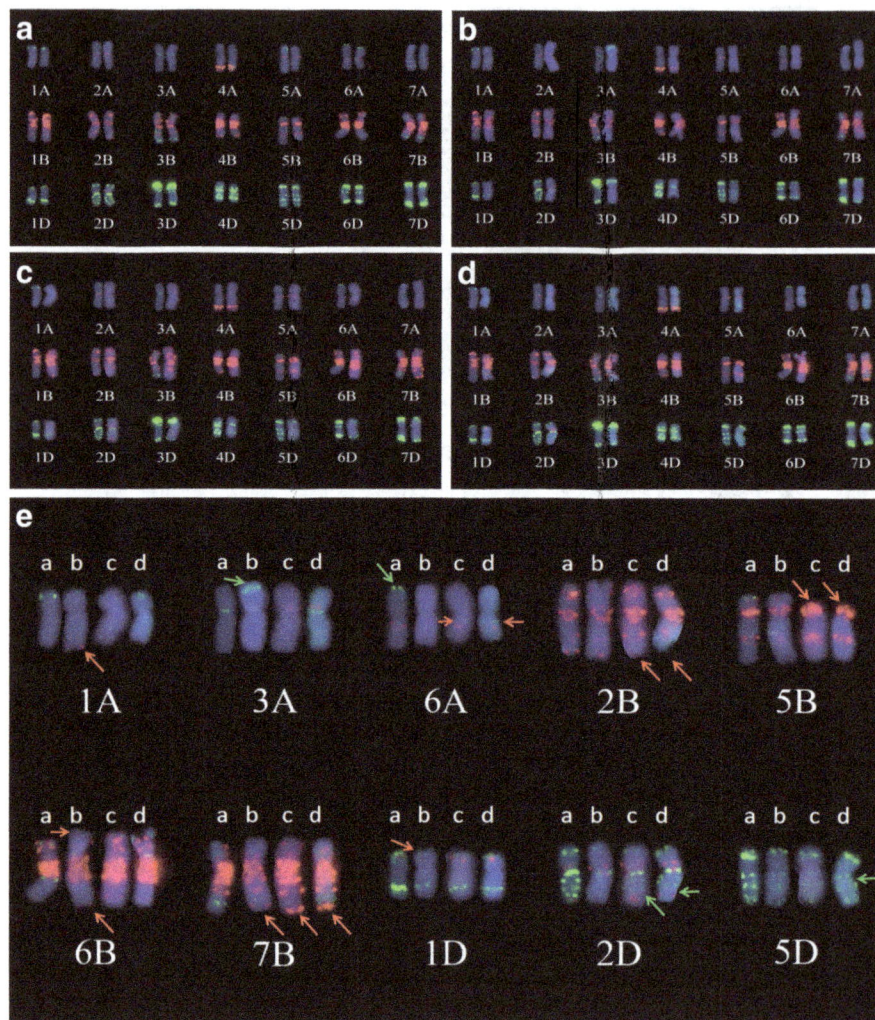

Fig. 3 FISH patterns of the wheat chromosomes in SN0389, SN0398 and SN0406 compared with the common wheat YN15. FISH patterns of YN15 (**a**), SN0389 (**b**), SN0398 (**c**), and SN0406 (**d**). In chromosomes H, I and J, on the left, were those in YN15, and those on the right were from the partial amphiploids. **e**, chromosome variations between YN15 and three partial amphiploids based on the FISH patterns. Among them, *a, b, c* and *d* indicated the corresponding chromosome of YN15, SN0389, SN0398 and SN0406 in turn

in the field. While its common wheat parent YN15 was susceptible to stripe rust and leaf rust and *Th. ponticum* was immune, we deduced that the resistance of partial amphiploids was derived from *Th. ponticum*.

Table 1 Stripe rust and leaf resistance evaluation of SN0389, SN0398 and SN0406

Materials	Stripe rust CYR32	Stripe rust	Leaf rust
	Seedling stage	Adult-plant stage	Adult-plant stage
Th. ponticum	0	0	0
YN15	4	4	4
SN0389	0;	0	0;
SN0398	0;	0	0;
SN0406	0;	0	0;

Discussion

Although *Th. ponticum* is closely related to wheat, it is difficult to obtain excellent germplasm materials directly by the hybridization between *Th. ponticum* and common wheat. Thus, wheat-*Th. ponticum* partial amphiploids, which contain the complete genomes of wheat but an incomplete genome (a set of chromosomes) of *Th. ponticum*, are used as crucial intermediate materials in the transfer of desirable genes from *Th. ponticum* to common wheat [3]. Several wheat-*Th. ponticum* amphiploids have been obtained, analyzed and exploited as alien sources of disease resistance in wheat improvement [3, 8, 12, 24, 31].

In this study, we identified three novel wheat-*Th. ponticum* partial amphiploids with good rust resistance indpendent of stage. These three octoploid *Trititrigia* were developed in the common wheat cultivar YN15 background, and they had good phenotypic characteristics, such as long spikes, advanced fluorescence, and higher cross-compatibility with wheat. Therefore, they could be used as bridge parents to cross with wheat to develop addition, substitution or translocation lines in order to provide new rust resistance germplasms for wheat breeding.

At both stages, YN15 was highly susceptible to stripe rust and leaf rust, whereas the three octoploid *Trititrigia* were immune at both stages. This indicated that SN0389, SN0398 and SN0406 possessed a resistant gene to rust that was derived from *Th. ponticum*. An analysis of the mitotic chromosomes showed that SN0389 had 42 wheat chromosomes and 12 *Th. ponticum* chromosomes, while SN0398 and SN0406 had 42 wheat chromosomes and 14 *Th. ponticum* chromosomes. The results indicated that the alien chromosome of SN0389 was $12J^S$. The alien chromosomes in SN0389 and SN0406 were not from a single genome of J^S or J, and the alien chromosome constitution of SN0398 and SN0406 was $12J^S + 2 J$. Since there were 12 or 14 alien chromosomes in these three octoploid *Trititrigia*, it was difficult to deduce which chromosome the rust resistance gene was located on. We had hybridized the amphiploid with YN15, thus try to screen addition lines with different alien chromosomes in the derivative generations. Then it will be easier to identify which alien chromosome carrying the rust resistance gene. As there were lack of specific FISH or GISH signals and specific molecular markers of each chromosomes in *Th. ponticum* now, more work is needed to make that conclusion.

It is generally believed that only euploid amphiploids are genetically stable, while aneuploids often result in the loss of the added alien chromosomes [20]. Nevertheless, our results here show that the chromosome number of SN0389 was 2n = 54, and it only contained 12 alien chromosomes. However, the meiotic studies showed that SN0389 had a regular meiotic behavior after it was self-pollinated for several generations, and its chromosome number was still 2n = 54. Similar phenomena are also observed in partial amphiploid lines obtained from wheat × *Th. ponticum* and wheat × *Th. intermedium* hybridizations [8, 10, 24]. For example, the partial amphiploid BE-1 contains 16 chromosomes derived from *Th. ponticum* and 40 wheat chromosomes, and the substituted wheat chromosome pair, as identified by FISH, was 7D [24]. Lines Zhong 1 (2n = 52) and Zhong 2 (2n = 54) both contain the complete wheat A, B and D genomes but with 10 and 12 *Th. intermedium* chromosomes, respectively [10]. Further research on the composition of these alien chromosomes and its compensation effect will be helpful in understanding the genetic relationship between the genome of *Th. ponticum* and wheat as well as be a benefit for transferring valuable traits from *Th. ponticum* into wheat.

Using the in situ hybridization pattern of FISH and McGISH, chromosome variations in wheat were also detected. In this study, the structural variations also occurred in chromosomes 1A, 3A, 6A, 2B, 5B, 6B, 7B, 1D and 5D of SN0389, SN0398 and SN0406. The results indicated that during the formation of the partial amphiploids, various intergenomic rearrangements occurred. Some of the chromosome recombinations were caused by introgressed chromosome segments from *Th. ponticum* into common wheat chromosomes, while the introgressed segments were too small to detect by GISH. The other reason for the structural variations in the wheat chromosomes might also be that they were generated by recombination between different wheat chromosomes, such as homeologous chromosome recombination between the A-, B-, and D- genome genomic chromosomes that was interfered by the existence of the *Th. ponticum* chromosomes.

Conclusions

Three partial amphiploids with good resistance and different phenotypic traits were obtained in this study. The chromosome composition of the wheat-*Th ponticum* partial amphiploid was studied by means of GISH, McGISH and FISH. As a good source for improving disease resistance, these amphiploids could be used as promising crossing partners in wheat breeding programs, and resistant progenies of this partial amphiploid could be used as rust resistance sources in wheat improvement.

Abbreviations

FISH: Fluorescence in situ hybridization; GISH: In situ hybridization; mcGISH: Multicolor GISH; MI: Metaphase I

Funding

This work was supported by the National Key Research and Development Program of China (2016YFD0102000), National Natural Science Foundation of China (31671675) and Shandong Provincial Natural Science Foundation (ZR2015CM034).

Authors' contributions

YP performed experiments and prepared the manuscript. YC and YZ performed partial experiments and assisted with the manuscript writing. HW and YB performed partial experiments. XLdesigned the experiment and prepared the manuscript. All the authors reviewed and approved the manuscript.

Competing interests

The authors declare that they have no competing interests.

References

1. Bao Y, Li X, Liu S, Cui F, Wang H. Molecular Cytogenetic Characterization of a new Wheat-*Thinopyrum intermedium* partial amphiploid resistant to powdery mildew and stripe rust. Cytogenet Genome Res. 2009;126(4):390–5.

2.   Bao Y, Wu X, Zhang C, Li X, He F, Qi X, Wang H. Chromosomal constitutions and reactions to powdery mildew and stripe rust of four novel wheat-*Thinopyrum intermedium* partial amphiploids. J Genet Genomics. 2014; 41(12):663–6.

3.   Chen Q, Conner R, Laroche A, Thomas J. Genome analysis of *Thinopyrum intermedium* and *Thinopyrum ponticum* using genomic in situ hybridization. Genome. 1998;41:580–6.

4.   Chen S, Xia G, Quan T, Xiang F, Jin Y, Chen H. Introgression of salt-tolerance from somatic hybrids between common wheat and Thinopyrum ponticum. Plant Sci. 2004;167(4):773–9.

5.   Dechyeva D, Schmidt T. Fluorescent in situ hybridization on extended chromatin fibers for high-resolution analysis of plant chromosomes. Plant Cytogenetics. 2016;1429:23–33.

6.   Draz I, Abou-Elseoud M, Kamara A, Alaa-Eldein O, El-Bebany A. Screening of wheat genotypes for leaf rust resistance along with grain yield. Ann Agric Sci. 2015;60(1):29–39.

7.   Dundas I, Zhang P, Verlin D, Graner A, Shepherd K. Chromosome engineering and physical mapping of the *Thinopyrum ponticum* translocation in wheat carrying the rust resistance gene *Sr26*. Crop Sci. 2015;55:648–57.

8.   Fedak G, Chen Q, Conner RL, Laroche A, Petroski R, Armstrong KW. Characterisation of wheat-*Thinopyrum* partial amphiploids by meiotic analysis and genomic in situ hybridization. Genome. 2000;43:712–9.

9.   Fu S, Lv Z, Qi B, Guo X, Li J, Liu B, Han F. Molecular cytogenetic characterization of wheat-*Thinopyrum elongatum* addition, substitution and translocation lines with a novel source of resistance to wheat Fusarium head blight. J Genet Genomics. 2012;39(2):103–10.

10. Han F, Liu B, Fedak G, Liu Z. Genomic constitution and variation in five partial amphiploids of wheat-*Thinopyrum intermedium* as revealed by GISH, multicolor GISH and seed storage protein analysis. Theor Appl Genet. 2004; 109(5):1070–6.

11. He F, Wang Y, Bao Y, Ma Y, Wang X, Li X, Wang H. Chromosomal constitutions of five wheat-*Elytrigia elongata* partial amphiploids as revealed by GISH, multicolor GISH and FISH. Comp Cytogenet. 2017;11(3):525–40.

12. Hu L, Li G, Zeng Z, Chang Z, Liu C, Yang Z. Molecular characterization of a wheat-*Thinopyrum ponticum* partial amphiploids and its derived substitution line for resistance to stripe rust. J Appl Genet. 2011;52(3):279–85.

13. Hu L, Li G, Zeng Z, Chang Z, Liu C, Zhou J, Yang Z. Molecular cytogenetic identification of a new wheat-*Thinopyrum* substitution line with stripe rust resistance. Euphytica. 2010;177(2):169–77.

14. Jauhar P, Peterson T, Xu S. Cytogenetic and molecular characterization of a durum alien disomic addition line with enhanced tolerance to Fusarium head blight. Genome. 2009;52(5):467–83.

15. Komuro S, Endo R, Shikata K, Kato A. Genomic and chromosomal distribution patterns of various repeated DNA sequences in wheat revealed by a fluorescence in situ hybridization procedure. Genome. 2013;56(3):131–7.

16. Kuzmanović L, Ruggeri R, Virili M, Rossini F, Ceoloni C. Effects of *Thinopyrum ponticum* chromosome segments transferred into durum wheat on yield components and related morpho-physiological traits in mediterranean rain-fed conditions. Field Crop Res. 2016;186:86–98.

17. Li H, Wang X. *Thinopyrum ponticum* and *Th. intermedium*: the promising source of resistance to fungal and viral diseases of wheat. J Genet Genomics. 2009;36(9):557–65.

18. Li X, Jiang X, Chen X, Song J, Ren C, Xiao Y, Gao X, Ru Z. Molecular cytogenetic identification of a novel wheat-*Agropyron elongatum* chromosome translocation line with powdery mildew resistance. PLoS One. 2017;12(9):e0184462.

19. Liu L, Luo Q, Teng W, Li B, Li H, Li Y, Li Z, Zheng Q. Development of *Thinopyrum ponticum*-specific molecular markers and FISH probes based on SLAF-seq technology. Planta. 2018;247(5):1099–108.

20. Matzke MA, Scheid OM, Matzke AJM. Rapid structural and epigenetic changes in polyploid and aneuploid genomes. Bioessays. 1999;21:761–7.

21. Monneveux P, Reynolds M, Aguilar J, Singh R. Effects of the 7DL.7Ag translocation from *Lophopyrum elongatum* on wheat yield and related morphophysiological traits under different environments. Plant Breed. 2003; 122:379–84.

22. Muramatsu M. Cytogenetics of decapoid *Agropyron elongatum* (*Elytrigia elongata*) (2n = 70). I . frequency of decavalent formation. Genome. 1990;33:811–7.

23. Niu Z, Klindworth D, Yu G, Friesen T, Chao S, Jin Y, Cai X, Ohm J, Rasmussen J, Xu SS. Development and characterization of wheat lines carrying stem rust resistance gene *Sr43* derived from *Thinopyrum ponticum*. Theor Appl Genet. 2014;127(4):969–80.

24. Sepsi A, Molnar I, Szalay D, Molnar-Lang M. Characterization of a leaf rust-resistant wheat-*Thinopyrum ponticum* partial amphiploids BE-1, using sequential multicolor GISH and FISH. Theor Appl Genet. 2008;116(6):825–34.

25. Sharma-Poudyal D, Chen X. Models for predicting potential yield loss of wheat caused by stripe rust in the U.S. pacific northwest. Phytopathology. 2011;101(5):544–54.

26. Shen X, Kong L, Ohm H. Fusarium head blight resistance in hexaploid wheat (*Triticum aestivum*)-*Lophopyrum* genetic lines and tagging of the alien chromatin by PCR markers. Theor Appl Genet. 2004;108(5):808–13.

27. Shen X, Ohm H. Molecular mapping of *Thinopyrum*-derived fusarium head blight resistance in common wheat. Mol Breed. 2007;20(2):131–40.

28. Wang M, Peng Z, Li C, Li F, Liu C, Xia G. Proteomic analysis on a high salt tolerance introgression strain of *Triticum aestivum/Thinopyrum ponticum*. Proteomics. 2008;8(7):1470–89.

29. Wang RRC, Zhang XY. Characterization of the translocated chromosome using fluorescence in situ hybridization and random amplified polymorphic DNA on two *Triticum aestivum-Thinopyrum intermedium* translocation lines resistant to wheat streak mosaic or barley yellow dwarf virus. Chromosome Res. 1996;4:583–7.

30. Yang Z, Ren Z. Chromosomal distribution and genetic expression of *Lophopyrum elongatum* (Host) A. Löve genes for adult plant resistance to stripe rust in wheat background. Genet Resour Crop Evol. 2001;48:183–7.

31. Zheng Q, Lv Z, Niu Z, Li B, Li H, Xu S, Han F, Li Z. Molecular cytogenetic characterization and stem rust resistance of five wheat-*Thinopyrum ponticum* partial amphiploids. J Genet Genomics. 2014;41(11):591–9.

11

Noninvasive prenatal diagnosis of fetal aneuploidy by circulating fetal nucleated red blood cells and extravillous trophoblasts using silicon-based nanostructured microfluidics

Chung-Er Huang[1,2†], Gwo-Chin Ma[3,4,5,6†], Hei-Jen Jou[7,8], Wen-Hsiang Lin[3,4], Dong-Jay Lee[3,4], Yi-Shing Lin[9], Norman A. Ginsberg[10], Hsin-Fu Chen[8,11], Frank Mau-Chung Chang[12,13,14] and Ming Chen[3,4,8,13,14,15,16*]

Abstract

Background: Noninvasive prenatal testing (NIPT) based on cell-free DNA in maternal circulation has been accepted worldwide by the clinical community since 2011 but limitations, such as maternal malignancy and fetoplacental mosaicism, preclude its full replacement of invasive prenatal diagnosis. We present a novel silicon-based nanostructured microfluidics platform named as "Cell Reveal™" to demonstrate the feasibility of capturing circulating fetal nucleated red blood cells (fnRBC) and extravillous cytotrophoblasts (EVT) for cell-based noninvasive prenatal diagnosis (cbNIPD).

Methods: The "Cell Reveal™" system is a silicon-based, nanostructured microfluidics using immunoaffinity to capture the trophoblasts and the nucleated RBC (nRBC) with specific antibodies. The automated computer analysis software was used to identify the targeted cells through additional immunostaining of the corresponding antigens. The identified cells were retrieved for whole genome amplification for subsequent investigations by micromanipulation in one microchip, and left in situ for subsequent fluorescence in situ hybridization (FISH) in another microchip. When validation, bloods from pregnant women (n = 24) at gestational age 11–13[+6] weeks were enrolled. When verification, bloods from pregnant women (n = 5) receiving chorionic villus sampling or amniocentesis at gestation age 11[+4]–21 weeks with an aneuploid or euploid fetus were enrolled, followed by genetic analyses using FISH, short tandem repeat (STR) analyses, array comparative genomic hybridization, and next generation sequencing, in which the laboratory is blind to the fetal genetic complement.

Results: The numbers of captured targeted cells were 1–44 nRBC/2 ml and 1–32 EVT/2 ml in the validation group. The genetic investigations performed in the verification group confirmed the captured cells to be fetal origin. In every 8 ml of the maternal blood being blindly tested, both fnRBC and EVT were always captured. The numbers of captured fetal cells were 14–22 fnRBC/4 ml and 1–44 EVT/4 ml of maternal blood.

Conclusions: This report is one of the first few to verify the capture of fnRBC in addition to EVT. The scalability of our automated system made us one step closer toward the goal of in vitro diagnostics.

Keywords: cbNIPD, Aneuploidy, fnRBC, EVT, NIPT, Fish, aCGH, NGS

* Correspondence: mingchenmd@gmail.com; mchen_cch@yahoo.com
†Equal contributors
[3]Department of Genomic Medicine and Center for Medical Genetics, Changhua Christian Hospital, Changhua, Taiwan
[4]Department of Genomic Science and Technology, Changhua Christian Hospital Healthcare System, Changhua, Taiwan
Full list of author information is available at the end of the article

Background

Noninvasive prenatal testing (NIPT) that uses cell-free DNA (cfDNA) in maternal circulation for fetal aneuploidy detection had already achieved widespread recognition and adoption by the clinician community worldwide since 2011 [1, 2]. On the other hand, the progress of cell-based noninvasive prenatal diagnosis (cbNIPD) is relatively not so promising or stagnant until very recently [3–8]. Scarcity of fetal cells in the maternal circulation poses a great hurdle to the progress of cbNIPD when compared with much more robust cfDNA-based NIPT. The cfDNA-based testing was conducted through the robust maximal parallel sequencing methods by utility of the high-sensitive, high-throughput, rapid-evolving platforms called next generation sequencing (NGS) technologies which can discriminate the trivial differences between the maternal blood who carry the euploid fetuses and those who carry the aneuploidy fetuses. The NIPT was successfully validated for common fetal chromosomal numerical disorders such as trisomy 13, 18, and 21 [1]. Recently some service providers claimed the repertoire of NIPT can be expanded to all autosomes, and even microdeletion syndromes [9], which is controversial. Most published statements, consensus, or recommendation from the professional societies now consider using NIPT to detect fetal microdeletion syndromes is not recommended [2, 10]. However, cfDNA-based screening heavily relied upon bioinformatics protected by intellectual property which is less easily accessible and thus mainly dominated by the commercial service providers, and had revolutionarily changed the landscape of prenatal diagnosis [2, 11]. Meanwhile, cfDNA-based tests need innovative algorithms to analyze the NGS data, and it is now well known that origins of the cfDNA, in addition to those from maternal, are from the placenta (trophoblasts) instead of from the fetus proper, indicating that fetoplacental mosaicism (namely, the chromosome complements of the fetus and the placenta are different), is an unarguable source of false-negatives and false-positives with the current NIPT [12, 13].

Since 2014, we have developed our in-house patent protected algorithms for cfDNA NIPT (called GWNS™) and the resolution, in some cases, can be even enhanced to a 3.21 Mb microduplication by simply using 20 M reads shallow-sequencing with 12.5% of fetal DNA fraction [14–16]. However, we also noticed the problem of fetoplacental mosaicism [12, 15, 17] and thus re-focused back our effort to cbNIPD since 2015. We believed with the utility of cbNIPD the issue of fetoplacental mosaicism in noninvasive prenatal diagnosis can be better tackled, if we can capture both cells from the fetal and placental origins, namely, the fetal nucleated red blood cells (fnRBC) and the extravillous cytotrophoblasts (EVT).

The major difficulty of cbNIPD is the extreme scarcity of fetal cells. It is estimated, by the best recent reports,

there were only 1–45 cells per 30 ml maternal blood. And most of the previous efforts captured EVT only, instead of fnRBC, which can truly represent the fetal genome [5]. How to find a feasible method to capture and enrich the fetal cells from the maternal blood become the major challenges of cbNIPD [5, 8]. However, the same technology, if being developed, can be used to capture not only the circulating fetal cells (CFC) but also other cells, including the circulating tumor cells (CTC), and the technologies devised for CTC are numerous: including PCR-based, flow cytometry, laser scanning cytometry, FDA-cleared Cell Search (Veridex, New Jersey, USA), EPISPOT assay [18], and microchip (microfluidics/lab-on-a-chip)-based technologies [19]. Among microchip technologies, the methods had been used to isolate single cells included immune-affinity, immune-magnetic, and size-based methodologies [20]. We selected microchip-based method by using immune-affinity approach which utilizes a microfluidic device (called PicoBioChip, the manufacturing flowchart of the chip was shown in Fig. 1) coated with antibodies which can capture the corresponding antigens on the targeted cells, due to the strength of the semiconductor industry in Taiwan, to devise our novel automated platform Cell Reveal™ to explore the feasibility of cbNIPD to capture CFC (including fnRBC and EVT), firstly by using a group of pregnant women at GA $11–13^{+6}$ weeks to demonstrate the capability of capturing nucleated RBC (nRBC) and EVT, followed by another group of pregnant woman to verify the captured cells are indeed fetal origin by subsequent genetic investigations, such as fluorescence in situ hybridization (FISH), array comparative genomic hybridization (aCGH), and NGS. The results of cbNIPD are compared with paralleled cfDNA NIPT, and confirmed with invasive procedures using karyotyping, aCGH, and if necessary, NGS. The aim of this small pilot series of proof-of-principle study is to demonstrate the feasibility of our platform with a performance comparable or even superior to the capture efficiencies of other designs previously reported in the literature (which ranged from <1 to 3–5 fetal cells per ml of maternal blood) [4, 6, 8]. Meanwhile, the need of manual handling is reduced to a minimum in our automated system.

Results

Circulating fnRBC and EVT captured by PicoBioChip

The scanning electron microscope (SEM) micrograph of the PicoBioChip is shown in Fig. 2a. The micrograph demonstrated that the PicoBioChip surface morphology is composed of patterned nanostructure with the same dimension and space, so that circulating cells could be captured by the chip surface (Fig. 2b). The processes of cells capture were automatically performed on a Cell Reveal™ system. By using a fluorescence microscope, the

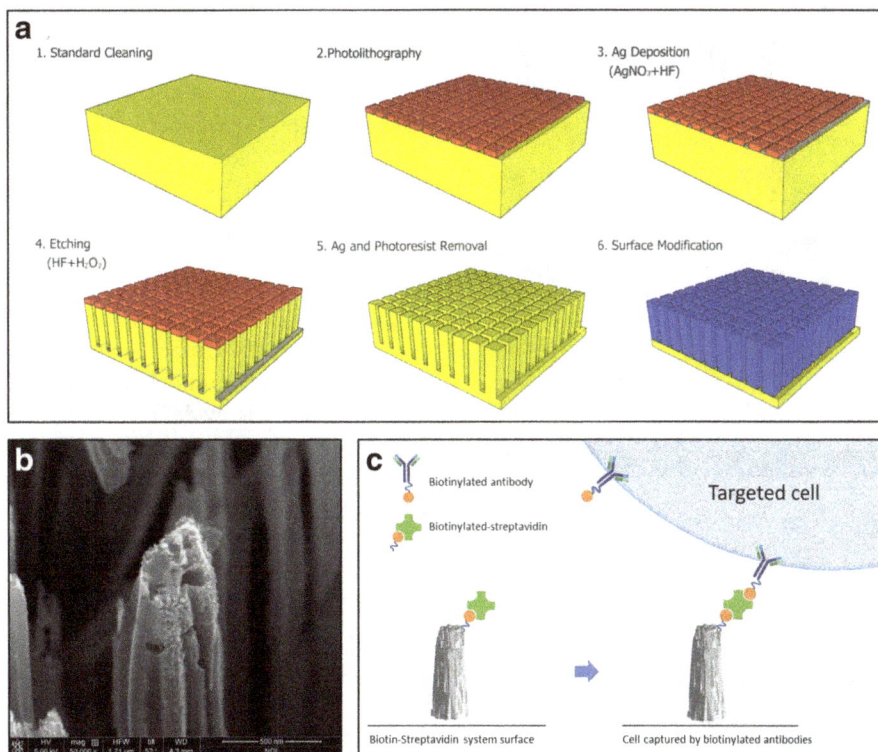

Fig. 1 a Flowchart of the PicoBioChip manufacture: 1. standard cleaning, 2. photolithography, 3. Ag deposition, 4. etching, 5. Ag and photoresist removal, and 6.surface modification. **b** The porous morphology on the PicoBioChip with a "nano-on-nano" structure. **c** Conceptual illustration of how an PicoBioChip can be employed to achieve significantly enhanced capture of targeted cell

nRBC and EVT can be unequivocally distinguished from the background packed with the WBC from the maternal origin (Fig. 3).

Capture efficiency

In every 4 ml of the maternal blood used for validation, circulating nRBC and EVT were always captured in all the 24 pregnant women with capture efficiencies as 1–44 nRBC/2 ml and 1-32EVT/ 2 ml (Additional file 1: Table S1). In every 8 ml of the maternal blood used for verification, circulating fnRBC (please refer to the below sections that the nRBCs we captured are indeed fetal origin) and EVT were always captured for all five pregnant women examined (Table 1). A total of 150 fetal cells (fnRBC + EVT) were successfully captured. The numbers of captured fetal cells were: 14–22 cells per 4 ml of maternal blood for fnRBC and 1–44 cells per 4 ml of maternal blood for EVT. The overall capture efficiency of the novel system is estimated as 2.38–7.25 fetal cells (fnRBC + EVT) per ml of maternal blood per individual (Table 2).

Fluorescence in situ hybridization (FISH)

Interphase FISH for the captured fetal cells from the blood of pregnant women with a fetus of trisomy 13, trisomy 18, or trisomy 21 revealed correct diagnoses in all

cases. The number of fnRBC and EVT examined ranged from one to ten for each case (Table 1). FISH for the trisomy 13 revealed nuc ish(RB1/D13S1195/D13S1155/D13S915x3, D21S270/D21S1867/D21S337/D21S1425/D21S1444/D21S341x2), for the trisomy 18 revealed nuc ish(D18Z1x3,DXZ1x2), and for the trisomy 21 revealed nuc ish(RB1/D13S1195/D13S1155/D13S915x2,D21S270/D21S1867/D21S337/D21S1425/D21S1444/D21S341x3) (Fig. 4).

Whole genome amplification (WGA)

All pooled captured cells underwent WGA successfully except those the total numbers of cells were too few (namely, less than 4 cells) to reach the amplified threshold for subsequent molecular genetic analyses by short tandem repeat (STR) analysis, aCGH, and NGS. Overall, fnRBC WGA from all the five cases and EVT WGA from two cases were obtained (Table 1). The WGA products were 50 µl in total with a concentration ranged from 290 to 844 ng/µl.

Short tandem repeat (STR) analysis

STR analyses were performed for the WGA DNA from captured fetal cells and maternal leukocytes as well as the DNA from the abortus tissue (if available). The results

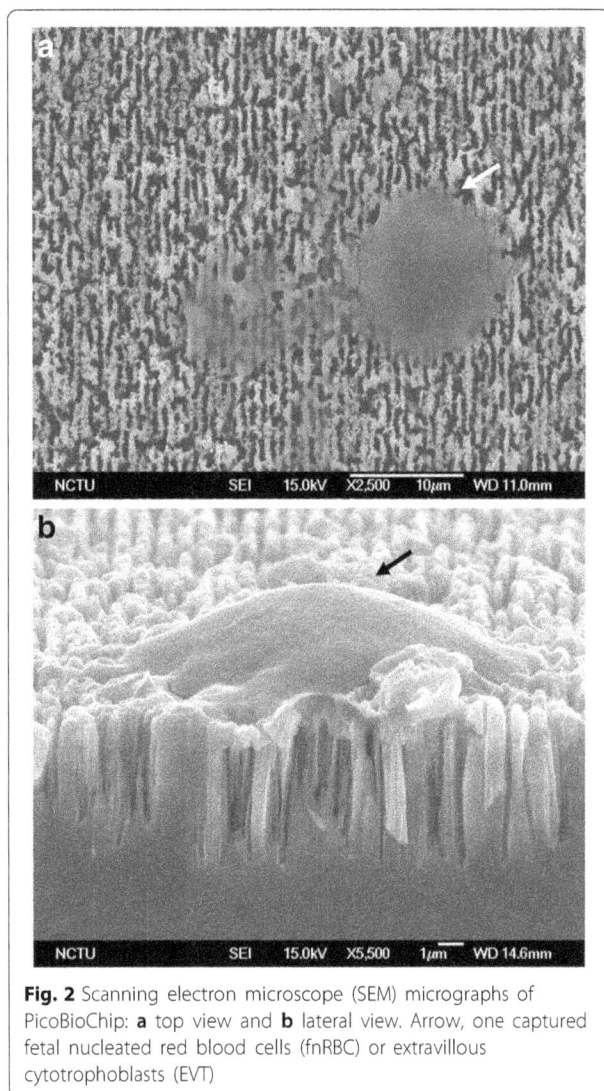

Fig. 2 Scanning electron microscope (SEM) micrographs of PicoBioChip: **a** top view and **b** lateral view. Arrow, one captured fetal nucleated red blood cells (fnRBC) or extravillous cytotrophoblasts (EVT)

demonstrated the captured fnRBC and/or EVT are indeed fetal origin in all the five cases examined. For each case, there are 4–8 informative STR makers containing non-maternal alleles that are feasible to distinguish the fetal cells from the maternal cells (Table 3).

Array comparative genomic hybridization (aCGH) and next generation sequencing (NGS)

Both of aCGH and NGS analyses were performed for the captured fnRBC from the five cases and all the cases were correctly diagnosed. The results of aCGH are comparable with that of NGS (Fig. 5), and are consistent with the karyotyping results.

Discussion

The quest to search for a true noninvasive prenatal diagnosis had been the Holy Grail of prenatal diagnosis since 1969 [5]. The major hurdle is the scarcity of fetal cells in maternal circulation, and therefore contributed

to the soaring cost of the technologies involved in the enrichment and isolation. Most previous reports found that the majority of nucleated red blood cells isolated from the maternal blood are actually maternal origin instead of fetal [5] whereas a recent published study did isolate fnRBC, confirmed by using chromosome Y-specific FISH [21]. Another group explored the monoclonal antibodies specific for fnRBC in addition to those specific for nucleated RBCs (including both fetal nucleated RBC and nucleated RBC from adult bone marrow origin) such as CD36, CD71, glycophorin-A, antigen-i, and galactose [22]. Unfortunately, it is not commercially available for such monoclonal antibodies claimed to be fetal specific. It is evident that our Cell Reveal™ system with PicoBioChip can capture both the fnRBC and EVT with capture efficiencies superior to or at least comparable to the previous reports (19–58 cells/8 ml v.s. 1–45 cells/30 ml maternal blood), especially all the NRBCs being captured in the verification group by our system are fnRBC. Therefore the feasibility of our platform to tackle the primary hurdle, the scarcity of fetal cells and the difficulty to successfully enrich and capture the very few fetal cells from a limited amount of maternal blood (i.e. 8 ml), is demonstrated. The importance to capture not only the trophoblasts (which is considered placental origin), but also the fnRBC is that the fetoplacental mosaicism can be overcome, otherwise cbNIPD adds not much additional value when being compared with the extremely successful cfDNA-based NIPT, since only fnRBC can genuinely represent the fetal origin instead of placenta origin, which NIPT has already managed [1, 23]. The nucleated red blood cells isolated through our platform are confirmed to be fetal origin by the subsequent analyses including STR analysis, FISH, aCGH, and NGS. Meanwhile, cbNIPD may clearly delineate which co-twin is affected (or much more uncommon, both co-twins are affected) by aneuploidy when the result of cfDNA-based NIPT showed high risk for aneuploidy in twin pregnancies.

In this proof-of-principle pilot study, we only demonstrated the feasibility of our Cell Reveal™ platform to detect fetal aneuploidy by using common trisomies (trisomy 13, 18, and 21). We admit it will be more persuasive if we included some genuine fetoplacental mosaicism cases as some of the cases we published before, and this will be included in our future studies [15, 17, 24]. Some researchers proposed that cbNIPD on EVT can be used to detect de novo copy number variations which can only be reliably diagnosed by microarray, since at the moment the claims by some commercial service providers to expand the repertoire of cfDNA-based NIPT to include microdeletions/microduplications are not widely endorsed by the academic community [5, 10]. However, the errors that may be

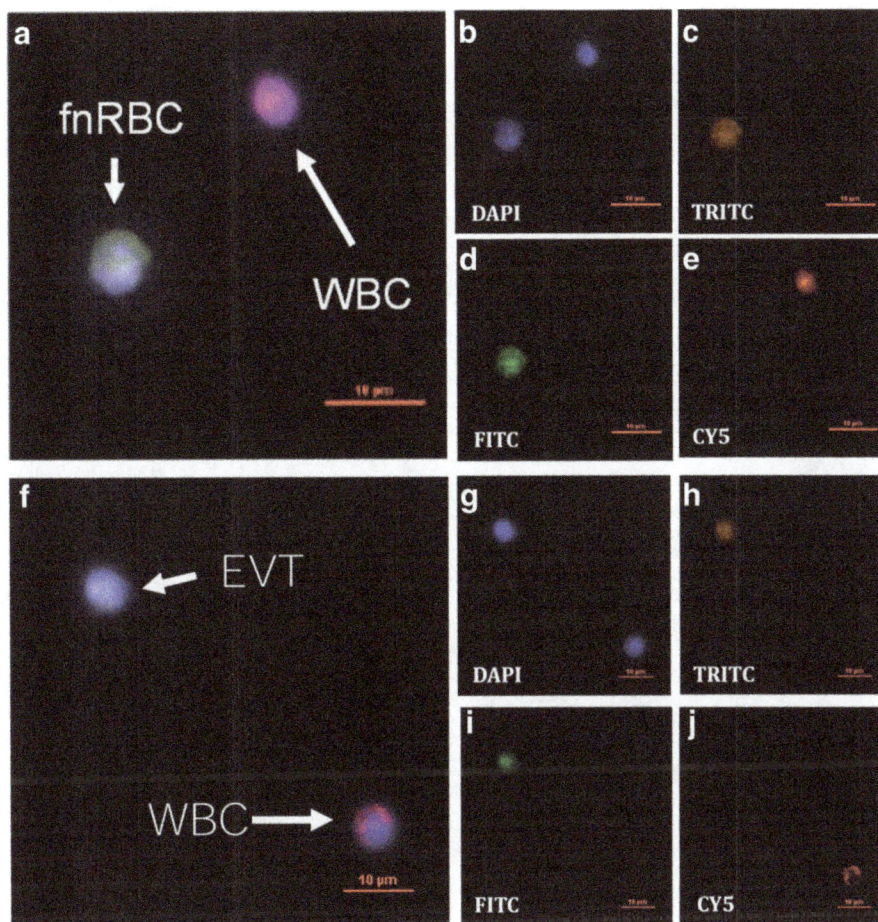

Fig. 3 Discrimination of **a-e** fnRBC and **f-j** EVT from maternal white blood cells (WBC) by fluorescence microscope. The fnRBC and EVT can be recognized by different antibodies labeled with TRITC (GPA and HLA-G) or FITC (CD71 and CK7). The maternal leukocytes can be recognized by antibody labeled with CY5 (CD45)

introduced by the indispensable WGA procedure had also been noticed recently from the experience obtained from the studies regarding preimplantation genetic screening. More and more reports were published since 2015 that euploid babies were born after transferring the aneuploid embryos into the womb [25] and the consistency of PGS across the laboratories adopting different genotyping technologies is questioned [26–29]. Thus, we considered aCGH and NGS can be used but should be interpreted with caution because WGA is the necessary step before using these technologies. A better capture efficiency to capture more cells and group them together for the subsequent analyses will be very helpful to minimize the errors introduced by WGA. In our laboratory, the previous experience on PGD/PGS made us only did WGA on at least four cells, therefore we did not do WGA on the EVT captured on Case no. 1, 4, 5 whereas we did WGA on the nRBC we captured on all the five cases in the verification group (Table 1). Remarkably, most previous reports in the literature

regarding cbNIPD using different methods such as immunoaffinity by magnetic enrichment [8] or NanoVelcro microchip [30], or isolation by size of tumor/trophoblast cells (ISET) [31] only successfully isolated trophoblasts instead of fnRBC. However, it is remarkable that ISET was reported to be able to isolate living cells [32].

On the other hand, it is now better known the trend of the variation of the fetal DNA fractions during the whole gestation, as well as the possible confounding factors, since the fetal fraction is one of the major factors affecting the accuracy of NIPT [10, 33]. Needless to say, such similar large-scale studies are mandatory for cbNIPD in order to better understand the variation as well as the confounding factors affecting the numbers of both types of the fetal cells (fnRBC and EVT), to facilitate its wider acceptance of clinical utility. The future studies will be ideal if including some fetoplacental mosaicism cases as well as twin pregnancies with one or two aneuploidy cases to better demonstrate its feasibility to supplement the current cfDNA-based NIPT. Lastly,

Table 1 The capture efficiency and related parameters of cell-based prenatal diagnosis by Cell Reveal™ platform with PicoBioChips for 5 pregnant women with an aneuploid or euploid fetus in the verification group

Case no.	Maternal age	Gestational age	Fetal karyotype	Type of fetal cell captured	Captured efficiency[a] Average (2 ml/2 ml)	FISH[b]	WGA[c]	cfDNA testing[d]
1	36	11[+6e]	47,XX,+13	fnRBC	11 (10/12)	10	11 (+)	High risk for T13:
				EVT	1 (1/1)	1	1 (−)	GWNS: p < 0.001
								Z score: Z = 8.74
2	34	18[+6]	47,XX,+18	fnRBC	7 (3/11)	3	11 (+)	High risk for T18:
				EVT	22 (11/33)	11	15 (+)	GWNS: p = 0.003
								Z score: Z = 4.29
3	37	21	47,XX,+21	fnRBC	11 (2/20)	2	15 (+)	High risk for T21:
				EVT	3.5 (3/4)	3	4 (+)	GWNS: p = 0.003
								Z score: Z = 3.91
4	30	13[+3]	46,XY	fnRBC	9 (8/10)	8	6 (+)	Low risk for T13, 18, 21
				EVT	1 (1/1)	1	2 (−)	
5	34	11[+4]	46,XX	fnRBC	9 (8/10)	8	9 (+)	Low risk for T13, 18, 21
				EVT	0.5 (0/1)	NP	1 (−)	

FISH fluorescence in situ hybridization, *fnRBC* fetal nucleated red blood cells, *GWNS* genome wide normalized score, *NP* Not be performed, *WGA* whole genome amplification

[a]Number of cell captured per 2 ml of maternal blood per PicoBioChip: mean of (chip1/chip2)

[b]Number of cells analyzed

[c]Number of cells pooled for DNA amplification. "+" and "-" indicated the successful amplification and unsuccessful amplification, respectively

[d]Cut-off values of high risk: p < 0.05 by GWNS algorithm and z < −3 or >3 by Z score algorithm [14]

[e]11[+6] denotes 11 weeks and 6 days. cfDNA: cell-free DNA; EVT: extravillous cytotrophoblasts

another critical issue affecting the uptake of cbNIPD by the clinical community in the future is the cost. A detailed cost-effective analysis is needed in the future for cbNIPD as it has been done in NIPT for fetal aneuploidy [34]. Nevertheless, this platform has the potential to be used for capturing the circulating tumor cells (CTC) as well [32]. It is arguably that the nRBC captured in the validation group (n = 24) may both include the fetal and the maternal nRBC (these cells are released from the adult bone marrow) since we did not use the fetal specific monoclonal antibodies such as those recognize the Epsilon hemoglobin [35]. However, the subsequent genetic investigations we performed (including FISH, aCGH, STR, and NGS) had verified the captured cells in the verification group (n = 5) are indeed fetal origin.

To the best of our knowledge, this report is one of the very few studies on the successful use of circulating fetal cells for noninvasive prenatal diagnosis. The strength of our study is that all the processes of cell capture are automatic which can be performed on a single individual case and completed within 15 h (Additional file 2: Table S2). The captured cells are available for a variety of genetic

Table 2 The characteristics of the 11 short tandem repeat (STR) loci and one gender-specific locus examined in this study. Primers are labeled with WellRED dye (Beckman Coulter, California, USA)

Locus	Chromosome location	Primer label	Repeat unit length
STR			
D3S1358	3p21.31	D4	4
TH01	11p15.5	D2	4
D13S317	13q31.1	D3	4
D8S1179	8q24.13	D4	4
D7S820	7q11.21–22	D3	4
TPOX	2p25.3	D4	4
D16S539	16q24.1	D3	4
D18S51	18q21.3	D2	4
CSF1PO	5q33.1	D4	4
Penta D	21q22.3	D4	5
Penta E	15q26.2	D3	5
Gender-specific			
AMEL	X and Y	D3	–

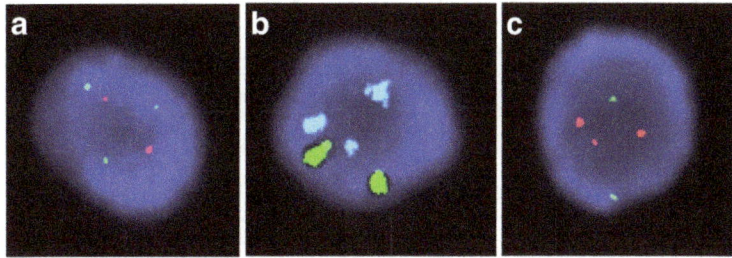

Fig. 4 Fluorescent in situ hybridization (FISH) for the captured fnRBC from 3 pregnant women with an aneuploid fetus of **a** trisomy 13, **b** trisomy 18, and **c** trisomy 21. In **a** and **c**, chromosome 13 was identified by a panel of probes (RB1, D13S1195, D13S1155, D13S915) in green and chromosome 21 was identified by a panel of probes (D21S270, D21S1867, D21S337, D21S1425, D21S1444, D21S341) in orange. In **b**, chromosome 18 was identified by a probe (D18Z1) in aqua and chromosome X was identified by a probe (DXZ1) in green

testing, such as FISH, aCGH and NGS. Overall, the turn-around time of the cbNIPD is less than 2 weeks, similar to that of NIPT as performed in our laboratory.

Conclusion

We demonstrated our silicon-based nanostructured microfluidics "The Cell Reveal™ system" can capture both the fnRBC and EVT. The scalability is greatly enhanced with the automation of the whole system, which may render cbNIPD from mainly a laboratory-developed-test (LDT) conducted only in a limited number of core laboratories, into an in-vitro-diagnostics (IVD) that can be applied in many research and clinical sites.

Methods
Samples

During 2016–2017, 24 women who carried the singleton pregnancy and received the first trimester serum screening for Down syndrome at GA 11–13 + 6 weeks or who decided to receive NIPT, was asked to donate blood sample to be used for validation. For each individual, 4 ml additional blood was stored in the BD vacutainer® with ACD solution A (Becton, Dickinson and Company, New Jersey, USA) for cbNIPD. When verification, at 2017 another five pregnant women carrying the singleton pregnancy at first or second trimester who decided to receive invasive procedures (chorionic villus sampling or amniocentesis) were recruited as a research basis to receive paralleled cfDNA testing (i.e. NIPT) and cbNIPD after informed consents (with the approved protocol CCH-IRB-141219) were signed. For each individual, approximately 20 ml of venous blood were collected. The blood was taken and stored in the Streck Cell-Free DNA BCT® (Streck, Nebraska, USA) for NIPT (12 ml) and in the BD vacutainer® with ACD solution A (Becton, Dickinson and Company, New Jersey, USA) for cbNIPD (8 ml). A total of

Table 3 Summary of the STR results for the captured fetal cells (fnRBC and/or EVT) from the 5 pregnant women. For each case, at least 4 informative STR loci are feasible to distinguish the fetal cells from the maternal cells (the non-maternal alleles are marked in bold)

Locus	Case 1 (Trisomy 13)		Case 2 (Trisomy 18)				Case 3 (Trisomy 21)			Case 4 (Disomy: 46,XY)		Case 5 (Disomy: 46,XX)	
	Maternal leukocyte	fnRBC	Maternal leukocyte	fnRBC	EVT	Abortus tissue	Maternal leukocyte	fnRBC	EVT	Maternal leukocyte	fnRBC	Maternal leukocyte	fnRBC
D3S1358	133, 137	**129**, 137	129, 137	129, 137	129, 137	129, 137	129, 137	129, 137	129, 137	129, 133	133, **137**	129, 133	129, 133
TH01	171, 179	171, **183**	167, 171	167, **179**	167, **179**	167, **179**	171, 179	171, 179	171, 179	179	179	179	**167**, 179
D13S317	182, 190	182, **198**	197	**181**, 197	**181**, 197	**181**, 197	181, 197	181, 197	181, 197	182, 194	**186**, 194	182, 186	182, 186
D8S1179	222, 234	**218**, 222	238	**218**, 238	**218**, 238	**218**, 238	230, 234	230	230	218, 230	218, 230	231, 239	231
D7S820	234, 238	**230**, 238	234	234, **238**	234, **238**	234, **238**	226, 238	226, 238	226, 238	242, 246	**234**, 242	231, 243	231, **235**
TPOX	272, 276	272	272	272, **284**	272, **284**	272, **284**	272	272, **276**	272, **276**	272, 284	272	272, 284	284
D16S539	285	285	285, 297	**289**, 297	**289**, 297	**289**, 297	284	284	284	289, 297	**293**, 297	285, 301	**297**, 301
D18S51	307, 311	311	303, 315	303, 315	303, 315	303, 315	307, 319	307, **315**	307, **315**	307	307	315, 337	**303**, 315
CSF1PO	315	315, **320**	344	**340**, 344	**340**, 344	**340**, 344	336, 344	336, 344	336, 344	344	**332**, 344	341	341, **349**
Penta D	404, 419	404, 419	405, 414	405, 414	405, 414	405, 414	400, 424	424, **433**	424, **433**	419, 433	419, 433	404, 414	404, **433**
Penta E	418, 451	418	429	**424**, 429	**424**, 429	**424**, 429	414, 419	419, **450**	419, **450**	445, 450	**424**, 450	414, 435	435, **451**
AMEL	105	105	105	105	105	105	105	105	105	105	105, **111**	105	105

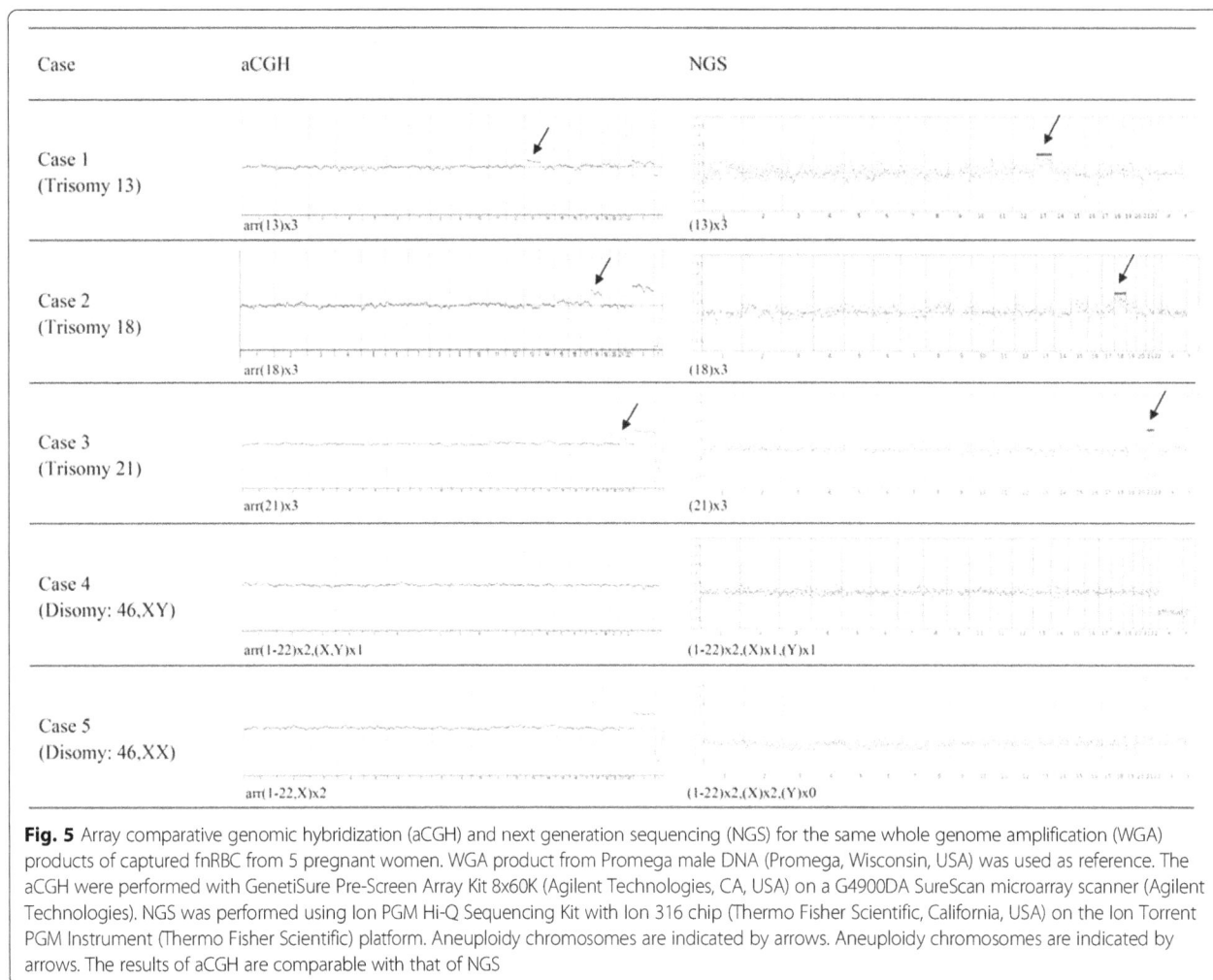

Fig. 5 Array comparative genomic hybridization (aCGH) and next generation sequencing (NGS) for the same whole genome amplification (WGA) products of captured fnRBC from 5 pregnant women. WGA product from Promega male DNA (Promega, Wisconsin, USA) was used as reference. The aCGH were performed with GenetiSure Pre-Screen Array Kit 8x60K (Agilent Technologies, CA, USA) on a G4900DA SureScan microarray scanner (Agilent Technologies). NGS was performed using Ion PGM Hi-Q Sequencing Kit with Ion 316 chip (Thermo Fisher Scientific, California, USA) on the Ion Torrent PGM Instrument (Thermo Fisher Scientific) platform. Aneuploidy chromosomes are indicated by arrows. Aneuploidy chromosomes are indicated by arrows. The results of aCGH are comparable with that of NGS

3 pregnant women who had singleton pregnancy affected with fetal aneuploidy were recruited, including trisomy 13 ($n = 1$), trisomy 18 (n = 1), and trisomy 21 (n = 1) fetuses respectively. Meanwhile, two women carrying the euploid fetuses (46,XX, n = 1 and 46,XY, n = 1) were also enrolled. The pregnant women were enrolled at first or second trimester ranged from gestational age 11^{+4} to 21 weeks (Table 1). It is noteworthy that the examiners of the cbNIPD lab have no prior knowledge of the karyotyping results, namely, they were blind to the results to avoid ascertainment bias. The recruitment of patients, collection of samples, and conduct of research projects, were approved by the Ethical Commitees of the medical institutions where the samples were collected (the Taiwan Adventist Hospital, Taipei, Taiwan, and the Changhua Christian Hospital, Changhua, Taiwan).

PicoBioChip manufacture

The PicoBioChip is a Si nanostructure with a porous morphology that is fabricated using the metal-assisted chemical etching (MACE) technology. The fabrication

sequence is described as followed: the starting materials are p-type (100) silicon wafers which followed standard cleaning procedures to remove environmental contaminants. The pattern of the PicoBioChip is defined by standard photolithographic techniques. The Ag film is deposited onto the silicon wafer in a $HF/AgNO_3$ mixture solution, and the wafers are etched in a HF/H_2O_2-mixture solution. Then, after the etching step and the Ag film removal, a Si nanostructure with a porous morphology is formed that is a "nano-on-nano" structure. To enhance the capturing effect, the potential targeted cells are pre-labeled with biotinylated antibodies and the PicoBioChip surface is made from a streptavidin material which has a specific binding interaction with biotin. The streptavidin-biotin is the strongest non-covalent biological interaction currently known. Via streptavidin-biotin interaction, biotinylated antibodies can be conjugated, enabling a high efficiency for targeted cells capture. The manufacturing flowchart, nano-on-nano structure and capture conception of the PicoBioChip are shown in Fig. 1.

Circulating fetal cells captured by cell reveal™ system with PicoBioChip

The whole blood sample (8 ml) is flown through the automated Cell Reveal™ system and then CFC are captured by PicoBioChips. For each run of test, four PicoBioChips were used: two for fnRBC capture and two for EVT capture. The antibodies used for primary capture of circulating fetal cells are CD71$^+$ for fnRBC and EpCAM$^+$ for EVT. PicoBioChips are examined using a fluorescence microscope equipped with a built-in automatic inspection and image analysis system, called the Cell Analysis Tool (CytoAurora CAT™), to filter out images of maternal white blood cells (WBC) for further analyses. The fnRBC and EVT can therefore be targeted, identified and enumerated. Image analyses with the count-in/filter-out criteria for different cell types are CD71(+)/GPA$^+$(glycophorin-A)/CD45$^-$/DAPI$^+$ for fnRBC and CK7$^+$(Cytokeratin-7)/HLA-G(+)/CD45$^-$/DAPI$^+$ for EVT, according to literatures and our in-house optimization [6, 21, 22, 35–40]. Namely, we first used one antibody to capture fnRBC and EVT separately, and then using other antibodies to stain the captured cells. Hence, the fnRBC were primarily captured by CD71 and then stained with CD71 and GPA, whereas the EVT were primarily captured by EpCAM and then stained with CK7 and HLA-G. Namely, we utilized dual antibodies (CD71 and GPA) to delineate the fnRBC and triple antibodies (EpCAM, CK7, HLA-G) to delineate EVT. It is noteworthy that in the validation group ($n = 24$) to validate the capture efficiency, only 4 ml maternal blood was used, in which 2 ml was for fnRBC (or more strictly, nRBC) and 2 ml was for EVT in each case. Only the five pregnant women enrolled for verification had 8 ml maternal blood to be withdrawn and used for cbNIPD.

Fluorescence in situ hybridization (FISH)

FISH was performed directly on one PicoBioChip capturing for fnRBC and one chip for EVT. Prior to hybridization, the formaldehyde on PicoBioChips were treated by 10 mM sodium citrate at 90 °C for 20 min, followed by being immersed in 0.1% Triton-X at room temperature for 10 min, then followed by serial washes of 0.2 N HCl at 25 °C for 20 min, purified water (double distilled) at 25 °C for 3 min and 2X SSC at 25 °C for 3 min, and an immersion of Vysis pretreatment solution (1 N NaSCN) (Abbott, IL, USA) at 25 °C overnight. Then, the PicoBioChips were deposited in purified water at 25 °C for 1 min, 2X SSC at 25 °C for 5 min (repeated two times), pepsin solution (10 μl 10% Pepsin / 40 ml 0.01 N HCl) at 37 °C for 3 min and 2X SSC at 25 °C for 5 min (repeated two times). Finally, the PicoBioChips were immersed in 70% ethanol at 4 °C for 1 min, 85% ethanol at 4 °C for 1 min and 100% ethanol at 4 °C for 1 min, and dried at 50 °C for 5 min. Interphase FISH for

chromosome 13, 18 and 21 on captured fnRBC and EVT was then conducted using Aquarius® FAST FISH Prenatal kit (Cytocell, Cambridge, UK). For hybridization experiment, the PicoBioChips were dehydrated in an ethanol series and hybridized overnight in a moist chamber at 37 °C. The chips were washed for 2 min in 0.4X SSC at 70 °C and for 5 min in 4X SSC, 0.1% Tween 20 at room temperature and blocked in 4X SSC, 3% bovine serum albumin (BSA), 0.1% Tween 20 at 37 °C for 30 min. The hybridization signal was detected with Nikon-Ni-E microscope system (Nikon, Tokyo, Japan). Chromosomes were counterstained with 0.125 μg/ml DAPI in Antifade (Vysis, Illinois, USA). FISH analyses were performed using the Aquarius® FAST FISH Prenatal kit (Cytocell). The chromosome 13 probe for RB1, D13S1195, D13S1155, and D13S915, the chromosome 18 probe for centromere of chromosome 18(D18Z1), the chromosome 21 probe for D21S270, D21S1867, D21S337, D21S1425, D21S1444, and D21S341, and the chromosome X probe for centromere of chromosome X (DXZ1) were labeled with green, aqua, orange, and green fluorophores, respectively.

Retrieval of captured cells by PicoBioChip

The captured fnRBC and EVT are separately released by with capillary micropipette from PicoBioChips which are destined for DNA analyses. The location of captured cells-on-chip is acquired by the CytoAurora CAT™. Capillary micropipette crashes the chip's nano structure of the target captured cells. The captured cells on the chip surface are followed by capillary micropipette picking up, which allows captured cells to escape from chip to be released for sequential analyses.

Whole genome amplification (WGA)

The captured fetal cells retrieved from the same PicoBioChip are pooled. The fnRBC and EVT were subjected separately to WGA, with 1.8 μg/μl BSA serving as the blocking agent to reduce the surface interaction from the silicon debris. WGA was performed using REPLI-g Single Cell Kit (Qiagen, Hilden, Germany) and following the manufacturer's instructions. Amplified DNA was purified using the QIAamp DNA Blood Mini Kit (Qiagen). The DNA purities and concentrations were examined by Qubit fluorometer (Thermo Fisher Scientific, Delaware, USA) and Nanodrop 2000 spectrophotometer (Thermo Fisher Scientific).

Short tandem repeat (STR) analysis

STR analysis was performed to confirm that the circulating cells captured and WGA DNA of fnRBC and EVT are indeed from fetuses instead of maternal origin. GenomeLab Human STR Primer Set kit (Beckman Coulter, California, USA) containing 12 primer pairs to amplify 11 STR loci and one gender-specific locus (Table 2) was used to analyze patterns of the STR by capillary electrophoresis according with the supplier's protocol. PCR products were run on GenomeLab™ GeXP Genetic Analysis System (Beckman Coulter). FRAGMENTS application program (Beckman Coulter) was used for data collection and allele sizing.

Array comparative genomic hybridization (aCGH)

Approximately 1000 ng of WGA DNA was subjected to aCGH by GenetiSure Pre-Screen Array Kit 8x60K (Agilent Technologies, CA, USA), following the manufacturer's instructions. The image on a chip was acquired with a G4900DA SureScan microarray scanner (Agilent Technologies, CA, USA) and analyzed with Agilent Cyto-Genomics software (Agilent Technologies) for chromosome gain or loss. Aberrations were detected by using default setting.

Next generation sequencing (NGS)

Approximately 1000 ng of WGA DNA was used for library construction using Ion Xpress Plus gDNA Fragment Library Preparation Kit Set (Thermo Fisher Scientific, California, USA) and following the manufacturer's instructions. The quantity of library was determined using Qubit dsDNA HS assay kits (Thermo Fisher Scientific) with Qubit fluorometer (Thermo Fisher Scientific). The template-positive Ion Sphere Particles were generated using Ion PGM Hi-Q Template Kits (Thermo Fisher Scientific) with the Ion OneTouch 2 Instrument (Thermo Fisher Scientific) and then enriched with the Ion OneTouch ES Instrument (Thermo Fisher Scientific). Sequencing was performed on the Ion Torrent PGM Instrument (Thermo Fisher Scientific) platform using the Ion PGM Hi-Q Sequencing Kit and Ion 316 chip (Thermo Fisher Scientific). Analysis of the WGA product being sequenced was performed by using the cloud-based the Ion Reporter™ Server System (https://ionreporter.thermofisher.com/ir/).

Abbreviations

aCGH: Array comparative genomic hybridization; BSA: Bovine serum albumin; cbNIPD: Cell-based noninvasive prenatal diagnosis; CFC: Circulating fetal cells; cfDNA: Cell-free DNA; CTC: Circulating tumor cells; EVT: Extravillous cytotrophoblasts; FISH: Fluorescence in situ hybridization; fnRBC: Fetal nRBC; GWNS: Genome wide normalized score; MACE: Metal-assisted chemical etching; NGS: Next generation sequencing; NIPT: Noninvasive prenatal testing; nRBC: Nucleated red blood cells; SEM: Scanning electron microscope; STR: Short tandem repeat; WBC: White blood cells; WGA: Whole genome amplification

Acknowledgements

The authors would like to thank Dr. Wan-Ju Wu, Department of Obstetrics and Gynecology, Changhua Christian Hospital, Taiwan, and Dr. Wei-Cheng Hsu, Mr. Sheng-Wen Chen and Mr. Hsin-Cheng Ho of Cytoaurora Biotechnologies, Inc., Hsinchu Science Park, Hsinchu, Taiwan, for their assistance in manuscript preparation. The "Cell Reveal™" system has been granted Taiwanese patent no. M539091.

Funding

Part of the study (the cfDNA part of the experiments) was funded by a grant (MOST 104–2314-B-371-009-MY3) from the Ministry of Science and Technology, Executive Yuan, Taiwan to MC.

Authors' contributions

CEH, GCM, MC designed the study. HJJ and MC recruited the patients. CEH, GCM, WHL, DJL, YSL did the experiments and performed the analyses. CEH, GCM, and MC wrote the manuscript. HJJ, NG, HFC, and FMCC provided critical review of the manuscript. MC revised the final version. All authors read and approved the final manuscript.

Competing interests

CEH is the founder, CEO and holds equity of the Cytoaurora Biotechnologies Inc., Hsinchu Science Park, Hsinchu, Taiwan. All other authors declare no conflict of interests.

Author details

[1]International College of Semiconductor Technology, National Chiao-Tung University, Hsinchu, Taiwan. [2]Cytoaurora Biotechnologies, Inc. Hsinchu Science Park, Hsinchu, Taiwan. [3]Department of Genomic Medicine and Center for Medical Genetics, Changhua Christian Hospital, Changhua, Taiwan. [4]Department of Genomic Science and Technology, Changhua Christian Hospital Healthcare System, Changhua, Taiwan. [5]Institute of Biochemistry, Microbiology and Immunology, Chung-Shan Medical University, Taichung, Taiwan. [6]Department of Medical Laboratory Science and Biotechnology, Central Taiwan University of Science and Technology, Taichung, Taiwan. [7]Department of Obstetrics and Gynecology, Taiwan Adventist Hospital, Taipei, Taiwan. [8]Department of Obstetrics and Gynecology, College of Medicine, National Taiwan University, Taipei, Taiwan. [9]Welgene Biotechnology Company, Nangang Business Park, Taipei, Taiwan. [10]Department of Obstetrics and Gynecology, Feinberg School of Medicine, Northwestern University Medical Center, Chicago, IL, USA. [11]Graduate Institute of Medical Genomics and Proteomics, College of Medicine, National Taiwan University, Taipei, Taiwan. [12]Department of Electrical Engineering, University of California Los Angeles, Los Angeles, CA, USA. [13]National Chiao-Tung University, Hsinchu, Taiwan. [14]Department of Obstetrics and Gynecology, Changhua Christian Hospital, Changhua, Taiwan. [15]Department of Medical Genetics, National Taiwan University Hospital, Taipei, Taiwan. [16]Department of Life Science, Tunghai University, Taichung, Taiwan.

References

1. Chitty LS, Lo YM. Noninvasive prenatal screening for genetic diseases using massively parallel sequencing of maternal plasma DNA. Cold Spring Harb Perspect Med. 2015;5:a023085.

2. Society for Maternal-Fetal Medicine, (SMFM) with the assistance of Norton ME, Biggio JR, Kuller JA, Blackwell SC. The role of ultrasound in women who undergo cell-free DNA screening. Am J Obstet Gynecol. 2017;216:B2–7.

3. Hatt L, Brinch M, Singh R, Møller K, Lauridsen RH, Schlütter JM, et al. A new marker set that identifies fetal cells in maternal circulation with high specificity. Prenat Diagn. 2014;34(11):1066–72.

4. Schlütter JM, Kirkegaard I, Petersen OB, Larsen N, Christensen B, Hougaard DM, et al. Fetal gender and several cytokines are associated with the number of fetal cells in maternal blood–an observational study. PLoS One. 2014;9(9):e106934.

5. Beaudet AL. Using fetal cells for prenatal diagnosis: history and recent progress. Am J Med Genet C Semin Med Genet. 2016;172(2):123–7.

6. Breman AM, Chow JC, U'Ren L, Normand EA, Qdaisat S, Zhao L, et al. Evidence for feasibility of fetal trophoblastic cell-based noninvasive prenatal testing. Prenat Diagn. 2016;36(11):1009–19.

7. Calabrese G, Fantasia D, Alfonsi M, Morizio E, Celentano C, Guanciali Franchi P, et al. Aneuploidy screening using circulating fetal cells in maternal blood by dual-probe FISH protocol: a prospective feasibility study on a series of 172 pregnant women. Mol Genet Genomic Med. 2016;4(6):634–40.

8. Kølvraa S, Singh R, Normand EA, Qdaisat S, van den Veyver IB, Jackson L, et al. Genome-wide copy number analysis on DNA from fetal cells isolated from the blood of pregnant women. Prenat Diagn. 2016;36(12):1127–34.

9. Wapner RJ, Babiarz JE, Levy B, Stosic M, Zimmermann B, Sigurjonsson S, et al. Expanding the scope of noninvasive prenatal testing: detection of fetal microdeletion syndromes. Am J Obstet Gynecol. 2015;212(3):332. e1-9

10. Gregg AR, Skotko BG, Benkendorf JL, Monaghan KG, Bajaj K, Best RG, et al. Noninvasive prenatal screening for fetal aneuploidy, 2016 update: a position statement of the AmericanCollege of medical genetics and genomics. Genet Med. 2016;18(10):1056–65.

11. Agarwal A, Sayres LC, Cho MK, Cook-Deegan R, Chandrasekharan S. Commercial landscape of noninvasive prenatal testing in the United States. Prenat Diagn. 2013;33(6):521–31.

12. Grati FR, Malvestiti F, Ferreira JC, Bajaj K, Gaetani E, Agrati C, et al. Fetoplacental mosaicism: potential implications for false-positive and false-negative noninvasive prenatal screening results. Genet Med. 2014;16(8):620–4.

13. Meck JM, Kramer Dugan E, Matyakhina L, Aviram A, Trunca C, Pineda-Alvarez D, et al. Noninvasive prenatal screening for aneuploidy: positive predictive values based on cytogenetic findings. Am J Obstet Gynecol. 2015;213(2):214. e1-5

14. Yeang CH, Ma GC, Hsu HW, Lin YS, Chang SM, Cheng PJ, et al. Genome-wide normalized score: a novel algorithm to detect fetal trisomy 21 during non-invasive prenatal testing. Ultrasound Obstet Gynecol. 2014;44(1):25–30.

15. Cheng HH, Ma GC, Tsai CC, WJ W, Lan KC, Hsu TY, et al. Confined placental mosaicism of double trisomies 9 and 21: discrepancy between non-invasive prenatal testing, chorionic villus sampling and postnatal confirmation. Ultrasound Obstet Gynecol. 2016;48(2):251–3.

16. WJ W, Ma GC, Lin YS, Yeang CH, Ni YH, Li WC, et al. Detection of 22q11.2 microduplication by cell-free DNA screening and chromosomal microarray in fetus with multiple anomalies. Ultrasound Obstet Gynecol. 2016;48(4):530–2.

17. WJ W, Ma GC, Lee MH, Chen YC, Chen M. Normal prenatal ultrasound findings reflect outcome in case of trisomy 14 confined placental mosaicism developing after preimplantation genetic diagnosis. Ultrasound Obstet Gynecol. 2017;50:128–30.

18. Ramirez JM, Fehm T, Orsini M, Cayrefourcq L, Maudelonde T, Pantel K, et al. Prognostic relevance of viable circulating tumor cells detected by EPISPOT in metastatic breast cancer patients. Clin Chem. 2014;60(1):214–21.

19. Gross A, Schoendube J, Zimmermann S, Steeb M, Zengerle R, Koltay P. Technologies for single-cell isolation. Int J Mol Sci. 2015;16(8):16897–919.

20. Sahmani M, Vatanmakanian M, Goudarzi M, Mobarra N, Azad M. Microchips and their significance in isolation of circulating tumor cells and monitoring of cancers. Asian Pac J Cancer Prev. 2016;17(3):879–94.

21. Byeon Y, Ki CS, Han KH. Isolation of nucleated red blood cells in maternal blood for non-invasive prenatal diagnosis. Biomed Microdevices. 2015;17(6):118.

22. Zimmermann S, Hollmann C, Stachelhaus SA. Unique monoclonal antibodies specifically bind surface structures on human fetal erythroid blood cells. Exp Cell Res. 2013;319(17):2700–7.

23. Norton ME, Jacobsson B, Swamy GK, Laurent LC, Ranzini AC, Brar H, et al. Cell-free DNA analysis for noninvasive examination of trisomy. N Engl J Med. 2015;372(17):1589–97.

24. Chen M, Yeh GP, Shih JC, Wang BT. Trisomy 13 mosaicism: study of serial cytogenetic changes in a case from early pregnancy to infancy. Prenat Diagn. 2004;24(2):137–43.

25. Greco E, Minasi MG, Fiorentino F. Healthy babies after intrauterine transfer of mosaic aneuploid blastocysts. N Engl J Med. 2015;373(21):2089–90.

26. Gleicher N, Vidali A, Braverman J, Kushnir VA, Barad DH, Hudson C, et al. International PGS consortium study group. Accuracy of preimplantation genetic screening (PGS) is compromised by degree of mosaicism of human embryos. Reprod Biol Endocrinol. 2016;14(1):54.

27. Orvieto R. Preimplantation genetic screening- the required RCT that has not yet been carried out. Reprod Biol Endocrinol. 2016;14(1):35.

28. Orvieto R, Gleicher N. Should preimplantation genetic screening (PGS) be implemented to routine IVF practice? J Assist Reprod Genet. 2016;33(11):1445–8.

29. Tortoriello DV, Dayal M, Beyhan Z, Yakut T, Keskintepe L. Reanalysis of human blastocysts with different molecular genetic screening platforms reveals significant discordance in ploidy status. J Assist Reprod Genet. 2016;33(11):1467–71.

30. Hou S, Chen JF, Song M, Zhu Y, Jan YJ, Chen SH, et al. Imprinted NanoVelcro microchips for isolation and characterization of circulating fetal trophoblasts: toward noninvasive prenatal diagnostics. ACS Nano. 2017; https://doi.org/10.1021/acsnano.7b03073.

31. Mouawia H, Saker A, Jais JP, Benachi A, Bussières L, Lacour B, et al. Circulating trophoblast cells provide genetic diagnosis in 63 fetuses at risk for cystic fibrosis or spinal muscular atrophy. Reprod BioMed Online. 2012;25(5):508–20.

32. Laget S, Broncy L, Hormigos K, Dhingra DM, BenMohamed F, Capiod T, et al. Technical insights into highly sensitive isolation and molecular characterization of fixed and live circulating tumor cells for early detection of tumor invasion. PLoS One. 2017;12(1):e0169427.

33. Ma GC, WJ W, Lee MH, Lin YS, Chen M. The use of low molecular weight heparin reduced the fetal fraction and rendered the cell-free DNA testing for fetal trisomy 21 false negative. Ultrasound Obstet Gynecol. 2017; https://doi.org/10.1002/uog.17473.

34. Sinkey RG, Odibo AO. Cost-effectiveness of old and new technology for aneuploidy screening. Clin Lab Med. 2016;36(2):237–48.

35. Sørensen MD, Gonzalez Dosal R, Jensen KB, Christensen B, Kølvraa S, Jensen UB, et al. Epsilon haemoglobin specific antibodies with applications in noninvasive prenatal diagnosis. J Biomed Biotechnol. 2009;2009:659219.

36. Iacono KT, Brown AL, Greene MI, Saouaf SJ. CD147 immunoglobulin superfamily receptor function and role in patheology. Exp Mol Pathol. 2007;83(3):283–95.

37. Nagao K, Zhu J, Heneghan MB, Hanson JC, Morasson MI, Tessarollo L, et al. Abnormal placental development and early embryonic lethality in EpCAM-null mice. PLoS One. 2009;4(12):e8543.

38. Hackmon R, Pinnaduwage L, Zhang J, Lye SJ, Geraghty DE, Dunk CE. Definitive class I human leukocyte antigen expression in gestational placentation: HLA-F, HLA-E, HLA-C, and HLA-G in extravillous trophoblast invasion on placentation, pregnancy, and parturition. Am J Reprod Immunol. 2017;77(6):e1264377.

39. Schreier S, Sawaison P, Udomsanpetch R, Triampo W. Advances in rare cell isolation: an optimization and evaluation study. J Transl Med. 2017;15:6.

40. Kanda E, Yura H, Kitagawa M. Practicability of prenatal testing using lectin-based enrichment of fetal erythroblasts. J Obstet Gynecol Res. 2016;42(8):918–26.

12

Cytogenetics and stripe rust resistance of wheat–*Thinopyrum elongatum* hybrid derivatives

Daiyan Li[1], Dan Long[1], Tinghui Li[1], Yanli Wu[1], Yi Wang[1], Jian Zeng[2], Lili Xu[1], Xing Fan[1], Lina Sha[1], Haiqin Zhang[1], Yonghong Zhou[1] and Houyang Kang[1*]

Abstract

Background: Amphidiploids generated by distant hybridization are commonly used as genetic bridge to transfer desirable genes from wild wheat species into cultivated wheat. This method is typically used to enhance the resistance of wheat to biotic or abiotic stresses, and to increase crop yield and quality. Tetraploid *Thinopyrum elongatum* exhibits strong adaptability, resistance to stripe rust and *Fusarium* head blight, and tolerance to salt, drought, and cold.

Results: In the present study, we produced hybrid derivatives by crossing and backcrossing the *Triticum durum–Th. elongatum* partial amphidiploid (*Trititrigia* 8801, $2n = 6\times = 42$, AABBEE) with wheat cultivars common to the Sichuan Basin. By means of cytogenetic and disease resistance analyses, we identified progeny harboring alien chromosomes and measured their resistance to stripe rust. Hybrid progenies possessed chromosome numbers ranging from 40 to 47 (mean = 42.72), with 40.0% possessing 42 chromosomes. Genomic in situ hybridization revealed that the number of alien chromosomes ranged from 1 to 11. Out of the 50 of analyzed lines, five represented chromosome addition ($2n = 44 = 42$ W + 2E) and other five were chromosome substitution lines ($2n = 42 = 40$ W + 2E). Importantly, a single chromosome derived from wheat–*Th. elongatum* intergenomic Robertsonian translocations chromosome was occurred in 12 lines. Compared with the wheat parental cultivars ('CN16' and 'SM482'), the majority (70%) of the derivative lines were highly resistant to strains of stripe rust pathogen known to be prevalent in China.

Conclusion: The findings suggest that these hybrid-derivative lines with stripe rust resistance could potentially be used as germplasm sources for further wheat improvement.

Keywords: Genomic in situ hybridization, Stripe rust, *Thinopyrum elongatum*, Hybrid progeny

Background

Sichuan is the largest wheat-producing region in southwest China, both in cultivatable land area and yield. Although many wheat varieties have been cultivated over the years, Sichuan currently faces a lack of breakthrough varieties that is mirrored in reduced grain quality and resistance to pathogens. Wheat stripe rust is one of the most serious wheat diseases. Therefore, stripe rust resistance gene *Yr26* has been widely used in wheat breeding

programs since its discovery in the early 1990s [1]. However, dependence on a single gene can be risky, as the rise of new virulent strains (such as the *Yr26*-virulent race V26/Gui 22) can easily lead to a significant decline in wheat production. *Yr26* virulence may represent a major threat to wheat production in the Sichuan Basin and other regions of China [1]. The use of cultivars harboring novel resistance is an efficient and economical alternative to control wheat stripe rust [2]. The yield and quality of common wheat (*Triticum aestivum* L., $2n = 6\times = 42$, AABBDD), which accounts for 95% of domesticated wheat in globally, can be improved by modifications of its genetic background [3]. Wild relatives of

---

* Correspondence: houyang.kang@sicau.edu.cn
[1]Triticeae Research Institute, Sichuan Agricultural University, 211 Huimin Road, Wenjiang, Chengdu, Sichuan 611130, China
Full list of author information is available at the end of the article

common wheat display numerous desirable agronomic traits, including strong adaptability, resistance to biotic and abiotic stress, and high-quality of wheat, and might thus potentially enrich the genetic repertoire of domesticated wheat species [4, 5]. Distant hybridization is a commonly used approach to modify the genetic background of common wheat in order to introduce the beneficial traits of wild species into the genome of domestic wheat [6, 7]. To date, numerous related species from the tribe *Triticeae*, including those from genera *Aegilops*, *Agropyron*, *Dasypyrum*, *Hordeum*, *Leymus*, *Lophopyrum*, *Psathyrostachys*, *Secale*, and *Thinopyrum*, have been successfully crossed with wheat, and the resulting cultivars have contributed significantly to wheat production worldwide [8–13].

Thinopyrum elongatum (syn. *Lophopyrum elongatum* or *Agropyron elongatum*) is a perennial herb of the tribe *Triticeae* that plays a prominent role as a gene pool source for genomic improvement of common wheat through hybridization. The taxon contains various cytotypes differing in genomic composition and ploidy level: diploid ($2n = 2\times = 14$, EE, syn. E^eE^e), tetraploid ($2n = 4\times = 28$, $E^eE^eE^bE^b$), hexaploid ($2n = 6\times = 42$, $E^eE^eE^bE^bE^bE^b$), and decaploid ($2n = 10\times = 70$, $E^eE^eE^bE^bE^xE^xStStStSt$) [14–16]. The E genome of the diploid *Th. elongatum* is the basal genome of the taxon [14, 15]. *Th. elongatum* has many agronomically desirable traits, including high-quality pasture resources, high protein content, and tolerance to salt, drought, and cold [17]. Several significant global advancements in wheat–*Th. elongatum* hybridization have been developed since the beginning of the twentieth century [18]. As example, Li and colleagues synthesized the first common wheat–*Th. elongatum* hybrids in China and developed a series of new wheat cultivars, such as allogeneic octoploid *Trititrigia* Xiaoyan 4, 5 and 6 [19, 20]. Subsequently, the Chinese Spring–*Th. elongatum* addition and substitution lines were successfully bred by Dvorak et al. [21]. Recent studies have uncovered that chromosomes 1E and 7E confer wheat resistance to *Fusarium* head blight (FHB), and the source of resistance was pinpointed to a gene located on chromosome 7ES [22, 23]. Most recently, multiple disease resistance genes were identified in the genus *Thinopyrum* and they were transferred successfully to common wheat, including genes conferring resistance to stem rust (*Sr24*, *Sr25*, *Sr26*, *Sr43*, and *Sr44*), leaf rust (*Lr19*, *Lr24*, *Lr29*, and *Lr38*), stripe rust (*Yr50*) and powdery mildew (*Pm40* and *Pm43*) [24–27].

The hexaploid *Trititrigia* 8801 ($2n = 6\times = 42$, AABBEE) is a genetically stable partial amphidiploid line induced by hybridization of *Triticum durum* with tetraploid *Th. elongatum* Ae41 ($2n = 4\times = 28$, $E_1E_1E_2E_2$) [28]. It harbors genes of *Th. elongatum* Ae41 that protect against many adverse conditions including stripe rust, powdery mildew, FHB, smut, cold, drought, and salinity [29]. However, owing to its extended growth period and the presence of many alien chromosomes, it is impractical for direct use in the wheat breeding industry. Instead, it is more commonly used as a genetic bridge to transfer alien genes and to create addition, substitution, and translocation lines that can be readily employed in wheat breeding [29]. Moreover, the genetic stability and compensatory effect of translocation lines are superior to those of the addition and substitution lines, thus a translocation line is of potentially greater value in breeding and is more highly regarded by breeders [30].

The objective of the present study was to identify the hybrid progenies derived from crosses between *Trititrigia* 8801 and prevalent *T. aestivum* cultivars grown in the Sichuan region. Using genomic in situ hybridization (GISH) and stripe rust resistance evaluation, we intend to perform a screen to identify genetically stable wheat–*Th. elongatum* progeny lines exhibiting enhanced resistance to stripe rust (Fig. 1). We identified several lines that have the potential to serve as genetic resources for breeding to improve the wheat yield and quality in the Sichuan Basin.

Methods

Plant material

The hexaploid *Trititrigia* 8801 ($2n = 6\times = 42$, AABBEE), which exhibits strong resistance to FHB, stripe rust, and powdery mildew, and wide adaptability including cold, drought, and salt tolerance, was kindly provided by Dr. George Fedak (Eastern Cereal and Oilseed Research Center, Ottawa, Canada). Here we used *T. aestivum* cultivars ($2n = 6\times = 42$, AABBDD) Shumai482 (SM482) and Chuannong16 (CN16) as the parental genotypes susceptible to stripe rust. Fifty progeny lines were derived by hybridization of SM482 and CN16 with *Trititrigia* 8801 (Table 1). The wheat line SY95–71 was used as a susceptible control in stripe rust resistance tests. For GISH analysis, the Sichuan wheat cultivar J-11 ($2n = 6\times = 42$, AABBDD) was used to generate blocking DNA, and the total genomic DNA of tetraploid *Th. elongatum* accession PI531750 ($2n = 4\times = 28$, EEEE) was used to generate probes for labeling.

Genomic in situ hybridization

Total genomic DNA of PI531750 and J-11 was isolated using the cetyltrimethylammonium bromide (CTAB) method [31]. PI531750 DNA was labeled with digoxigenin-11-dUTP (or biotin-11-dUTP) by nick translation (Roche, Mannheim, Germany) and used as a probe. Unlabeled J-11 DNA was fragmented to 300–500 base pairs by autoclaving at 100 kPa, 115 °C for 10 min and subsequently was used for a competitor to block A, B, and D-genome sequences from hybridization.

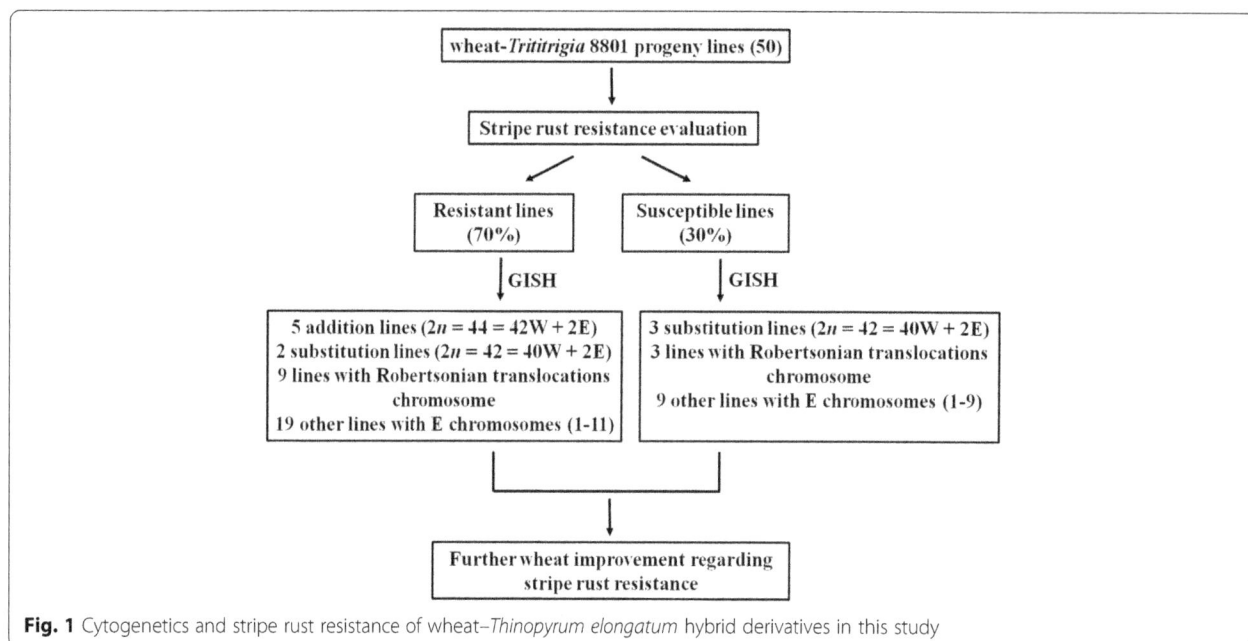

Fig. 1 Cytogenetics and stripe rust resistance of wheat–*Thinopyrum elongatum* hybrid derivatives in this study

Seedling root tips were collected and treated with nitrous oxide for 4 h, 90% acetic acid for 10 min, and digestion by pectinase and cellulase, using the procedure of Komuro et al. [32]. Slides for GISH were prepared as previously described by Han et al. [33], with slight modifications. The hybridization mixture was composed of 37.5% deionized formamide, 15% dextran sulfate, 7.5% 20 × SSC, and 75 µg salmon sperm DNA (initial concentration 10 µg/µL), as well as 50 ng probe DNA (initial concentration 100 ng/µL) and 7.5 µg blocking agent DNA (initial concentration 1250 ng/µL), and the proportion was 1:150 of probe and competitive DNA. A total volume 20 µL of solution was loaded per slide and were denatured together by heating at 80 °C for 5 min, incubated for 8–12 h at 37 °C. Digoxigenin was detected using anti-digoxigenin-rhodamine Fab fragments (Roche, Mannheim, Germany) and biotin was detected with streptavidin-FITC (Roche). Chromosomes were counterstained with 4-6-diamino-2-phenylindole (DAPI) or propidium iodide (PI) solution (Vector Laboratories, Inc., Burlingame, CA, USA). Chromosome images were taken with an Olympus BX-51 microscope equipped with a DP-70 CCD camera. All images were processed using Adobe Photoshop CS 5.0.

Stripe rust resistance screening
Parental species 8801, SM482 and CN16, derived offspring lines, and the control line SY95–71 were each evaluated for seedling and adult plant responses to stripe rust. Stripe rust tests were performed at the Wenjiang experimental station of Sichuan Agricultural University, Chengdu, Sichuan, China. For each line, plants were grown annually in 2 m rows, with inter-plant spacing of

10 cm and inter-row spacing of 30 cm. The stripe rust susceptible spreader line SY95–71 was planted on both sides of each experimental row. The SY95–71 rows were inoculated at the two-leaf stage with a mixture of fresh urediniospores and talc (1:20 ratio). The *Pst* races (CYR-32, CYR-33, V26/Gui22–9, V26/Gui22–14, Su4, and Su5) were supplied by the Research Institute of Plant Protection, Gansu Academy of Agricultural Sciences, Gansu, China. Stripe rust infection types (IT) were recorded on a scale of 0–4. The plants scored with IT 2 or lower were considered as resistant, whereas the plants with IT 3 or 4 were considered as susceptible. Infection was scored three times, when uniform rust stripe severity was observed on SY95–71 during the booting, flowering, and milky stages [34].

Results
GISH analysis of hybrid progenies
Chromosome numbers for 50 randomly selected progeny are presented in Table 1. The mean chromosome number of all hybrid progenies was $2n = 42.72$, with a range of 40–47. Most lines (94.0%) were $2n = 41$–45. Of these, progenies with 42 chromosomes were predominant (40%), whereas the remainder of the progeny displayed various degrees of aneuploidy ($2n = 44, 43, 45, 41, 40, 47$) where the order reflects the decreasing proportion of incidence (16.0%, 14.0%, 12.0%, 12.0%, 4.0% and 2.0%). Among these lines with 42 chromosomes, K13–415-3, K14–480-2 and K15–1016-12 derived from the crosses of *Trititrigia* 8801 with SM482 showed the greatest degree of cytological stability. By contrast, some lines exhibited loss of chromosomes, such as K13–415-1 and K15–1007-5 (from 43 to 42). Collectively, these

Table 1 Chromosome number and stripe rust response of hybrid progenies

Lines	Materials	Generation	Chromosome Numbers				Infection type	Resistance/ susceptibility
			2n	E	W	W/E		
	SY95–71		42		42		4	S
	SM482		42		42		4	S
	CN16		42		42		4	S
	8801		42	14	28		0	R
K13–415-1	8801 × SM482	F_2	43	5	37	1	4	S
K13–415-2	8801 × SM482	F_2	42	6	35	1	4	S
K13–415-3	8801 × SM482	F_2	42	9	33		4	S
K13–415-4	8801 × SM482	F_2	42	5	37		4	S
K13–422-1	8801 × CN16	F_2	43	7	36		0	R
K13–437-3	8801/ SM482// SM482	BC_1F_1	40	3	37		3	S
K13–437-4	8801/ SM482// SM482	BC_1F_1	41	7	33	1	0	R
K13–438-4	8801/ SM482//11 N21	F_1	40	3	37		0	R
K13–439-1	8801/ SM482// SM969	F_1	45	3	42		4	S
K13–439-4	8801/ SM482// SM969	F_1	42	4	38		4	S
K13–440-2	8801/ SM482//N08–51	F_1	42	3	39		0	R
K14–478-6	8801 × SM482	F_3	42	5	36	1	0	R
K14–479-4	8801 × SM482	F_3	44	1	42	1	4	S
K14–480-2	8801 × SM482	F_3	42	2	40		4	S
K14–485-1	8801 × CN16	F_2	43	8	35		0	R
K14–490-4	8801 × CN16	F_2	42	11	31		0	R
K14–499-3	8801/ SM482// SM482	BC_1F_2	44	3	41		3	S
K14–500-4	8801/ SM482// SM482	BC_1F_2	42	2	39	1	0	R
K14–501-3	8801 / SM482 // 11 N21	F_2	44	2	42		2	R
K14–501-4	8801 / SM482 // 11 N21	F_2	42	2	40		1	R
K14–501-5	8801 / SM482 // 11 N21	F_2	41	1	40		1	R
K14–502-1	8801 / SM482 // 11 N21	F_2	43	3	40		0	R
K14–502-3	8801 / SM482 // 11 N21	F_2	43	1	41	1	0	R
K14–502-5	8801 / SM482 // 11 N21	F_2	47	5	42		0	R
K14–509-1	8801 / SM482 // SM969	F_2	42	1	41		3	R
K14–511-9	8801 / SM482 // SM51	F_2	42	1	41		4	S
K14–516-2	8801 / SM482 // SM51	F_2	44	5	39		0	R
K14–516-4	8801 / SM482 // SM51	F_2	45	6	39		0	R
K14–528-1	8801 / SM482 F_2 //SM482	F_1	45	4	41		4	S
K14–528-4	8801 / SM482 F_2 //SM482	F_1	42	2	40		4	S
K14–562-1	8801 / CN16 // CN16	BC_1F_1	42	3	39		2	R
K14–637-2	8801 / SM482 // SM482 /// SM482	BC_2F_1	43	1	42		0	R
K15–1007-1	8801 × SM482	F_4	41	4	36	1	1	R
K15–1007-3	8801 × SM482	F_4	42	5	37		1	R
K15–1007-5	8801 × SM482	F_4	42	4	37	1	1	R
K15–1016-12	8801 × SM482	F_4	42	2	40		3	S
K15–1033-8	8801/ SM482 // SM482	BC_1F_3	43	3	39	1	0	R
K15–1035-11	8801/ SM482 // 11 N21	F_3	44	2	42		2	R
K15–1035-12	8801/ SM482 // 11 N21	F_3	42	2	40		2	R

Table 1 Chromosome number and stripe rust response of hybrid progenies *(Continued)*

Lines	Materials	Generation	Chromosome Numbers				Infection type	Resistance/ susceptibility
			2n	E	W	W/E		
K15–1035-13	8801/ SM482 // 11 N21	F_3	44	2	42		2	R
K15–1036-13	8801/ SM482 // 11 N21	F_3	45	3	42		1	R
K15–1049-1	8801 / SM482 // SM51	F_3	45	6	39		1	R
K15–1049-4	8801 / SM482 // SM51	F_3	45	2	42	1	2	R
K15–1048-10	8801 / SM482 // SM51	F_3	41	4	37		0	R
K15–1058-5	8801 /CN16 //CM104	F_2	41	1	40		3	S
K15–1020-4	8801 × CN16	F_3	42	10	31	1	0	R
K15–1053-3	8801 /CN16 // aobaimai3	F_2	41	1	40		1	R
K15–1083-1	8801/ SM482 // SM482 F_2 /// SM482	F_1	44	2	42		1	R
K15–1035-4	8801/ SM482 // 11 N21	F_3	44	2	42		2	R
K15–1005-3	8801 × SM482	F_4	42	6	36		1	R

Abbreviations: E E-genome chromosomes of *Th. elongatum, W* A, B, and D-genome chromosomes of wheat, *W/E* translocation chromosome of wheat–*Th. elongatum.* The wheat line SY95–71 was used as a susceptible control. Infection type was based on a scale of 0–4, where 0 = resistant, and 1–4 indicate increasing sporulation and decreasing necrosis or chlorosis, considered highly resistant, resistant, susceptible, and highly susceptible, respectively

observations indicated that the chromosome number of 8801-derived hybrid progeny tended to conform with the chromosome number of common wheat ($2n = 42$).

To identify the alien chromosomes derived from *Trititrigia* 8801 in the 50 progeny lines, we performed GISH using genomic DNA of tetraploid *Th. elongatum* accession PI531750 as a probe. The number of *Th. elongatum* chromosomes in the progeny lines ranged from 1 to 11 (Table 2). Figure 2 provides representative examples of chromosome substitution (Fig. 2a–d), addition (Fig. 2e, f), addition-substitution (Fig. 2g–i), and translocation (Fig. 2j–l) in the progeny. Most of the resulting daughter plants (42%) represent substitution lines, in which from one up to 11 chromosomes of common wheat were replaced by E-specific chromosomes (Fig. 2a–d). Among the lines possessing 42 chromosomes, five exhibited substitution with two E chromosomes (Fig. 2b). Chromosome addition ($2n > 42$) was detected in nine lines, with up to five E chromosomes being added (Fig. 2e, f). Five lines possessed 44 chromosomes, with two additional E chromosomes (Fig. 2e). We also identified eight

Table 2 Chromosome constitutions of hybrid progenies

Chromosome number	Number of lines	Number of E chromosomes (number of lines)
40	2	3 (2)
41	6	1 (3), 4 (1), 4.5 (1), 7.5 (1)
42	20	1 (2), 2 (5), 2.5 (1), 3 (2), 4 (1), 4.5 (1), 5 (2), 5.5 (1), 6 (1), 6.5 (1), 9 (1), 10.5 (1), 11 (1)
43	7	1 (1), 1.5 (1), 3 (1), 3.5 (1), 5.5 (1), 7 (1), 8 (1)
44	8	1.5 (1), 2 (5), 3 (1), 5(1)
45	6	2.5 (1), 3 (2), 4 (1), 6 (2)
47	1	5 (1)

addition-substitution lines (Fig. 2g–i). In line K13–422-1 ($2n = 43 = 36$ W + 7E), for example, six common wheat chromosomes were replaced and one additional E chromosome was inserted. Most importantly, a single product of intergenomic (wheat–*Th. elongatum*) Robertsonian (Rb) translocation was observed uniformly in 12 progeny lines (Fig. 2j–l). In addition, during the process of selfing (e.g. K13–415-2) or backcrossing (e.g. K13–422-1), majority of the alien chromisomes have been lost and, in some plants, they were completely lacking. The above-mentioned examples indicated that lines with $2n = 42$ or $2n = 44$ may be cytologically stable, and those with a Rb translocation may loose the chromosomes in the process of transmission to the next generation, or form a new pair of stable translocation chromosomes by recombination.

Stripe rust resistance evaluation

Each of the 50 derivative lines, the parental lines (8801, SM482 and CN16), and a stripe rust-sensitive control line (SY95–71) was evaluated for stripe rust resistance using a mixture of *Pst* races (see Materials and Methods). Representative examples of stripe rust resistance are provided in Fig. 3. At the seedling and adult plant stages, the 8801 parental line was highly resistant to stripe rust (IT = 0). By contrast, SM482, CN16, and SY95–71 showed IT scores of 4, indicating susceptibility to stripe rust (Table 1). Of the 50 derivative lines, 35 (70.0%) exhibited resistance to stripe rust, whereas the remaining 15 (30%) were susceptible.

Discussion

Distant hybridization is a promising method to transfer agronomically valuable genes from wild relatives to

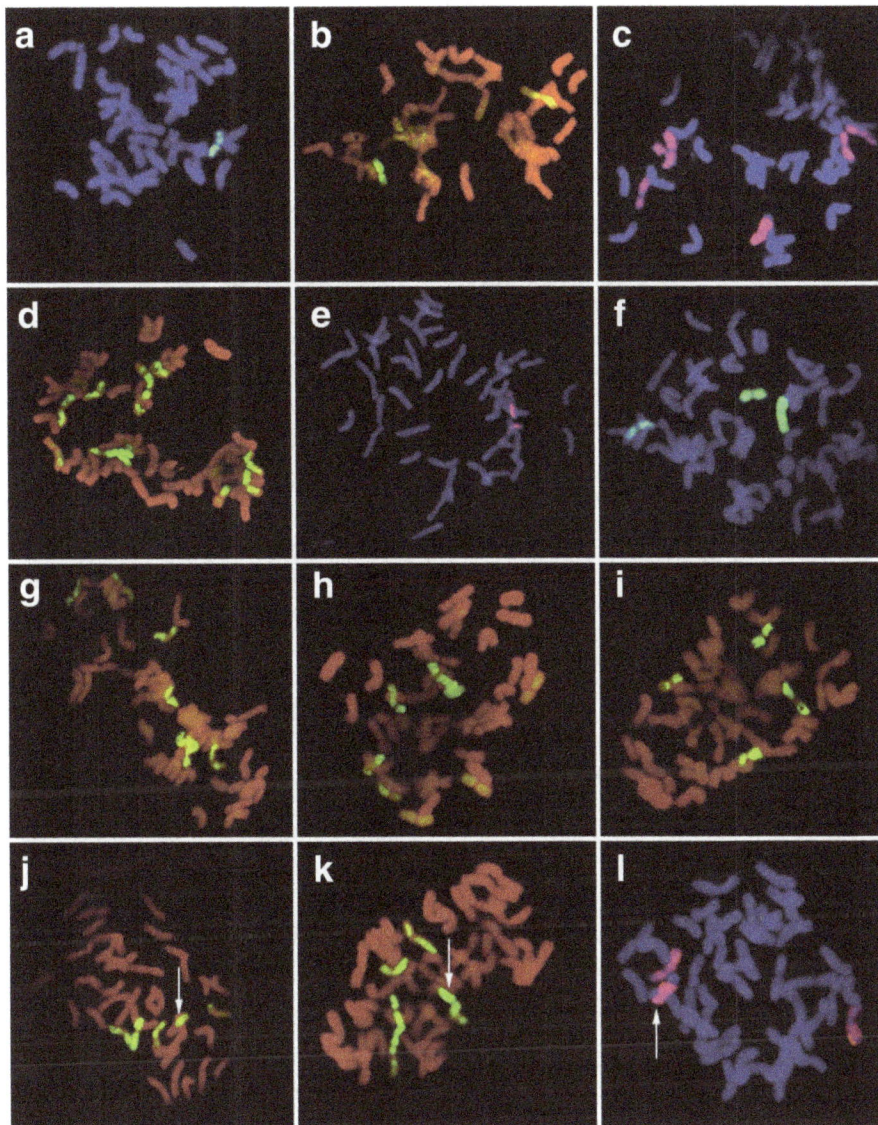

Fig. 2 GISH analysis of hybrid progenies at mitotic metaphase. *Thinopyrum elongatum* genomic DNA was used as a probe for in situ hybridization. Chromosomes in red and blue are derived from wheat (W); chromosomes in yellow-green, green, and pink are derived from *Th. elongatum* (E). Arrows indicate Robertsonian translocations. **a** K15–1058-5, $2n = 41 = 1E + 40$ W; (**b**) K14–480-2, $2n = 42 = 2E + 40$ W; (**c**) K15–1005-3, $2n = 42 = 6E + 36$ W; (**d**) K14–490-4, $2n = 42 = 11E + 31$ W; (**e**) K15–1083-1, $2n = 44 = 2E + 42$ W; (**f**) K15–1036-13, $2n = 45 = 3E + 42$ W; (**g**) K13–422-1, $2n = 43 = 7E + 36$ W; (**h**) K14–485-1, $2n = 43 = 8E + 35$ W; (**i**) K14–528-1, $2n = 45 = 4E + 41$ W; (**j**) K15–1007-1, $2n = 41 = 4E + 1$ W/E + 36 W; (**k**) K14–478-6, $2n = 42 = 5E + 1$ W/E + 36 W; (**l**) K15–1049-4, $2n = 45 = 2E + 1$ W/E + 42 W

common wheat. Creating intermediate lines carrying alien chromosomes provides a basis for using germplasm resources of wheat relatives to improve domesticated wheat [35, 36]. *Th. elongatum* harbors many beneficial genes that protect against adverse conditions such as disease, cold, drought, and salinity, and thus represents a promising gene donor to improve tolerance to biotic or abiotic stresses in common wheat [37–39]. In the current study, we produced hybrid progenies by crossing a *Triticum durum–Th. elongatum* partial amphidiploid (*Trititrigia* 8801, $2n = 6 \times = 42$, AABBEE) with prevalent

wheat cultivars grown in the Sichuan area. A previous study demonstrated that the chromosome number of derivative progeny is gradually reaching back the natural chromosome number of *T. aestivum* ($2n = 42$) with each subsequent generation, and a similar phenomenon has been observed in both inbred and backcross lines [40]. In the present study, we provided another evidence that the number of chromosomes in hybrid progenies approaches 42 (*T. aestivum* L., $2n = 42$). It is often observed that chromosomes of different parental subgenomes segregate unequally to daughter cells in

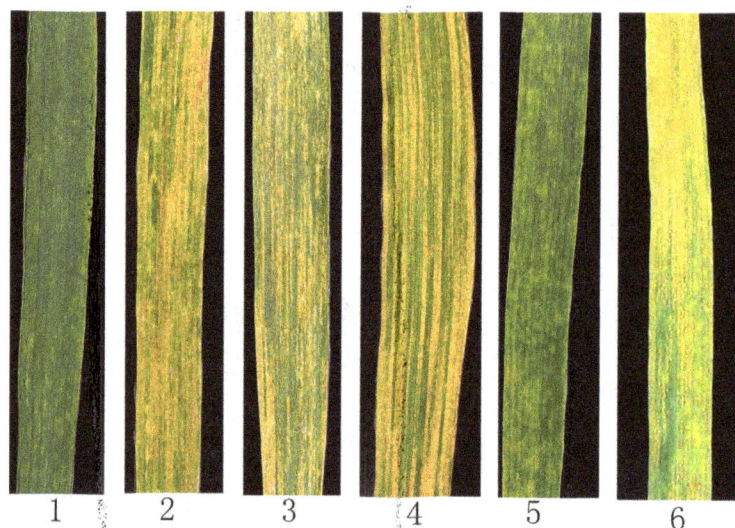

Fig. 3 Representative examples of stripe rust resistance in parental lines, hybrid progeny, and controls. (1) *Trititrigia* 8801; (2) *T. aestivum* Shumai482; (3) *T. aestivum* Chuannong16; (4) *T. aestivum* SY95–71; (5) resistant derivative line K15–1007-1; (6) susceptible derivative line K15–1016-12

progeny derived from distant hybridization. Such observation may result from the chromosome elimination during mitosis [41, 42]. Also in our study, we observed unequal chromosome divisions. For example, K13–415-1, K13–415-2, K13–415-3, and K13–415-4 are derived from the same individual parental lines but differed in chromosome number. Likewise, K14–485-1 and K14–490-4 were derived from the same parental lines (*Trititrigia* 8801 and CN16) and also differed in chromosome number.

Identification of alien chromosomes against the wheat chromosome background is an essential step in utilizing alien genetic resources. The Rb translocations typically result from erroneous repair of double strand breaks (by NHEJ pathway), where the p-arms and possibly also one centromere from the original monoarmed chromosome are lost [43]. In the wheat meiosis the process, sister centromeres often lose their coordination in metaphase I and lead to stable bipolar attachment and frequent separation of sister chromatids or to misdivision in the progression of anaphase I, and misdivision may occur across the centromere region or across thepericentric chromatin and subsequent fusion of broken centromeres [44]. In the present study, GISH revealed that all translocated chromosomes had undergone Rb translocation. The line K13–415-1 had a Rb translocation chromosome transmitted to the following generation by single-seed descent, which indicated that this translocation chromosome may remain stable in future generations. Furthermore, some generations derived by single-seed descent from the same parental lines, such as line K13–438-4, showed an elevated number of chromosomes produced by Rb translocations, which indicated that continuous

selfing favors the inheritance of alien chromosomes in future generations and contributes to the appearance of new alien types. A similar phenomenon was observed in a previous study by Guan [45]. The formation of a new translocation is probably due to multiple chromosomes breakages in late meiosis at the same time fracture, and chromosomal fragments are misjoined to form aberrant novel chromosome [46]. In addition, the present GISH analysis showed that during the process of selfing or backcrossing, alien chromosomes are predominantly lost or (in some individuals) completely lost. Our findings are in agreement with previous study of Wu et al. [47] in the sense that the plants from the earlier generations tend to sustain/retain more alien chromosomes in comparison to those of later generations. With increase in number of selfing or backcrossing generations, alien chromosome differentiation occurs. In the present study, we identified five relatively stable addition lines ($2n = 44 = 42$ W + 2E) and five substitution lines ($2n = 42 = 40$ W + 2E). Furthermore, a previous study indicated that partial homology exists between wheat and *Th. elongatum* [48], and Cai et al. [49] identified genes that promote partial homologous chromosome pairing in *Th. elongatum*. In addition, in wheat, *Ph1* is a major chromosome pairing locus facilitating correct pairing of homologous, and in wheat hybrids *Ph1* prevents pairing between related chromosomes [35, 50, 51]. This may be another important reason for the chromosome pairing diversity of *Th. elongatum* and different wheat-derived hybrids observed in the present study.

The Sichuan Basin is one of the most important regions for wheat production in China, but it has suffered a serious stripe rust epidemy in recent years. In this study, a series of stripe rust-resistant strains was obtained through distant hybridization with strains carrying E-genome chromosomes. Further work is needed to identify the genomic composition of these lines by fluorescence in situ hybridization (FISH) and to evaluate their agronomic performance. Nevertheless, these lines provide novel and valuable bridge resources for improvement of stripe rust resistance in wheat.

Conclusion

The use of amphiploid provides a facile method to transfer alien genes to common wheat compared with the direct use of wild species [52]. In this study, we selected and identified substitution, addition, and translocation lines that exhibited high resistance to stripe rust. Although the experimental lines are still in early generation, these lines have the potential to serve as primary material for wheat genetic improvements. Further work is needed to identify the genomic composition of these lines by FISH and to evaluate their agronomic performance. In conclusion, genes with desirable traits were transferred to wheat, thereby extending the genetic source of wheat breeding, enriching genetic diversity and improving the yield and quality of wheat.

Acknowledgments

We thank Dr. George Fedak, Eastern Cereal and Oilseed Research Center, Ottawa, Canada, for kindly supplying the *Trititrigia* 8801 material used in this study. We thank Robert McKenzie, PhD, from Liwen Bianji, Edanz Group China (https://www.liwenbianji.cn), for editing the English text of a draft of this manuscript. We thank the anonymous reviewers of the manuscript for their useful comments.

Funding

This work was funded by the National Key Research and Development Program of China (2016YFD0102000, 2017YFD0100905), the National Natural Science Foundation of China (No. 31501311, 31771781), and the Science and Technology Bureau of Sichuan Province (No. 2016HH0048).

Authors' contributions

HYK conceived and designed the research. DYL, DL, THL, and YLW conducted the experiments. YW, JZ, LLX, XF, and LNS participated in the preparation of the reagents and materials. HQZ, YHZ and HYK analyzed the data. DYL and DL wrote the manuscript. All the authors read and approved the manuscript.

Competing interests

The authors declare that they have no competing interests.

Author details

[1]Triticeae Research Institute, Sichuan Agricultural University, 211 Huimin Road, Wenjiang, Chengdu, Sichuan 611130, China. [2]College of Resources, Sichuan Agricultural University, 211 Huimin Road, Wenjiang, Chengdu, Sichuan 611130, China.

References

1. Han DJ, Wang QL, Chen XM, Zeng QD, Wu JH, Xue WB, et al. Emerging *Yr26*-virulent races of *Puccinia striiformis f. tritici* are threatening wheat production in the Sichuan Basin, China. Plant Dis. 2015;99(6):754–60.
2. Ren Y, Li S, Xia X, Zhou Q, He Y, Wei Y, et al. Molecular mapping of a recessive stripe rust resistance gene *YrMY37* in Chinese wheat cultivar Mianmai 37. Mol Breeding. 2015;35(3):97.
3. Dubcovsky J, Dvorak J. Genome plasticity a key factor in the success of polyploid wheat under domestication. Science. 2007;316:1862–6.
4. Dong YS, Zhou RH. Xu SJ, Cauderon Y, Wang RC. Desirable characteristics in perennial Triticeae collected in China for wheat improvement. Hereditas. 1992;116:175–8.
5. Mujeeb-Kazi A, Kazi AG, Dundas I, Rasheed A, Ogbonnaya F, Kishii M, et al. Chapter four-genetic diversity for wheat improvement as a conduit to food security. In: Advances in agronomy. Edited by Dr. Sparks. Vol. 122. Burlington: academic press; 2013. p. 179–257.
6. Qi L, Friebe B, Zhang P, Gill BS. Homoeologous recombination, chromosome engineering and crop improvement. Chromosom Res. 2007; 15(1):3–19.
7. Qi W, Tang Y, Zhu W, Li D, Diao C, Xu L, et al. Molecular cytogenetic characterization of a new wheat-rye 1BL·1RS translocation line expressing superior stripe rust resistance and enhanced grain yield. Planta. 2016;244(2): 405–16.
8. Cabrera A, Martin A. A trigeneric hybrid between *Hordeum*, *Aegilops*, and *Secale*. Genome. 1992;35(4):647–9.
9. Li LH, Dong YS. A self-fertile trigeneric hybrid, *Triticum aestivum* × *Agropyron michnoi* × *Secale cereale*. Theor Appl Genet. 1993;87(3):361–8.
10. Sun GL, Yen C, Yang JL, Wu BH. Production and cytogenetics of intergeneric hybrids between *Triticum durum-Dasypyrum villosum* amphidiploid and *Psathyrostachys huashanica*. Euphytica. 1995;81(1):7–11.
11. Mujeeb-Kazi A. Apomixis in Trigeneric hybrids of *Triticum aestivum/Leymus racemosus//Thinopyrum elongatum*. Cytologia. 1996;61(1):15–8.
12. Kang HY, Wang H, Huang J, Wang YJ, Li DY, Diao CD, et al. Divergent development of hexaploid triticale by a wheat – *Rye* –*Psathyrostachys huashanica* trigeneric hybrid method. PLoS One. 2016;11(5):e0155667.
13. Kang HY, Tang L, Li DY, Diao CD, Zhu W, Tang Y, et al. Cytogenetic study and stripe rust response of the derivatives from a wheat-*Thinopyrum intermedium - Psathyrostachys huashanica* trigeneric hybrid. Genome. 2016; 60:393–401.
14. Dewey DR. The genomic system of classification as a guide to intergeneric hybridization with the perennial triticeae. In *Gene Manipulation in Plant Improvement*. Edited by Gustafson, J. P. New York: Plenum Press; 1984. p. 209–210.
15. Lou H, Dong L, Zhang K, Wang DW, Zhao M, et al. High throughput mining of E-genome specific SNPs for characterizing Thinopyrum elongatum introgressions in common wheat. Mol Ecol Resour 2017; doi:https://doi.org/ 10.1111/1755-0998.12659.
16. Mao PS, Huang Y, Wang XG, Lin M, Mao PC, Zhang GF. Cytological evaluation and karyotype analysis in plant germplasms of *Elytrigia* Desv. Agric Sci China. 2010;9(11):1553–60.
17. Guo Q, Meng L, Mao PC, Tian XX. Salt tolerance in two tall wheatgrass species is associated with selective capacity for K $^+$ over Na $^+$. Acta Physiol Plan. 2015;37(1):1708.
18. Dvorak J, Phylogenetic CKC. Relationships between chromosomes of wheat and chromosome. Genome. 1984;26(2):128–32.
19. Li Z, Li B, Tong Y. The contribution of distant hybridization with decaploid *Agropyron elongatum* to wheat improvement in China. J Genet Genomics. 2008;35(8):451–6.
20. Zhang X, Dong Y, Wang RR. Characterization of genomes and chromosomes in partial amphiploids of the hybrid *Triticum aestivum* × *Thinopyrum ponticum* by in situ hybridization, isozyme analysis, and RAPD. Genome. 1996;39(6):1062–71.

21. Dvorak J, Sosulski FW. Effects of additions and substitutions of *Agropyron elongatum* chromosomes on quantitative characters in wheat. Can J Genet Cytol. 1974;16(3):627–37.

22. Jauhar PP, Peterson TS, Xu SS. Cytogenetic and molecular characterization of a durum alien disomic addition line with enhanced tolerance to fusarium head blight. Genome. 2009;52(5):467–83.

23. Fu S, Lv Z, Qi B, Guo X, Li J, Liu B, et al. Molecular cytogenetic characterization of wheat-*Thinopyrum elongatum* addition, substitution and translocation lines with a novel source of resistance to wheat fusarium head blight. J Genet Genomics. 2012;39(2):103–10.

24. Zhang X, Shen X, Hao Y, Cai J, Ohm HW, Kong L. A genetic map of *Lophopyrum ponticum* chromosome 7E, harboring resistance genes to fusarium head blight and leaf rust. Theor Appl Genet. 2011;122(2):263–70.

25. Niu Z, DL K, Yu G, Friesen TL, Chao S, Jin Y, et al. development and characterization of wheat lines carrying stem rust resistance gene *Sr43* derived from *Thinopyrum ponticum*. Theor Appl Genet. 2014;127(4):969–80.

26. Tang X, Shi D, Xu J, Li Y, Li W, Ren Z, et al. Molecular cytogenetic characteristics of a translocation line between common wheat and *Thinopyrum intermedium* with resistance to powdery mildew. Euphytica. 2014;197:201–10.

27. Li G, Wang H, Lang T, Li J, La S, Yang E, et al. New molecular markers and cytogenetic probes enable chromosome identification of wheat-*Thinopyrum intermedium* introgression lines for improving protein and gluten contents. Planta. 2016;244:865–76.

28. Guo X, Shi Q, Wang J, Hou Y, Wang Y, Han F. Characterization and genome changes of new amphiploids from wheat wide hybridization. J Genet Genomics. 2015;42(8):459–61.

29. Xin WL. Cytogenetic study on crosses between octoploid Trititrigia and hexaploid Trititrigia. Heilongjiang agricultural. Science. 1998;3:4–7.

30. Sears ER. Chromosome engineering in wheat. Stadler Symposia, University of Missouri, Columbia. 1972;4:23-38.

31. Allen GC, Flores-Vergara MA, Krasynanski S, Kumar S, Thompson WF. A modified protocol for rapid DNA isolation from plant tissues using cetyltrimethylammonium bromide. Nat Protoc. 2006;1(5):2320–5.

32. Komuro S, Endo R, Shikata K, Kato A. Genomic and chromosomal distribution patterns of various repeated DNA sequences in wheat revealed by a fluorescence in situ hybridization procedure. Genome. 2013;56(3):131–7.

33. Han F, Liu B, Fedak G, Liu Z. Genomic constitution and variation in five partial amphiploids of wheat–*Thinopyrum intermedium* as revealed by GISH, multicolor GISH and seed storage protein analysis. Theor Appl Genet. 2004; 109(5):1070–6.

34. Study LXK. On the yellow rust resistance to common wheat (*T.aestivum*). Plant Prot. 1988;15:33–9.

35. Liu D, Zhang H, Zhang L, Yuan Z, Hao M, Zheng Y. Distant hybridization: a tool for interspecific manipulation of chromosomes. Springer New York. 2014;9(1):e86667.

36. Kwiatek M, Belter J, Majka M, Wiśniewska H. Allocation of the S-genome chromosomes of *Aegilops variabilis* powdery mildew resistance in triticale (×*Triticosecale*Wittmack). Protoplasma. 2016;253(2):329–43.

37. Lammer D, Cai X, Arterburn M, Chatelain J, Murray T, Jones S. A single chromosome addition from *Thinopyrum elongatum* confers a polycarpic, perennial habit to annual wheat. J Exp Bot. 2004;55(403):1715–20.

38. Chen S, Huang Z, Dai Y, Qin S, Gao Y, Zhang L, et al. The development of 7E chromosome-specific molecular markers for *Thinopyrum elongatum* based on SLAF-seq technology. PLoS One. 2013;8(6):e65122.

39. Dai Y, Duan Y, Liu H, Chi D, Cao W, Xue A, et al. Molecular cytogenetic characterization of two *Triticum-Secale-Thinopyrum* trigeneric hybrids exhibiting superior resistance to fusarium head blight, leaf rust, and stem rust race Ug99. Front Plant Sci. 2017;8:797.

40. Wang MX, Zhang CZ, Cytology WCY. Of the progenies derived from hybrid between wheat and octoploid agroticum. Journal of Shanxi. Agric Sci. 2008; 36(2):26–7.

41. Tu Y, Sun J, Ge X, Li Z. Chromosome elimination, addition and introgression in intertribal partial hybrids between Brassica Rapa and Isatis Indigotica. Ann Bot. 2009;103(7):1039–48.

42. Tang Z, Fu S, Yan B, Zhang H, Ren Z. Unequal chromosome division and inter-genomic translocation occurred in somatic cells of wheat–rye allopolyploid. J Plant Res. 2012;125(2):283–90.

43. WMRB R. Chromosome studies. I. Taxonomic relationships shown in the chromosomes of Tettegidae and Acrididiae: V-shaped chromosomes and their significance in Acrididae, Locustidae and Grillidae: chromosomes and variations. J Morphol. 1916;27:179–331.

44. Lukaszewski AJ. Behavior of centromeres in univalents and centric misdivision in wheat. Cytogenet Genome Res. 2010;129(1–3):97–109.

45. Guan Q. Formation, meiotic stability and karyotype analysis of octoploid agrotriticum hybrids. Acta Agron Sin. 1980;6(3):129–37.

46. Zhang X, Dong Y, Li Z. Cytogenetic Research on hybrids between *Trilicum* and Decaploid *Thinopyrum ponticum* and their derivatives I. Chromosome pairing in Decaploid Th. ponticum and F₁ hybrids of it with both *T. aeativum* and *T. durum*. J Genet Genomics. 1993;20(5):439–47.

47. Wu J, Zhao JX, Chen XH, Liu SH, Yang QH, Liu WX, et al. Cytology characteristic and GISH analysis on the progenies derived from common wheat (*T.aestivum* L.) ×*Psathyrostachys huashanica*. Journal of Triticeae Crops. 2007;27(5):772–5.

48. Dvorak J. Homoeology between *Agropyron elongatum* chromosomes and *Triticum aestivum* chromosomes. Can J Genet Cytol. 1980;22(2):237–59.

49. Cai X, Jones S. Direct evidence for high level of autosyndetic pairing in hybrids of *Thinopyrum intermedium* and *Th. ponticum* with *Triticum aestivum*. Theor Appl Genet. 1997;95(4):568–72.

50. Martinezperez E, Shaw P, Moore G. The *Ph1* locus is needed to ensure specific somatic and meiotic centromere association. Nature. 2001; 411(6834):204–7.

51. Griffiths S, Sharp R, Foote TN, et al. Molecular characterization of *Ph1* as a major chromosome pairing locus in polyploid wheat. Nature. 2006; 439(7077):749–52.

52. Feldman M, Levy AA. Allopolyploidy–a shaping force in the evolution of wheat genomes. Cytogenet Genome Res. 2005;109(2):250–8.

13

Formation of upd(7)mat by trisomic rescue: SNP array typing provides new insights in chromosomal nondisjunction

Sandra Chantot-Bastaraud[1,2,3,4], Svea Stratmann[5], Frédéric Brioude[1,2,3], Matthias Begemann[5], Miriam Elbracht[5], Luitgard Graul-Neumann[6], Madeleine Harbison[7], Irène Netchine[1,2,3] and Thomas Eggermann[5*]

Abstract

Background: Maternal uniparental disomy (UPD) of chromosome 7 (upd(7)mat) accounts for approximately 10% of patients with Silver-Russell syndrome (SRS). For upd(7)mat and trisomy 7, a significant number of mechanisms have been proposed to explain the postzygotic formation of these chromosomal compositions, but all have been based on as small number of cases. To obtain the ratio of isodisomy and heterodisomy in UPDs (hUPD, iUPD) and to determine the underlying formation mechanisms, we analysed a large cohort of upd(7)mat patients ($n = 73$) by SNP array typing. Based on these data, we discuss the UPDs and their underlying trisomy 7 formation mechanisms.

Results: A whole chromosome 7 maternal iUPD was confirmed in 28.8%, a mixture or complete maternal hUPD in 71.2% of patients.

Conclusions: We could demonstrate that nondisjunction mechanism affecting chromosome 7 are similar to that of the chromosomes more frequently involved in trisomy (and/or UPD), and that mechanisms other than trisomic rescue have a lower significance than previously suspected. Furthermore, we suggest SNP array typing for future parent- and cell-stage-of origin studies in human aneuploidies as they allow the definite classification of trisomies and UPDs, and provide information on recombinational events and their suggested association with aneuploidy formation.

Keywords: Maternal uniparental Disomy 7, Formation mechanism, Chromosome 7, Trisomic rescue

Background

With a frequency of 0.5% among newborns and up to 50% among abortions, human trisomies significantly contribute to human malformations and human reproduction failure. Therefore comprehensive studies have been focused on the origin and formation mechanisms of human aneuploidies, and their etiological factors. For the common autosomal trisomies 13, 18 and 21, it has been shown that they are mainly caused by meiotic errors in oogenesis, whereas the number of trisomic cases originating from missegregation in paternal meiosis or postzygotic mitosis is low [1]. Increased maternal age as well as altered numbers and the distribution of recombination sites have been identified as risk factors for errors in the maternal meiosis (for review: [2]). Naturally, the majority of data have been obtained from the frequent human numerical aberrations, whereas studies on the other chromosomes are hampered because they are not compatible with live and therefore only randomly ascertained, e.g. in prenatal diagnosis or in abortions. As a result, it is difficult to assess whether general formation mechanisms and factors exist which contribute to chromosomal nondisjunction and trisomy, or whether these factors are specific for each chromosome as suggested by Hassold et al. [1].

With the increasing number of reported cases with uniparental disomies (UPDs), this ascertainment problem could at least in part be circumvented for some of the rare trisomies in particular those which significantly contribute to the high reproductive failure in humans and/or can frequently be detected in prenatal testing

---

* Correspondence: teggermann@ukaachen.de
[5]Institute of Human Genetics, RWTH University Hospital Aachen, Pauwelsstr 30, D-52074 Aachen, Germany
Full list of author information is available at the end of the article

(e.g. chromosomes 7, 16, 20). UPD as the exceptional inheritance of both homologues of a chromosomal pair from the same parent has been reported for nearly every human chromosome [3]. In case the affected chromosome harbors imprinted genes, an imprinting disorder will arise (e.g Prader-Willi syndrome, Silver-Russell syndrome) [4], but for many chromosomes a specific UPD phenotype does not exist as they do not harbor imprinted genes. Several mechanisms of UPD formation have been identified or suggested, with trisomic rescue as the most important one [5]: here the supernumerary chromosome of an originally trisomic zygote is lost, a mechanism which has been confirmed in-vivo (e.g. [6–9]) (Fig. 1). In contrast, other mechanisms of UPD formation are conceivable but are rare because they require a lot of events.

The parental origin and the cell-stage of formation of trisomy and UPD can be determined by polymorphic DNA markers consisting of at least two different alleles

(Fig. 1). In case of a normal biparental transmission, an individual inherits one allele from each parent. In case of UPD, only alleles from one parent can be observed in the offspring. In case the contributing parent is heterozygous for two different alleles and both are transferred, the child has a uniparental heterodisomy (hUPD) for this marker. In case only one allele is inherited twice, the offspring is carrier of a uniparental isodisomy (iIUPD). By considering the physical localization of polymorphic DNA markers on a chromosome and the type of UPD (iUPD or hUPD), the stage of meiotic nondisjunction can be inferred (Fig. 1). In case pericentromeric markers show hUPD, a meiosis I error is probably the major step of UPD formation, in case of iUPD for these markers a meiosis II nondisjunction can be assumed. In contrast, a iUPD of a whole chromosomes is rather compatible with a postzygotic mitotic nondisjunction mechanism, for this constitution three different modes of formation have been postulated: (i) gamete complementation (fertilization of a

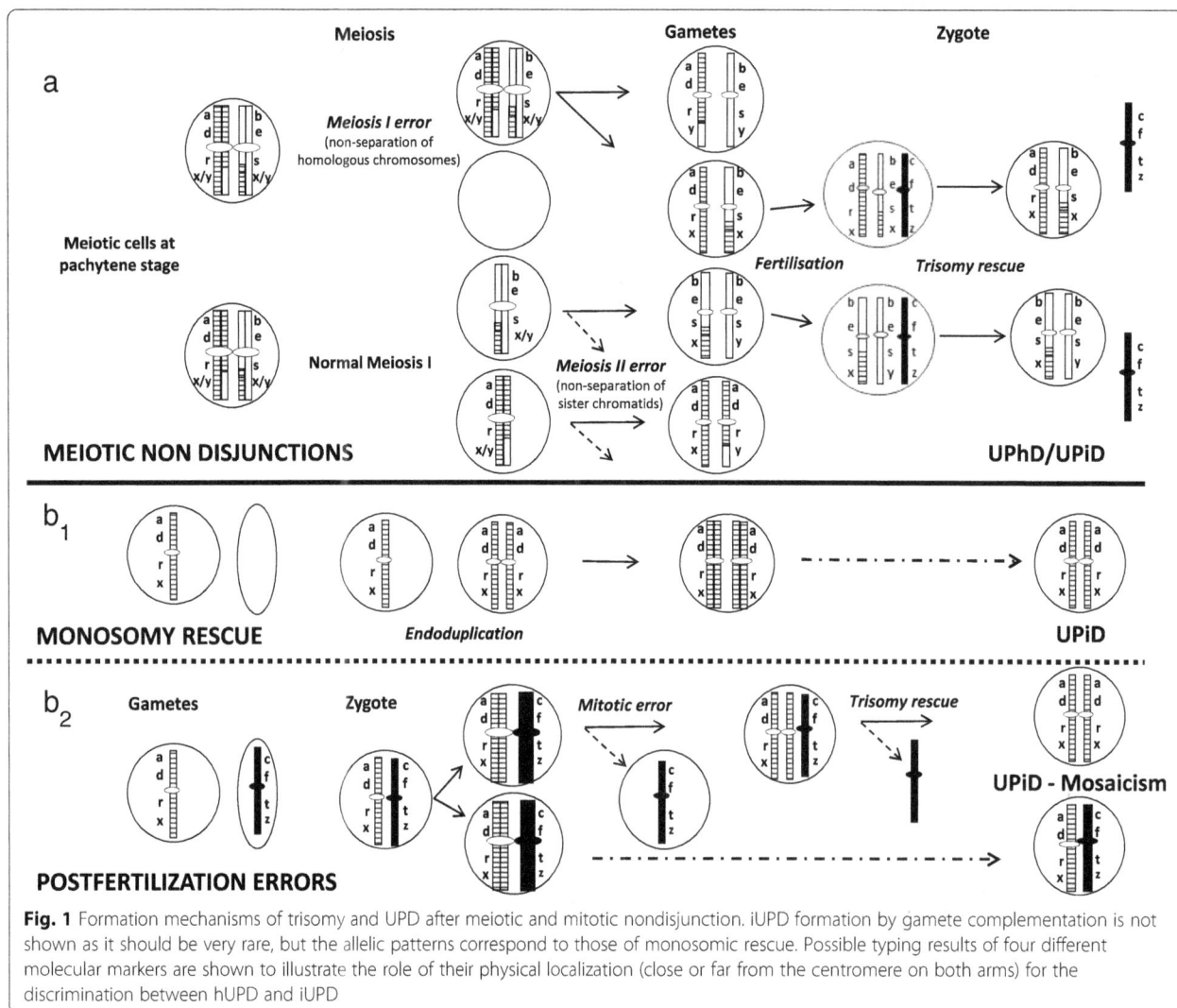

Fig. 1 Formation mechanisms of trisomy and UPD after meiotic and mitotic nondisjunction. iUPD formation by gamete complementation is not shown as it should be very rare, but the allelic patterns correspond to those of monosomic rescue. Possible typing results of four different molecular markers are shown to illustrate the role of their physical localization (close or far from the centromere on both arms) for the discrimination between hUPD and iUPD

nullisomic by a disomic gamete), (ii) monosomic rescue (fertilization of a nullisomic by a monosomic gamete with subsequent endoduplication), and (iii) postfertilization errors (nondisjunction in a originally disomic zygote resulting in a trisomy mosaicism and rescue in a subsequent mitosis, associated with a mosaic constitution) [5].

Until recently, nearly all studies on UPD formation have been based on microsatellite analyses (short tandem repeat markers, short sequence repeat markers), i.e. on a group of polymorphic markers consisting of alleles of different repeat numbers. The high information content of microsatellite markers and their chromosomal position allow the delineation of the parental origin of the supernumerary chromosome as well as determination of the cell-stage in which the nondisjunction occurs. However, the use of microsatellites is limited by their number and the incomplete coverage in the genome. In contrast single nucleotide polymorphisms, despite their limitation to two alleles, have the advantage of extreme frequency and wide distribution over the human genome. With the application of SNP array analysis for molecular karyotyping and the possibility to differentiate between a homozygosity and heterozygosity as well as uniparental isodisomy and heterodisomy, SNP arrays have become a valuable tool to enlighten the formation mechanisms of trisomies and UPDs [2, 10].

A relevant UPD in humans is maternal UPD of chromosome 7 (upd(7)mat), which accounts for approximately 10% of patients with Silver-Russell syndrome (SRS, [11]). It has been suggested that a considerable number of cases are the result from a postzygotically occurring trisomy 7, [1, 12], in that case trisomy 7 would be different from other autosomal trisomies. To obtain a representative overview on the ratio of isodisomy and heterodisomy in UPDs and the underlying formation mechanisms, we analysed a large cohort of upd(7)mat individuals by SNP array microsatellite typing. Based on these data, we discuss their formation mechanism and that of their underlying trisomy 7.

Study population

Our study cohort was derived from patients who had been referred for routine testing for Silver-Russell syndrome (SRS) to either the French or the German laboratories. Some of them have already been reported [11–16]. Our final cohort consisted of the 76 patients who were confirmed to have upd(7)mat. In three patients, a segmental UPD restricted to the long arm had been reported previously [13, 14]. The others 73 patients carried a UPD of the whole chromosome 7. Upd(7)mat/upd(7q)mat was identified molecularly by microsatellite typing and methylation-specific assays targeting loci on both arms of chromosome 7.

To compare the distribution of recombination breakpoints between the German upd(7)mat carriers and controls, we used data from 28 unrelated German controls of normal growth.

The study was approved by the ethics review boards of the University Hospital of the RWTH Aachen and the Hôpitaux de Paris. Written informed consent for participation was received for all patients, either from the patients themselves or their parents.

Methods

Upd(7)mat was identified in the routine diagnostic workup by methylation-specific tests (methylation-specific (MS)-PCR, MS single nucleotide primer extension (MS-SNuPE), MS multiplex ligation probe-dependent amplification (MS-MLPA), or ASMM RTQ-PCR (TaqMan Allele-Specific Methylated Multiplex Real-Time Quantitative PCR)), the upd(7)mat was then confirmed by microsatellite typing. Further information on the markers used and PCR conditions are available on request.

From three of the patients with a mixed hUPD/iUPD, fibroblasts were available and tested by MS-MLPA.

For genome-wide copy number analysis and to determine the size of isodisomic regions, the patients were typed by SNP array analysis.

In the 34 German patients, Affymetrix SNP6.0 array analysis (Affymetrix, Santa Clara, California/USA) was carried out following the manufacturer's protocol. Data analysis was performed with the Genotyping Console and Chas software (Affymetrix). For iUPD detection, the software option "LOH" (loss of heterozygosity) was used, indicating all regions with a loss of heterozygosity (LOH) (default: >1 kb, >50 marker) (Fig. 2). Chromosomal regions were classified as iUPD in case of a LOH, the non-LOH parts of the chromosomes 7 were defined as hUPD. The number of recombinations was delineated from the number of hUPD and iUPD stretches per patient. Furthermore, mosaicism for trisomy 7 was determined by SNP array typing, using a test that had been validated for a mosaic detection level of 5%.

The 42 patients samples analysed in France were processed using Infinium assays (HumanCytoSNP-12 or Omniexpress-24BeadChips, Illumina, San Diego, California/USA) as previously described [17]. Results were analysed with the Illumina Genome Studiosoftware. For iUPD detection, CNV partition 3.1.6 software were used, indicating all regions with a loss of heterozygosity with a minimum size of 1,000,000 and a minimum 3 Probe Count.

Results

In the group of 73 carriers of whole chromosome upd(7)mat tested by SNP array analysis, we determined

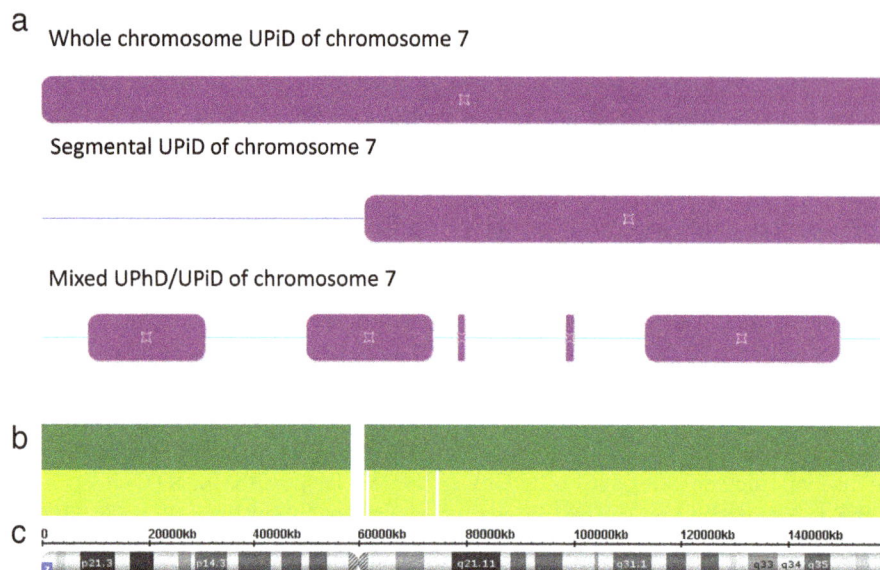

Fig. 2 Local Affymetrix GenomeWideSNP_6.0 Array signal distribution pattern (**a**) showing total upd(7)mat, segmental iUPD(7q)mat and mixed hUPD/iUPDiUPD. Note that only a differentiation between hUPD and iUPD is possible, whereas the parental origin as well as the identification of segmental UPD is only possible by including the results of microsatellite typing. **b** Distribution of SNP (light green) and oligo probes (*dark green*). **c** Physical map of chromosome 7

a complete iUPD in 28.8% (21/73) and a mixture of complete hUPD or iUPD/hUPD in 71.2% (52/73) of patients (Table 1). Mean maternal age in the hUPD cohort (n = 33) was 36.24+/−5.77, in the iUPD group (n = 16) it was 31.33+/−5.39 years, the difference was statistically significant (p = 0.006).

SNP array analysis in the three segmental upd(7q)mat carriers revealed a iUPD for the whole uniparental regions and confirmed the sizes of the UPD segments obtained from previous microsatellite studies [13, 14].

The frequency of recombination events was determined in 20 German hUPD carriers by the Affymetrix SNP 6.0 array analysis. On average, 9.2 recombinations/chromosome 7 could be observed per individual, this frequency did not differ significantly from that in the control population (9.8/individual). Furthermore, the

Table 1 Origin and (postulated) formation mechanisms of the most frequent autosomal trisomies and UPDs. (°only UPD cases with a definite classification as hUPD or iUPD from [18] are listed)

Chromosome	N=	Trisomy					N=	UPD°				Reference
		Maternal		Paternal		PZM		Maternal		Paternal		
		MI	MII	MI	MII			UPhD	UPiD	UPhD	UPiD	
2	18	53.4%	13.3%	27.8%		5.6%	11	45.4%	36.4%	9.1%	9.1%	Reviewed by [1, 3]
6							18	-	11.1%		88.8%	Reviewed by [3]
7	14	27.2%	25.7%			57.1%	55	61.8%	38.2%		4.3%	Reviewed by [1, 18]
							73	71.2%	28.8%			Own data: [11, 12]
8	12	50.0%	50.0%			50.0%	4	50.0%	25.0%		25.0%	Reviewed by [1, 3]
13	74	56.6%	33.9%	2.7%	5.4%	1.4%	10	30.0%	20.0%	10.0%	40.0%	Reviewed by [1, 3]
14	26	36.5%	36.5%		19.2%	7.7%	48	45.8%	28.8%	10.4%	17.7%	Reviewed by [1, 3]
15	34	76.3%	9.0%		14.7%		62	80.6%	6.5%	1.6%	11.3%	Reviewed by [1, 8]
16	104	100.0%					35	91.4%	5.7%		2.8%	Reviewed by [1, 3]
18	150	33.3%	58.7			8.0%	2					Reviewed by [1, 3]
20	3	2		1		-	5	60.0%	20.0%		20.0%	Reviewed by [3]
21	782	69.6%	23.6	1.7%	2.3%	2.7%	12	33.3%	33.3%		33.3%	Reviewed by [1, 3]
22	130	86.4%	10.0	1.8%		1.8%	17	52.9%	11.8%		35.3%	Reviewed by [1, 3]

recombination events showed a similar distribution over the whole chromosome 7 in both cohorts.

In the hUPD cohort, there was no common isodisomic region but the isodisomic regions were randomly distributed (Fig. 3).

Array typing in lymphocytes as well as MS-MLPA in fibroblasts from three out of these cases did not provide evidence for a trisomy 7/upd(7)mat mosaicism.

As expected, molecular karyotyping revealed several apathogenic copy number variations, but there was no evidence for any pathogenic genomic imbalances in this cohort.

Discussion

Previous reports suggested that in upd(7)mat and trisomy 7 formation postzygotic mitotic nondisjunction plays a significant role, accounting for 40 to 57% of cases, respectively (Table 1), [1, 3, 12, 18, 19] Based on the heterogeneous findings in trisomies and UPDs of other chromosomes it has been suggested that three chromosome-specific nondisjunction mechanisms should exist: a) those accounting for all chromosomes, b) those affecting a subset of chromosomes, and c) those responsible for aneuploidies of single chromosomes [1]. However, some of these assumptions were based on single case reports or small cohorts, and a standardized set of markers covering a whole chromosome has not been applied. With the present study we can show

for chromosome 7 that the majority of whole chromosome upd(7)mat cases are hUPD or mixed hUPD/iUPD and thus originates from maternal meiosis nondisjunction. With a percentage of ~71%, maternal meiotic errors are the dominant cause of upd(7)mat formation, corresponding to that of the common autosomal trisomies (Table 1). In fact, this number is probably higher, as some iUPD might originate from a meiotic II error without precedent recombination. Additionally, the major role of maternal meiosis in upd(7)mat formation is corroborated by the increased maternal age in the hUPD group in comparison to the iUPD cohort. Altered numbers and locations of recombination events as further factor contributing to nondisjunction in trisomy 21 could not be confirmed for upd(7)mat.

Interestingly, we did not get any evidence for trisomy 7 mosaicism in three hUPD carriers, although the upd(7)mat formation by trisomic rescue has been proven directly or indirectly in single studies [6, 7, 12, 20, 21]. In fact, low-level mosaicism can hardly be detected by SNP array analysis, but we think that trisomy 7 cell lines should be extremely rare in the body as this constitution is not compatible with life. The situation seems to be different in the placenta as the presence of extraembryonic trisomy 7 cells does obviously not affect fetal growth [22]. As a result, it is obvious that the SRS phenotype is associated with the upd(7)mat and not with an undetectable trisomy 7.

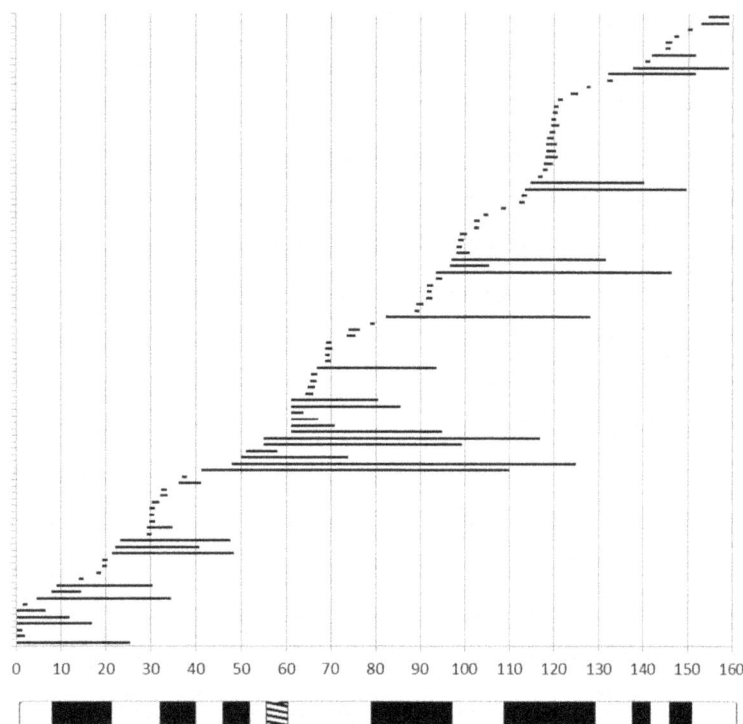

Fig. 3 Analysis of the data from the array typing in hUPD carriers: Distribution of uniparental isodisomy stretches in the 20 hUPD cases analysed by the Affymetrix SNP6.0 arrays

Trisomic rescue after meiotic nondisjunction is probably the major mode of upd(7)mat formation in case of hUPD. However, in case of iUPD the formation mechanism is difficult to determine. At first glance, the reports on extraembryonic trisomy 7 mosaicism in upd(7)mat indicate that a postzygotic nondisjunction followed by a trisomic rescue might have occurred. In that case mosaicism for a normal biparental disomic, a trisomic and iUPD cell line can be expected. As there is no functional reason for the elimination of the biparental disomic cells, iUPD should therefore be associated with a mosaicism for at least iUPD and normal cells. However, there is no evidence for a iUPD/biparental cell lines mosaicism, we therefore assume that whole iUPD of chromosome 7 rather occurs by monosomy rescue than by a postfertilization error.

In the three carriers of a segmental upd(7q)mat we could confirm that the uniparental segments were totally isodisomic. This finding is in agreement with similar studies on segmental UPDs of chromosomes 6 and 11 representing the major fraction of reported segmental UPDs in humans [23] (for review: [24, 25]). Interestingly, mosaicism for segmental UPD can be observed only in BWS, caused by postzygotic mitotic errors. In case of segmental upd(6q)mat and upd(7q)mat a mosaic distribution has not yet been reported, it therefore remains unclear whether they are also caused mitotically or by meiotic errors.

In our cohort of 73 upd(7)mat carriers we did not detect any further uniparental (iso)disomies or pathogenic copy number variations, as reported recently for a maternal upd(6)mat and a upd(11p)pat carrier [10, 14]. Furthermore, there was no evidence for a common isodisomic segment on chromosome 7 in all patients (Fig. 3). Thus, an autosomal recessive factor on this chromosome causing SRS can be excluded, and we thereby support the microsatellite-based data from Preece et al. [26].

Our results confirm the power of SNP array typing to characterize hUPDs and to determine UPD formation mechanisms. As Keren et al. [23] recently demonstrated, SNP array analysis is also a valuable tool to determine the mosaic distribution of upd(11)pat and partial trisomy 11 cell lines in BWS. However, in case of upd(7)mat mosaicism both of UPD and trisomic cell lines is extremely rare. Therefore for routine diagnosis, it is sufficient to perform methylation-specific tests and microsatellite typing.

Conclusions

Our data illustrate the limitations of microsatellite-based formation studies, thus results based on this type of markers should be considered with caution as they depend on the distribution of the used markers over the chromosome. Rather we suggest SNP array typing for future parent- and cell-stage-of origin studies in human aneuploidies, because they allow the definite classification of trisomies and UPDs. Additionally, they provide information on recombinational events and their suggested association with aneuploidy formation [2].

Using this approach, we demonstrated that nondisjunction mechanisms affecting chromosome 7 are similar to those affecting chromosomes more frequently involved in trisomy (and/or UPD), and that mechanisms other than trisomic rescue have a lower significance than previously suspected.

Acknowledgements
Not applicable.

Funding
The authors are supported by the Bundesministerium für Bildung und Forschung (Network "Imprinting Diseases", 01GM1513B) and members of the COST Action BM1208 and EUCID.net (European congenital imprinting disorders network; www.imprinting-disorders.eu).

Authors' contributions
SCB has analysed and interpreted the array data of the French cohort and was a major contributor in writing the manuscript. SS and MB have performed and interpreted the molecular data in the German cohort, and revised the draft of the paper. FB, ME, LGN, MH have diagnosed the patients, supervised the sample drawing, linked the molecular data with the clinical data, and revised the draft of the paper. IN and TE have supervised the study, and prepared the paper. All authors read and approved the final manuscript.

Competing interests
The authors declare that they have no competing interests.

Author details
[1]INSERM, UMR_S 938, CDR Saint-Antoine, F-75012 Paris, France. [2]UMR_S 938, CDR Saint-Antoine, Sorbonne Universities, UPMC Univ Paris, 06 Paris, France. [3]APHP, Armand Trousseau Hospital, Pediatric Endocrinology, Paris, France. [4]APHP, Hôpital Armand-Trousseau, Département de Génétique, UF de Génétique Chromosomique, Paris, France. [5]Institute of Human Genetics, RWTH University Hospital Aachen, Pauwelsstr 30, D-52074 Aachen, Germany. [6]Institute of Human Genetics, Charité University Hospital, Berlin, Germany. [7]Department of Pediatrics, Icahn School of Medicine at Mount Sinai, New York, NY, USA.

References
1. Hassold T, Hall H, Hunt P. The origin of human aneuploidy: where we have been, where we are going. Hum Mol Genet. 2007; Spec No. 2:R203–8.
2. Oliver TR, Middlebrooks CD, Tinker SW, Allen EG, Bean LJ, Begum F, et al. An examination of the relationship between hotspots and recombination associated with chromosome 21 nondisjunction. PLoS One. 2014;9:e99560.

3. Kotzot D, Utermann G. Uniparental disomy (UPD) other than 15: phenotypes and bibliography updated. Am J Med Genet A. 2005;136:287–305.

4. Eggermann T, Netchine I, Temple K, Tümer Z, Monk D, Mackay D, Grønskov K, Riccio A, Linglart A, Maher ER. Congenital imprinting disorders: EUCID.Net – a network to decipher their aetiology and Congenital imprinting disorderic and clinical care. Clin. Epigenetics. 2015;7:123.

5. Eggermann T, Soellner L, Buiting K, Kotzot D. Uniparental Disomy and mosaicism in context with pregnancy. Trends Mol Med. 2015;21(2):77–87.

6. Sharp A, Moore G, Eggermann T. Evidence from skewed X inactivation for trisomy mosaicism in silver-Russell syndrome. Eur J Hum Genet. 2001;9:887–91.

7. Petit F, Holder-Espinasse M, Duban-Bedu B, Bouquillon S, Boute-Benejean O, Bazin A, Rouland V, et al. Trisomy 7 mosaicism prenatally misdiagnosed and maternal uniparental disomy in a child with pigmentary mosaicism and Russell-silver syndrome. Clin Genet. 2012;81:265–71.

8. Robinson WP, Bernasconi F, Mutirangura A, Ledbetter DH, Langlois S, Malcolm S, Morris MA, et al. Nondisjunction of chromosome 15: origin and recombination. Am J Hum Genet. 1993;53:740–51.

9. Robinson WP, Kuchinka BD, Bernasconi F, Petersen MB, Schulze A, Brondum-Nielsen K, et al. Maternal meiosis I non-disjunction of chromosome 15: dependence of the maternal age effect on level of recombination. Hum Mol Genet. 1998;7:1011–9.

10. Schroeder C, Sturm M, Dufke A, Mau-Holzmann U, Eggermann T, Poths S, et al. UPDtool: a tool for detection of iso- and heterodisomy in parent-child trios using SNP microarrays. Bioinformatics. 2013;29:1562–4.

11. Eggermann T, Wollmann HA, Kuner R, Eggermann K, Enders H, Kaiser P, Ranke MB. Molecular studies in 37 silver-Russell syndrome patients: frequency and etiology of uniparental disomy. Hum Genet. 1997;100:415–9.

12. Mergenthaler S, Wollmann HA, Burger B, Eggermann K, Kaiser P, Ranke MB, Schwanitz G, Eggermann T. Formation of uniparental disomy 7 delineated from new cases and a UPD7 case after trisomy 7 rescue. Presentation of own results and review of the literature. Ann Genet. 2000;43:15–21.

13. Eggermann T, Schönherr N, Jäger S, Spaich C, Ranke MB, Wollmann HA, Binder G. Segmental maternal UPD(7q) in silver-Russell syndrome. Clin Genet. 2008;74:486–9.

14. Begemann M, Spengler S, Kordass U, Schröder C, Eggermann T. Segmental maternal uniparental disomy 7q associated with DLK1/GTL2 (14q32) hypomethylation. Am J Med Genet A. 2012;158A:423–8.

15. Netchine I, Rossignol S, Dufourg MN, Azzi S, Rousseau A, Perin L, Houang M, et al. 11p15 Imprinting center region 1 loss of methylation is a common and specific cause of typical Russell-silver syndrome: clinical scoring system and epigenetic-phenotypic correlations. J Clin Endocrinol Metab. 2007;92: 3148–54.

16. Azzi S, Salem J, Thibaud N, Chantot-Bastaraud S, Lieber E, Netchine I, Harbison MD. A prospective study validating a clinical scoring system and demonstrating phenotypical-genotypical correlations in silver-Russell syndrome. J Med Genet. 2015;52:446–53.

17. Steemers FJ, Chang W, Lee G, Barker DL, Shen R, Gunderson KL. Whole-genome genotyping with the single-base extension assay. Nat Methods. 2006 Jan;3:31–3.

18. Kotzot D. Maternal uniparental disomy 7 and silver-Russell syndrome - clinical update and comparison with other subgroups. Eur J Med Genet. 2008;51:444–51.

19. Gardner RJ, Sutherland GR, Shaffer LG. Chromomal aberrations in men, 4th ed. Oxford Monographs on Medical Genetics. 2011;

20. Mergenthaler S, Sharp A, Ranke MB, Kalscheuer VM, Wollmann HA, Eggermann T. Gene dosage analysis in silver-Russell syndrome: use of quantitative competitive PCR and dual-color FISH to estimate the frequency of duplications in 7p11.2-p13. Genet Test. 2001;5:261–6.

21. Monk D, Hitchins M, Russo S, Preece M, Stanier P, Moore GE. No evidence for mosaicism in silver-Russell syndrome. J Med Genet. 2001;38:E11.

22. Kalousek DK, Langlois S, Robinson WP, Telenius A, Bernard L, Barrett IJ, Howard-Peebles PN, Wilson RD. Trisomy 7 CVS mosaicism: pregnancy outcome, placental and DNA analysis in 14 cases. Am J Med Genet. 1996;65:348–52.

23. Keren B, Chantot-Bastaraud S, Brioude F, Mach C, Fonteneau E, Azzi S, Depienne C, Brice A, Netchine I, Le Bouc Y, Siffroi JP, Rossignol S. SNP arrays in Beckwith-Wiedemann syndrome: an improved diagnostic strategy. Eur J Med Genet. 2013;56:546–50.

24. Poke G, Doody M, Prado J, Gattas M. Segmental maternal UPD6 with prenatal growth restriction. Mol Syndromol. 2013;3:270–3.

25. Andrade RC, Nevado J. De Faria Domingues de lima MA, Saad T, Moraes L, Chimelli L, Lapunzina P, Vargas FR. Segmental uniparental isodisomy of chromosome 6 causing transient diabetes mellitus and merosin-deficient congenital muscular dystrophy. Am J Med Genet A. 2014;164A(11):2908–13.

26. Preece MA, Abu-Amero SN, Ali Z, Abu-Amero KK, Wakeling EL, Stanier P, Moore GE. An analysis of the distribution of hetero- and isodisomic regions of chromosome 7 in five mUPD7 Silver-Russell syndrome probands. J Med Genet. 1999;36:457–60.

14

Can telomere shortening be the main indicator of non-viable fetus elimination?

Nataliya Huleyuk[1*], Iryna Tkach[1], Danuta Zastavna[1,2] and Miroslaw Tyrka[2]

Abstract

Background: Telomeres are transcriptionally inactive genomic areas, which, if shortened, are associated with pathological processes, unsuccessful fertilization, aging, and death. Telomere dysfunction has also been linked to chromosomal rearrangements and genomic instability. The role of telomeres in postnatal life has been extensively studied and discussed both in physiological as well as in pathological processes. However, the role of telomere length in prenatal development is still poorly understood, and mainly concerns the preimplantation stage. The aim of this study was to estimate relative telomere length in spontaneously eliminated human embryos between 5th and 12th week of gestation.

Results: Relative telomere length was measured from total genomic DNA using a real-time polymerase chain reaction approach. In this study, we examined relative telomere length in 80 spontaneously eliminated embryos and in 25 embryos eliminated due to induced abortions. Relative telomere length in spontaneous abortions was significantly lower ($P = 0.000001$) compared to the induced abortions. Spontaneous abortions with aneuploid anomalies (monosomy X, trisomy 21, trisomy 16 and triploidy) were characterized by shorter telomeres, compared to spontaneous abortions, subgroup with euploid (46,XN) karyotype.

Conclusion: Spontaneously lost pregnancies are characterized by shortened telomeres, especially in embryos with aneuploidies. We hypothesize that the shortening of telomeres is involved in the processes leading to spontaneous abortions.

Keywords: Relative telomere length, Spontaneous abortions, Aneuploidy, Euploidy

Background

Telomeres are transcriptionally inactive areas of the human genome, involved in maintenance of genomic integrity. Telomere DNA consists of 10–15 kb long hexamer iterations (TTAGGG)n [1, 2], which end with a 3′-single-helixed area, creating a D-loop [3, 4]. Formation of telomeric loop takes place with support of the shelterin complex, which consists of 6 proteins (TRF1, TRF2, TIN2, RAP1, TPP1 and POT1). The main function of this complex is to prevent degradation of telomeres [5]. During each cellular division, telomeric DNA is shortened by 50–200 bp [6–8]. As soon as the length of telomeres becomes critically low, the cells stop dividing and enter apoptosis [9, 10]. Thus, telomeres are believed to be the so-called cellular clock, which controls division

and cellular death. Moreover, telomere dysfunction is linked to chromosomal rearrangements, genomic instability, tumorigenesis and cellular senescence [11, 12].

Telomere length (TL) is proposed to be an indicator of biological age of an organism, and a significant correlation between age and TL has been shown [13]. Role of telomeres during postnatal development was intensely studied and discussed both for normal and pathological conditions. In particular, telomere length is decreased in diabetes mellitus [14], cardiovascular disease [15], liver disorders [16, 17], cancer [18], and severe premature aging phenotypes [19]. Decreased TL has also been linked to adiposity [20, 21], low social and economic status [22], chronic emotional stress [23], smoking [24], increased mortality [25] and others.

However, the role of telomere length in prenatal human development remains mostly unknown, both under pathological as well as under physiological conditions, and the available data is contradictory [26–29]. Few recent studies mainly focused on preimplantation stages of

* Correspondence: huleyuk@yahoo.com
[1]Institute of Hereditary Pathology, NAMS of Ukraine, Lysenko Str. 31a, Lviv 79008, Ukraine
Full list of author information is available at the end of the article

human embryonic development available due to preimplantation diagnostic procedures [30–33]. According to the recent data, aneuploid human polar bodies possess significantly shorter telomeres than euploid polar bodies from sibling oocytes, although, at the blastocyst stage, telomeres did not differ in euploid and aneuploid embryos [30, 31]. It is also likely that the chance of successful in vitro fertilization decreases along with the decrease in TL in oocytes. In particular, it has been shown by Keefe et al. [32, 33] that oocytes from women who did not conceive after in vitro fertilization had shorter telomeres compared to those who did. In addition, oocytes from cycles that produced fragmented embryos also had shorter telomeres.

In summary, shortened telomeres were already associated with pathological processes, unsuccessful fertilization, aging, and death. In this regard, here we estimated the relative telomere length in spontaneously aborted human embryos at 5–12 weeks of gestation (w.o.g). In addition, the results of this pioneering study were interpreted taking into account the presence of chromosomal anomalies.

Methods

In this work, we have studied relative telomere lengths (RTL) in 80 chorionic villi samples (CVS) from spontaneously eliminated product of conception at 5–12 weeks of gestational age (spontaneous abortions - SA) and from 25 induced abortions (IA) due to personal reasons at the same term of gestation. All studied pregnancies occurred naturally. Maternal age ranged from 20 to 34 years.

Collection of chorionic villi samples

A total of 105 chorionic villi samples (CVS) at 5–12 weeks of gestation were obtained from pregnant women, 80 of them from spontaneous abortions with the following selected karyotype:

- 46,XX or 46,XY – 32 samples;
- 69,XXN – 13 samples;
- trisomy 16–13 samples;
- trisomy 21–10 samples;
- monosomy X – 12 samples;

and 25 samples from induced abortions with euploid karyotype 46,XN (46,XX or 46,XY).

All CVS samples were tested for absence of maternal deciduae by histological analysis. Samples were washed twice with PBS and stored at – 20 °C until DNA extraction.

DNA extraction

Genomic DNA was extracted using salting-out or phenol/chloroform method, and dissolved in Tris-EDTA pH 8.0. DNA concentration and purity was assessed using Qubit® 2.0 Fluorometer (Thermo Fisher Scientific).

All DNA samples were stored at – 20 °C until telomere length analysis.

RTL measurement by real-time PCR

Relative telomere length was measured from total genomic DNA using a real-time PCR assay [34]. PCR reactions were performed in the Eco Real-Time PCR System (Illumina, Inc), using 1X GoTaq® qPCR Master Mix (Promega) and specific primers (Table 1) in recommended concentrations [34].

Two reaction mixes of PCR reagents were prepared, one for amplification of telomere repeats (T), the other for gene *36B4* (S). Each PCR reaction contained 12 µl of the reaction mix (GoTaq® qPCR Master Mix and primers) and 7 µl (14 ng/aliquot) DNA. Tel1 and tel2 primers for telomeres were added to the final concentrations 270 nM and 900 nM, respectively. The final *36B4* gene primer concentrations were: 36B4u - 300 nM and 36B4d - 500 nM. For each sample in whom T/S ratio was measured, tree identical aliquots of DNA were added to plate T (telomere) and another tree aliquots were added to the same well positions in plate SCG (single copy gene). Reference DNA was included into each PCR run.

The reference DNA for measurement standardization was obtained from whole blood of two healthy individuals (male and female). Standard curves for telomere length and for the single copy gene were generated by performing serial dilutions (dilution factor 1.68) from a reference DNA sample to produce concentrations of DNA ranging from 0.63 to 5 ng/µl in two parallel reactions – one for the telomeric sequences and the other for the reference gene (36B4) (Fig. 1). The data obtained from reference DNA measurement were used to setup calibration curves needed to estimate reaction efficiency and the average RTL. The relative ratio of telomere repeats copy number to *36B4* gene copy number (T/S ratio) in experimental samples were compared to the reference DNA sample. Telomere length was expressed as a relative T/S ratio, based on the calculation of the ΔCt [$Ct_{(telomere)}/Ct_{(single\ gene)}$] value, which was normalized to the average T/S ratio of the reference sample [$2^{-(\Delta Ct(sample)-\ \Delta Ct(control))} = 2^{-\Delta\Delta Ct}$].

Illumina Eco Software v4.1.11.2 was used to generate curves for the telomere signal (T) or the single copy

Table 1 List of specific primers used for determination of telomere length

Primer name	Sequence (5'-3')
Tel 1	GGTTTTTGAGGGTGAGGGTGAGGGTGAGGGTGAGGGT
Tel 2	TCCCGACTATCCCTATCCCTATCCCTATCCCTA
36B4u	CAGCAAGTGGGAAGGTGTAATCC
36B4d	CCCATTCTATCATCAACGGGTACAA

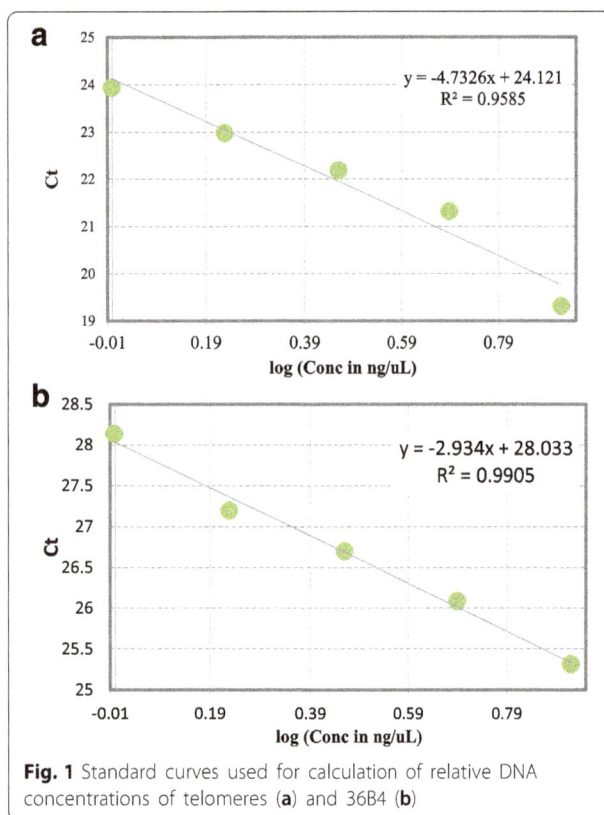

Fig. 1 Standard curves used for calculation of relative DNA concentrations of telomeres (**a**) and 36B4 (**b**)

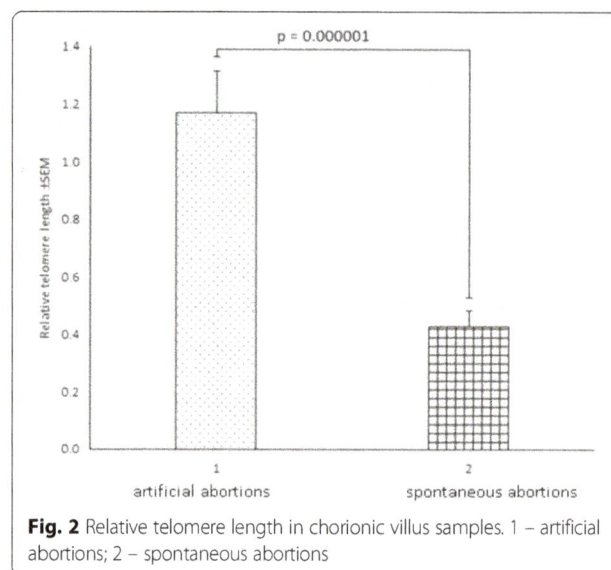

Fig. 2 Relative telomere length in chorionic villus samples. 1 – artificial abortions; 2 – spontaneous abortions

gene signal (S) and to determine quantity of DNA for our research.

The coefficient of variation (standard deviation/mean) was calculated to be 0.89% for within plate measurements and 0.77% for measurement between plates.

Statistical analysis

The data acquired from RLT measurement was normally distributed (Shapiro-Wilk test, $p = 0.00001$). Statistical differences between means were tested with ANOVA and t-test using Statistica 12 (StatSoft, Inc., USA).

Results

The average RTL in the combined group was 0.60 and was characterized by inter-individual variations within the range of 0.03 to 2.94. In the IA group, the average RTL was 1.17 with inter-individual variations ranging from 0.14 to 2.94. In the main SA investigated group, the mean of RTL was 0.43 with inter-individual variations ranging from 0.03 to 2.40 (Table 2).

Statistical analysis showed that RTL were significantly lower in SA group compared to IA group (SA: 0.43 ± 0.06 vs IA: 1.17 ± 0.14, $P = 0.000001$) (Fig. 2).

The SA group was further divided into subgroups depending on the karyotype. Molecular cytogenetic (interphase mFISH with centromeric probe panels for chromosomes 13, 21, 14, 22, 15, 16, 17, 18, X and Y) and cytogenetic studies showed the following results in this group: 32 cases with euploid karyotype (46,XX or 46,XY) and 48 with aneuploid karyotype (autosomal trisomy 21 or 16, triploidy, monosomy X). Variability of the mean RTL for SA with or without chromosome number abnormalities are shown in Table 3.

As indicated in Table 3, the aneuploid SA was characterized by shorter telomeres in comparison to the euploid SA with interindividual variations from 0.07 to 1.66 and from 0.03 to 2.40, respectively.

Statistical analysis showed a highly significant difference in RTL between SA with aneuploid and SA with euploid karyotype (aneuploid: 0.29 ± 0.03 vs euploid: 0.64 ± 0.12, $P = 0.0015$) (Fig. 3).

Further, we compared RTL in SA with different types of aneuploidy - trisomy chromosome 21, trisomy chromosome 16, triploidy and monosomy X (Table 4). The results showed no significant variation in RTL length among the various aneuploid groups (monosomy X: 0.36 ± 0.12; trisomy 21: 0.26 ± 0.03; trisomy 16: 0.28 ± 0.04; and triploidy: 0.27 ± 0.02, $P > 0.05$) (Fig. 4). Consequently, the telomere

Table 2 Relative telomere length ratios in spontaneous and artificial abortions overall and within each group

Overall		Spontaneous abortions		Artificial abortions	
Mean (max-min)	N	Mean (max-min)	n	Mean (max-min)	n
0.60 (0.03–2.94)	105	0.43 (0.03–2.40)	80	1.17 (0.14–2.94)	25

n- number of samples

Table 3 Relative telomere length ratios in spontaneous abortions with euploid or aneuploid karyotype

Overall		Euploid karyotype		Aneuploid karyotype	
Mean (max-min)	n	Mean (max-min)	n	Mean (max-min)	n
0.43 (0.03–2.40)	80	0.64 (0.03–2.40)	32	0.29 (0.07–1.66)	48

n- number of samples

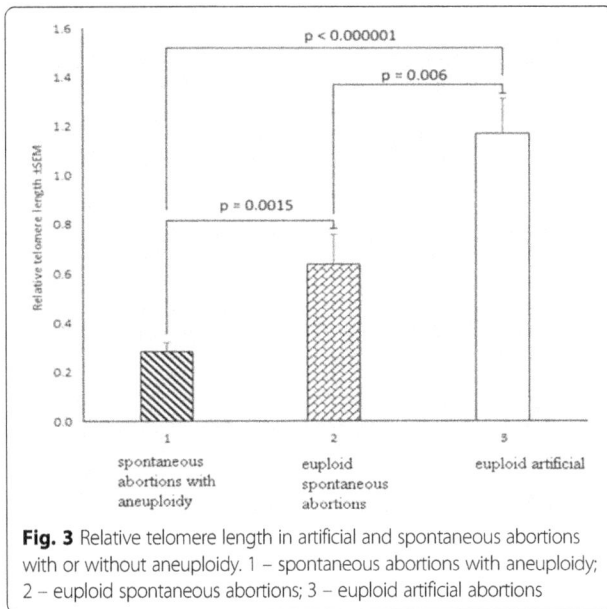

Fig. 3 Relative telomere length in artificial and spontaneous abortions with or without aneuploidy. 1 – spontaneous abortions with aneuploidy; 2 – euploid spontaneous abortions; 3 – euploid artificial abortions

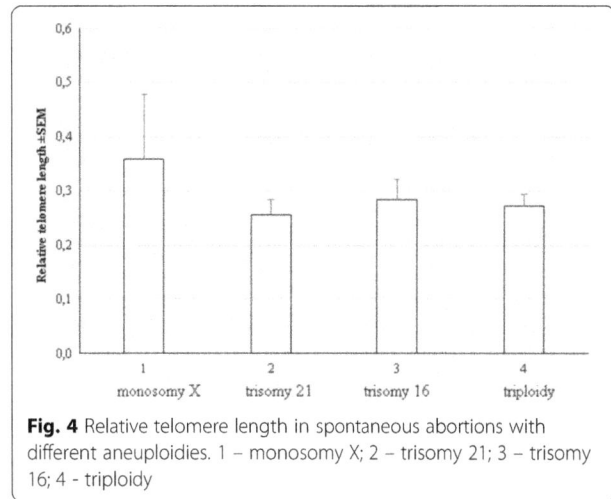

Fig. 4 Relative telomere length in spontaneous abortions with different aneuploidies. 1 – monosomy X; 2 – trisomy 21; 3 – trisomy 16; 4 - triploidy

length does not depend on the kind of aneuploidy in CVS of spontaneously lost pregnancies.

It should be noted that aneuploidy was not detected in IA group. In fact, euploid karyotype (46,XX or 46,XY) was found in all 25 samples. Therefore, we compared relative telomere length between euploid SAs and IAs and observed a highly significant difference in RTL (0.64 ± 0.12 and 1.17 ± 0.14 respectively, $P = 0.006$). These results indicate that the shortening of telomeres seems to play a role in the early human intrauterine interruption of further growth and development (Fig. 3).

In addition, aware of the possibility of contamination of embryonic material with maternal cells, we compared the groups only with male karyotypes (Table 5, Fig. 5, Fig. 6). A total of 48 male embryos were examined: 14 - IA, 15 - euploid SA, 19 - aneuploid SA. Apparently, a significant difference is maintained when comparing the XY-euploid IA to XY-euploid SA embryos ($P = 0.0012$) and even increased ($P = 0.00002$) when comparing IA to aneuploid SA, further strengthening our hypothesis.

Discussion

Based on our and data obtained by others [35–46], it can be stated that telomere length is characterized by interindividual variability both in prenatal and in the postnatal human development. To date, very few studies focus on telomere length in the early stages of human prenatal development. Therefore, our study provides a unique example of studying RTL in early (5–12 w.o.g.) prenatal development and evaluate it according to anamnesis (SA and IA) and in association with aneuploid (autosomal trisomy, monosomy X and triploidy) and euploid karyotype.

Our results show, with a high degree of reliability ($P = 0.000001$), that spontaneously lost pregnancies are characterized by short telomeres in comparison to induced abortions. Therefore, we report a strong correlation between telomere length and the viability of embryos. In particular chronic stress in pregnant women is associated with short telomeres in posterity [41, 43, 44]. In addition, a lower maternal folate concentration in early pregnancy is associated with shorter telomeres in the newborn [45]. Genomic instability is commonly found in newborns with short telomeres, which increases the risk of cancer and age-related diseases [46]. Our data shows significantly shorter RTL in spontaneously eliminated embryos with aneuploid (with trisomy of chromosome 21 or 16, triploidy and monosomy X) karyotype, regardless of the type of aneuploidy. Similar results were shown [30, 31] for aneuploid oocytes and embryos at the cleavage stage, although the telomere length was aligned at the blastocyst stage. The results of studies of telomere length in newborns with trisomy 21 (Down syndrome) are conflicting - from the claim of shortening [47] or lack of a likely difference in telomere length [48] to a

Table 4 Relative telomere length ratios in spontaneous abortions with different form of aneuploidy

Monosomy X		Trisomy 21		Trisomy 16		Triploidy	
Mean (max-min)	n	Mean (max-min)	n	Mean (max-min)	n	Mean (max-min)	n
0.36 (0.08–1.66)	12	0.26 (0.11–0.35)	10	0.28 (0.07–0.49)	13	0.27 (0.11–0.37)	13

n- number of samples

Table 5 Relative telomere length ratios in chorionic villus samples with Y-chromosome

Spontaneous abortions with euploid karyotype		Spontaneous abortions with aneuploid karyotype		Artificial abortions	
Mean (max-min)	n	Mean (max-min)	n	Mean (max-min)	n
0.37(0.30–1.13)	15	0.24(0.07–0.49)	19	1.86(0.14–2.94)	14

n- number of samples

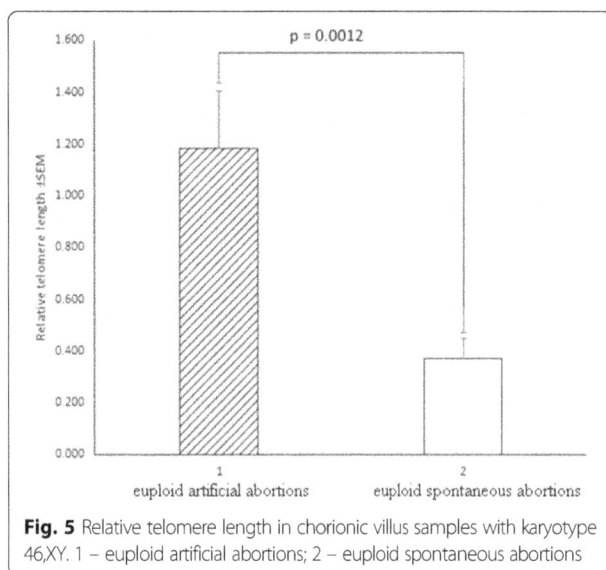

Fig. 5 Relative telomere length in chorionic villus samples with karyotype 46,XY. 1 – euploid artificial abortions; 2 – euploid spontaneous abortions

probable elongation of telomeres in newborns with trisomy 21 versus newborns without chromosomal anomalies [49]. Similarly, ambiguous results are obtained in adults with monosomy X (Turner syndrome) [50], which indicate rather that there is no difference in the length of telomeres in Turner syndrome cells compared to individuals without chromosomal abnormalities.

Conclusion

Spontaneously lost pregnancies are characterized by shortened telomeres, especially in embryos with aneuploidies.. We hypothesize that the shortening of telomeres is involved in the complex elimination machinery leading to early embryo death.

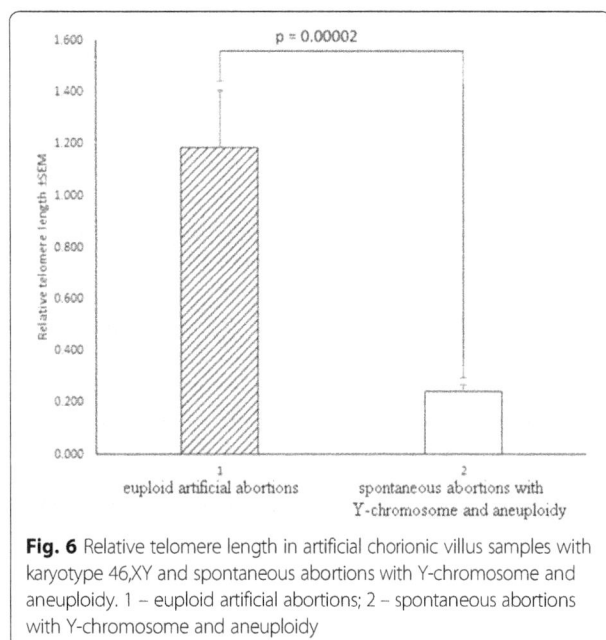

Fig. 6 Relative telomere length in artificial chorionic villus samples with karyotype 46,XY and spontaneous abortions with Y-chromosome and aneuploidy. 1 – euploid artificial abortions; 2 – spontaneous abortions with Y-chromosome and aneuploidy

Abbreviations
CVS: Chorionic villi samples; IA: Induced abortions; RTL: Relative telomere length; RT-PCR: Real-time polymerase chain reaction; S: Single copy gene; SA: Spontaneous abortions; T: Telomere repeat; TL: Telomere length; w.o.g: Weeks of gestation

Acknowledgments
Prof. Liehr T. (Universitätsklinikum Jena, Institut für Humangenetik) for comprehensive advisory and corrective assistance in writing and interpreting the results.
Prof. Yashchenko A. (Lviv National Medical University, Department of Histology, Cytology and Embryology) for histological evaluation and approval of uncontaminated by maternal cells and tissues chorionic villi.
Kuzyk O. (University of Vienna, Department of Microbial Ecology) for help with the design of studies of relative telomere length.

Funding
Not applicable.

Authors' contributions
NH, DZ - study concepts. IT, NH - collected of samples. NH, MT – performed measuring of RTL, data analyzes and interpretation. NH, IT, DZ, MT - manuscript preparation. All authors read and approved the final manuscript.

Competing interests
The authors declare that they have no competing interest.

Author details
Institute of Hereditary Pathology, NAMS of Ukraine, Lysenko Str. 31a, Lviv 79008, Ukraine. [2]Department of Biotechnology and Bioinformatics, Faculty of Chemistry, Rzeszow University of Technology, Al. Powstańców Warszawy 6, 35-959 Rzeszow, Poland.

References
1. Blackburn EH. Structure and function of telomeres. Nature. 1991;350(6319): 569–73. https://doi.org/10.1038/350569a0.
2. Cairney CJ, Keith WN. Telomerase redefined: integrated regulation of hTR and hTERT for telomere maintenance and telomerase activity. Biochimie. 2008;90(1):13–23. https://doi.org/10.1016/j.biochi.2007.07.025.
3. Griffith JD, Comeau L, Rosenfield S, Stansel RM, Bianchi A, Moss H, de Lange T. Mammalian telomeres end in a large duplex loop. Cell. 1999;97(4):503–14. https://doi.org/10.1016/S0092-8674(00)80760-6.
4. De Lange T. Protection of mammalian telomeres. Oncogene. 2002;21(4): 532–40. https://doi.org/10.1038/sj.onc.1205080.
5. De Lange T. Shelterin: the protein complex that shapes and safeguards human telomeres. Genes Dev. 2005;19(18):2100–10. https://doi.org/10.1101/gad.1346005.
6. Zhao Y, Sfeir AJ, Zou Y, Buseman CM, Chow TT, Shay JW, Wright WE. Telomere extension occurs at most chromosome ends and is uncoupled from fill-in in human cancer cells. Cell. 2009;138(3):463–75. https://doi.org/10.1016/j.cell.2009.05.026.
7. Watson JD. Origin of concatemeric T7 DNA. Nat New Biol. 1972;239(94):197–201. PMID:4507727
8. Sfeir AJ, Chai W, Shay JW, Wright WE. Telomere-end processing the terminal nucleotides of human chromosomes. Mol Cell. 2005;18(1):131–8. https://doi.org/10.1016/j.molcel.2005.02.035.
9. Hayflick L. The limited in vitro lifetime of human diploid cell strains. Exp Cell Res. 1965;37:614–36. PMID:14315085
10. Arkus N. A mathematical model of cellular apoptosis and senescence through the dynamics of telomere loss. J Theor Biol. 2005;235:13–32. https://doi.org/10.1016/j.jtbi.2004.12.016.
11. Mai S, Garini Y. The significance of telomeric aggregates in the interphase nuclei of tumor cells. J Cell Biochem. 2006;97:904–15. https://doi.org/10.1002/jcb.20760.

Can telomere shortening be the main indicator of non-viable fetus...

137

12. Bernadotte A, Mikhelson VM, Spivak IM. Markers of cellular senescence. Telomere shortening as a marker of cellular senescence. Aging (Albany NY). 2016;8(1):3–11. https://doi.org/10.18632/aging.100871.

13. Hunt SC, Chen W, Gardner JP, Kimura M, Srinivasan SR, Eckfeldt JH, Berenson GS, Aviv A. Leukocyte telomeres are longer in African Americans than in whites: the National Heart, Lung, and Blood Institute family heart study and the Bogalusa heart study. Aging Cell. 2008;7(4):451–8. https://doi.org/10.1111/j.1474-9726.2008.00397.x.

14. Murillo-Ortiz B, Albarran-Tamayo F, Arenas-Aranda D, Benitez-Bribiesca L, Malacara-Hernandez J, Martinez-Garza S, Hernández-González M, Solorio S, Garay-Sevilla ME, Mora-Villalpando C. Telomere length and type 2 diabetes in males, a premature aging syndrome. Aging Male. 2012;15(1):54–8. https://doi.org/10.3109/13685538.2011.593658.

15. Fitzpatrick AL, Kronmal RA, Kimura M, Gardner JP, Psaty BM, Jenny NS, Tracy RP, Hardikar S, Aviv A. Leukocyte telomere length and mortality in the cardiovascular health study. J Gerontol A Biol Sci Med Sci. 2011;66A(4):421–9. https://doi.org/10.1093/gerona/glq224

16. Hartmann D, Srivastava U, Thaler M, Kleinhans KN, N'Kontchou G, Scheffold A, Bauer K, Kratzer RF, Kloos N, Katz SF, Song Z, Begus-Nahrmann Y, Kleger A, von Figura G, Strnad P, Lechel A, Günes C, Potthoff A, Deterding K, Wedemeyer H, Ju Z, Song G, Xiao F, Gillen S, Schrezenmeier H, Mertens T, Ziol M, Friess H, Jarek M, Manns MP, Beaugrand M, Rudolph KL. Telomerase gene mutations are associated with cirrhosis formation. Hepatology. 2011; 53(5):1608–17. https://doi.org/10.1002/hep.24217.

17. Calado RT, Brudno J, Mehta P, Kovacs JJ, Wu C, Zago MA, Chanock SJ, Boyer TD, Young NS. Constitutional telomerase mutations are genetic risk factors for cirrhosis. Hepatology. 2011;53(5):1600–7. https://doi.org/10.1002/hep.24173.

18. Martinez-Delgado B, Yanowsky K, Inglada-Perez L, Domingo S, Urioste M, Osorio A, Benitez J. Genetic anticipation is associated with telomere shortening in hereditary breast cancer. PLoS Genet. 2011;7(7):e1002182. https://doi.org/10.1371/journal.pgen.1002182

19. Calado RT, Young NS. Telomere diseases. N Engl J Med. 2009;361(24):2353–65. https://doi.org/10.1056/NEJMra0903373. PMCID: PMC3401586

20. Nordfjall K, Eliasson M, Stegmayr B, Lundin S, Roos G, Nilsson PM. Increased abdominal obesity, adverse psychosocial factors and shorter telomere length in subjects reporting early ageing; the MONICA northern Sweden study. Scand J Public Health. 2008;36(7):744–52. https://doi.org/10.1177/1403494808090634

21. Njajou OT, Cawthon RM, Blackburn EH, Harris TB, Li R, Sanders JL, Newman AB, Nalls M, Cummings SR, Hsueh W-C. Shorter telomeres are associated with obesity and weight gain in the elderly. Int J Obes. 2012;36(9):1176–9. https://doi.org/10.1038/ijo.2011.196.

22. Cherkas LF, Hunkin JL, Kato BS, Richards JB, Gardner JP, Surdulescu GL, Kimura M, Lu X, Spector TD, Aviv A. The association between physical activity in leisure time and leukocyte telomere length. Arch Intern Med. 2008;168(2):154–8. https://doi.org/10.1001/archinternmed.2007.39.

23. Epel ES, Blackburn EH, Lin F, Dhabhar FS, Adler NE, Morrow JD, Cawthon RM. Accelerated telomere shortening in response to life stress. Proc Natl Acad Sci U S A. 2004;101(49):17312–5. PMCID: PMC534658. https://doi.org/10.1073/pnas.0407162101.

24. Valdes AM, Andrew T, Gardner JP, Kimura M, Oelsner E, Cherkas LF, Aviv A, Spector TD. Obesity, cigarette smoking, and telomere length in women. Lancet. 2005;366(9486):662–4. https://doi.org/10.1016/S0140-6736(05)66630-5.

25. Cawthon RM, Smith KR, O'Brien E, Sivatchenko A, Kerber RA. Association between telomere length in blood and mortality in people aged 60 years or older. Lancet. 2003;361(9355):393–5. https://doi.org/10.1016/S0140-6736(03)12384-7.

26. Ferrari F, Facchinetti F, Saade G, Menon R. Placental telomere shortening in stillbirth: a sign of premature senescence? J Matern Fetal Neonatal Med. 2016;29(8):1283–8. https://doi.org/10.3109/14767058.2015.1046045.

27. Menon R, Yu J, Basanta-Henry P, Brou L, Berga SL, Fortunato SJ, Taylo RN. Short fetal leukocyte telomere length and preterm prelabor rupture of the membranes. PLoS One. 2012;7(2):e31136. PMCID: PMC3278428. https://doi.org/10.1371/journal.pone.0031136.

28. Biron-Shental T, Sukenik-Halevy R, Sharon Y, Goldberg-Bittman L, Kidron D, Fejgin MD, Amiel A. Short telomeres may play a role in placental dysfunction in preeclampsia and intrauterine growth restriction. Am J Obstet Gynecol. 2010;202(4):381 .e1-7. https://doi.org/10.1016/j.ajog.2010.01.036.

29. Davy P, Nagata M, Bullard P, Fogelson NS, Allsopp R. Fetal growth restriction is associated with accelerated telomere shortening and increased expression of cell senescence markers in the placenta. Placenta. 2009;30(6):539 42. PMCID:PMC2692289 https://doi.org/10.1016/j.placenta.2009.03.005

30. Treff NR, Su J, Taylor D, Scott RT Jr. Telomere DNA deficiency is associated with development of human embryonic aneuploid. PLoS Genet. 2011;7(6):e1002161. PMCID: PMC3128107. https://doi.org/10.1371/journal.pgen.1002161.

31. Mania A, Mantzouratou A, Delhanty JD, Baio G, Serhal P, Sengupta SB. Telomere length in human blastocysts. Reprod BioMed Online. 2014;28(5):624–37. https://doi.org/10.1016/j.rbmo.2013.12.010.

32. Keefe DL, Franco S, Liu L, Trimarchi J, Cao B, Weitzen S, Agarwal S, Blasco MA. Telomere length predicts embryo fragmentation after in vitro fertilization in women—toward a telomere theory of reproductive aging in women. Am J Obstet Gynecol. 2005;192(4):1256–60. https://doi.org/10.1016/j.ajog.2005.01.036.

33. Keefe DL, Liu L, Marquard K. Telomeres and aging-related meiotic dysfunction in women. Cell Mol Life Sci. 2007;64(2):139–43. https://doi.org/10.1007/s00018-006-6466-z.

34. Cawthon RM. Telomere measurement by quantitative PCR. Nucleic Acids Res. 2002;30(10):e47. PMCID: PMC115301

35. Holmes DK, Bellantuono I, Walkinshaw SA, Alfirevic Z, Johnston TA, Subhedar NV, Chittick R, Swindell R, Wynn RF. Telomere length dynamics differ in foetal and early post-natal human leukocytes in a longitudinal study. Biogerontology. 2009;10(3):279–84. https://doi.org/10.1007/s10522-008-9194-y.

36. Cheng G, Kong F, Luan Y, Sun C, Wang J, Zhang L, Jiang B, Qi T, Zhao J, Zheng C, Xu D. Differential shortening rate of telomere length in the development of human fetus. Biochem Biophys Res Commun. 2013;442(1–2):112-5. https://doi.org/10.1016/j.bbrc.2013.11.022.

37. Youngren K, Jeanclos E, Aviv H, Kimura M, Stock J, Hanna M, Skurnick J, Bardeguez A, Aviv A. Synchrony in telomere length of the human fetus. Hum Genet. 1998;102(6):640–3. PMID: 9703424

38. Turner S, Wong HP, Rai J, Hartshorne GM. Telomere lengths in human oocytes, cleavage stage embryos and blastocysts. Mol Hum Reprod. 2010;16(9):685–94. https://doi.org/10.1093/molehr/gaq048.

39. Okuda K, Bardeguez A, Gardner JP, Rodriguez P, Ganesh V, Kimura M, Skurnick J, Awad G, Aviv A. Telomere length in the newborn. Pediatr Res. 2002;52(3):377–81. https://doi.org/10.1203/00006450-200209000-00012.

40. Akkad A, Hastings R, Konje JC, Bell SC, Thurston H, Williams B. Telomere length in small for gestational age babies. BJOG Int J Obstet Gynaecol. 2006;113:318–23. https://doi.org/10.1111/j.1471-0528.2005.00839.x.

41. Entringer S, Epel ES, Lin J, Buss C, Shahbaba B, Blackburn EH, Simhan HN, Wadhwa PD. Maternal psychosocial stress during pregnancy is associated with newborn leukocyte telomere length. Am J Obstet Gynecol. 2013; 208(2):134.e1–134.e7. https://doi.org/10.1016/j.ajog.2012.11.033.

42. Armanios M, Blackburn EH. The telomere syndromes. Nat Rev Genet. 2012; 13(10):693–704. PMCID: PMC3548426. https://doi.org/10.1038/nrg3246.

43. Marchetto NM, Glynn RA, Ferry ML, Ostojic M, Wolff SM, Yao R, Haussmann MF. Prenatal stress and newborn telomere length. Am J Obstet Gynecol. 2016;215(1):94.e1-8. https://doi.org/10.1016/j.ajog.2016.01.177.

44. Entringer S, Epel ES, Kumsta R, Lin J, Hellhammer DH, Blackburn EH, Wüst S, Wadhwa PD. Stress exposure in intrauterine life is associated with shorter telomere length in young adulthood. Proc Natl Acad Sci U S A. 2011;108(33):E513–8. PMCID:PMC3158153. https://doi.org/10.1073/pnas.1107759108.

45. Entringer S, Epel ES, Lin J, Blackburn EH, Buss C, Shahbaba B, Gillen DL, Venkataramanan R, Simhan HN, Wadhwa PD. Maternal Folate concentration in early pregnancy and newborn telomere length. Ann Nutr Metab. 2015; 66(4):202–8. PMCID: PMC5457533. https://doi.org/10.1159/000381925.

46. Moreno-Palomo J, Creus A, Marcos R, Hernández A. Genomic instability in newborn with short telomeres. PLoS One. 2014;9(3):e91753. https://doi.org/10.1371/journal.pone.0091753.

47. Wenger SL, Hansroth J, Shackelford AL. Decreased telomere length in metaphase and interphase cells from newborns with trisomy 21. Gene. 2014;542(1):87. https://doi.org/10.1016/j.gene.2014.03.019.

48. Nakamura K, Ishikawa N, Izumiyama N, Aida J, Kuroiwa M, Hiraishi N, Fujiwara M, Nakao A, Kawakami T, Poon SS, Matsuura M, Sawabe M, Arai T, Takubo K. Telomere lengths at birth in trisomies 18 and 21 measured by Q-FISH. Gene. 2014;533(1):199–207. https://doi.org/10.1016/j.gene.2013.09.086.

49. Bhaumik P, Bhattacharya M, Ghosh P, Ghosh S, Kumar DS. Telomere length analysis in down syndrome birth. Mech Ageing Dev. 2017;164:20–6. https://doi.org/10.1016/j.mad.2017.03.006.

50. Kveiborg M, Gravholt CH, Kassem M. Evidence of a normal mean telomere fragment length in patients with Ullrich-turner syndrome. Eur J Hum Genet. 2001;9(11):877–9. https://doi.org/10.1038/sj.ejhg.5200722.

15

Scattered genomic amplification in dedifferentiated liposarcoma

Nils Mandahl[1*], Linda Magnusson[1], Jenny Nilsson[1], Björn Viklund[2], Elsa Arbajian[1], Fredrik Vult von Steyern[3], Anders Isaksson[2] and Fredrik Mertens[1]

Abstract

Background: Atypical lipomatous tumor (ALT), well differentiated liposarcoma (WDLS) and dedifferentiated liposarcoma (DDLS) are cytogenetically characterized by near-diploid karyotypes with no or few other aberrations than supernumerary ring or giant marker chromosomes, although DDLS tend to have somewhat more complex rearrangements. In contrast, pleomorphic liposarcomas (PLS) have highly aberrant and heterogeneous karyotypes. The ring and giant marker chromosomes contain discontinuous amplicons, in particular including multiple copies of the target genes *CDK4*, *HMGA2* and *MDM2* from 12q, but often also sequences from other chromosomes.

Results: The present study presents a DDLS with an atypical hypertriploid karyotype without any ring or giant marker chromosomes. SNP array analyses revealed amplification of almost the entire 5p and discontinuous amplicons of 12q including the classical target genes, in particular *CDK4*. In addition, amplicons from 1q, 3q, 7p, 9p, 11q and 20q, covering from 2 to 14 Mb, were present. FISH analyses showed that sequences from 5p and 12q were scattered, separately or together, over more than 10 chromosomes of varying size. At RNA sequencing, significantly elevated expression, compared to myxoid liposarcomas, was seen for *TRIO* and *AMACR* in 5p and of *CDK4*, *HMGA2* and *MDM2* in 12q.

Conclusions: The observed pattern of scattered amplification does not show the characteristics of chromothripsis, but is novel and differs from the well known cytogenetic manifestations of amplification, i.e., double minutes, homogeneously staining regions and ring chromosomes. Possible explanations for this unusual distribution of amplified sequences might be the mechanism of alternative lengthening of telomeres that is frequently active in DDLS and events associated with telomere crisis.

Keywords: Liposarcoma, Chromosomes, Amplification, 5p, 12q, Gene expression

Background

Cytogenetic analyses of more than 3200 benign and malignant soft tissue tumors have revealed that different patterns of chromosomal aberrations exist among these lesions [1, 2]. Several tumor entities are characterized by specific, sometimes pathognomonic, structural rearrangements, mostly translocations, giving rise to oncogenic fusion genes, often with no or few other changes of chromosome number or morphology. Another set of tumors displays a moderate number of chromosomal imbalances, whereas still another set of tumors shows highly complex karyotypic rearrangements with extensive cytogenetic heterogeneity. Both losses

and gains of sequences may be of pathogenetic importance. While losses affect one or both copies of one or more genes, gains can range from one to hundreds of extra gene copies. Moderate and high level gene amplification manifest cytogenetically as intrachromosomal homogeneously staining regions (hsr), extrachromosomal double minutes (dmin) or ring chromosomes (r); other mechanisms behind amplification are presumed to be rare and are not easily recognized by chromosome banding analysis. Among soft tissue tumors, ring chromosomes are much more abundant than dmin, and hsr is even more infrequent (Additional file 1). Ring chromosomes, allowing for gene amplification through breakage-fusion-bridge cycles [3], constitute the characteristic cytogenetic feature of some soft tissue tumors, including atypical lipomatous tumor/well differentiated liposarcoma (ALT/WDLS) and dedifferentiated liposarcoma (DDLS).

---

* Correspondence: nils.mandahl@med.lu.se
[1]Division of Clinical Genetics, Department of Laboratory Medicine, Lund University, SE-221 84 Lund, Sweden
Full list of author information is available at the end of the article

Modern array technologies have revealed that gene amplification is more common among neoplastic cells than detected by banding analyses. Such technologies, however, do not reveal the chromosomal organization of multiplied sequences, which might provide some clues about how they originated and their evolutionary potential. In the present study, amplification through scattering over many chromosomes is described in a case of dedifferentiated liposarcoma.

Methods

As part of a study of soft tissue sarcomas that at G-banding analysis showed aberrations including add(5)(p15), FISH analyses were performed in order to find out if the breakpoint in 5p was localized to a restricted position that could indicate the involvement of a particular gene. No consistent pattern was found, but one case showed a peculiar distribution of chromosome 5 sequences, which prompted further investigation.

The patient was a 67-year-old man with a deep-seated tumor in the left thigh. The largest diameter of the highly necrotic, infiltratively growing tumor was 24 cm. Two samples – an open biopsy and the resected specimen – were obtained with an interval of five weeks. The diagnosis was dedifferentiated liposarcoma with atypical fat cells, sclerosis, a spindle cell component, as well as a component of spindle cells with rhabdoid differentiation; no region compatible with a well-differentiated liposarcoma was seen. Postoperative radiation therapy was given. X-ray two years later revealed no apparent lung metastases. Five years after diagnosis, metastases to the lungs and soft tissues on the back appeared. The patient died soon after.

Chromosome preparations were made from short-term cultured cells obtained from disaggregated tumor tissue from both samples and stained for G-banding as previously described [4].

FISH analyses were performed using whole chromosome painting probes wcp5 (green) and wcp12 (blue) (Vysis, Downers Grove, IL). Site-specific probes were CTD-2074D8 (5p14.1–14.3), RP11-509B9 (5p15.1), RP11-35 K22 (5p15.32), CTD-3080P12 (5p15.33), hereafter referred to as D8, B9, K22 and P12, respectively, as well as RP11–1137 N1 (12q14.3–15) for detection of the *MDM2* gene (BACPAC Resource Center; https://bacpacresource-s.org). The following fluorophores were used for labelling: red, Cy3 dUTP (VWR), green, Chromatide Alexa Fluor 488–5-dUTP (Thermo Fisher Scientific). Hybridizations were performed as described [5]. No material was available for further analyses.

SNP array analysis of the two samples was performed as described [6]. In brief, tumor DNA (250 ng) was extracted and analyzed using the Affymetrix CytoScan HD array (Affymetrix, Santa Clara, CA, USA). Genomic

aberrations were identified by visual inspection using the Chromosome Analysis Suite version 1.2 (Affymetrix). The human reference sequence used for alignment was the GRCh37/hg19 assembly. Constitutional copy number variations were excluded through comparison with the Database of Genomic Variants (http://dgv.tcag.ca/dgv/app/home). Further bioinformatic analysis regarding copy numbers and segmentation was performed using Rawcopy and the Tumor Aberration Prediction Suite (TAPS), as described [7, 8]. Since the chromosome number was at the triploid level, only copy numbers of at least 6 were considered true amplification. Mean and median copy numbers were calculated as well as the total length of amplified sequences.

RNA sequencing (RNA-Seq) was performed on the excised tumor biopsy, as described [9]. Identification of potential fusion transcripts was performed on fastq files using FusionCatcher [10]. The GRCh37/hg19 build was used as the human reference genome. Expression of some selected candidate target genes in 5p and known targets in 12q was compared with their expression in a set of myxoid liposarcomas.

Results

A hypertriploid, complex karyotype was found in both samples (Fig. 1). The only difference between the two samples was a slight variation in chromosome number, 70–74 and 73–76, respectively. Based on both samples the composite karyotype was interpreted as 70–76,XX,-Y, +1,del(1)(-q12)×2,add(2)(p1?),+del(3)(q11),-4,-5,add(5)(p15),?add(5)(p 11),-7,add(7)(p11)×2,-8,-10, −11,?add(11)(q22),?ins(12;?)(q1 3;?)×2,der(12)add(12)(p11)add(12)(q24),add(14)(p11),add(1 9) (q13)×2,?der(19)add(19)(p11)del(19)(q12),-20,+21,+22,in c[cp24].

FISH analyses revealed that chromosome 5 sequences were spread to several chromosomes (Fig. 2). Using wcp5, no intact chromosome 5 was found, but wcp5-positive segments were detected in 14–19 chromosomes, at least 17 of which were clonal (Fig. 3a). Large segments were seen in four chromosomes (designated A-D in Fig. 3a) and three of these most likely contained the centromere of chromosome 5. Two identical chromosomes (L and M) could represent i(5)(p10). One chromosome (E) was identified, based on the DAPI staining pattern, as a derivative chromosome 9 with chromosome 5 material added to the truncated 9p. FISH using the more proximal probes D8 and B9 revealed 9–11 and 9–13 signals, respectively, per metaphase. The corresponding number of signals for K22 and P12 were 11–15 and 11–16 respectively. Similar signal patterns for all four probes of the two probe sets were seen in chromosomes E, H, L, M, and Q.

Chromosome 12 sequences were identified in 12 chromosomes (Fig. 3b). In most metaphases there were 10 signals for *MDM2* located in eight chromosomes.

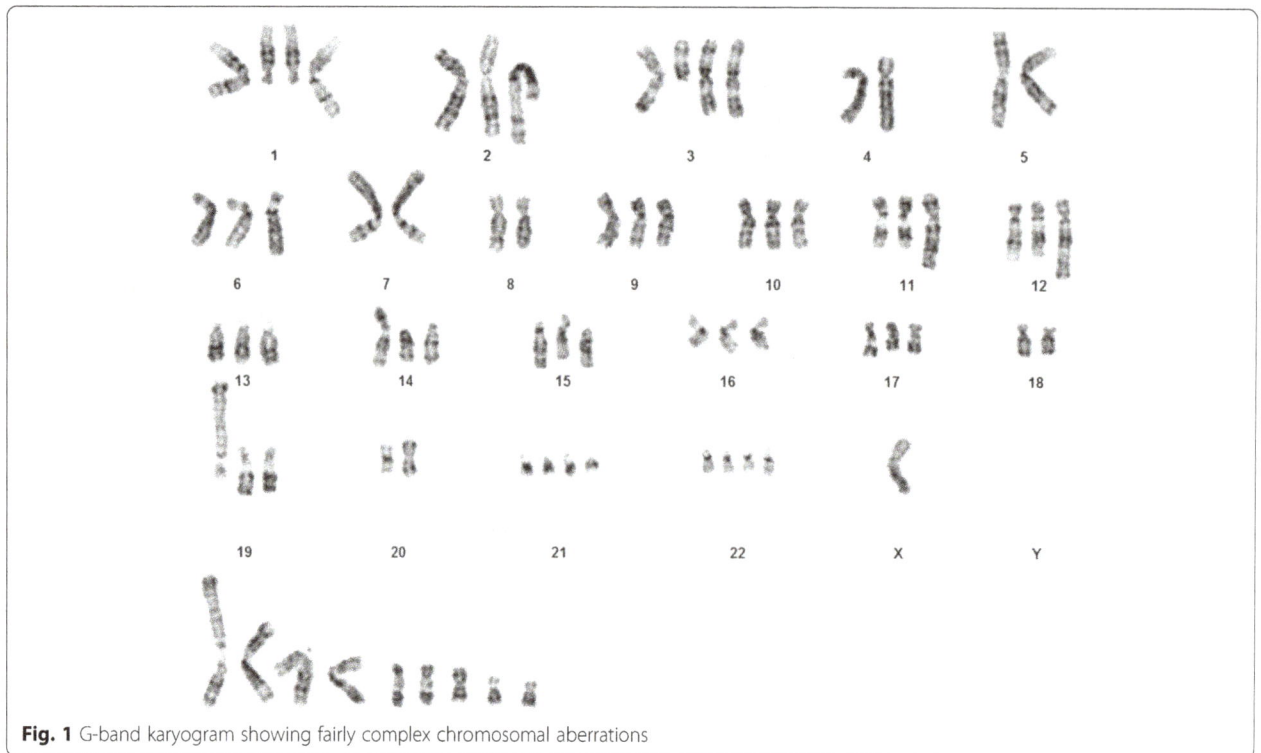

Fig. 1 G-band karyogram showing fairly complex chromosomal aberrations

Sequences from both chromosomes 5 and 12 were present in seven chromosomes (B, C, H, I, K, R, and S); in R and S no signals for the site-specific 5p probes were detected. Twelve chromosomes were positive for wcp5 but not for wcp12 (A, D-G, J, and L-Q), whereas five chromosomes were wcp5 negative but wcp12 positive (T-X). A summary of several FISH analyses is shown in Fig. 3c.

At SNP array analysis, amplified sequences were found on chromosome arms 1q, 3q, 5p, 7p, 9p, 11q, 12q, and 20q (Table 1, Additional file 2). Few differences were found between the two samples (Fig. 4). The chromosome 5 amplicons emanated from almost the entire short arm, with peak copy numbers from p15.33-p15.32, p15.31-p15.2, p14.3, and p14.1-p12. The major parts of 5q were estimated to 4 copies. In chromosome 12, discontinuous high level amplicons were found from q12 to q24.21. There were about 10 copies of sequences covering the *HMGA2* and *MDM2* genes, whereas *CDK4* was estimated to 17 copies. In general, amplified

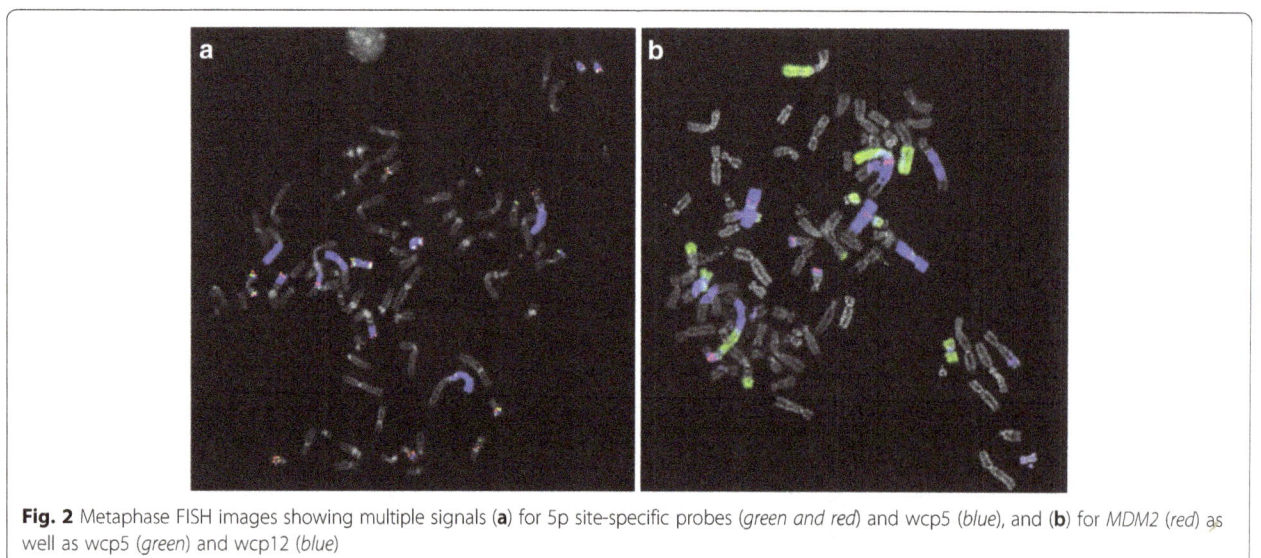

Fig. 2 Metaphase FISH images showing multiple signals (**a**) for 5p site-specific probes (*green and red*) and wcp5 (*blue*), and (**b**) for *MDM2* (*red*) as well as wcp5 (*green*) and wcp12 (*blue*)

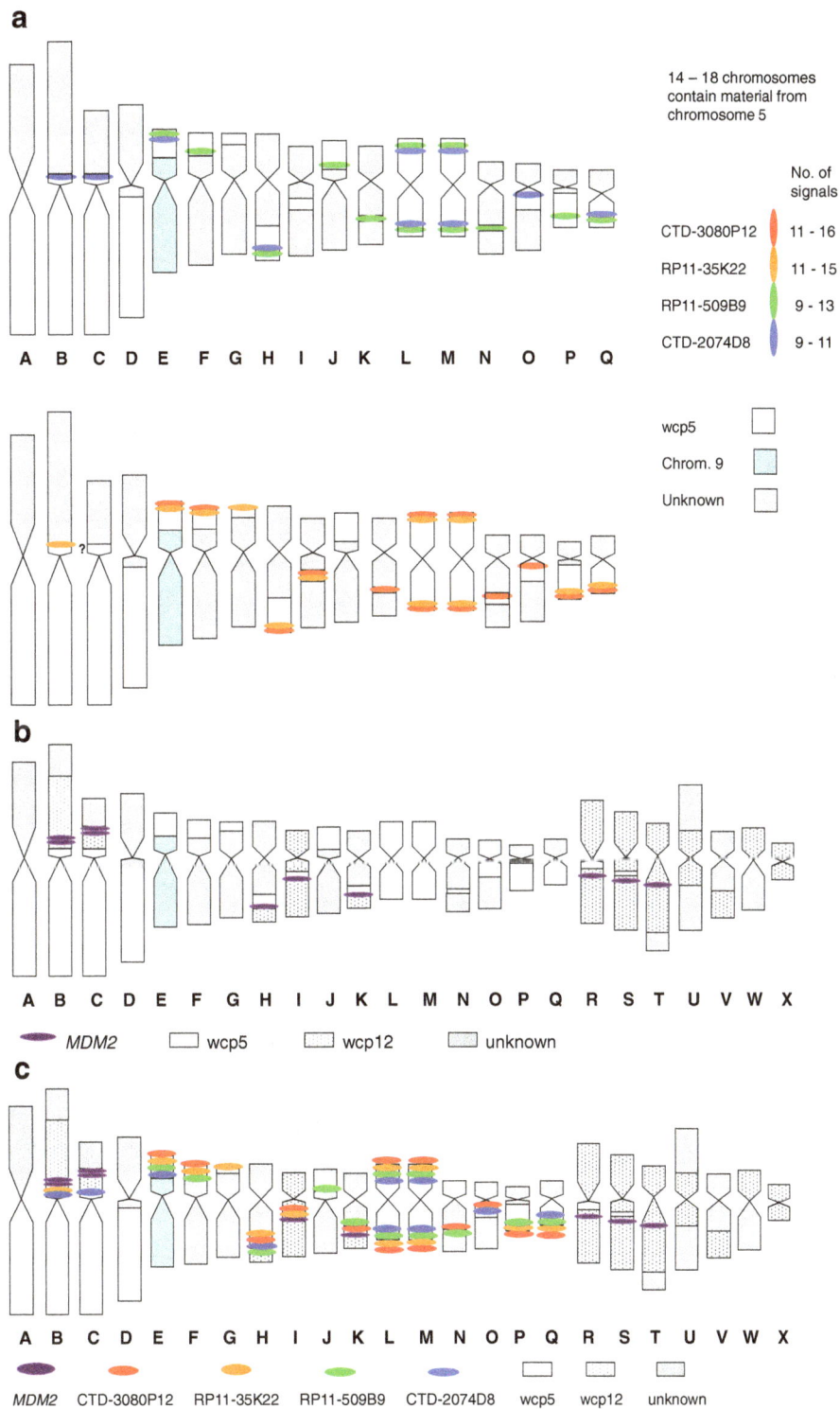

Fig. 3 Schematic representations of the FISH results. **a** analysis using four site-specific 5p probes and wcp5; **b** analysis using a probe detecting *MDM2* as well as wcp5 and wcp12; **c** summary of all FISH analyses. Letters A to X are used as identification of different aberrant chromosomes

sequences in 12q showed higher copy numbers than those in 5p. The size of increased copy numbers in 5p and 12q corresponded to 46.3 Mb and 17.2 Mb

representing about 94% and 17% of the length of these chromosome arms, respectively. Gain/amplification in other chromosomes was found for sequences within

Table 1 Distribution and size of chromosome segments showing amplification

Chromosome arm	Mean copy number	Median copy number	Extension (Mb)	Fraction of arm with amplification
1q	8.1	8	8.462	6.8%
3q	7.2	7	2.013	1.9%
5p	9.9	10	46.273	93.6%
7p	6.8	6	13.772	23.2%
9p	8.1	8	13.905	31.5%
11q	12.0	9	3.866	4.8%
12q	12.4	11	17.159	17.4%
20q	13.3	12.5	13.212	36.6%
Total			118.662	

Only copy numbers of at least 6 are included

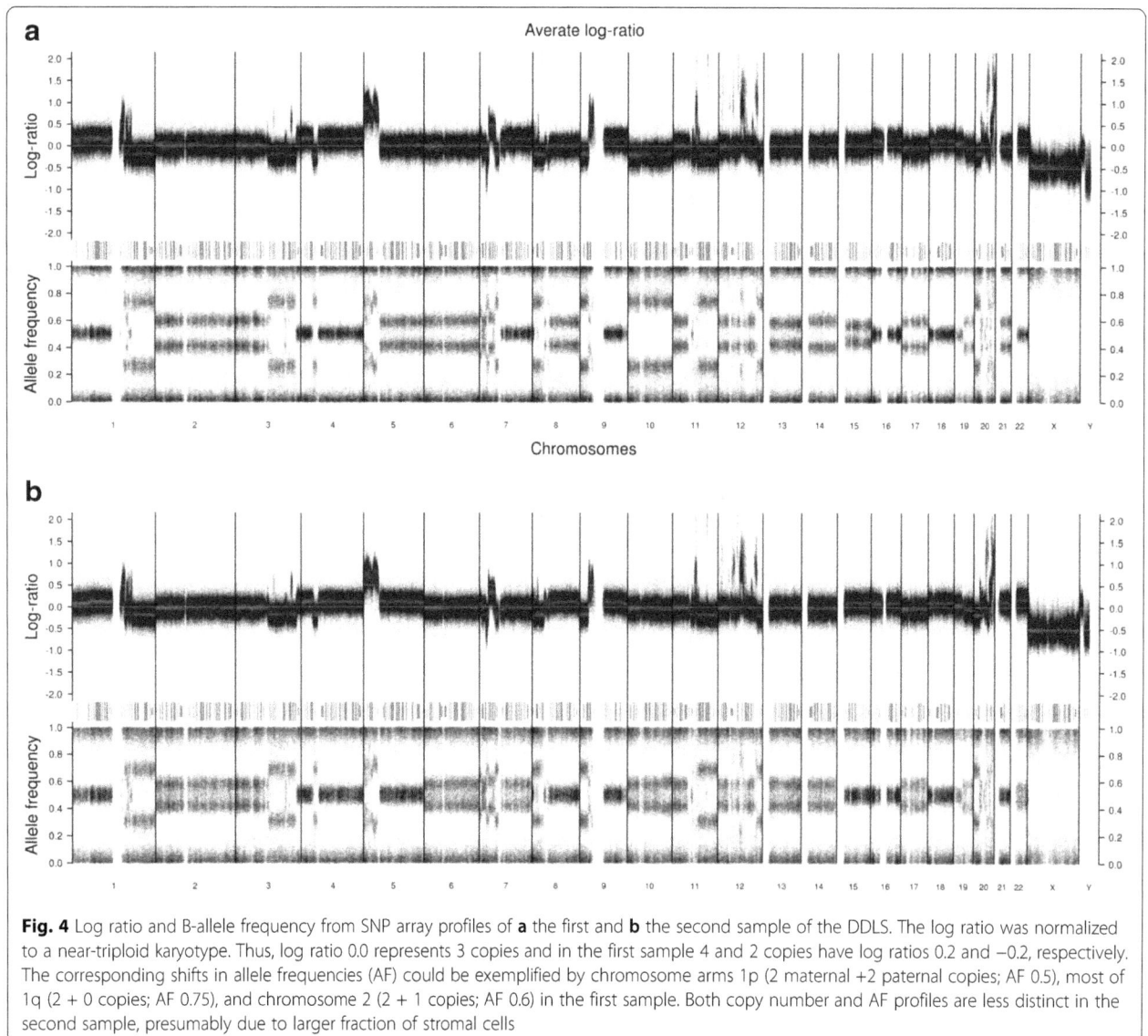

Fig. 4 Log ratio and B-allele frequency from SNP array profiles of **a** the first and **b** the second sample of the DDLS. The log ratio was normalized to a near-triploid karyotype. Thus, log ratio 0.0 represents 3 copies and in the first sample 4 and 2 copies have log ratios 0.2 and −0.2, respectively. The corresponding shifts in allele frequencies (AF) could be exemplified by chromosome arms 1p (2 maternal +2 paternal copies; AF 0.5), most of 1q (2 + 0 copies; AF 0.75), and chromosome 2 (2 + 1 copies; AF 0.6) in the first sample. Both copy number and AF profiles are less distinct in the second sample, presumably due to larger fraction of stromal cells

1q21.2-q22 and 1q24.1, 3q26.2, 7p15.2-p12.3, 9p21.3-p13.1, 11q13.2-q13.4 and 11q22.1, and 20q11.23-q13.33, representing about 7%, 2%, 23%, 32%, 5% and 37%, respectively, of the chromosome arms. Among these chromosomes, only chromosome 20 displayed more extensive high level amplification (12 copies), in particular confined to 20q13.2-q13.33.

None of the potential fusion transcripts that were detected at RNA-Seq was considered significant (Additional file 3). Of the selected target genes, *AMACR* and *TRIO* in 5p and *CDK4*, *HMGA2* and *MDM2* in 12q showed significantly ($p < 0.05$) elevated expression in relation to myxoid liposarcomas (Fig. 5).

Discussion

ALT/WDLS share many cytogenetic characteristics with DDLS - supernumerary ring chromosomes and/or giant marker chromosomes constitute the hallmark of the reported karyotypes from ALT/WDLS (n = 174) and DDLS (n = 27). On average, DDLS tend to have somewhat more complex karyotypes than ALT/WDLS, whereas the 15 published karyotypes of pleomorphic liposarcomas (PLS) are distinctly more complex and ring chromosomes are much less frequent [2] (Additional file 1). Similarly, near-diploid stemline chromosome numbers predominate in ALT/WDLS and DDLS, but are rare in PLS. The ring and giant marker chromosomes in ALT/WDLS and DDLS always contain sequences from 12q, typically with several separate amplicons that invariably include *MDM2* (and often also *CDK4* and *HMGA2*), and frequently also segments from one or more other chromosomes [11–17]. Available data show that sequences from almost all chromosome arms may be co-amplified with 12q; the only exceptions - Yp, Yq and the p-arms of the acrocentric chromosomes - could be due to the methods of detection. The most commonly involved chromosome arms are 1q (46%), 6q (22%), 7p, 8q, 9q (13%), 1p, 4p, 14q (12%), 5p, 12p, 20q (11%) and 16q (10%). The non-random co-amplification of certain regions suggests that they harbour genes of potential pathogenetic significance, or that they contain sequences prone to recombine with 12q amplicons.

DDLS usually also show more copy number changes than ALT/WDLS [16]. A comparison between the well-differentiated and dedifferentiated components of the same tumor revealed more aberrations among the latter, but no particular sequence(s) could account for the dedifferentiation process [12, 18]. Even more extensive genomic reorganization is found among PLS. The dominating (>15% of cases) amplifications include sequences from 1q and 12q in WDLS, from 1p, 1q, 6q, 8q and 12q in DDLS, and from 5p and 20q in PLS (Table 2). A conspicuous difference is the paucity of 12q amplification in PLS. A clear trend of increasing frequencies in WDLS to

DDLS to PLS is seen for amplifications in 5p and 20q – 3%, 13%, 23% and 0%, 6%, 23%, respectively. Such a trend is not seen for amplifications in any other chromosome arm. Possibly, these differences indicate that some gene(s) in 5p and 20q are of importance for tumor aggressiveness.

Amplification of 5p segments is not confined to adipocytic tumors, but has been reported in other soft tissue sarcomas, as well as in epithelial neoplasms. Among sarcomas, it is preferentially seen in tumors typically characterized by complex chromosomal aberrations, such as myxofibrosarcomas, undifferentiated pleomorphic sarcomas, leiomyosarcomas and angiosarcomas, some of which are difficult to distinguish from PLS [19–28]. Also some other non-mesenchymal tumors, such as urinary bladder cancer, non-small cell lung cancer, cervical cancer and multiple myeloma, show 5p amplification with amplicons to some extent overlapping those found in sarcomas (e.g., [29–32]). These data further support the suggestion that amplification of genes in 5p may be associated with aggressive tumor growth. Information on concomitant amplification of 5p and 12q sequences is only available in some of the tumor types listed above, but data indicate that it is not common among PLS, leiomyosarcoma, or myxofibrosarcoma. Findings from array analyses support the paucity of extra copies of both 5p and 12q in PLS; it is rare in WDLS, but found in about one-fourth of DDLS (Table 3).

Apart from amplified 12q sequences, regularly confined to ring and giant marker chromosomes, the chromosomal distribution of other amplified sequences is less well documented. Co-amplified chromosomal material, in particular from 1q, has, however, been shown to be intermingled with 12q sequences in rings and giant markers [13, 33–35]. The present case, showing both 5p and 12q amplicons, fits well with a minor subset of DDLS, but is atypical in the sense that it displays a near-triploid chromosome complement without any ring or giant marker chromosomes. Moreover, the complex pattern of amplification of 5p and 12q sequences, together in the same chromosomes and separately in different chromosomes, is unusual. Admittedly, there is no definition of what should be regarded as a giant marker, but those described in the literature are typically at least twice as large as chromosome 1. The size of the largest aberrant chromosome (B) containing 5p and 12q sequences in the present case was 1.5 times the length of chromosome 1, as estimated from G-banding (Fig. 3c). The vast majority of the 24 chromosomes with wcp5 and/or wcp12 signals were much smaller than chromosome 1. Only rare cases of ALT/WDLS with amplification in medium-sized linear chromosomes have been reported [36, 37]. No similar pattern of amplified sequences scattered over so many chromosomes has been reported before.

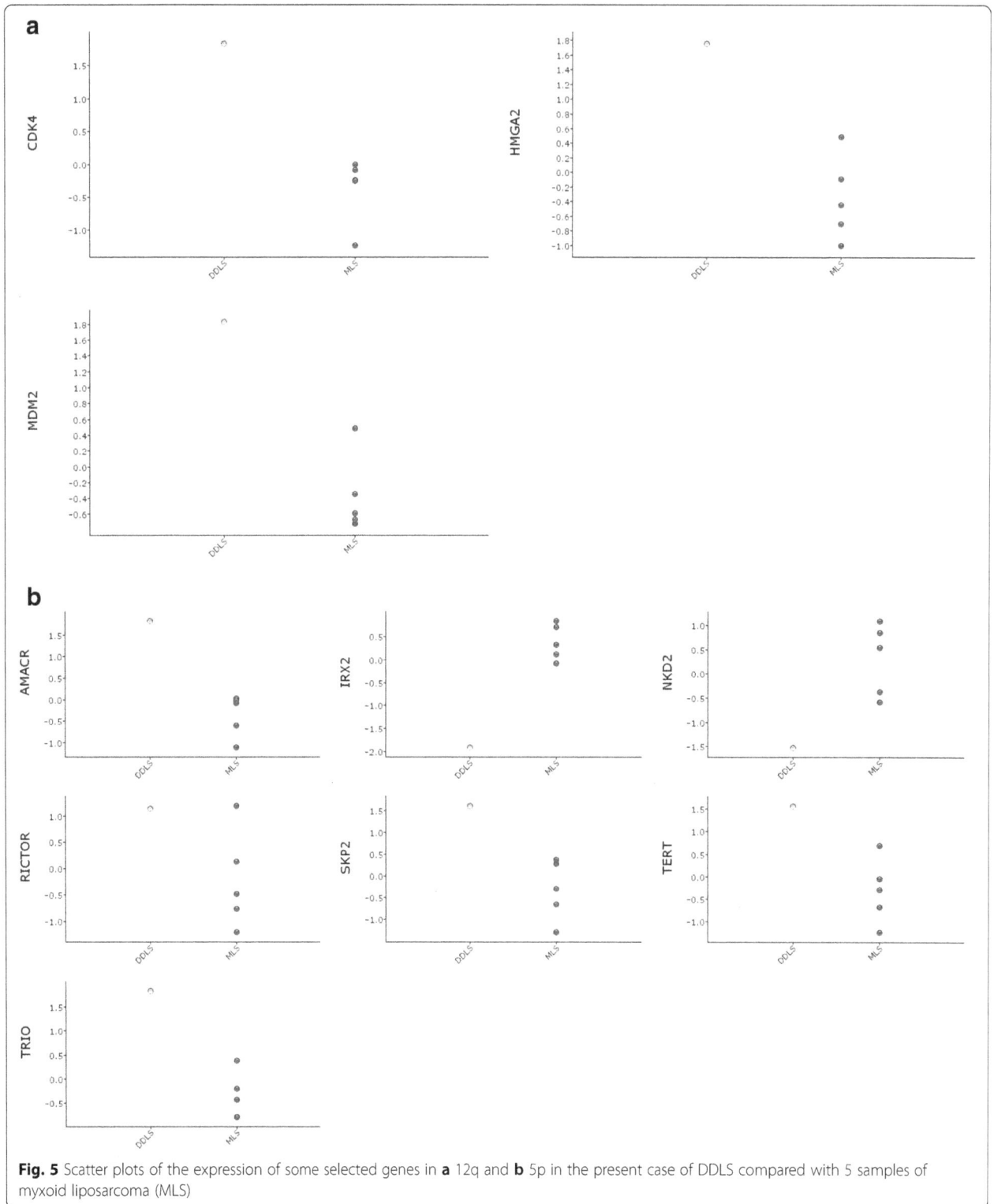

Fig. 5 Scatter plots of the expression of some selected genes in **a** 12q and **b** 5p in the present case of DDLS compared with 5 samples of myxoid liposarcoma (MLS)

Genes located in 5p that have been suggested as possible amplicon targets in sarcomas include *NKD2*, *TERT*, *IRX2*, *TRIO*, *AMACR*, *SKP2* and *RICTOR* (e.g., [24, 38–40]). In the present case, these genes were amplified at similar levels (about 10 copies), but with a slightly lower level for *IRX2* and a slightly higher level for *TRIO*. On average, the amplification levels of sequences covering almost the entire 5p were lower than the levels seen in 12q and 20q, In particular, one of the well documented targets in 12q, *CDK4*, was highly amplified (about 17

Table 2 Amplification of sequences from chromosome arms in WDLS, DDLS and PLS, based on literature data

Chromosome arm	Ampl. WDLS (%) $n = 79$	Ampl. DDLS (%) $n = 32$	Ampl. PLS (%) $n = 22$	Chromo-some arm	Ampl. WDLS (%) $n = 79$	Ampl. DDLS (%) $n = 32$	Ampl. PLS (%) $n = 22$
1p	0	19	9	11q	0	6	0
1q	30	28	9	12p	3	6	0
2p	3	0	0	12q	76	88	0
2q	0	9	0	13q	0	9	5
3p	0	3	0	14q	4	13	5
3q	3	3	5	15q	0	9	0
4p	5	9	0	16p	0	0	0
4q	3	3	0	16q	0	3	0
5p	3	13	23	17p	0	0	5
5q	0	0	0	17q	0	0	0
6p	0	6	0	18p	1	0	0
6q	5	31	14	18q	3	3	0
7p	3	9	5	19p	1	3	0
7q	1	3	0	19q	4	9	0
8p	4	6	0	20p	0	3	5
8q	4	16	0	20q	0	6	23
9p	0	3	5	21q	4	0	5
9q	3	9	0	22q	0	0	5
10p	0	9	0	Xp	0	3	0
10q	0	0	0	Xq	0	0	0
11p	1	9	0	Yp, Yq	0	0	0

Table 3 Fraction of borderline and malignant adipose tissue tumors with copy number changes in 5p and 12q13–21

Chromosome segment[a]		WDLS	DDLS	PLS
5p	12q13–21			
0	0	0.01	0	0.14
0	G	0.21	0.09	0.09
0	A	0.73	0.63	0
G	0	0	0.03	0.36
A	0	0	0	0.23
G	G	0.01	0	0.18
G	A	0.01	0.13	0
A	A	0.03	0.13	0

Summary of the figures above, making no distinction between gain and amplification

0	G/A	0.94	0.72	0.09
G/A	0	0	0.03	0.59
G/A	G/A	0.05	0.26	0.18

These calculations are based on available literature data
[a]0 = no copy number change; G = gain; A = amplification; G/A = gain or amplification

copies). Also, in 5p there were very few and short intervening sequences showing a copy number corresponding to the ploidy level, in contrast to 12q and 20q where such intervening sequences were more abundant and mostly much larger, resulting in a more discontinuous amplicon pattern. This could indicate that the gene gains in 5p are less important, or merely passengers, or that 5p contains no or few genes that, if amplified, would counteract cell survival or proliferative advantages conferred by the amplified target genes. Negatively acting genes, from the tumor cell's perspective, would be selected against. Also neutral passenger genes would gradually be lost since they represent a replication cost affecting the tumor cells' fitness. However, it is not necessarily so that higher copy numbers are a sign of pathogenetic impact. First, the copy number is not always directly correlated with expression at the protein level [41]. Second, the tuning of protein co-expression is delicate. Amplified genes can affect the activity of many non-amplified genes and too many copies of some genes could be counterproductive for the cancer cell fitness.

The origin of the observed scattered pattern of amplified 5p and 12q sequences is obscure. Most probably, there was an early rearrangement involving substantial parts of chromosomes 5 and 12 resulting in a mitotically unstable, possibly dicentric, structure. Through further structural reorganization, *MDM2/CDK4* and 5p genes may have been positioned close to each other and then spread to other chromosomes, sometimes together and sometimes separately. The many chromosomes involved indicate a stage of karyotypic instability, which may have been transient. Although the observed karyotype may represent a sideline in the tumor cell population that was preferentially dividing in vitro, or biased sampling, it did not, despite its complexity, show signs of extensive heterogeneity. A possible initial event could be chromothripsis, a phenomenon that in itself does not result in copy number changes, but can be a starting point [42, 43]. However, some of the aberrant chromosomes, in particular B but also C, containing large segments of both chromosomes 5 and 12 are hardly compatible with amplification following chromothripsis. An alternative scenario might be related to the mechanism of telomere length maintenance active in the tumor. Instead of activation of the telomerase-associated mechanism many sarcomas use alternative lengthening of telomere mechanisms. This is rare in WDLS and myxoid liposarcomas, but fairly common in DDLS and the dominating mechanism in PLS [44]. Part of the alternative lengthening of telomeres confers a destabilization of the genome through nuclear receptor binding to telomeres resulting in multiple inserted interstitial telomere sequences that are fragile and thus recombination prone [45]. This mechanism alone or, more likely, combined with an early mitotically unstable structure including 5p and 12q sequences as alluded to above could lead to amplification and a spreading of these sequences to a variety of chromosomes. Indeed, other mechanisms may be responsible for the observed pattern of scattered amplification. Recent studies have demonstrated that telomere crisis and telomere healing can have dramatic and multiple effects on the genome [46, 47]. These include polyploidization as well as chromosome instability that may lead to kataegis or chromothripsis-like aberrations.

Whether the present tumor represents an exceptional case remains unknown since few similar studies of liposarcomas without ring or giant marker chromosomes have been reported.

Conclusions

The finding of genomic amplification through distribution of 5p and 12q sequences, together and separately, to many chromosomes in a DDLS lesion represents a novel cytogenetic pattern of copy number gains. This contrasts with amplification through formation of ring or giant marker chromosomes commonly seen in WDLS and DDLS. The amplicons of 12q were discontinuous, whereas those of 5p comprised almost the entire arm. Apart from *CDK4*, *HMGA2* and *MDM2* in 12q,

candidate target genes in 5p contributing to pathogenesis include *TRIO* and *AMACR* that showed elevated expression.

Additional files

Additional file 1: Fraction of lesions with cytogenetically detectable structures associated with gene amplification among soft tissue tumors. (DOC 104 kb)

Additional file 2: SNP array results from the two tumor samples. (ZIP 720 kb)

Additional file 3: Putative fusion transcripts detected at mRNA sequencing. (XLSX 26 kb)

Acknowledgements
Not applicable.

Funding
This work was supported by the Swedish Cancer Society.

Authors' contributions
NM and FM designed the study and wrote the manuscript. LM and NM performed karyotyping and FISH analyses. FVvS provided patient data. JN, FM, BV, AI and NM performed the SNP array analyses. FM and EA performed the RNA-seq analyses. All authors read and approved the manuscript.

Competing interests
The authors declare that they have no competing interest.

Author details
[1]Division of Clinical Genetics, Department of Laboratory Medicine, Lund University, SE-221 84 Lund, Sweden. [2]Array and Analysis Facility, Uppsala University, Uppsala, Sweden. [3]Department of Orthopedics, Clinical Sciences, Lund University and Skåne University Hospital, Lund, Sweden.

References
1. Mandahl N, Mertens F. Soft tissue tumors. In: Heim S, Mitelman F, editors. Cancer cytogenetics: chromosomal and molecular genetic aberrations of tumor cells, 4th ed. Oxford: Wiley Blackwell; 2015. p. 583-614.
2. Mitelman F, Johansson B, Mertens F (Eds.). Mitelman database of chromosome aberrations and Gene fusions in cancer. 2017. http://cgap.nci.nih.gov/Chromosomes/Mitelman.
3. Gisselsson D, Pettersson L, Höglund M, Heidenblad M, Gorunova L, Wiegant J, et al. Chromosomal breakage-fusion-bridge events cause genetic intratumor heterogeneity. Proc Natl Acad Sci U S A. 2000;97:5357–62.
4. Mandahl N, Heim S, Arheden K, Rydholm A, Willén H, Mitelman F. Three major cytogenetic subgroups can be identified among chromosomally abnormal solitary lipomas. Hum Genet. 1988;79:203–8.
5. Jin Y, Möller E, Nord KH, Mandahl N, Vult von Steyern F, Domanski HA, et al. Fusion of the *AHRR* and *NCOA2* genes through a recurrent translocation t(5;8)(p15;q13) in soft tissue angiofibroma results in upregulation of aryl hydrocarbon receptor target genes. Genes Chromosomes Cancer. 2012;51:510–20.
6. Walther C, Mayrhofer M, Nilsson J, Hofvander J, Jonson T, Mandahl N, et al. Genetic heterogeneity in rhabdomyosarcoma revealed by SNP array analysis. Genes Chromosomes Cancer. 2016;55:3–15.
7. Rasmussen M, Sundström M, Göransson Kultima H, Botling J, Micke P, Birgisson H, et al. Allelespecific copy number analysis of tumor samples with aneuploidy and tumor heterogeneity. Genome Biol. 2011;12:R108.
8. Mayrhofer M, Viklund B, Isaksson A, Rawcopy: improved copy number analysis with Affymetrix arrays http://www.nature.com/articles/srep36158
9. Hofvander J, Tayebwa J, Nilsson J, Magnusson L, Brosjö O, Larsson O, et al. RNA sequencing of sarcomas with simple karyotypes: identification and enrichment of fusion transcripts. Lab Investig. 2015;95:603–9.
10. Nicorici D, Satalan M, Edgren H, Kangaspeska S, Murumagi A, Kallioniemi O, Virtanen S, Kilkku O. Fusion catcher - a tool for finding somatic fusion genes in paired-end RNA-sequencing data. 2014. http://dx.doi.org/10.1101/011650.

11. Szymanska J, Tarkkanen M, Wiklund T, Virolainen M, Blomqvist C, Asko-Seljavara S, et al. Gains and losses of DNA sequences in liposarcomas evaluated by comparative genomic hybridization. Genes Chromosomes Cancer. 1996;15:89–94.

12. Chibon F, Mariani O, Derre J, Malinge S, Coindre J-M, Guillou L, et al. A subgroup of malignant fibrous histiocytomas is associated with genetic changes similar to those of well-differentiated liposarcomas. Cancer Genet Cytogenet. 2002;139:24–9.

13. Micci F, Teixeira MR, Bjerkehagen B, Heim S. Characterization of supernumerary rings and giant marker chromosomes in well-differentiated lipomatous tumors by a combination of G-banding, CGH, M-FISH, and chromosome- and locus specific FISH. Cytogenet Genome Res. 2002;97:13–9.

14. Rieker RJ, Joos S, Bartsch C, Willeke F, Schwarzbach M, Otano-Joos M, et al. Distinct chromosomal imbalances in pleomorphic and in high-grade dedifferentiated liposarcomas. Int J Cancer. 2002;99:68–73.

15. Schmidt H, Bartel F, Kappler M, Würl P, Lange H, Bache M, et al. Gains of 13q are correlated with a poor prognosis in liposarcoma. Modern Pathol. 2005;18:638–44.

16. Tap WD, Eilber FC, Ginther C, Dry SM, Reese N, Barzan-Smith K, et al. Evaluation of well-differentiated/de-differentiated liposarcomas by high-resolution oligonucleotide array-based comparative genomic hybridization. Genes Chromosomes Cancer. 2011;50:95–112.

17. Garsed DW, Marshall OJ, Corbin VDA, Hsu A, Di Stefano L, Schröder J, et al. The architecture and evolution of cancer neochromosomes. Cancer Cell. 2014;26:653–67.

18. Horvai AE, DeVries S, Roy R, O'Donnell RJ, Waldman F. Similarity in genetic alterations between paired well-differentiated and dedifferentiated components of dedifferentiated liposarcoma. Modern Pathol 2009;22:1477-1488.

19. Wang R, Titley JC, Lu Y-J, Summersgill BM, Bridge JA, Fisher C, et al. Loss of 13q14-q21 and gain of 5p14-pter in the progression of leiomyosarcoma. Mod Pathol. 2003;16:778–85.

20. Idbaih A, Coindre J-M, Derre J, Mariani O, Terrier P, Ranchere D, et al. Myxoid malignant fibrous histiocytoma and pleomorphic liposarcoma share very similar genomic imbalances. Lab Investig. 2005;85:176–81.

21. Adamowicz M, Radlwimmer B, Rieker RJ, Mertens D, Schwarzbach M, Schraml P, et al. Frequent amplifications and abundant expression of TRIO, NKD2, and IRX2 in soft tissue sarcomas. Genes Chromosomes Cancer. 2006; 45:829–38.

22. Larramendy ML, Gentile M, Soloneski S, Knuutila S, Böhling T. Does comparative genomic hybridization reveal distinct differences in DNA copy number sequence patterns between leiomyosarcoma and malignant fibrous histiocytoma? Cancer Genet Cytogenet. 2008;187:1–11.

23. Ohguri T, Hisaoka M, Kawauchi S, Sasaki K, Aoki T, Kanemitsu S, et al. Cytogenetic analysis of myxoid liposarcoma and myxofibrosarcoma by array-based comparative genomic hybridization. J Clin Pathol. 2009;59:978–83.

24. Barretina J. And 45other authors. Subtype-specific genomic alterations define new targets for soft tissue sarcoma therapy. Nat Genet. 2010;42:715–21.

25. Guillou L, Aurias A. Soft tissue sarcomas with complex genomic profiles. Virchows Arch. 2010;456:201–17.

26. Gibault L, Perot G, Chibon F, Bonnin S, Lagarde P, Terrier P, et al. New insights in sarcoma oncogenesis: a comprehensive analysis of a large series of 160 soft tissue sarcomas with complex genomics. J Pathol. 2011;223:64–71.

27. Li C-F, Wang J-M, Kang H-Y, Huang C-K, Wang J-W, Fang F-M, et al. Characterization of amplification-driven SKP2 overexpression in myxofibrosarcoma: potential implications in tumor progression and therapeutics. Clin Cancer Res. 2012;18:1598–610.

28. Nord KH, Macchia G, Tayebwa J, Nilsson J, Vult von Steyern F, Brosjö O, et al. Integrative genome and transcriptome analyses reveal two distinct types of ring chromosome in soft tissue sarcomas. Hum Mol Genet. 2014;23:878–88.

29. Zheng M, Simon R, Mirlacher M, Maurer R, Gasser T, Forster T, et al. TRIO amplification and abundant mRNA expression is associated with invasive growth and rapid tumor cell proliferation in urinary bladder cancer. Am J Pathol. 2004;165:63–9.

30. Kang JU, Koo SH, Kwon KC, Park JW, Kim JM. Gain at chromosomal region 5p15.33, containing TERT, is the most frequent genetic event in early stages of non-small cell lung cancer. Cancer Genet Cytogenet. 2008;182:1–11.

31. Scotto L, Narayan G, Nandula SV, Subramaniyam S, Kaufmann AM, Wright JD, et al. Integrative genomics analysis of chromosome 5p gain in cervical cancer reveals target over-expressed genes, including Drosha. Mol Cancer. 2008;7:58.

32. Tapper W, Chiecchio L, Dagrada GP, Konn ZJ, Stocley DM, Szubert AJ, et al. 2011. Heterogeneity in the prognostic significance of 12p deletion and chromosome 5 amplification in multiple myeloma. J Clin Oncol. 2011;29: e37–9.

33. Pedeutour F, Forus A, Coindre J-M, Berner J-M, Nicolo G, Michiels J-F, et al. Structure of the supernumerary ring and giant rod chromosomes in adipose tissue tumors. Genes Chromosomes Cancer. 1999;24:30–41.

34. Meza-Zepeda LA, Berner J-M, Henriksen J, South AP, Pedeutour F, Dahlberg AB, et al. Ectopic sequences from truncated HMGIC in liposarcomas are derived from various amplified chromosomal regions. Genes Chromosomes Cancer. 2001;31:264–73.

35. Snyder EL, Sandstrom DJ, Law K, Fiore C, Sicinska E, Brito J, et al. C-Jun amplification and overexpression are oncogenic in liposarcoma but not always sufficient to inhibit the adipocytic differentiation programme. J Pathol. 2009;218:292–300.

36. Forus A, Bjerkehagen B, Sirvent N, Meza-Zepeda LA, Coindre J-M, Berner J-M, et al. A well-differentiated liposarcoma with a new type of chromosome 12-derived markers. Cancer Genet Cytogenet. 2001;131:13–8.

37. Nilsson M, Domanski H, Mertens F, Mandahl N. Atypical lipomatous tumor with rare structural rearrangements involving chromosomes 8 and 12. Oncol Rep. 2005;13:649–52.

38. Santarius T, Shipley J, Brewer D, Stratton MR, Cooper CS. A census of amplified and overexpressed human cancer genes. Nat Rev Cancer. 2010;10: 59–64.

39. Gibault L, Ferreira C, Perot G, Audebourg A, Chibon F, Bonnin S, et al. From PTEN loss of expression to RICTOR role in smooth muscle differentiation: complex involvement of the mTOR pathway in leiomyosarcomas and pleomorphic sarcomas. Modern Pathol. 2012;25:197–211.

40. Okada T, Lee AY, Qin L-X, Agaram N, Mimae T, Shen Y, et al. Integrin-α10 dependency identifies RAC and RICTOR as therapeutic targets in high-grade myxofibrosarcoma. Cancer Discov. 2016;6:1148–65.

41. Dürrbaum M, Storchova Z. Effects of aneuploidy on gene expression: implications for cancer. FEBS J. 2016;283:791–802.

42. Kloosterman WP, Koster J, Molenaar JJ. Prevalence and clinical implications of chromotripsis in cancer genomes. Current Opinion. 2014;26:64–72.

43. Rode A, Maass KK, Willmund KV, Lichter P, Ernst A. Chromothripsis in cancer cells: an update. Int J Cancer. 2015;138:2322–33.

44. Lee J-C, Jeng Y-M, Liau J-Y, Tsai J-H, Hsu H-H, Yang C-Y. Alternative lengthening of telomeres and loss of ATRX are frequent events in pleomorphic and dedifferentiated liposarcomas. Modern Pathol. 2015;28: 1064–73.

45. Marzec P, Armenise C, Perot G, Roumelioti F-M, Basyuk E, Gagos S, et al. Nuclear-receptor-mediated telomere insertion leads to genome instability in ALT cancers. Cell. 2015;160:913–27.

46. Maciejowski J, de Lange T. Telomeres in cancer: tumour suppression and genome instability. Nat Rev Mol Cell Biol. 2017;18:175–86.

47. Hannes F, Van Houdt J, Quarrell OW, Poot M, Hochstenbach R, Fryns J-P, et al. Telomere healing following DNA polymerase arrest-induced breakages is likely the main mechanism generating chromosome 4p terminal deletions. Hum Mut. 2010;31:1343–51.

16

Karyotype features of trematode *Himasthla elongata*

Anna I. Solovyeva[1*], Vera N. Stefanova[1], Olga I. Podgornaya[1,2,3] and Serghei Iu. Demin[1]

Abstract

Background: Trematodes have a complex life cycle with animal host changes and alternation of parthenogenetic and hermaphrodite generations. The parthenogenetic generation of the worm (rediae) from the first intermediate host *Littorina littorea* was used for chromosome spreads production. Karyotype description of parasitic flatworm *Himasthla elongata* Mehlis, 1831 (Digenea: Himasthlidae) based on fluorochrome banding and 18S rDNA mapping.

Results: Chromosome spreads were obtained from cercariae embryos and redial tissue suspensions with high pressure squash method.74.4 % of the analysed spreads contained 12 chromosome pairs (2n = 24). Chromosome classification was performed according to the morphometry and nomenclature published. *H. elongata* spread chromosomes had a rather bead-like structure. Ideograms of DAPI-banded chromosomes contained 130 individual bands. According to flow cytometry data, the *H. elongata* genome contains 1.25 pg of DNA, so one band contains, on average, 9.4 Mb of DNA. Image bank captures of individual high-resolution DAPI-banded chromosomes were provided. Differential DAPI- and CMA₃-staining revealed the chromatin areas that differed in AT- or GC-content. Both dyes stained chromosomes all along but with varying intensities in different areas. FISH revealed that vast majority (95.0 %) of interphase nuclei contained one signal for 18S rDNA. This corresponded to the number of nucleoli per cell detected by observations *in vivo*. The rDNA signal was observed on one or two homologs of chromosome 10 in 72.2 % of analysed chromosome spreads, therefore chromosome 10 possessed the main rDNA cluster and minor ones on chromosomes 3 and 6, that corresponds with AgNOR results.

Conclusions: *Himasthla elongata* chromosomes variations presented as image bank. Differential chromosome staining with fluorochromes and FISH used for 18S rDNA mapping let us to conclude: (1) *Himasthla elongata* karyotype is 2n = 24; (2) chromosome number deviates from the previously studied echinostomatids (2n = 14–22); (3). Chromosome 10 possesses the main rDNA cluster with the minor ones existing on chromosomes 3 and 6.

Keywords: *Himasthla elongata*, Digenea, Karyotype, 18S rDNA mapping

Background

The digenetic trematodes, or flukes, are ones of the most common and abundant of parasitic worms. They act as parasites on all classes of vertebrates, especially marine fishes, and nearly every organ of the vertebrate body can be parasitised by some kind of trematode, adult or juvenile [1]. Many trematode species are the causative agents for massive zoonosises. The list of flukes infectious to humans is quite large, and because of their importance, numerous investigations have been initiated, especially regarding parasite-host interactions [1]. Human parasites as model objects require appropriate laboratory conditions. The subclass Digenea comprises about 18000 species and it is possible to find a safe alternative for parasite research. Genus *Himasthla* is an example of a safe research option. There are 25 presently described species of *Himasthla Mehlis*, 1831 (Digenea: Himasthlidae [2]). Just two of them were found in fishes and one in humans; all three cases seemed to be accidental infections [3]. However, most are studied quite insufficiently, excepting *Himasthla elongata* (Mehlis, 1831), which became a new model for ecological, immunologic and molecular investigations [4–7].

H. elongata is common in the coastal ecosystems of northern European seas. Like other trematodes, it has a complex lifecycle dependent on of host and parthenogenetic (redia, cercaria) and hermaphrodite generations.

* Correspondence: orcinuca@gmail.com
[1]Institute of Cytology RAS, St. Petersburg 194064, Russia
Full list of author information is available at the end of the article

The first intermediate hosts of this parasite are intertidal snails of the *Littorina* (Gastropoda, Prosobranchia) genus and the second intermediate hosts are the intertidal bivalves, *Mytilus edulis* and *Cerastoderma edule*; gulls are its final hosts [8].

Trematode metacercariae parasitising bivalve molluscs may influence the vital functions of the hosts, lowering their resistance to unfavourable environmental factors and, in the case of intensive infection, even causing their death and resulting in mass mollusc mortality [4].

Cytogenetic studies of parasites are useful not only for understanding systematics, but also the basic mechanisms underlying parasitic agents. Among invertebrates, chromosome mapping has been carried out for a few model organisms due to methodological difficulties.

H. elongata becomes a model for zoological and molecular studies, but it has not been studied at the cytogenetic level. The lack of knowledge about karyotype makes problems for genomic investigation. Moreover, propelled by ever-increasing throughput and decreasing costs, next generation sequencing (NGS) has produced a growing number of genomes and transcriptomes sequenced (existing in databases) and it looks like the *H. elongata* genome will be sequenced soon. Newly sequenced genome should be assembled and attached to a chromosome's physical map, thus it is necessary to acquire the data on its karyotype. The purpose of the current study is the description of *H. elongata* chromosomes. DNA sequence mapping is most convenient for carrying out counterstaining chromosome bands with fluorochromes. DAPI excitation emission varies in proportion to the AT-content of DNA and chromatin condensation level [9]. We elaborated protocols for chromosome preparation and fluorescence *in situ* hybridisation (FISH), enabling conservation of the typical pattern of DAPI-banding for all components of the karyotype. To establish the position of GC-rich bands on individual chromosome sets, a GC-specific fluorochrome, chromomycin A_3 (CMA$_3$), was used for staining in addition to DAPI counterstaining. The present study is focused on karyotype description of the parasitic flatworm, *H. elongata*, based on fluorochrome banding and 18S rDNA mapping.

Methods

Sampling site and collection of parasites

A collection of periwinkles infected with *H. elongata* was obtained from, along with cell suspension preparation carried out at the White Sea Biological Station of the Zoological Institute of the Russian Academy of Sciences situated in the Chupa Inlet, the Kandalaksha Bay of the White Sea (66°20′N; 33°38′E) during July and early August in 2012 and 2013. Digeneans were identified on the basis of their mollusc hosts and their morphological [3] and molecular (18S rDNA) features. At least 8 snails with only *H. elongata* infection i.e. 8 populations of *H. elongata* parthenogenetic larvae obtained from their hosts were used in cytogenetic experiments.

Intravital observations

Live materials were observed under a Leika DM2500 microscope. Dark field illumination at low magnification (objective 10×) was realised by use of the Ph3 phase diaphragm in combination with closed differential interference contrast (DIC) prisms. DIC was utilized for observations under the 100× DIC objective.

Metaphase chromosome spread preparation

H. elongata parthenitae - rediae were obtained in amount of several hundreds individuals from each *L. littorea* snails and washed from the host tissue by three exchanges of seawater filtered through a 0.22 mm Millipore filter. The worms were incubated in Leiboviz L-15 (Sigma) medium with 0,01 mg/ml gentamycin (PanECO, Russia) and 0.1 % colchicine (PanECO, Russia) for 4 h at room temperature and treated with hypotonic solution (5 mM KCl) for 40 min, then fixed with Carnoy's solution (methanol:glacial acetic acid mixture; 3:1). Fixed rediae were repeatedly passed through the syringe with a 22 G needle. The suspension was placed in 15 ml tubes and kept still for 3–5 min to sediment large fragments. The top phase was collected and centrifuged three times at 2.5 krpm for 10 min with the three changes of fixative and stored at −20 °C until slide preparation. Chromosome spreads were prepared according to classic cytogenetical protocols used for trematodes [10–15] with convenient air-drying method, along with more recent techniques, such as high-pressure squash preparation [16, 17]. The convenient air-drying method was performed as follows: 4 or 5 drops of cell suspension were carefully placed onto slides which had been previously chilled in ice water for maintaining a thin film of water at the time when the drops fall on the slide from a height of about 20 cm. Slides were air-dried and then stored at −20 °C until staining. A modified protocol from Deng et al. [14] was performed the next way: the washed slides were placed an a stainless steel bar inside a moist chamber. 30 µl of cell suspension were dropped on each slide Then the moist chamber was at 50 °C in thermostat until fixative drying.

High-pressure squash preparation

Whole *H. elongata* rediae were fixed after colchicine and hypotonic solution treatment and used for spreading chromosomes. On average 50 rediae from different snails were used for slides preparations. The suspension of dissociated into small pieces worms' tissues was dropped on slides containing Carnoy's solution on the surface. The spread cells were coated with a 50.0 % propionic acid drop and then covered by 24 × 24 mm cover slips immediately after fixative evaporation. A mechanical vise was used to evenly apply pressure to further flatten chromosomes on the preparation. Approximately 150 kg/cm^2 of pressure through the precision vise was gradually applied during 90–120 second intervals. At that point, the slides were placed into liquid nitrogen and the cover slips were removed. Afterwards, the slides were dehydrated in a series of ethanol (70.0, 80.0, and 100.0 %), air-dried and kept in –20 °C until staining.

Giemsa staining

The slides were stained in a 3.0 % solution of Giemsa dye (Merck, USA) in phosphate buffer solution (pH 6.8) for 12 min and flushed with flowing water.

Fluorescent *in situ* hybridization with 18S rDNA probe

As the *H. elongata* genome is not yet sequenced and 18S rDNA is quite conservative, a small subunit ribosomal probe was generated by polimerase chain reaction (PCR) using the 18Sa forward primer (AACCTGGTTGAT CCTGCCA) and the 18Sb reverse primer (GATCCTT CTGCAGGTTCACCTAC) [18]. The PCR product was sequenced in order to confirm its attribution to 18S rDNA and submitted to GenBank (KU886143). The analysis of a 18S rDNA probe sequence was performed with the BLAST tool [19]. Isolation of genomic DNA was performed according to Winnenpeninx [20]. The probes were labelled with biotin-14-dUTP under appropriate conditions. Slide pretreatment was performed according to Khodyuchenko et al. [21] with modifications: chromosome preparations were digested with 100 µg/ml RNase A in 2 × SSC for 1 h at 37 °C and washed twice in 2 × SSC for 5 min each, then prefixed with 2.0 % PFA for 15 min, and then washed with 1 × PBS three times for 5 min at a time and incubated in 0.1 % Triton X-100 for 10 min and washed again with 1 × PBS. Hybridisation at 37 °C for 18 h was followed by the washes, which included 0.2 × SSC (3 × 5 min, 60 °C) and 2 × SSC (3 × 5 min, 42 °C). Probe signals were detected with streptavidin – Alexa Fluor 594 conjugate (Life technologies, USA) in blocking solution. The slides were counterstained with Slow Fade Gold Antifade with DAPI (Molecular Probes, USA).

Double Chromomycin A₃ - DAPI staining

The slides were stained with Chromomycin A$_3$ (CMA$_3$) based on Schweizer [22] with several modifications. The stock solution of chromomycin A$_3$ (Sigma-Aldrich) (1 mg/ml) was prepared by dissolution in deionised water without stirring for several days at 4 °C in the dark.

Older solutions tend to stain better. Working solution of CMA$_3$ (0.5 mg/ml) was prepared by dissolving (1:1) the stock solution in McIlvaine's buffer (pH = 7.0) with 5 mM MgCl$_2$. Slides were rinsed in McIlvaine's buffer and placed in CMA$_3$ working solution under a coverslip and stained in the dark at RT for 1 to 2 hours. To remove the coverslip, the slides were briefly washed in McIlvaine's buffer and air-dried. After that a few drops of DAPI solution are placed on slides and covered with a coverslips. Slides are stained in the dark for 20–30 min at RT, rinsed in McIlvaine's buffer and air-dried. DAPI stock solution (1 mg/ml) is prepared on deionized water and can be stored frozen in dark for a year. DAPI working solution (0.8mkg/ml) is prepared on McIlvaine's buffer (pH = 7.0) usually fresh before use. Then the slides were mounted in ProLongR Gold antifade (Invitrogen) and sealed with nail polish. Stained slides were aged for 3 to 5 days in the dark at 4 °C to stabilise CMA$_3$ fluorescence before examination.

Fluorescence microscopy

Chromosome spreads were examined with a Leica Fluorescence Microscope DMI 6000B (Leica Wetzlar GmbH, Germany) at the Development of Molecular and Cellular Technologies Resource Centre at Saint-Petersburg State University. Images were taken with a 100×/1.4 oil immersion objective using appropriate filter cubes fluorescent dyes, like CMA$_3$(430–480 nm), Alexa 594 and DAPI(360–390 nm), and recorded using a monochrome-cooled CCD camera. Karyological data of *H. elongata* (relative length and centromeric index) were calculated in 64 best spreads out of 100 evaluated spreads with Image Tool 3.0 software [23]. The centromere position on the chromosomes was classified according to the nomenclature of Levan et al. [24]. Negative images of DAPI-stained chromosomes were enhanced in Adobe Photoshop version 4 as described before [25].

Results

Identification of a prometaphase and metaphase chromosome source among larval cells was carried out by comparing cell morphology at preparations of shredded and fixed rediae tissues with preparations of live juvenile cercariae or embryos at different developmental stages. Cytological preparations stained with Giemsa contained cells of various sizes and morphology (Fig. 1a, b). All slides contained large amounts of resting cells, which contained a round or oval 6–8 µm diameter nuclei, uniformly filled with condensed chromatin, and possessed a narrow cytoplasm rim with a width of 1 µm. The vast majority of chromosome spreads were determined among the large round or oval cells with a 10–20 µm core diameter, representing no more than 1.0–5.0 % of all cells in

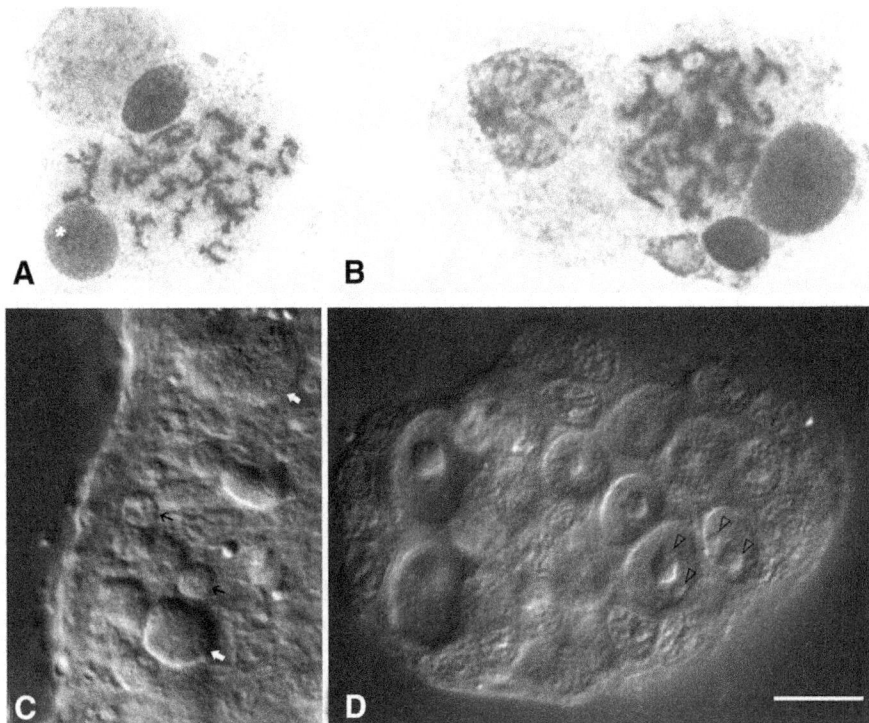

Fig. 1 a, b flattened small pieces of tissues with large sized prometaphase-metaphase and interphase cells in association with small sized, probably senescent or stem cells (asterisk), dissociated mature rediae (Giemsa staining). **c, d** DIC images of alive juvenile cercaria (lateral fragment of the body) and its embryo; (**c**) – tegumental margin with large subtegumental glandular cells (white arrows) and small, probably senescent or stem cells (black arrows); (**d**) cercarial embryo, nucleoli are visible (arrowheads). Scale bar – 10 μm

the preparation. These cells had either an acentric core and a developed cytoplasm or a centrally located nucleus and a narrow (no wider than 3 μm) layer of cytoplasm (Fig. 1c, d). According to histological and cytological features, the large cells located near the tegument may correspond to subtegumental glandular cells – socalled cyton precursors, – the tegument nucleus-bearing compound [26]. This source was used for chromosome preparations. The prometaphase spreads were obtained with a high pressure (~150 kg/cm^2) spreading technique [16] applied to the cell suspension, made from shredded rediae and cercariae embryos. Compared with a convenient air-drying method and a complexed protocol described by Deng et al. [14], the chromosomes, treated with pressure had a much better bands resolution, therefore we considered to call them "high-resolution" chromosomes. An example of a metaphase chromosomes' DAPI-banding pattern is shown in Fig. 2.

About 74.4 % of the spreads analysed contained 12 chromosome pairs (2n = 24), while the others were aneuploid. Generally, *H. elongata* chromosomes had a rather bead-like structure than a banded one. Prometaphase-metaphase chromosomes of *H. elongata* large sized cells relatively rare had conjugated sister chromatids (SCs). Usually their SCs were dissociated elsewhere

for the exception of centromeric region. X- or Λ-shaped chromosome figures that is considered typical only for metaphase, formed as the result. Sister chromatids were associated only in the centromere region in approximately half of the typical prometaphase-metaphase chromosomes with dissociated SCs. In the other half, they had a conjugated SCs yielding to a rod-shaped or I-shaped form. Chromomeric patterns of sister chromatids for the chromosomes with dissociated SCs were similar but not the same. Such chromosomes consisted of two 0.5–2 μm collaterally-associated chromatin strands with clearly visible primary (centromeric) constriction. Such primary constriction was observed quite rarely in chromosomes with conjugated SCs. The frequencies chromosomes with different type of SCs association observed in prometaphase-metaphase spreads are summarised in Table 1.

The difference in chromosome shapes may reflect the dynamics of sister chromatid segregation during cell division (Table 1). Not a single spread exhibited complete segregation, i.e. in all the set (24) with 2 chromatids, usually about half of the set already went through segregation. Metaphase DAPI-banded karyotype of *H. elongata* (2n = 24, Fig. 2) allows chromosomes' classification. Table 2 demonstrates the morphometric data for each

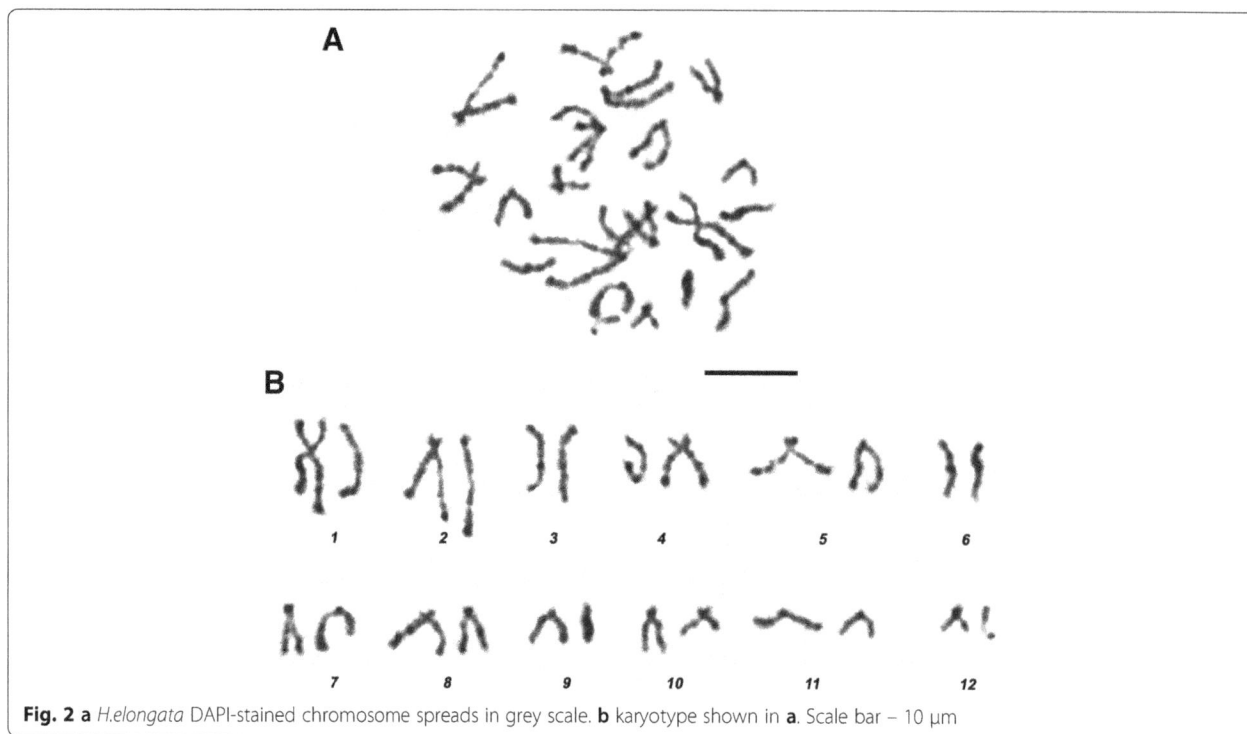

Fig. 2 a H.elongata DAPI-stained chromosome spreads in grey scale. **b** karyotype shown in **a**. Scale bar – 10 µm

set of chromosomes. All measurements and centromeric index calculations were performed for metaphase chromosomes with dissociated SCs. Pairs 2, 4–7 and 11 and 12 can accurately be classified as subtelocentric, pair 3 – metacentric. The classification of chromosomes 1 (m-sm) and 8–10 (sm-st) is uncertain for centromeric index values SD is on the border of two types [24].

High-resolution DAPI-banded H. elongata chromosome ideogram construction was based on the results of relative chromosome length and the centromeric index counted (Table 2) as well as morphology. Graphic ideograms were based on the negative image of DAPI-banded chromosomes with maximum bands resolution. H. elongata chromosomes possess a typical chromomere (necklace-like) structure. Such morphology is characteristic of human and animal pachytene meiotic chromosomes, but not mitotic chromosomes [27, 28]. All chromosomes contained a block of centromeric heterochromatin. Homologous chromosomes within a single cell could possess centromeric heterochromatin of different sizes; they also vary at different metaphase plates. Ideograms of H. elongata high-resolution DAPI-banded

chromosomes contain 130 individual bands resolved in haploid chromosomes set (Fig. 3). According to flow cytometry data, the H. elongata genome contains 1.25 pg of DNA [29] (for a detailed information see Additional file 1: Figure S1 and Additional file 2: Supplementary methods). Simple recalculation (1 pg DNA = 978 Mb) [30] shows that one band in H. elongata chromosome contains, on average 9.4 Mb of DNA.

The image bank of individual DAPI-banded H. elongata chromosomes consists of 12 chromosome rows: each row represents one of the 12 chromosomes of the set (Fig. 4). Each chromosome row shows the basic structural variations typical for the similar sets. Chromosomes are arranged in row according to decreasing length and, consequently, band visibility (i.e. they have morphological differences). Each row shows all two types of chromosome morphology: chromosomes with conjugated or dissociated SCs. Sister chromatid heteromorphism is related to secondary constrictions of chromosomes with dissociated SCs. Nomenclature used for the description of the individual bands is traditional for animal cytogenetics [31]. Chromatid heteromorphism as

Table 1 Frequencies of chromosomes with dissociated sister chromatids in H. elongata chromosome spreads (N = 100)

Number of chromosomes with dissociated SCs in each spread	4	5	6	7	8	9	10	11	12	13	14	15	16	17	18	19	20	21	23
% of spreads with chromosomes with dissociated SCs	1.0	3.0	1.0	2.0	4.0	11.0	7.0	13.0	6.0	9.0	8.0	9.0	10.0	3.0	4.0	3.0	3.0	2.0	1.0

The top row of the table indicates the number of chromosomes with dissociated sister chromatids (SCs) detected in each spread. The bottom row of the table indicates the percent of corresponding cells among 100 spreads analysed

Table 2 Relative length (means ± SD) and centromeric index of *H. elongata* chromosomes

Chromosome №	Relative length, %	Centromeric index, %	Classification
1	14.6 ± 1.7	37.2 ± 2.8	m-sm
2	12.6 ± 2.1	14.9 ± 2.3	st
3	10.8 ± 2.0	42.2 ± 3.8	m
4	9.4 ± 1.4	20.2 ± 3.1	st
5	8.4 ± 1.5	21.4 ± 2.9	st
6	8.3 ± 1.6	15.8 ± 2.6	st
7	8.2 ± 1.4	14.8 ± 2.8	st
8	7.0 ± 1.1	24.2 ± 3.4	sm-st
9	6.5 ± 1.0	24.5 ± 2.9	sm-st
10	5.6 ± 1.0	27.1 ± 3.6	sm-st
11	5.2 ± 0.9	20.2 ± 2.8	st
12	4.1 ± 1.9	20.7 ± 2.3	st

m metacentric, *sm* submetacentric, *st* subtelocentric (= acrocentric)

a consequence of chrommere difference is displayed on the ideograms as circles (Fig. 3, legend). The banding pattern of chromosomes with conjugated SCs corresponds to those of one or another dissociated chromatids.

Sister chromatid variability was observed in the majority of analysed chromosome sets. Interchromosomal variability of premature sister chromatid segregation, leading to the appearance of chromosomes with dissociated SCs, can

be characterised by data from 100 randomly selected spreads (Table 3).

The chromosome pairs are distinguished by different types of sister chromatid segregation patterns: e.g. pairs 4, 5, and 8–11 are represented mostly in form with dissociated SCs, while some pairs are represented mostly by forms with conjugated SCs – pairs 3, 7, and 12. It appears that chromosomes prefer to segregate in the approximate order: 10 > 9 > 8, and so on.

Differential chromosome DAPI- and CMA$_3$-staining revealed the chromatin areas that varied in AT- and GC-content. Both dyes stained the chromosomes all along but with fluctuating intensities in different areas. Staining differences were observed between homologues of several chromosomes (Fig. 5, Arrows). A number of terminal bands, dark with AT-specific fluorochrome DAPI, were stained quite pronouncedly by GC-specific fluorochrome CMA$_3$, namely chromosomes 2, 4, 9 and 10. On the contrary, terminal and centromeric regions of chromosome 5 stained more intensive with DAPI than with CMA$_3$ (Fig. 5).

There was variability in staining between homologs and sister chromatids. A clear example is seen on chromosome 4 (Fig. 5d). This kind of chromosome variability could be associated with the recombination that takes place during the sexual process between adult worms inside definitive host birds.

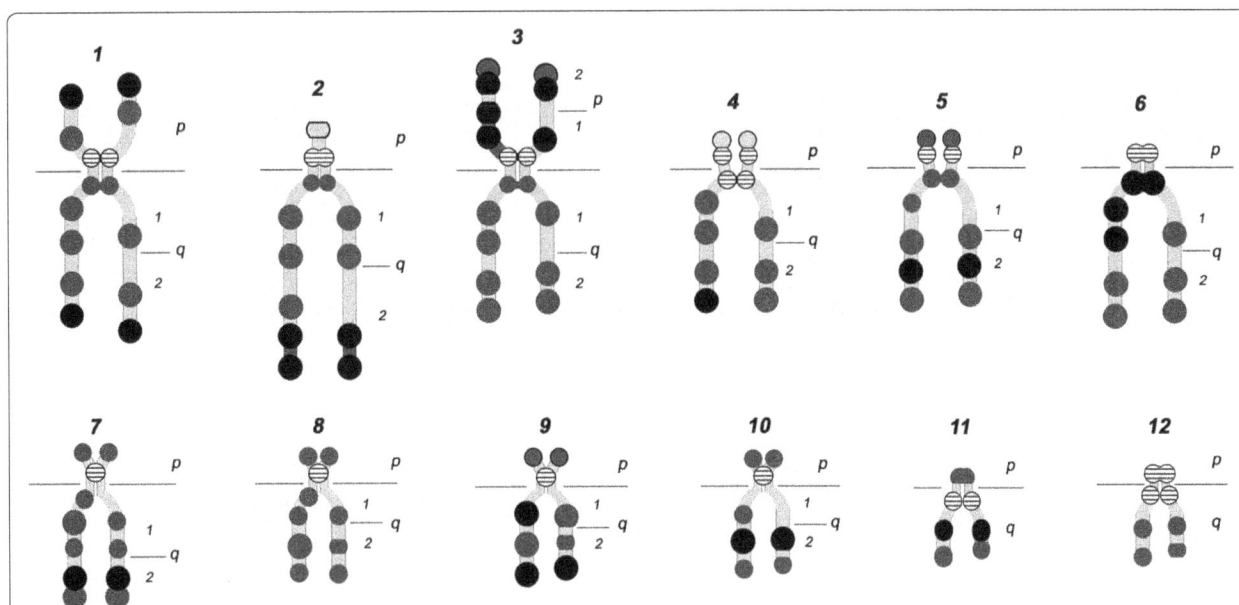

Fig. 3 *H. elongata* chromosomes ideogram. Left chromatid on each ideogram represents the summary of chromosome bands with the best resolution and maximum amount of bands visible; the right chromatid represent chromatid often observed; p and q arms are marked. Differences between sizes of DAPI-bands are indicated by circles of two sizes, fluorescence intensity are marked by three shades in grey scale. The terminal bands (chromosomes 2–5, 9) which are designated as black line bordered circles, are not always detected after DAPI-staining. Heterochromatin containing bands are designated with hatching. The straight lines adjacent to the chromosome on both sides indicate the centromere position

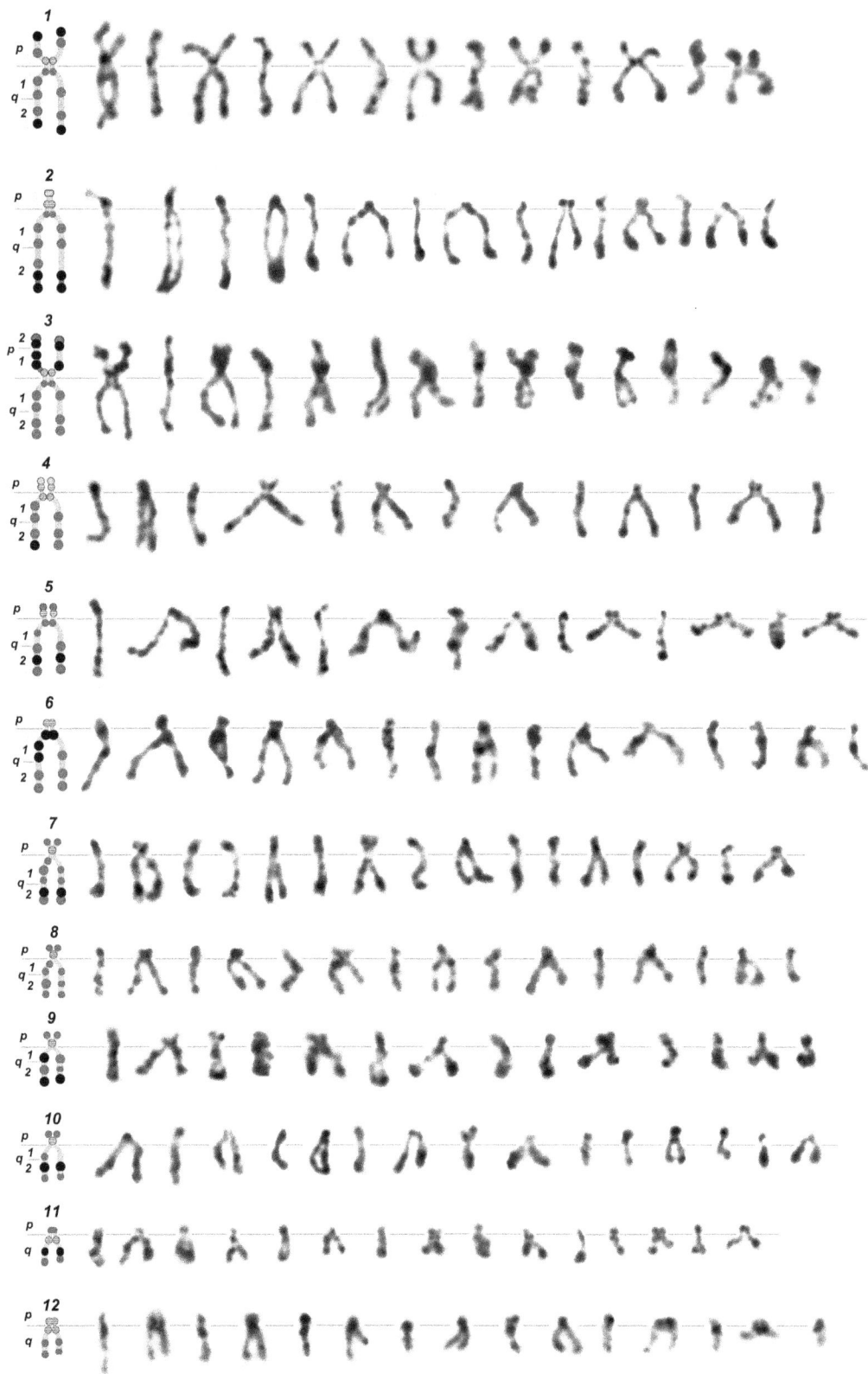

Fig. 4 (See legend on next page.)

Fig. 4 Representative rows of individual DAPI-banded *H. elongata* chromosomes. Each row begins with the ideogram of chromosome ; p and q arms marked; Differences between sizes of DAPI-bands are indicated by circles of two sizes, fluorescence intensity are marked by three shades in grey scale. The following row shows the main chromosome structural variations. Chromosomes are arranged according to decrease of their length and bands' resolution. The straight lines adjacent to the chromosome on both sides indicate the centromere position

FISH of 18S rDNA probe revealed that the vast majority (95.0 %) of interphase nuclei contained one signal (Fig. 6 a, 1). One signal corresponds to the number of nucleoli per cell *in vivo* (Fig. 1). Sometimes one or two small nucleoli were also observed in addition to one large nucleolus (Fig. 6 a, 1). A maximum five signals were detected for 18S rDNA in interphase nuclei. That corresponded to NORs number, detected by Ag-staining (see Additional file 2: Supplementary methods and Additional file 3: Figure S2). The same was true for the chromosome spreads – most of them contained signal on two chromosomes. Three signals were detected in several cases. The rDNA clusters were located on chromosomes 3, 6 and 10. Physical mapping of 18S rDNA clusters on high-resolution *H. elongata* chromosomes (Fig. 6b) uncovered that chromosomes 3 and 10 could contain up to two loci simultaneously on the same arm or on the p and q arm of chromosomes. At the same time only one rDNA signal was detected in chromosome 6. Chromosome mapping of 18S rDNA in *H. elongata* (Fig. 6) revealed rDNA clusters in chromosome pairs 3, 6 and 10. Two labelled chromosome pairs were detected in 82.0 % of cells observed and three were singly labelled in 18.0 %. Only five combinations of two labeled chromosomes (of the six possible) per cell were seen, and a combination of

chromosomes 3 and 6 was not observed. Approximately 78.9 % of evaluated spreads contained signals on chromosome 10 – 42.1 % with signal on pair 10 only, 26.3 % in combination with chromosome 3 and 10.5 % in combination with chromosome 6. Signals on chromosome 6 were found in 28.9 % of spreads (18.4 % with signal only on chromosome 6 and 10.5 % in combination with chromosome 10), and on chromosome 3 in 28.9 % of spreads (2.6 % of only chromosome 3 signal and 26.3 % in combination with chromosome 10). The size of signals at different chromosome pairs was generally equal. Ag-staining revealed 5 signals at chromosomes 3, 6 and 10 (Additional file 4: Figure S3). So at this stage of studies we suppose that chromosome 10 possesses the main rDNA cluster with the minor ones existing on chromosomes 3 and 6.

Discussion

The goal of the work was the description of the *H. elongata* chromosome spreads, good enough for further cytogenetic and molecular researches.

In case of using conventional methods, metaphase cell accumulation observed only after prolonged 4–6 h of colchicine treatment of redia in culture medium and only clumpy metaphases unsuitable for future cytogenetic investigations obtained. It was impossible to determine more than one half of the metaphase chromosome set, while separate chromosomes were too condensed for bands identification. Up to 0.5 % per preparations of prometaphase cells suitable for band detection were obtained by suspending rediae after 4 h and 6 h of colchicine treatment. Thus, it was necessary to find the appropriate method for obtaining a larger amount of a better prometaphase or metaphase spreads. So *in vivo* observations helped to detect multiple dividing cells in several rediae tissues and cercarial embryos. High-pressure squash preparation used to improve chromosome spreads resolution. This delicate approach allows to get unbroken even fragile structures of polytene chromosomes. The results reproduced in multiple experiments at *H. elongata* spreads without significant chromosome damages.

There are morphologic polymorphisms in the number of spreads revealed varying levels of sister chromatid segregation (Tables 1 and 3) and discordance among homologous chromosomes. Partial sister chromatid segregation in *H. elongata* cells is always accompanied by a

Table 3 Distribution of different types of homologous sister chromatid segregation in *H. elongata* chromosomes (100 spreads analysed)

Chromosome №	Homologous chromosomes combinations		
	Dissociated SCs	Dissociated and conjugated SCs	Conjugated SCs
1	15.0	45.0	40.0
2	17.0	47.0	36.0
3	13.0	30.0	57.0
4	59.0	26.0	15.0
5	53.0	30.0	17.0
6	45.0	32.0	33.0
7	16.0	35.0	49.0
8	56.0	33.0	11.0
9	66.0	21.0	12.0
10	74.0	20.0	6.0
11	58.0	23.0	19.0
12	10.0	17.0	73.0

Columns represent % of spreads with amount of homologs dissociated or conjugated for correspondent chromosomes

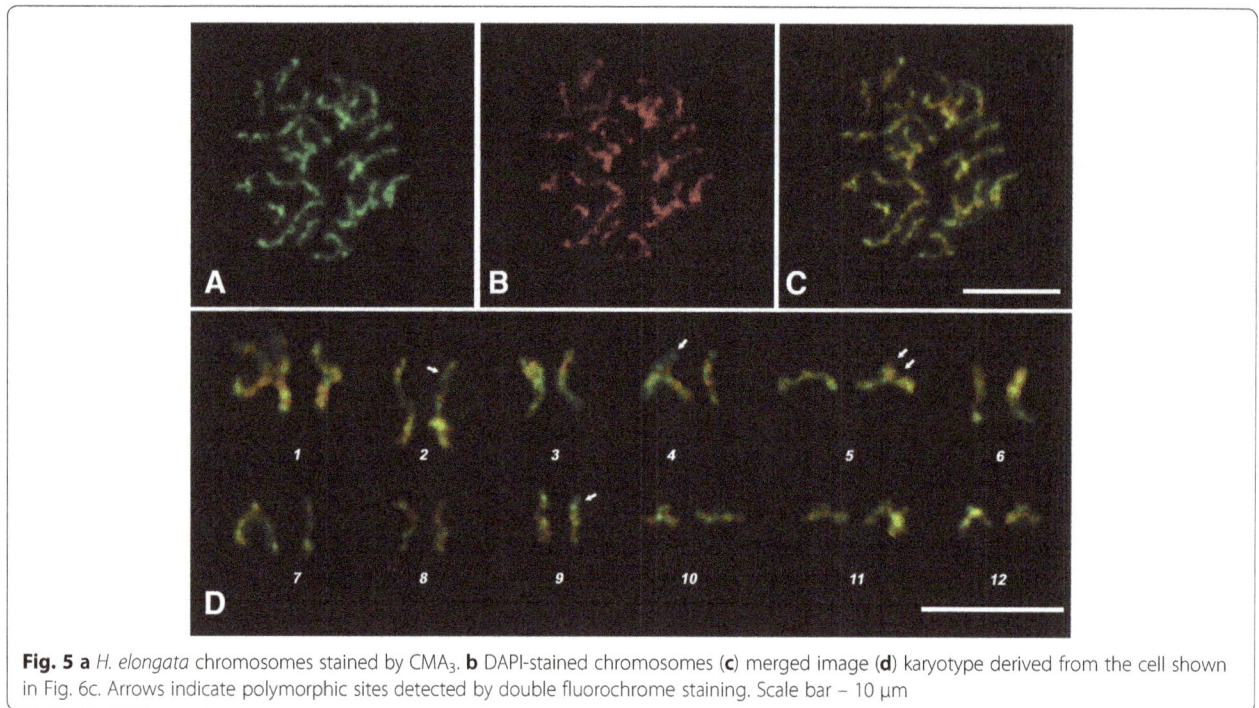

Fig. 5 a *H. elongata* chromosomes stained by CMA$_3$. **b** DAPI-stained chromosomes (**c**) merged image (**d**) karyotype derived from the cell shown in Fig. 6c. Arrows indicate polymorphic sites detected by double fluorochrome staining. Scale bar – 10 µm

pronounced asymmetry in the level of chromatin condensation and (or) the band pattern. The phenomenon of homologue discordance is well established for human chromosomes. It was shown that the discordance minimum values (6.7 – 14.2 %) were observed at metaphase after GTG chromosome banding (G-banding with trypsin-Giemsa), whereas prometaphase chromosomes varied in size and had greater homolog discordance – up to 29.8 % after GTG and 64.2 % RBG (R-banding using bromodeoxyuridine and Giemsa) banding [32].

Homologue discordance has been widely discussed in the literature in terms of embryogenesis [33] and tissue specific stem cell differentiation [34], as well as asymmetry in cell division and tissue differentiation during embryogenesis [35–37]. Thus, the image bank for *H. elongata* karyotype component was made in order to detect all probable variabilities in chromosome morphology.

Representative rows for *H. elongata* individual chromosomes (Fig. 4) served for identification of individual

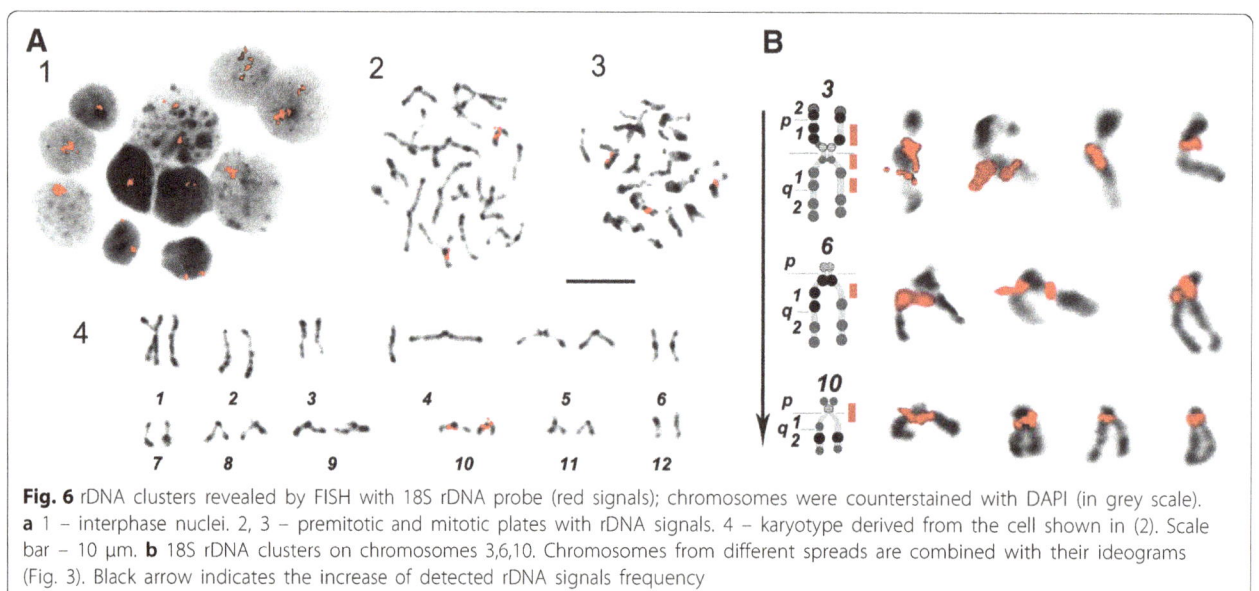

Fig. 6 rDNA clusters revealed by FISH with 18S rDNA probe (red signals); chromosomes were counterstained with DAPI (in grey scale). **a** 1 – interphase nuclei. 2, 3 – premitotic and mitotic plates with rDNA signals. 4 – karyotype derived from the cell shown in (2). Scale bar – 10 µm. **b** 18S rDNA clusters on chromosomes 3,6,10. Chromosomes from different spreads are combined with their ideograms (Fig. 3). Black arrow indicates the increase of detected rDNA signals frequency

chromosomes of prometaphase and metaphase sets. Individual chromosome variation was estimated by the following criteria: cohesion and incomplete sister chromatid segregation, banding pattern, centromeric heterochromatin and the possibility of distinguishing terminal bands by DAPI-staining. A more detailed description of homologs discordance and sister chromatids' segregation variability requires additional study. Right now, we point out that one spread can contain homologs with resolutions corresponding to the extreme right and left positions in the chromosome identification rows (Fig. 5). The chromosome shapes are the superposition of two events: (1) the degree of condensation, which reflects mitosis advance; (2) the extent of sister chromatids' segregation.

Centromeric heterochromatin blocks' size variations, different from other morphological changes, may potentially reflect population variability. The source of such polymorphism could be found with the determination of species major tandem repeat, the main constituent of heterochromatic regions. It is possible that the first steps of H. elongata genome sequencing will bring up a major tandem repeat of this species. Such a repeat will serve as a reliable probe to assess heterochromatin block variability. Right now, it may only be supposed that possible heterozygosity of large heterochromatin blocks visible in many chromosome sets could be associated with cross fertilisation in adult flukes. The intercellular variation observed in heterochromatin does not exclude the possibility of polymorphism in parthenogenetic clonal populations.

Noticeable banding pattern along H. elongata chromosome arms visible after differential DAPI- and CMA_3-staining. It is widely accepted that clear G- and R-blocks, typical for higher vertebrate chromosomes, are heterochromatic and euchromatic regions, respectively [38]. In the current work such banding is obtained for the flatworm karyotype for the first time. Echinostoma caproni is the nearest H. elongata relative, whose genome size is known – 0.85 pg [39]. Unfortunately, E. caproni karyotype is performed by Giemsa staining and C bands (centromeric) were described [10] and no detailed ideograms were made.

From 40.0 to 95.0 % of ribosomal DNA is in the inactive state in animal cells [40]. FISH identification of genes in heterochromatin requires increased chromosome deproteinisation to improve hybridization conditions. Chromosome mapping of inactive rDNA clusters is a common problem of animals cytogenetics with no universal solution so far. Even short-term treatment with pepsin and proteinase K led to the complete disappearance of the chromomere patterns on H. elongata chromosomes. We used the 18S rDNA FISH protocol without any protease treatment. All signals detected with rDNA FISH were also revealed by Ag-staining. Thus, there are at least 3 nucleoli organizing chromosomes in H. elongata karyotype.

Before very recent phylogenetic update [2] H. elongata belonged to Echinostomatidae Looss, 1899 family and following discussion focuses at "old" family state. Karyological data for the Echinostomatidae Looss, 1899 family was available for a rather small number of species whose intermediate hosts are freshwater molluscs and final hosts are birds, pets and humans. The diploid number of chromosomes in the Echinostomatidae family varies from 14 to 22 according to the literature available (Table 4). There is debate about the existence of an evolutionary tendency in the Digenea to maintain the diploid number equal to 20, which seems to be ancestral [11]. No karyological data on any of Himasthla species have been described yet. Based on chromosome number (2n = 24) H. elongata slightly deviates from the previously studied echinostomatids (2n = 14–22). H. elongata karyotype consists of two pairs of large chromosomes and 10 pairs of smaller-sized chromosomes. In contrast with a previous reports collected and analysed by

Table 4 Chromosome number described for Echinostomatidae Looss, 1899 family representatives before recent phylogenetic update [2]

Species	Chromosome number (2n)	Reference
Echinochasmus baleocephalus	14	Barsiene, Kiseliene, 1990 [12]
Echinochasmus sp	20	Staneviciute et al. 2015 [43]
Echinoparyphium aconiatum	20	Mutafova, Kanev, 1984 [44]
Echinoparyphium recurvatum	20	Mutafova et al. 1987 [45]
Echinoparyphium pseudorecurvatum	20	Barsiene et al. 1990 [46]
Echinostoma barbosai	22	Mutafova, Kanev, 1983 [47]
Echinostoma caproni	22	Richard, Voltz, 1987 [10]
Echinostoma echinatum	22	Mutafova, Kanev, 1983; 1986 [47, 48]
Echinostoma revolutum	22	Mutafova, Kanev, 1983; 1986 [47, 48]
Echinostoma cinetorchis	22	Terasaki et al. 1982 [49]
Echinostoma hortense	20	Terasaki et al. 1982 [49]
Episthmium bursicola	20	Barsiene, Kiseliene, 1990 [42]
Hypoderaeum conoideum	20	Mutafova et al. 1986 [50]
Isthmiophora melis	20	Mutafova, et al. 1991 [12]
Moliniela anceps	20	Barsiene et al. 1990 [51]
Neoacantoparyphium echinoides	20	Mutafova, 1994 [13]
Paryphostomum radiatum	16	Mutafova, 1994 [13]
Pegosomum asperum	20	Aleksandrova, Podgornova, 1978 [52]
Pegosomum saginatum	20	Aleksandrova, Podgornova, 1978 [52]
Sphaeridiotrema globulus	22	Mutafova et al. 2001 [53]

Garcia-Souto and J. Pasantes [41] where single loci of major rDNA clusters are described in several digeneans, we revealed multiple signals of rDNA at 3 chromosome pairs in *H. elongata* karyotype. The lack of karyological data on the other *Himasthla* species doesn't allow any speculation about chromosome number characteristic for this genus. More precise evaluation of karyotype components could be performed by geographic population of *H. elongata* expansion and involvement of other *Himasthla* species.

Conclusions

In the current work karyotype of the first representative of *Himastla* genus determined. It is shown that *H. elongata* karyotype consists of two pairs of large chromosomes and 10 pairs of smaller-sized chromosomes. Differential DAPI- and CMA$_3$-staining revealed the AT- and GC-rich chromosome bands. The identification of nucleoli organizing chromosomes was performed with 18S rDNA FISH and Ag-staining. The main rDNA cluster was observed on chromosome 10 with minor examples on chromosomes 3 and 6.

Additional files

Additional file 1: Figure S1. Flow cytometry profile of 2C peaks for the species indicated. X axis - the relative pripidium iodide (PI) fluorescence intensity at FL3 channel; Y-axis, the number of events. (TIF 88 kb)

Additional file 2: Supplementary methods. (DOC 16 kb)

Additional file 3: Figure S2. Ag-staining of *H. elongata* nuclei. Nuclei with more than two Ag-NORs detected are shown in B, C, E, F, G. Scale bar – 10 μm. (TIF 4102 kb)

Additional file 4: Figure S3. Correspondence of Ag-NOR-staining and rDNA FISH signals at aneuploid metaphase spread of *H. elongata*. A – metaphase spread. B – karyotype of the metaphase spread shown in A. Asterisks mark the correspondent chromosomes with rDNA FISH signals at (main text, Fig. 6). Scale bar – 10 μm. (TIF 481 kb)

Competing interests

The authors declare that they have no competing interests.

Authors' contributions

Research concept and design: AS, DS, OP. Material collection AS. Performed the experiments: AS, DS, VS. Image and data analysis: DS, AS. Wrote the paper: DS, AS, OP, VS. All authors read and approved the final version of the manuscript.

Acknowledgements

This work was supported by the Russian Foundation for Basic Research (grants № 05-04-49156-a, 11-04-01700, 15-04-01857), the Russian Science Foundation (grant no.15-15-20026), and the granting program for "Molecular and Cell Biology" of the Presidium of Russian Academy of Sciences (№ 01.2.00 955639). Editing and publishing costs have been paid for by a grant from the Russian Science Foundation (grant №15-15-20026). We deeply appreciate our colleagues, especially Prof. Kirill Galaktionov and Dr. Ivan Levakin, of the Zoological Institute RAS White Sea Biological Station "Kartesh" for provided support and constant attention. We also thank Dr. Nikolai Aksenov of the Flow cytometry and sorting group at Institute of Cytology RAS for kind advises and help with genome size evaluation. The work was partially carried out at the Development of Molecular and Cellular Technologies Resource Center at St. Petersburg University (project № 1.50.1042.2014).

Author details

[1]Institute of Cytology RAS, St. Petersburg 194064, Russia. [2]Saint Petersburg State University, St. Petersburg 199034, Russia. [3]Far Eastern Federal University, Vladivostok 690922, Russia.

References

1. Schmidt GD, Roberts LS. Foundations of parasitology, 6th ed. Boston: McGraw-Hill Comp; 2000. p. 209–33.
2. Tkach VV, Kudlai O, Kostadinova A. Molecular phylogeny and systematics of the Echinostomatoidea Looss, 1899 (Platyhelminthes: Digenea). Int J Parasitol. 2016;46(3):171–85.
3. Stunkard HW. Further studies on the trematode genus *Himasthla* with descriptions of *H. mcintoshi* n. sp., *H. piscicola* n. sp., and stages in the life-history of *H. compacta* n. sp. Biol Bull. 119(3):529. doi: 10.2307/1539266
4. Nikolaev KE, Sukhotin AA, Galaktionov KV. Infection patterns in White Sea blue mussels *Mytilus edulis* L. of different age and size with metacercariae of *Himasthla elongata*(Mehlis, 1831) (Echinostomatidae) and *Cercaria parvicaudata* Stunkard & Shaw, 1931 (Renicolidae). Dis Aquat Organ. 2006;71:51–8.
5. Levakin IA, Losev EA, Nikolaev KE, Galaktionov KV. In vitro encystment of *Himasthla elongata* cercariae (Digenea, Echinostomatidae) in the hemolymph of blue mussels Mytilus edulis as a tool for assessing cercarial infectivity and molluscan susceptibility. J Helminthol. 2012;87:180–8.
6. Solovyeva AI, Galaktionov NK, Podgornaia OI. LINE class retroposon is the component of the DNA polymorphic fragments pattern of trematode *Himasthla elongata* parthenitae. Cell Tissue Biol. 2013;7(6):563–72.
7. Gorbushin AM, Borisova EA. *Himasthla elongata*: implantation of rediae to the specific iteroparous long-living host, *Littorina littorea*, results in the immune rejection. Fish Shellfish Immunol. 2014;39(2):432–8.
8. Werding B. Morphologie, Entwicklung und Okologie digener Trematoden-Larven der Strandschnecke *Littorina littorea*. Marine Biol. 1969;3:306–33.
9. Kapuscinski J. DAPI: a DNA-specific fluorescent probe. Biotech Histochem. 1995;70(5):220–33.
10. Richard J, Voltz A. Preliminary data on the chromosomes of *Echinostoma caproni* Richard, 1964 (Trematoda: Echinostomatidae). Syst Parasitol. 1987;9:169–72.
11. Birstein VJ, Mikhailova NA. On the karyology of trematodes of the genus *Microphallus* and their intermediate gastropod host, *Littorina saxatilis* I.Chromosome analysis of three *Microphallus* species. Genetica. 1990;80:159–66.
12. Mutafova T, Kanev I, Eizenhut U. Karyological studies of *Isthmiophora melis*(Schrank, 1788) from its type locality. J Helminthol. 1991;65:255–8.
13. Mutafova T. Karyological studies on some species of the families Echinostomatidae and Plagiorchiidae and aspects of chromosome evolution in trematodes. Syst Parasitol. 1994;28:229–38.
14. Deng W, Tsao SW, Lucas JN, Leung CS, Cheung AL. A new method for improving metaphase chromosome spreading. Cytometry Part A. 2003;51(1):46–51.
15. Hirai H, Hirai Y. FISH mapping for Helminth genomes. Methods Mol Biol. 2004;270:379–94.
16. Novikov DV, Kireev I, Belmont AS. High-pressure treatment of polytene chromosomes improves structural resolution. Nat Methods. 2007;4(6):483–5.
17. George P, Sharakhova MV, Sharakhov IV. High-resolution cytogenetic map for the African malaria vector anopheles gambiae. Insect Mol Biol. 2010;19(5):675–82.
18. Bayha KM, Dawson MN, Collins AG, Barbeitos MS, Haddock SH. Evolutionary relationships among scyphozoan jellyfish families based on complete taxon sampling and phylogenetic analyses of 18S and 28S ribosomal DNA. Integr Comp Biol. 2010;50(3):436–55.
19. Altschul SF, Gish W, Miller W, Myers EW, Lipman DJ. Basic local alignment search tool. J Mol Biol. 1990;5:403–10.
20. Winnepenninckx B, Backeljau T, De Wachter R. Extraction of high molecular weight DNA from molluscs. Trends Genet. 1993;9:407.
21. Khodyuchenko T, Gaginskaya E, Krasikova A. Non-canonical Cajal bodies form in the nucleus of late stage avian oocytes lacking functional nucleolus. Histochem Cell Biol. 2012;138(1):57–73.

22. Scweizer D. Reverse fluorescent chromosome banding with chromomycin and DAPI. Chromosoma. 1976;58:307–24.

23. UTHSCSA ImageTool Version 3.0 Final. Available from: http://www.uthscsa.edu/academics/dental/departments/comprehensive-dentistry/imagetool/downloads. Accessed 5 Nov 2014.

24. Levan A, Fredga K, Sandberg AA. Nomenclature for centromeric position on chromosomes. Hereditas. 1964;52(2):201–20.

25. Demin S, Pleskach N, Svetlova M, Solovjeva L. High-resolution mapping of interstitial telomeric repeats in Syrian hamster metaphase chromosomes. Cytogenet Genome Res. 2011;132(3):151–5.

26. Whitfield PJ. Trematoda: form, function, and classification of digeneans. In: Foundations of Parasitology. 6th ed. Boston: McGraw-Hill Comp; 2000. p. 209–33.

27. Jhanwar SC, Burns JP, Alonso ML, Hew W, Chaganti RS. Mid-pachytene chromomere maps of human autosomes. Cytogenet Cell Genet. 1982;33(3):240–8.

28. Jhanwar SC, Chaganti RS. Pachytene chromomere maps of Chinese hamster autosomes. Cytogenet Cell Genet. 1981;31(2):70–6.

29. Galaktionov NK, Solovyeva AI, Fedorov AV, Podgornaya OI. Trematode H. elongata mariner element (Hemar): structure and applications. J Exp Biol B. 2014;322(3):142–55.

30. Dolezel J, Bartos J, Voglmayr H, Greilhuber J. Nuclear DNA content and genome size of trout and human. Cytometry A. 2003;51(2):127–8.

31. Nesbitt MN, Francke U. A system of nomenclature for band patterns of mouse chromosomes. Chromosoma. 1973;41:145–58.

32. Schwartz S, Palmer CG. High-resolution chromosome analysis: I. Applications and limitations. Am J Med Genet. 1984;19(2):291–9.

33. Patkin EL. Epigenetic mechanisms for primary differentiation in mammalian embryos. Int Rev Cytol. 2002;216:81–129.

34. Tran V, Feng L, Chen X. Asymmetric distribution of histones during Drosophila male germline stem cell asymmetric divisions. Chromosome Res. 2013;21:255–69.

35. Bell CD. Is mitotic chromatid segregation random? Histol Histopathol. 2005;20:1313–20.

36. Tajbakhsh S, Rocheteau P, Le Roux I. Asymmetric cell divisions and asymmetric cell fates. Ann Rev Cell Dev Biol. 2009;25:671–99.

37. Lansdorp PM, Falconer E, Tao J, Brind'Amour J, Naumann U. Epigenetic differences between sister chromatids? Ann NY Acad Sci. 2012;1266:1–6.

38. Rodionov AV. Evolution of differential chromosome banding. Genetika. 1999;35(2):277–90.

39. WormBase ParaSite release 3. EMBL-EBI & WTSI, 2015 http://parasite.wormbase.org/Echinostoma_caproni_prjeb1207/Info/Annotation/. Accessed 12 Dec 2015.

40. Grummt I. Life on a planet of its own: regulation of RNA polymerase I transcription in the nucleolus. Genes Dev. 2003;17(14):1691–702.

41. Garcia-Souto D, Pasantes JJ. Molecular cytogenetics in Digenean parasites: linked and unlinked major and 5S rDNAs, B chromosomes and karyotype diversification. Cytogenet Genome Res. 2015;147(2–3):195–207.

42. Barsiene J, Kiseliene V. Karyological studies of trematodes within the families Psilostomidae and Echinochasmidae. Helminthologia. 1990;27:99–108.

43. Stanevičiūtė G, Stunžėnas V, Petkevičiūtė R. Phylogenetic relationships of some species of the family EchinostomatidaeOdner, 1910 (Trematoda), inferred from nuclear rDNA sequences and karyological analysis. Comp Cytogenet. 2015;9(2):257–70.

44. Mutafova T, Kanev I. Studies on the karyotype of Echinoparyphium aconiatum Diez, 1909 (Trematoda:Echinostomatidae). Helminthology (Bulg). 1984;17:37–40.

45. Mutafova T, Kanev I, Vassilev I. Comparative karyological investigations of Echinoparyphium aconiatum Dietz, 1909, and Echinoparyphium recuriatum (Linstow, 1873) Dietz, 1909 (Trematoda: Echinostomatidae). Helminthology (Bulg). 1987;24:32–6.

46. Barshene YV, Pyatkyavichyute RB, Stanyavichyute GI, Orlovskaya OM. Karyological studies of trematodes from the families Notocotylidae, Echinostomatidae and Strigeidae in north-western Chukotka. Parazitologiya. 1990;24(1):3–11.

47. Mutafova T, Kanev I. Studies on the karyotype of the echinostome Echinostoma barbosai Lie et Basch, 1966 (Trematoda: Echinostomatidae) from Bulgaria. Helminthology (Bulg). 1983;16:42–6.

48. Mutafova T, Kanev I. Studies on the karyotype of Echinostoma revolutum (Fre1ich, 1802) and Echinostoma echinatum (Zeder, 1803) (Trematoda: Echinostomatidae). Helminthology (Bulg). 1986;22:37–41.

49. Terasaki K, Moriyama N, Tanis S, Ishida K. Comparative studies on the karyotypes of Echinostoma cinetorchis and E. hortense (Echinostomatidae: Trematoda). Jpn J Parasitol. 1982;31:569–74.

50. Mutafova T, Kanev I, Angelova R. Studies on the karyotype of Hypoderaeum concideum (Blanch, 1782) Dietz, 1909 (Trematoda: Echinostomatidae). Helminthology. 1986;22:33–6.

51. Barsiene J, Kiseliene V. Grabda - Kazubska B. Karyotypes of Isthmiophora melis (Schrank, 1788) and Moliniella anceps (Molin, 1858) (Trematoda: Echinostomatidae). Acta Parasitol Polonica. 1990;35:265–9.

52. Aleksandrova OV, Podgornova GP. Taxonomic analysis of Pegosomum asperum and P. saginatum (Trematoda: Echinostomatidae). Parazitologiia. 1978;12(5):413–7.

53. Mutafova T, Kanev I, Panaiotova M. A cytological study of Sphaeridiotrema globulus (Rudolphi, 1819) Odhner, 1913. Exp Pathol Parasitol. 2001;4(5):24–5.

17

A report of nine cases and review of the literature of infertile men carrying balanced translocations involving chromosome 5

Hong-Guo Zhang, Rui-Xue Wang, Yuan Pan, Han Zhang, Lei-Lei Li, Hai-Bo Zhu and Rui-Zhi Liu*

Abstract

Background: Balanced translocations may cause the loss of genetic material at the breakpoints and may result in failure of spermatogenesis. However, carriers of reciprocal translocation may naturally conceive. Genetic counseling of male carriers of translocations remains challenging. This study explores the clinical features of carriers of chromosome 5 translocations, enabling informed genetic counseling of these patients.

Results: Of 82 translocation carriers, 9 (11%) were carriers of a chromosome 5 translocation. One case had azoospermia, while three cases had experienced recurrent spontaneous abortions, two cases had each experienced stillbirth, and three cases produced a phenotypically normal child confirmed by amniocentesis. A literature review identified 106 patients who carried chromosome 5 translocations. The most common chromosome 5 translocation was t(4,5), observed in 13 patients. Breakpoint at 5p15 was observed in 11 patients. All breakpoints at chromosome 5 were associated with gestational infertility.

Conclusion: In genetic counseling, physicians should consider chromosome 5 and its breakpoints. Carriers of chromosome 5 translocations may continue with natural conception or use assisted reproductive technologies, such as preimplantation genetic diagnosis.

Keywords: Male infertility, Chromosome 5, Balanced translocation, Breakpoint, Genetic counseling

Background

Known chromosomal alterations play a major role in perturbing male fertility [1]. Reciprocal chromosomal translocations are the most common structural rearrangement, with an incidence in infertile males up to ten times higher than in fertile men [2]. Balanced chromosomal translocations may cause the loss of genetic material at breakpoints and may result in failure of spermatogenesis [3]. Individuals affected by such translocations exhibit reproductive problems such as infertility, recurrent pregnancy loss, and malformed offspring [4, 5]. These effects are related to the specific chromosomes and breakpoints involved in the translocation [6, 7]. Some breakpoints can disrupt the structure of an important gene, leading to spermatogenic or maturation disorders, and male infertility [5]. Important genes associated with male infertility are located on

chromosome 5. For example, *Camk4* (encoding Ca^{2+}/calmodulin-dependent protein kinase IV) is located on chromosome 5q22.1, and is expressed in spermatids and associated with chromatin and nuclear matrix [8]. Disrupted *CAMK4* expression may be associated with human male infertility [8]. In addition, the *Spink13* gene (encoding serine protease inhibitor, Kazal-type 13), mapped on chromosome 5 at 5q32, was reported to be associated with sperm maturation [9]. The breakpoint of 5p13 was shown to be related to impaired spermatogenesis [10].

However, genetic counseling of male carriers of chromosomal translocations remains challenging. Preimplantation genetic diagnosis (PGD) is recommended for those exhibiting a balanced translocation. Microdissection testicular sperm extraction and in vitro fertilization accompanied by PGD increases the chance of these carriers fathering a healthy child [11, 12]. Clinical characteristics, including spontaneous abortion, do not differ between those couples who accept and those who decline PGD [13]. A systematic review showed there was

* Correspondence: lrz410@126.com
Center for Reproductive Medicine and Center for Prenatal Diagnosis, First Hospital, Jilin University, 71 Xinmin Street, Chaoyang District, Changchun, Jilin Province 130021, China

Table 1 Karyotypes of chromosome 5 translocation carriers and their clinical features

Infertility causes	Clinical findings	Karyotype	Giemsa banding
Pregestational infertility	Azoospermia	46,XY,t(5;21)(q13;p12)	Figure 1a
Gestational infertility	Normal sperm density; a history of miscarriage, or normal fertility	46,XY,t(4;5)(q31;p15)	Figure 1b
		46,XY,t(5;11)(p14;p15)	Figure 1c
		46,XY,t(5;13)(q13;q12)	Figure 1d
		46,XY,t(5;18)(p13;p11)	Figure 1e
		46,XY,t(5;18)(p15;q11.2)	Figure 1f
		46,XY,t(5;20)(q13;q12)	Figure 1g
		46,XY,t(5;21)(p13;q22)	Figure 1h
		46,XY,t(5;22)(p11;p11)	Figure 1i

insufficient evidence that PGD improves the live birth rate in couples with repeated miscarriage and carrying a structural chromosome abnormality [14]. In addition, the live birth rate in patients refused PGD and choosing to conceive naturally was reported to be 37–63% for the first pregnancy, and then a cumulative rate of 65–83% [4]. Natural pregnancy success rates for couples in which the male carries a chromosomal translocation ranged from 30% to 70% [15]. This suggests that continued attempts to conceive naturally are a viable option for successful pregnancy, however, the relationship between clinical features and chromosome structural abnormality warrants further study.

The present study was established to explore the clinical features and translocation breakpoints in carriers of balanced translocations involving chromosome 5. This paper also highlights the importance of genetic counseling for infertile men.

Methods

Patients

Between July 2010 and December 2016, 82 male carriers of chromosomal translocations who were experiencing infertility, or receiving counseling, were recruited from the outpatient's department at the Center for Reproductive Medicine, the First Hospital of Jilin University, Changchun, China. All patients underwent a thorough physical examination and semen analysis, and were required to complete a detailed questionnaire regarding their smoking habits, marital status, medical history, and working conditions. The study protocol was approved by the Ethics Committee of the First Hospital of Jilin University, and written informed consent was obtained from all participants.

Semen analysis

Semen analysis was performed according to procedures recommended by the World Health Organization guidelines. If no sperm was found, sperm was analyzed by sedimenting semen samples through centrifugation. Patients with oligozoospermia were diagnosed as a sperm count less than 15×10^6/ml in their last three semen samples (taken at intervals of 1–3 weeks). Azoospermia and oligozoospermia were defined as previously described [5]. All analyses were performed at the same laboratory, and all data were accessed from medical records.

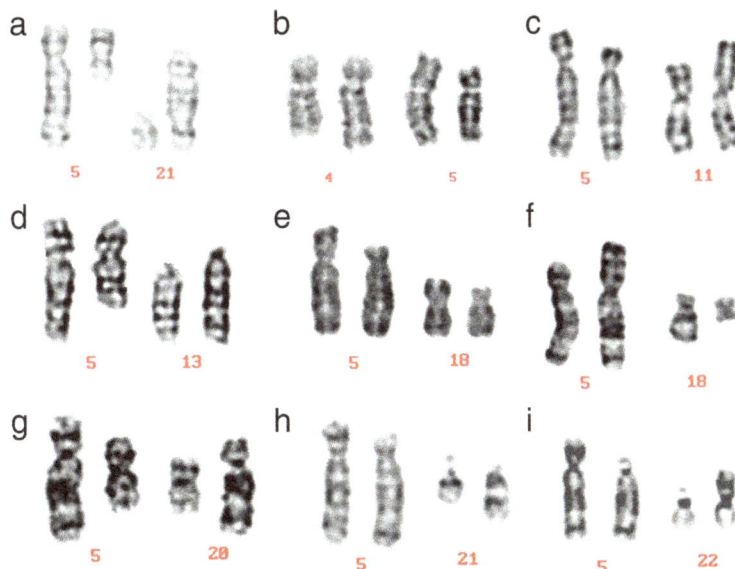

Fig. 1 G-banding karyotype of the nine cases identified as possessing chromosome 5 translocations. **a**: t(5;21), **b**: t(4;5), **c**: t(5;11), **d**:t(5;13), **e**: t(5;18)(p13;p11), **f**: t(5;18)(p15;q11.2), **g**: t(5; 20), **h**: t(5;21), **i**: t(5;22)

Table 2 Breakpoints in chromosome 5 translocation carriers and clinical features

Case	Karyotype	Breakpoints	Clinical findings	Reference
1	t(1;5)	1p32;5q31	Severe oligoasthenoteratozoospermia	Peschka et al., 1999 [27]
2	t(1;5)	1p31.1;5q33.3	Normozoospermia	Brugnon et al., 2006 [28]
3	t(1;5)	1p22;5q11	Malformed/stillborn children	Meza-Espinoza et al., 2008 [29]
4	t(1;5)	1q36.1;5q31	2 miscarriage, PGD and 2 term delivery	Ikuma et al., 2015 [4]
5	t(1;5)	1q41;5q33	Miscarriage and PGD	Kyu Lim et al., 2004 [30]
6	t(1;5)	1qter;5p14	Recurrent miscarriage	Goud et al., 2009 [31]
7	t(2;5)	2p25;5p12	Teratozoospermia, Habitual abortions	Vegetti et al., 2000 [32]
8	t(2;5)	2p21;5p15	Recurrent spontaneous abortion	Gada Saxena et al., 2012 [33]
9	t(2;5)	2p13;5p15	Recurrent fetal wastage	Fryns et al., 1998 [34]
10	t(2;5)	2p11;5q15	Abortion	Templado et al., 1988 [35]
11	t(2;5)	2p11;5q31	Recurrent abortion	Portnoï et al., 1988 [36]
12	t(2;5)	2q12;5q35.3	Recurrent pregnancy loss	Kochhar et al., 2013 [22]
13	t(2;5)	2q13.1;5q35.1	6 miscarriage, PGD and 1 term delivery	Ikuma et al., 2015 [4]
14	t(3;5)	3p27;5p14	4 fetal losses	Adamoli et al., 1986 [37]
15	t(3;5)	3q13;5q35	Repeated abortions	Venkateshwari et al., 2011 [21]
16	t(3;5)	3q26.2;5p15.1	Miscarriage	Sugiura-Ogasawara et al., 2008 [38]
17	t(3;5)	3q27;5p15	Normospermic, A boy 46,XY,t(3;5)pat	Vozdova et al., 2013 [11]
18	t(3;5)	3q28;5p13	Recurrent spontaneous abortion	Gada Saxena et al., 2012 [33]
19	t(3;5)	3q29;5q13	Multiple abortions	Castle et al., 1988 [39]
20	t(3;5)	3q29;5q33.2	PGD	Findikli et al., 2003 [40]
21	t(4;5)	4p15.2;5p12	Normozoospermia	Wiland et al., 2007 [41]
22	t(4;5)	4p15;5q12	Oligozoospermia	Perrin et al., 2010 [42]
23	t(4;5)	4p14;5q13.1	recurrent miscarriage	Pundir et al., 2016 [43]
24	t(4;5)	4q21;5p15	Habitual miscarriage	Li et al., 2012 [23]
25	t(4;5)	4q21;5p15	Recurrent spontaneous abortion	Zhang M et al., 2015 [44]
26	t(4;5)	4q21;5q11.2	Severe oligoasthenoteratozoospermia	Peschka et al., 1999 [27]
27	t(4;5)	4q22;5q35	2 fetal losses	Adamoli et al., 1986 [37]
28	t(4;5)	4q25;5p15.2	4 abortions	Ghazaey et al., 2015 [45]
29	t(4;5)	4q31;5p15	Recurrent spontaneous abortions	Zhang et al., 2011 [46]
30	t(4;5)	4q31;5q13	normozoospermia	Huang et al., 2007 [47]
31	t(4;5)	4q32;5q14	Oligoasthenoteratozoospermia	Dohle et al., 2002 [48]
32	t(4;5)	4q32;5q14	Miscarriage	Dul et al., 2012 [49]
33	t(4;5)	4q35;5p15	Recurrent miscarriages	Dutta et al., 2011 [50]
34	t(5;6)	5p15.3;6q13	recurrent abortion	Kiss et al., 2009 [51]
35	t(5;6)	5p13.3;6q27	Recurrent spontaneous abortion	Gada Saxena et al., 2012 [33]
36	t(5;6)	5q21;6q33	Recurrent fetal wastage	Fryns et al., 1998 [34]
37	t(5;6)	5q33.1;6p11.2	Miscarriage	Sugiura-Ogasawara et al., 2008 [38]
38	t(5;6)	5q35;6p21.3	PGD	Ko et al., 2010 [52]
39	t(5;7)	5p15.2;7p14	Recurrent spontaneous abortion	Gada Saxena et al., 2012 [33]
40	t(5;7)	5p13;7p15	Recurrent pregnancy loss	Kochhar et al., 2013 [22]
41	t(5;7)	5p13;7p15	Spontaneous abortion	Stephenson et al., 2006 [53]
42	t(5;7)	5p11;7q11	8 abortions	Al-Hussain et al., 2000 [54]
43	t(5;7)	5q13;7p15.1	2 miscarriages	Estop et al., 1995 [55]
44	t(5;7)	5q21;7q32	Normozoospermia	Cifuentes et al., 1999 [56]

Table 2 Breakpoints in chromosome 5 translocation carriers and clinical features *(Continued)*

Case	Karyotype	Breakpoints	Clinical findings	Reference
45	t(5;7)	5q33;7q22	Miscarriage and PGD	Kyu Lim et al., 2004 [30]
46	t(5;8)	5p14;8q22	Asthenozoospermia	Godo et al., 2013 [7]
47	t(5;8)	5q22;8q24.1	Oligoasthenoteratozoospermia	Meschede et al., 1998 [57]
48	t(5;8)	5q22.1;8q23.2	PGD	Ko et al., 2010 [52]
49	t(5;8)	5q23.1;8p23.2	4 miscarriage,1 term delivery	Ikuma et al., 2015 [4]
50	t(5;8)	5q33.3;8q11.21	Recurrent miscarriage	Pundir et al., 2016 [43]
51	t(5;8)	5q33;8q13	Normozoospermia	Blanco et al., 1998 [58]
52	t(5;8)	5q33;8q13	Normozoospermia	Estop et al., 2000 [59]
53	t(5;8)	5q33;8q13	Normozoospermia	Godo et al., 2013 [7]
54	t(5;8)	5q33;8q13	Normozoospermia	Anton et al., 2008 [60]
55	t(5;8)	5q35.1;8p11.2	Astenozoospermia	Anton et al., 2008 [60]
56	t(5;8)	5q35.3;8q22.1	Recurrent fetal wastage	Fryns et al., 1998 [34]
57	t(5;9)	5p15.1;9q22.1	Normospermic, Primary infertility	Vozdova et al., 2013 [11]
58	t(5;9)	5p13;9q22	PGD	Zhang et al., 2014 [61]
59	t(5;9)	5q10;9q10	Recurrent spontaneous abortions	Rouen et al., 2017 [62]
60	t(5;9)	5q21;9q34	2 fetal losses	Adamoli et al., 1986 [37]
61	t(5;9)	5q23.2;9q22.3	Spontaneous abortion	Stephenson et al., 2006 [53]
65	t(5;9)	5q23.3;9p24	Recurrent miscarriage	Iyer et al., 2007 [63]
63	t(5;10)	5p13.3;10p12.2	PGD	Ko et al., 2010 [52]
64	t(5;10)	5q22;10q11.2	PGD	Ko et al., 2010 [52]
65	t(5;10)	5q22;10q22	Miscarriage	Sugiura-Ogasawara et al., 2008 [38]
66	t(5;10)	5q34;10p12.1	Recurrent spontaneous abortions	Rouen et al., 2017 [62]
6/	t(5;10)	5q35;10q22	Spontaneous abortions	Bourrouillou et al., 1986 [64]
68	t(5;10)	5q35;10q24	Recurrent miscarriage	Goud et al., 2009 [31]
69	t(5;11)	5p14;11p15	Normozoospermia	Zhang HG et al., 2015 [5]
70	t(5;12)	5p15.1;12p12.2	Spontaneous abortion	Stephenson et al., 2006 [53]
71	t(5;12)	5p15.1;12q21	Infertility	Ravel et al., 2006 [65]
72	t(5;12)	5p14;12q15	Recurrent spontaneous abortion	Gada Saxena et al., 2012 [33]
73	t(5;12)	5q11;12p13	10 abortions	Al-Hussain et al., 2000 [54]
74	t(5;12)	5q13;12q13	Recurrent spontaneous abortions	Rouen et al., 2017 [62]
75	t(5;12)	5q35.1;12q24.1	Repeated miscarriage	Goddijn et al., 2004 [66]
76	t(5;13)	5p13;13q34	Neonatal death	Zhang et al., 2006 [67]
77	t(5;13)	5q11;13q33	3 spontaneous abortions	Pellestor et al., 1989 [68]
78	t(5;13)	5q13;13q12	Normozoospermia	Zhang HG et al., 2015 [5]
79	t(5;13)	5q15;13p12	Oligozoospermia	Matsuda et al., 1992 [69]
80	t(5;13)	5q21;13q12.1	2 miscarriage, no conception	Ikuma et al., 2015 [4]
81	t(5;13)	5q33;13q12	Infertility	Mikelsaar et al., 2012 [20]
82	t(5;13)	5q34;13q33	Recurrent miscarriage	Iyer et al., 2007 [63]
83	t(5;14)	5p13;14q11.2	PGD	Zhang et al., 2014 [61]
84	t(5;14)	5p13;14q23	Spontaneous abortions	Bourrouillou et al., 1986 [64]
85	t(5;14)	5q11.2;14q32.1	Spontaneous abortion	Stephenson et al., 2006 [53]
86	t(5;15)	5p15.2;15q21.1	PGD	Ko et al., 2010 [52]
87	t(5;15)	5p13.3;15q15.3	PGD	Ko et al., 2010 [52]
88	t(5;15)	5q35;15q22	Pregnancy of PGD	Escudero et al., 2003 [70]

Table 2 Breakpoints in chromosome 5 translocation carriers and clinical features *(Continued)*

Case	Karyotype	Breakpoints	Clinical findings	Reference
89	t(5;15)	5q35;15q26.2	Abnormal semen, 2 IVF-ET	Vozdova et al., 2013 [11]
90	t(5;16)	5q13; 16p13.1	Normozoospermia	Haapaniemi Kouru et al., 2017 [71]
91	t(5;16)	5q33;16p13	Recurrent pregnancy loss	Kochhar et al., 2013 [22]
92	t(5;16)	5q33.3;16p13.3	Recurrent miscarriages	Dutta et al., 2011 [50]
93	t(5;17)	5q13.2;17q21.2	infertility	Mau et al., 1997 [72]
94	t(5;17)	5q31;17p13	Normozoospermia	Anton et al., 2008 [60]
95	t(5;17)	5q33.1;17q25.3	Repeated miscarriage	Goddijn et al., 2004 [66]
96	t(5;18)	5p15;18q11.2	Spontaneous abortion	Zhang HG et al., 2015 [5]
97	t(5;18)	5p15;18q21	Malformed children	Balkan et al., 1983 [73]
98	t(5;18)	5q15;18q22	Spontaneous abortions	Soh et al., 1984 [74]
99	t(5;18)	5q15;18q23	2 fetal loss	Smith et al., 1990 [75]
100	t(5;18)	5q31.1;18q21.1	PGD	Ko et al., 2010 [52]
101	t(5;19)	5q15;19p12	Normospermic, A boy 46,XY,t(5;19)pat	Vozdova et al., 2013 [11]
102	t(5;20)	5q22;20p13	Asthenozoospermia, Habitual abortions	Vegetti et al., 2000 [32]
103	t(5;20)	5q13;20q12	Normozoospermia	Zhang HG et al., 2015 [5]
104	t(5;20)	5q22;20p12	Recurrent fetal wastage	Fryns et al., 1998 [34]
105	t(5;20)	5q31;20p13	Azoospermia	Poli et al., 2016 [18]
106	t(X;5)	Xp22.1;5p11	Azoospermia	Peschka et al., 1999 [27]

Cytogenetic analysis

Cytogenetic analysis was carried out on all patients. Peripheral blood (0.5 mL) was collected in sterile tubes containing 30 U/mL heparin. Lymphocytes were then cultured in appropriate culture medium (Yishengjun; Guangzhou Baidi Biotech, Guangzhou, China) for 72 h, and subsequently treated with 20 μg/mL colcemid for 1 h. G-banding of metaphase chromosomes and karyotype analysis were performed using previously described methods [5]. Twenty metaphases were counted and 6 karyotypes were analyzed per patient. Karyotype nomenclature was described in accordance of ISCN2009. The resolution level of chromosome analysis was 400–550 band levels.

Analysis of the identified translocation breakpoints

A search of translocations identified in chromosome 5 from infertile males was performed using PubMed. The keywords "chromosome / translocation / sperm" and "chromosome / translocation / abortion" were used for the PubMed search. The relationships of translocation breakpoints with male infertility and recurrent pregnancy loss were analyzed. Such searches were performed for a total of 106 carriers of chromosomal 5 translocations. This study included the cases of reciprocal chromosomal translocations involving chromosome 5 in reported papers, and excluded cases without breakpoints, females, newborns, and bone marrow detection involving chromosome 5.

Results

A total of 82 translocation carriers were detected in this study. Of these, nine (11%) were carriers of a chromosome 5 translocation, in which other chromosome abnormality had been excluded. Karyotype results and G-banding karyotypes from these nine patients are respectively summarized in Table 1 and Fig. 1. One case had azoospermia (pregestational infertility), while eight cases had normal semen. For the former, no AZF gene deletion was found. Of the later eight cases, it was evident that their partners were able to conceive, but had a tendency to miscarry (gestational infertility): three cases had experienced recurrent spontaneous abortions, two cases each experienced stillbirths, and three cases produced a phenotypically normal child confirmed by amniocentesis. For the other 73 cases of translocations, we will describe or have published in another study.

A literature review was also performed, from which karyotype results, clinical manifestations, and breakpoints on chromosome 5 were collected, as shown in Table 2. A total of 106 karyotypes included chromosome 5 translocations. The most common translocation was t(4;5), observed in 13 patients, followed t(5;8) ($N = 11$). Chromosomes 4($N = 13$), 8($N = 11$), 2,3,7,13($N = 7$), 1,9,10,12($N = 6$), 6, 18($N = 5$), 15,20($N = 4$),14,16,17($N = 3$) and 11,19, X ($N = 1$) were respectively involved in the balanced translocation with chromosome 5.

The most common breakpoint, at 5p15, was observed in 11 patients, followed by 5q13 ($N = 10$).

Breakpoints at 5p14, 5p11, 5q13, 5q14, 5q15, 5q22, 5q31, 5q35 and 5q35.1 were found with cases of both pregestational and gestational infertility. All breakpoints were associated with gestational infertility (Table 3).

Discussion

In clinical practice, male infertility can be broadly divided into two types of reproductive failure: pregestational and gestational infertility [16]. In the present

Table 3 Incidence of breakpoints on chromosome 5

Breakpoints	Number of patients with pregestational infertility	Number of patients with gestational infertility
p15.3		1
p15.2		3
p15.1		4
p15		11
p14	1	5
p13.3		3
p13		9
p12		2
p11	1	2
q10		1
q11		3
q11.2		2
q12		1
q13	1	9
q13.1		1
q13.2		1
q14	1	1
q15	1	4
q21		4
q22	2	3
q22.1		1
q23.1		1
q23.2		1
q23.3		1
q31	2	3
q31.1		1
q33		8
q33.1		2
q33.2		1
q33.3		3
q34		2
q35	1	6
q35.1	1	2
q35.3		2

study, nine of our cases were identified as carriers of chromosome 5 translocations, and we also reviewed 106 cases of chromosome 5 translocation reported in the literature. The breakpoints that we identified on chromosome 5 were found to be associated with pregestational or gestational infertility. One case was associated with pregestational infertility and eight cases were related to gestational infertility. Mikelsaar et al. [17] and Venkateshwari et al. [18] reported that the breakpoints at 5q33 and 5q35 in male carriers were associated with infertility. Kim et al. [19] reported that the breakpoint at 5p13 could interfere with spermatogenesis, and that breakpoints at 5q15, 5q21.2, 5q22 and 5q32 were related to recurrent abortion. To study the relationship of these breakpoints on chromosome 5 with male infertility, we analyzed recent published literature and revealed clinical features in carriers of chromosome 5 translocations. The karyotype results and clinical findings at chromosome 5 are summarized in Table 2. A common clinical feature associated with the breakpoints at 5p13, 5q33 and 5q35 was recurrent miscarriage, which was not consistent with the above reports.

Male infertility affects about 50% of couples unable to achieve pregnancy [20]. Chromosomal abnormalities are closely related to male infertility [21], and cytogenetic detection can provide valuable information for genetic counseling of infertile males [22]. Previous reports have shown that infertile men have an 8–10-fold higher prevalence of chromosomal abnormalities than fertile men [19]. Chromosomal translocation alters the complex and vital process of spermatogenesis, and leads to male infertility [20]. Chromosome 5 translocation has often been associated with male infertility or recurrent pregnancy loss [17, 18, 23].

Table 3 shows that all breakpoints were associated with gestational infertility. These cases indicated that such breakpoints were not responsible for pregestational infertility, so another breakpoint of translocation must be responsible in these individuals. For instance, two individuals with the breakpoint 5q22 were associated with pregestational infertility, and exhibited clinical features of oligoasthenoteratozoospermia and asthenozoospermia (case 47 and 102, respectively, Table 2). The corresponding breakpoints of translocation in case 47 and 102 were 8q24.1 and 20p13, respectively. Kott et al. [24] reported that the primary ciliary dyskinesia-19 (*CILD19*) gene (OMIM: 614,935), mapped to chromosome 8q24, was associated with asthenospermia in infertile males. Previous studies have shown that the sperm flagellar protein 1 (*SPEF1*) gene (OMIM: 610,674) located on chromosome 20p13 was be associated with curvature of microtubule bundles and the axoneme of sperm flagella [25]. Previous studies suggested that disruptions of *CAMK4* located on chromosome 5q22.1, *SPINK13* located on chromosome5q32 and the testis-specific serine/threonine kinase (*TSSK1B*) gene mapped to chromosome 5q22.2 were associated with loss of sperm function and human male infertility [8, 9, 26]. In addition, the most common breakpoint, mapped to 5p15, was associated with gestational infertility. Other breakpoints were also identified as being associated with gestational infertility. For those affected by these breakpoints, natural conception remained possible with the potential to have normal children. For example, Ikuma et al. [4] reported that the live birth rate with natural conception for translocation carriers was 65%–83% cumulatively. However, natural conception has a greater risk. The number of chromosomal unbalanced gametes is large, leading to repetitive pregnancy loss, and may have repercussions on the fertility of translocation carriers. For these carriers, informed choice should be provided during genetic counseling.

The major limitation of our present study was the relatively small number of carriers of chromosome 5 translocations. Furthermore, we did not investigate the specific molecular effects of the translocations by molecular-cytogenetic methods.

Conclusions

In the present study, 115 carriers of chromosome 5 translocations were reviewed. The most common translocation and breakpoint were t(4;5) and 5p15, respectively. All breakpoints at chromosome 5 were associated with gestational infertility. In genetic counseling, physicians should consider chromosome 5 and its breakpoints. Carriers of chromosome 5 translocations maybe choose to continue with natural conception or use available assisted reproductive technologies, such as preimplantation genetic diagnosis.

Abbreviations

AZF: Azoospermia factor; CAMK4: Ca^{2+}/calmodulin-dependent protein kinase IV; CILD19: Ciliary dyskinesia-19; ISCN: International System for Human Cytogenetic Nomenclature; PGD: Preimplantation genetic diagnosis; SPEF1: Sperm flagellar protein 1; Spink13: Serine protease inhibitor, Kazal-type 13; TSSK1B: Testis-specific serine/threonine kinase

Acknowledgments

We thank Charles Allan, PhD, from Liwen Bianji, Edanz Editing China (http://www.liwenbianji.cn), for editing the English text of a draft of this manuscript.

Funding

This work was supported by the Special Funds of Jilin Province Development and Reform Commission, China (2017C025).

Authors' contributions

HGZ, LLL and HBZ performed the literature search, analyzed the data and wrote the manuscript. RXW, YP and HZ collected the clinical cases and patients. HGZ and RZL are responsible for the content and writing of the paper. All authors read and approved the final manuscript.

Competing interests

The authors declare that they have no competing interests.

References

1. Ventimiglia E, Capogrosso P, Boeri L, et al. When to perform karyotype analysis in infertile men? Validation of the European Association of Urology guidelines with the proposal of a new predictive model. Eur Urol. 2016;70:920–3.
2. Hotaling J, Carrell DT. Clinical genetic testing for male factor infertility: current applications and future directions. Andrology. 2014;2:339–50.
3. Song SH, Chiba K, Ramasamy R, et al. Recent advances in the genetics of testicular failure. Asian J Androl. 2016;18:350–5.
4. Ikuma S, Sato T, Sugiura-Ogasawara M, et al. Preimplantation genetic diagnosis and natural conception: a comparison of live birth rates in patients with recurrent pregnancy loss associated with translocation. PLoS One. 2015;10:e0129958.
5. Zhang HG, Wang RX, Li LL, et al. Male carriers of balanced reciprocal translocations in Northeast China: sperm count, reproductive performance, and genetic counseling. Genet Mol Res. 2015;14:18792–8.
6. Harton GL, Tempest HG. Chromosomal disorders and male infertility. Asian J Androl. 2012;14:32–9.
7. Godo A, Blanco J, Vidal F, et al. Accumulation of numerical and structural chromosome imbalances in spermatozoa from reciprocal translocation carriers. Hum Reprod. 2013;28:840–9.
8. Wu JY, Ribar TJ, Cummings DE, et al. Spermiogenesis and exchange of basic nuclear proteins are impaired in male germ cells lacking Camk4. Nat Genet. 2000;25:448–52.
9. Ma L, Yu H, Ni Z, et al. Spink13, an epididymis-specific gene of the Kazal-type serine protease inhibitor (SPINK) family, is essential for the acrosomal integrity and male fertility. J Biol Chem. 2013;288:10154–65.
10. Kim JW, Chang EM, Song SH, et al. Complex chromosomal rearrangements in infertile males: complexity of rearrangement affects spermatogenesis. Fertil Steril. 2011;95:349–52. 352.e1–5
11. Vozdova M, Oracova E, Kasikova K, et al. Balanced chromosomal translocations in men: relationships among semen parameters, chromatin integrity, sperm meiotic segregation and aneuploidy. J Assist Reprod Genet. 2013;30:391–405.
12. Vloeberghs V, Verheyen G, Haentjens P, et al. How successful is TESE-ICSI in couples with non-obstructive azoospermia? Hum Reprod. 2015;30:1790–6.
13. De Krom G, Arens YH, Coonen E, et al. Recurrent miscarriage in translocation carriers: no differences in clinical characteristics between couples who accept and couples who decline PGD. Hum Reprod. 2015;30:484–9.
14. Franssen MT, Musters AM, van der Veen F, et al. Reproductive outcome after PGD in couples with recurrent miscarriage carrying a structural chromosome abnormality: a systematic review. Hum Reprod Update. 2011; 17:467–75.
15. Ozawa N, Maruyama T, Nagashima T, et al. Pregnancy outcomes of reciprocal translocation carriers who have a history of repeated pregnancy loss. Fertil Steril. 2008;90:1301–4.
16. Li D, Zhang H, Wang R, et al. Chromosomal abnormalities in men with pregestational and gestational infertility in northeast China. J Assist Reprod Genet. 2012;29:829–36.
17. Mikelsaar R, Nelis M, Kurg A, et al. Balanced reciprocal translocation t(5; 13)(q33;q12) and 9q31.1 microduplication in a man suffering from infertility and pollinosis. J Appl Genet. 2012;53:93–7.
18. Venkateshwari A, Srilekha A, Begum A, et al. De novo chromosomal translocation t(3;5)(q13;q35) in an infertile man. Andrologia. 2011;43:428–30.
19. RI ML, O'Bryan MK. Clinical Review#: State of the art for genetic testing of infertile men. J Clin Endocrinol Metab. 2010;95:1013–24.
20. Stouffs K, Seneca S, Lissens W. Genetic causes of male infertility. Ann Endocrinol (Paris). 2014;75:109–11.
21. Naasse Y, Charoute H, El Houate B, et al. Chromosomal abnormalities and Y chromosome microdeletions in infertile men from Morocco. BMC Urol. 2015;15:95.
22. Poli MN, Miranda LA, Gil ED, et al. Male cytogenetic evaluation prior to assisted reproduction procedures performed in mar del Plata, Argentina. JBRA Assist Reprod. 2016;20:62–5.
23. Kochhar PK, Ghosh P. Reproductive outcome of couples with recurrent miscarriage and balanced chromosomal abnormalities. J Obstet Gynaecol Res. 2013;39:113–20.
24. Kott E, Duquesnoy P, Copin B, et al. Loss-of-function mutations in LRRC6, a gene essential for proper axonemal assembly of inner and outer dynein arms, cause primary ciliary dyskinesia. Am J Hum Genet. 2012;91:958–64.

25. Dougherty GW, Adler HJ, Rzadzinska A, et al. CLAMP, a novel microtubule-associated protein with EB-type calponin homology. Cell Motil Cytoskeleton. 2005;62:141–56.

26. Hao Z, Jha KN, Kim YH, et al. Expression analysis of the human testis-specific serine/threonine kinase (TSSK) homologues. A TSSK member is present in the equatorial segment of human sperm. Mol Hum Reprod. 2004;10:433–44.

27. Peschka B, Leygraaf J, Van der Ven K, et al. Type and frequency of chromosome aberrations in 781 couples undergoing intracytoplasmic sperm injection. Hum Reprod. 1999;14:2257–63.

28. Brugnon F, Van Assche E, Verheyen G, et al. Study of two markers of apoptosis and meiotic segregation in ejaculated sperm of chromosomal translocation carrier patients. Hum Reprod. 2006;21:685–93.

29. Meza-Espinoza JP, Anguiano LO, Rivera H. Chromosomal abnormalities in couples with reproductive disorders. Gynecol Obstet Investig. 2008;66:237–40.

30. Kyu Lim C, Hyun Jun J, Mi Min D, et al. Efficacy and clinical outcome of preimplantation genetic diagnosis using FISH for couples of reciprocal and Robertsonian translocations: the Korean experience. Prenat Diagn. 2004;24:556–61.

31. Goud TM, Mohammed Al Harassi S, Khalfan Al Salmani K, et al. Cytogenetic studies in couples with recurrent miscarriage in the Sultanate of Oman. Reprod BioMed Online. 2009;18:424–9.

32. Vegetti W, Van Assche E, Frias A, et al. Correlation between semen parameters and sperm aneuploidy rates investigated by fluorescence in-situ hybridization in infertile men. Hum Reprod. 2000;15:351–65.

33. Gada Saxena S, Desai K, Shewale L, et al. Chromosomal aberrations in 2000 couples of Indian ethnicity with reproductive failure. Reprod BioMed Online. 2012;25:209–18.

34. Fryns JP, Buggenhout G. Structural chromosome rearrangements in couples with recurrent fetal wastage. Eur J Obstet Gynecol Reprod Biol. 1998;81:171–6.

35. Templado C, Navarro J, Benet J, et al. Human sperm chromosome studies in a reciprocal translocation t(2;5). Hum Genet. 1988;79:24–8.

36. Portnoï MF, Joye N, van den Akker J, et al. Karyotypes of 1142 couples with recurrent abortion. Obstet Gynecol. 1988;72:31–4.

37. Adamoli A, Bernardi F, Chiaffoni G, et al. Reproductive failure and parental chromosome abnormalities. Hum Reprod. 1986;1:99–102.

38. Sugiura-Ogasawara M, Aoki K, Fujii T, et al. Subsequent pregnancy outcomes in recurrent miscarriage patients with a paternal or maternal carrier of a structural chromosome rearrangement. J Hum Genet. 2008;53:622–8.

39. Castle D, Bernstein R. Cytogenetic analysis of 688 couples experiencing multiple spontaneous abortions. Am J Med Genet. 1988;29:549–56.

40. Findikli N, Kahraman S, Kumtepe Y, et al. Embryo development characteristics in Robertsonian and reciprocal translocations: a comparison of results with non-translocation cases. Reprod BioMed Online. 2003;7:563–71.

41. Wiland E, Midro AT, Panasiuk B, et al. The analysis of meiotic segregation patterns and aneuploidy in the spermatozoa of father and son with translocation t(4;5)(p15.1;p12) and the prediction of the individual probability rate for unbalanced progeny at birth. J Androl. 2007;28:262–72.

42. Perrin A, Morel F, Douet-Guilbert N, et al. A study of meiotic segregation of chromosomes in spermatozoa of translocation carriers using fluorescent in situ hybridisation. Andrologia. 2010;42:27–34.

43. Pundir J, Magdalani L, El-Toukhy T. Outcome of preimplantation genetic diagnosis using FISH analysis for recurrent miscarriage in low-risk reciprocal translocation carriers. Eur J Obstet Gynecol Reprod Biol. 2016;203:214–9.

44. Zhang M, Fan HT, Zhang QS, et al. Genetic screening and evaluation for chromosomal abnormalities of infertile males in Jilin Province, China. Genet Mol Res. 2015;14:16178–84.

45. Ghazaey S, Keify F, Mirzaei F, et al. Chromosomal analysis of couples with repeated spontaneous abortions in northeastern iran. Int J Fertil Steril. 2015;9:47–54.

46. Zhang Z, Gao H, Li S, et al. Chromosomal abnormalities in patients with recurrent spontaneous abortions in northeast China. J Reprod Med. 2011;56:321–4.

47. Huang XF, Xiao SQ, Fei QJ, et al. Meiotic segregation results of male reciprocal chromosome translocations. Zhonghua Yi Xue Yi Chuan Xue Za Zhi. 2007;24:217–20.

48. Dohle GR, Halley DJ, Van Hemel JO, et al. Genetic risk factors in infertile men with severe oligozoospermia and azoospermia. Hum Reprod. 2002;17:13–6.

49. Dul EC, van Echten-Arends J, Groen H, et al. Chromosomal abnormalities in azoospermic and non-azoospermic infertile men: numbers needed to be screened to prevent adverse pregnancy outcomes. Hum Reprod. 2012;27:2850–6.

50. Dutta UR, Rajitha P, Pidugu VK, et al. Cytogenetic abnormalities in 1162 couples with recurrent miscarriages in southern region of India: report and review. J Assist Reprod Genet. 2011;28:145–9.

51. Kiss A, Rosa RF, Dibi RP, et al. chromosomal abnormalities in couples with history of recurrent abortion. Rev Bras Ginecol Obstet. 2009;31:68–74.

52. Ko DS, Cho JW, Park SY, et al. Clinical outcomes of preimplantation genetic diagnosis (PGD) and analysis of meiotic segregation modes in reciprocal translocation carriers. Am J Med Genet A. 2010;152A:1428–33.

53. Stephenson MD, Sierra S. Reproductive outcomes in recurrent pregnancy loss associated with a parental carrier of a structural chromosome rearrangement. Hum Reprod. 2006;21:1076–82.

54. Al-Hussain M, Al-Nuaim L, Abu Talib Z, et al. Cytogenetic study in cases with recurrent abortion in Saudi Arabia. Ann Saudi Med. 2000;20:233–6.

55. Estop AM, Van Kirk V, Cieply K. Segregation analysis of four translocations, t(2;18), t(3;15), t(5;7), and t(10;12), by sperm chromosome studies and a review of the literature. Cytogenet Cell Genet. 1995;70:80–7.

56. Cifuentes P, Navarro J, Blanco J, et al. Cytogenetic analysis of sperm chromosomes and sperm nuclei in a male heterozygous for a reciprocal translocation t(5;7)(q21;q32) by in situ hybridisation. Eur J Hum Genet. 1999;7:231–8.

57. Meschede D, Lemcke B, Exeler JR, et al. Chromosome abnormalities in 447 couples undergoing intracytoplasmic sperm injection–prevalence, types, sex distribution and reproductive relevance. Hum Reprod. 1998;13:576–82.

58. Blanco J, Egozcue J, Clusellas N, et al. FISH on sperm heads allows the analysis of chromosome segregation and interchromosomal effects in carriers of structural rearrangements: results in a translocation carrier, t(5; 8)(q33;q13). Cytogenet Cell Genet. 1998;83:275–80.

59. Estop AM, Cieply K, Munne S, et al. Is there an interchromosomal effect in reciprocal translocation carriers? Sperm FISH studies. Hum Genet. 2000;106:517–24.

60. Anton E, Vidal F, Blanco J. Reciprocal translocations: tracing their meiotic behavior. Genet Med. 2008;10:730–8.

61. Zhang Y, Zhu S, Wu J, et al. Quadrivalent asymmetry in reciprocal translocation carriers predicts meiotic segregation patterns in cleavage stage embryos. Reprod BioMed Online. 2014;29:490–8.

62. Rouen A, Carlier L, Heide S, et al. Potential selection of genetically balanced spermatozoa based on the hypo-osmotic swelling test in chromosomal rearrangement carriers. Reprod BioMed Online. 2017;35:372–8.

Iyer P, Wani L, Joshi S, et al. Cytogenetic investigations in couples with repeated miscarriages and malformed children: report of a novel insertion. Reprod BioMed Online. 2007;14:314–21.

64. Bourrouillou G, Colombies P, Dastugue N. Chromosome studies in 2136 couples with spontaneous abortions. Hum Genet. 1986;74:399–401.

65. Ravel C, Chantot-Bastaraud S, Siffroi JP, et al. Tail stump syndrome associated with chromosomal translocation in two brothers attempting intracytoplasmic sperm injection. Fertil Steril. 2006;86(719):e1–7.

66. Goddijn M, Joosten JH, Knegt AC, et al. Clinical relevance of diagnosing structural chromosome abnormalities in couples with repeated miscarriage. Hum Reprod. 2004;19:1013–7.

67. Zhang YP, Xu JZ, Yin M, et al. Pregnancy outcomes of 194 couples with balanced translocations. Zhonghua Fu Chan Ke Za Zhi. 2006;41:592–6.

68. Pellestor F, Sèle B, Jalbert H, Jalbert P. Direct Segregation analysis of reciprocal translocations: a study of 283 sperm karyotypes from four carriers.

63. Am J Hum Genet. 1989;44:464–73.

69. Matsuda T, Horii Y, Ogura K, et al. Chromosomal survey of 1001 subfertile males: incidence and clinical features of males with chromosomal anomalies. Hinyokika Kiyo. 1992;38:803–9.

70. Escudero T, Abdelhadi I, Sandalinas M, et al. Predictive value of sperm fluorescence in situ hybridization analysis on the outcome of preimplantation genetic diagnosis for translocations. Fertil Steril. 2003; 79(Suppl 3):1528–34.

71. Haapaniemi Kouru K, Malmgren H, White I, et al. Meiotic segregation analyses of reciprocal translocations in spermatozoa and embryos: no support for predictive value regarding PGD outcome. Reprod BioMed Online. 2017;34:645–52.

72. Mau UA, Bäckert IT, Kaiser P, et al. Chromosomal findings in 150 couples referred for genetic counselling prior to intracytoplasmic sperm injection. Hum Reprod1997; 12:930–937.

73. Balkan W, Martin RH. Chromosome segregation into the spermatozoa of two men heterozygous for different reciprocal translocations. Hum Genet. 1983;63:345–8.

74. Soh K, Yajima A, Ozawa N, et al. Chromosome analysis in couples with recurrent abortions. Tohoku J Exp Med. 1984;144:151–63.

75. Smith A, Gaha TJ. Data on families of chromosome translocation carriers ascertained because of habitual spontaneous abortion. Aust N Z J Obstet Gynaecol. 1990;30:57–62.

18

Molecular characterization of a novel ring 6 chromosome using next generation sequencing

Rui Zhang[1*], Xuan Chen[1], Peiling Li[2], Xiumin Lu[1], Yu Liu[1], Yan Li[1], Liang Zhang[3], Mengnan Xu[4] and David S. Cram[4*]

Abstract

Background: Karyotyping is the gold standard cytogenetic method for detection of ring chromosomes. In this study we report the molecular characterization of a novel ring 6 (r6) chromosome in a six-year-old girl with severe mental retardation, congenital heart disease and craniofacial abnormalities.

Methods: Cytogenetic analysis was performed by conventional karyotyping. Molecular genetic analyses were performed using high-resolution chromosome microarray analysis (CMA) and next generation sequencing (NGS). OMIM, UCSC and PubMed were used as reference databases to determine potential genotype to phenotype associations.

Results: Peripheral blood and skin fibroblast karyotyping revealed the presence of a dominant cell line, 46,XX,(r6)(p25.3;q27) and a minor cell line 45,XX,-6. Molecular karyotyping using NGS identified 6p25.3 and 6q27 subtelomeric deletions of 1.78 Mb and a 0.56 Mb, respectively. Based on the known genes located within the r6 deletion interval 6q25.3-pter, genotype to phenotype association studies found compelling evidence to suggest that hemizygous expression of disease genes *FOXC1*, *FOXF2*, *IRF4* and *GMDS* was the main underlying cause of the patient's phenotype. We further speculate that the severity of the patient's symptoms may have been exacerbated by low-level instability of the r6 chromosome.

Conclusion: This is the first report of a novel r6 chromosome characterized at the molecular level using NGS.

Keywords: Karyotyping, Ring chromosome, Chromosome microarray analysis, Copy number variation, Next generation sequencing

Background

Human ring chromosomes were first reported in 1956 from cytogenetic analyses of tumor cells [1]. Ring chromosomes can involve any of the 24 chromosomes and are recognized in approximately 1 in 25,000 conceptions by karyotyping [2]. Random de novo recombination events during gametogenesis or early pre-implantation embryo development are believed to be responsible for the formation of ring chromosomes. The most common mechanism of ring chromosome formation usually either involves breakage near the termini of the short and long arms or breakage of one of the arms, followed by a subsequent fusion to generate a circular shortened chromosome with two or one terminal deletions [3, 4]. Occasionally, telomere-telomere fusions can also occur without the loss of any significant chromosomal material to generate complete ring chromosomes [3, 5, 6]. In general, the overall phenotype of the patients with ring chromosomes are highly variable, but generally overlap with phenotypes of known chromosome disease syndromes associated with similar interstitial copy number variations (CNVs) [4].

De novo ring chromosome 6 (r6) is a rarely observed structural abnormality compared to other types of ring chromosomes, with just over 30 case reports published in the literature [7]. Several r6 cases have been serendipitously detected by karyotyping during routine prenatal

* Correspondence: zhangrui@hrbmu.edu.cn; david.cram@berrygenomics.com
[1]Center for Obstetrics and Prenatal Diagnosis, The Second Affiliated Hospital of Harbin Medical University, 150000 Harbin, China
[4]Berry Genomics Corporation, Building 9, No 6 Court Jingshun East Road, Chaoyang District, Beijing 100015, China
Full list of author information is available at the end of the article

diagnosis [8, 9]; however, the majority of cases have been revealed postnatally following genetic investigation of children with unexplained clinical features. The most common r6 variants reported involve terminal 6p deletions extending to p25 or p24 in addition to 6q deletions extending to q26 or q27 [10–15]. In a review of selected r6 cases [7], phenotypes were highly variable, with the most consistent clinical features involving mental and developmental retardation, in association with facial dysmorphic features including microcephaly, microgathia, short neck, flat or broad nasal bridge, epicanthus bilateral and malformations of the ocular and auditory systems.

Apart from karyotyping and fluorescent in situ hybridization with 6p and 6q probes, most reported cases pre-date the availability of high resolution molecular techniques such as array comparative genomic hybridization (CGH) and next generation sequencing (NGS) and thus determination of precise genotype to phenotype associations has been limited. Recently, by applying an NGS method called copy number variation sequencing (CNV-Seq), we were able to identify the precise terminal deletion intervals in three cases of r14, r22 and r18 chromosomes [16]. In this study, using both array CGH and CNV-Seq, we report a comprehensive molecular characterization of a novel r6 chromosome in a six-year-old girl with severe intellectual disability, congenital heart disease and dysmorphic craniofacial features.

Results

Clinical evaluation of the patient

A 31-year-old father and mother presented at our prenatal diagnostic department for clinical assessment of their six-year-old daughter with unexplained dysmorphic facial features and severe intellectual disability. In review of the family, both parents were healthy and there was no history of genetic diseases or birth defects. Their daughter was born at the gestational age of 40 weeks via emergency caesarian section with a low birth weight of 2200 grams.

When examined at the age of 6.5 years, her weight was 14.00 kg (< third percentile), length 103 cm (< third percentile), head circumference 42 cm and chest circumference 51 cm. A thorough physical examination revealed microcephaly, a low posterior hairline, dysmorphic facial features including microphthalmia, epicanthus, leukoma, nystagmus, iridogoniodysgenesis, a down slanting brow and canthus, a flat nasal bridge and tooth agenesis. She also had a short neck and flat occiput, widely spaced nipples, short and an inturned recurved little finger (Fig. 1). By two-dimensional color-doppler echocardiography, congenital heart disease was detected involving an ostium secundum defect (left to right shunt), patent ductus arteriosus (left to right shunt), pulmonary stenosis, left superior vena cava residues and coronary sinus distention. In addition, the girl exhibited developmental delay, mental

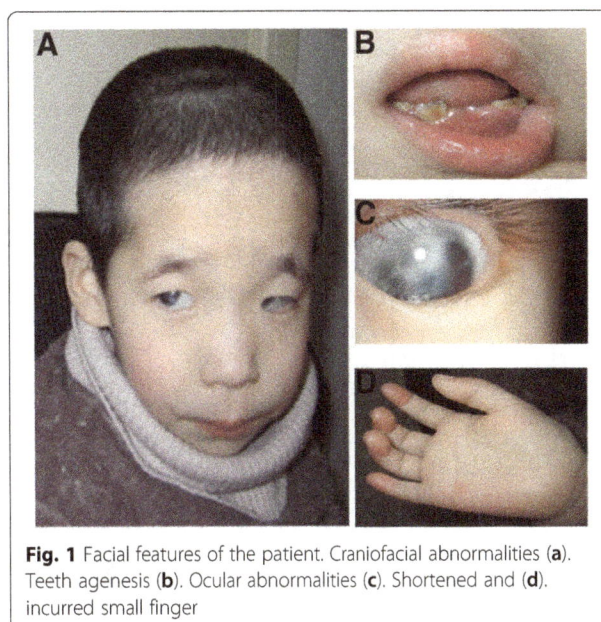

Fig. 1 Facial features of the patient. Craniofacial abnormalities (**a**). Teeth agenesis (**b**). Ocular abnormalities (**c**). Shortened and (**d**). incurred small finger

retardation and speech difficulties, and her overall intellectual ability was judged to be equivalent to that of a one-year old infant. The girl was able to walk, but her gait was unsteady. She also presented with hyperactivity and gatism.

Genetic investigation of the child

Conventional cytogenetic analysis of peripheral blood collected from the parents revealed normal karyotypes. Unexpectedly, their daughter returned a 46,XX,r(6) (p25.3q27) karyotype, involving one copy of a ring 6 chromosome and one copy of a normal chromosome 6. A further blood sample and a skin punch biopsy sample was collected from the patient to investigate the possibility of tissue mosaicism. From testing 88 lymphocytes, the karyotype was 46,XX,r(6)(p25.3;q27)[81]/45,XX,-6[7], revealing 8 % of cells without the r6 chromosome (Fig. 2a). Similarly, from testing 50 skin fibroblasts, the karyotype was 46,XX,r(6)(p25.3;q27)[47]/45,XX,-6[3] indicating that 6 % of cells had lost the r6 chromosome (Fig. 2b).

To determine the molecular structure of the r6 chromosome in more detail, high-resolution array CGH was performed on genomic DNA extracted from peripheral blood (Fig. 3). Genome-wide profiling for pathogenic copy number changes by array CGH detected a 1.78 Mb 6p25.3-pter deletion. However, on chromosome 6, there was also evidence of a small intra-chromosomal deletion at 6q22.31 and a small terminal 6q27 deletion, respectively, although the "call" by the software was not confident due to the lack of informative probes in these two regions. To confirm the array CGH results, we also performed NGS using copy number variation sequencing (CNV-Seq). Sequence data analysis revealed four CNVs, namely a 0.66 Mb 5q11-12 duplication, a 1.78

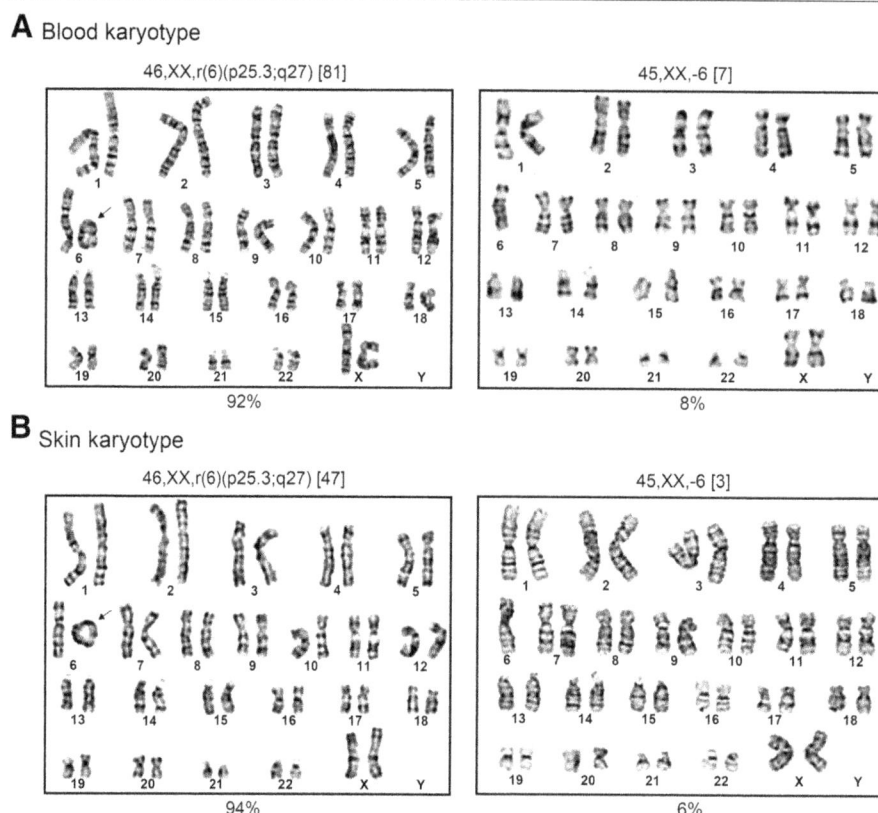

Fig. 2 Tissue karyotyping. **a** Blood lymphocytes, 46,XX,r6(p25.3;q27)[81]/45,XX,-6[7]. **b** Skin fibroblasts, 46,XX,r6(p25.3;q27)[47]/45,XX,-6[3]. Loss of the r6 chromosome was seen in 8 % of blood lymphocytes and 6 % of skin fibroblasts

Mb 6p25-pter deletion, a 0.26 Mb 6q22.31 deletion and a 0.56 Mb 6q27-qter deletion (Fig. 4).

Searches of the UCSC and OMIM databases for reference and disease genes were performed for the four CNVs defined by CNV-Seq to identify the genes encoded in these intervals (Fig. 3). Within the 6p25-pter deletion interval 13 reference genes were identified; namely, *LOC285766*, *DUSP22*, *IRF4*, *EXOC2*, *HUS1B*, *LOC101927691*, *LOC285768*, *FOXQ1*, *FOXF2*, *MIR6720*, *FOXCUT*, *FOXC1* and *GMDS*, where *IRF4* and *FOXC1* have been classified as OMIM disease genes. The 6q22.31 deletion interval encoded the gene *NKAIN2*, which has no known disease association. Within the 6q27-qter deletion interval there were 10 genes identified, namely; *LOC102724511*, *LOC154449*, *LOC285804*, *FLJ38122*, *DLL1*, *FAM120B*, *MIR4644*, *PSMB1*, *TBP* and *PDCD2*, where only *TBP* has been classified as an OMIM disease gene. The 5q11-12 duplication region contained no known genes. Literature searches found no evidence that this region is associated with pathogenicity, and on this basis, the 5q11-12 duplication was deemed to be benign.

Discussion

This study presents detailed cytogenetic and molecular analyses to characterize a novel r6 chromosome originally detected by conventional karyotyping in a six-year-old girl. More extensive karyotyping of blood and skin cells showed that while the vast majority of cells had one copy of chromosome 6 and one copy of the r6 chromosome, a minority of cells in both tissues (6–8 %) had lost the r6 chromosome, resulting in monosomy 6. Since the blood karyotyping was performed on short-term cultures, and that long term cultures of skin fibroblasts did not increase the incidence of r6 chromosome loss, we conclude that the mosaic karyotype most likely originated in vivo due to r6 instability. High-resolution genomic analysis by array CGH and CNV-Seq was used to survey genome-wide CNVs and, simultaneously analyze the terminal CNVs associated with the r6 chromosome. The most significant CNVs identified were 1.76 Mb (6p) and 0.56 Mb (6q) subtelomeric deletions of the r6 chromosome. In comparison to other cytogenetically defined r6 chromosomes, this novel variant has the smallest 6p deletion involving p25.3-pter, whereas all other r6 variants reported to date have more extensive deletions, involving 25p-pter or 24p-pter [7].

By comparison, NGS provided a much higher resolution analysis of the patient's DNA than array CGH, allowing precise definition of genome-wide CNVs and the subtelomeric CNVs associated with the r6 chromosome. While both

A Array and CNV-Seq analysis of Chr6

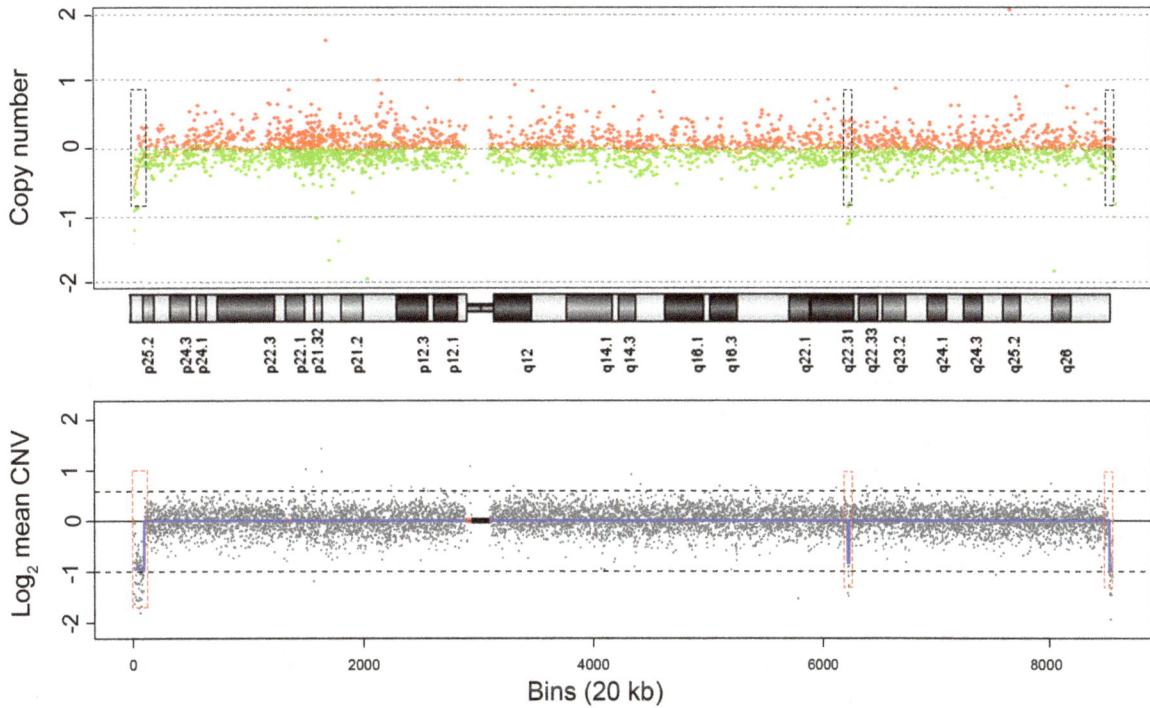

B Deletion intervals and genes

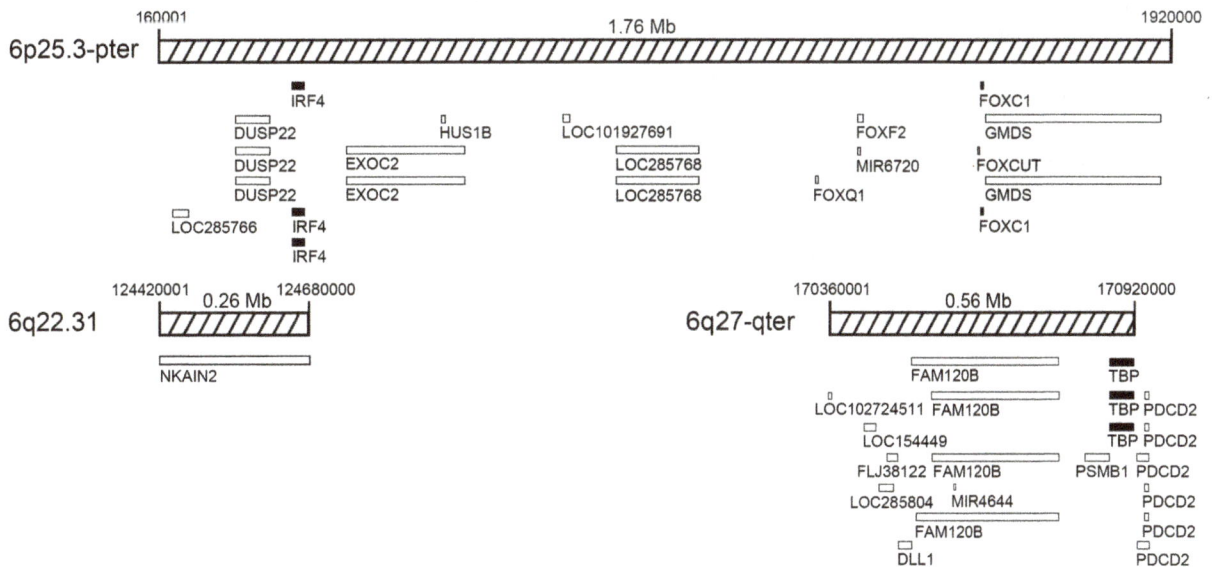

Fig. 3 (See legend on next page.)

(See figure on previous page.)
Fig. 3 High-resolution analysis of r6 microdeletions and associated genes. **a** CMA and NGS copy number plots for chromosome 6. The array CGH plot is shown as copy number (Y-axis) versus cytogenetics co-ordinates. Red dots indicate chromosomal gain and green dots indicate chromosomal loss. The NGS chromosome 6 plot is shown as $\log_2$ mean CNV (Y-axis) versus 20 kb sequencing bins (X-axis). The blue line along chromosome 6 tracks the mean CNV. The upper dashed line represents a 100 % chromosome gain [$\log_2(1.5)$] and the lower dashed line represents a 100 % chromosome loss [$\log_2(0.5)$]. Red lines indicate regions of repetitive sequences and the black box marks the centromere. Three microdeletions were identified (red dashed boxes); 6p25.3-pter (detected by CMA and NGS), 6q22.31 (detected by NGS) and 6q27-qter (detected by NGS). **b** Gene deletion intervals. The relative size and position of UCSC database reference genes in the three intervals is shown. Open boxes represent non-disease genes and solid black boxes represent disease-genes, according to OMIM database

NGS and array CGH identified the 1.76 Mb 6p subtelomeric deletion, array CGH missed the 0.56 Mb 6q subtelomeric deletion. In addition, NGS was able to accurately quantitate the copy number changes of the deletions. The difference in resolving power between the two techniques for the subtelomeric regions of chromosome 6 was attributable to the increased data points generated by NGS, which is based on analysis of randomly distributed sequencing reads whereas array CGH probes are more targeted to disease genes located throughout the genome. For example, to detect the 0.56 Mb 6q deletion, NGS utilized multiple data points provided by 28 contiguous 20 kb sequencing bins, which contain on average of 30–35 reads per bin [16]. In contrast, within this region, the array CGH platform only contained five probes and, collectively, the individual probe results were not informative for confidently calling a deletion. Thus, based on these findings, we speculate that NGS will not only be a useful technique for detecting additional genome-wide CNVs contributing to disease phenotypes, but also a preferable technology for precisely delineating CNVs at the terminal ends of chromosomes, with particular application to the analysis of all types of ring chromosomes. Further, based on similar principles, NGS technology may also have useful application for the diagnosis of unbalanced translocations with small subtelomeric duplications and deletions and, aid in defining more precise phenotypes associated with these structural re-arrangements.

The cytogenetic and molecular karyotypes defined provided a sound basis for exploring possible genotype to phenotype correlations in the patient studied. The 6p25.3 microdeletion syndrome is a known chromosome disease with well-described clinical features, consisting of developmental delay, mental retardation, language impairment, hearing loss, and ophthalmologic, cardiac, and craniofacial abnormalities [17–20]. Further, patients with unbalanced translocations involving deletion of the 6p 25.3 region, also display a similar phenotype [21]. These clinical features of all patients with interstitial deletions of 6p25.3 closely overlap with the clinical features of patients that carry a r6 chromosome [7] and strongly suggest that the main phenotypes displayed are primarily due to hemizygous expression of genes within the 6p25.3-pter interval. Therefore, in order to explore genotypic associations with congenital heart disease,

mental retardation and craniofacial abnormalities observed in the six-year-old girl, we specifically analyzed the known function of the genes encoded within the subtelomeric 6p25.3 region (Table 1).

The FOX family are a group of transcription factors characterized by a conserved 110 amino acid DNA binding domain that play an important synergistic role in embryonic development, tissue-specific gene expression, morphogenesis [22] as well as cardiovascular development [23]. Four members of the FOX gene family *FOXC1*, *FOXF2*, *FOXQ1* and *FOXCUT* are encoded by genes within the 6p25.3-pter interval (Fig. 4). RNA studies found that both FOXC1 and FOXF2 are highly expressed in the left ventricle [24, 25] whereas FOXQ1 was not expressed in the heart [22]. Loss of function studies comparing different models with normal or abnormal heart development have also shown that lower levels of several FOX proteins, including FOXC1, is strongly associated with the pathogenesis of heart failure. Further, studies of compound *FOXC1* and *FOXC2* mutant embryos identified a wide spectrum of cardiac abnormalities, including cardiac inflow and outflow dysplasia and abnormal formation of the epicardium [26]. Moreover, patients with *FOXC1* specific mutations often have identifiable cardiac abnormalities [27]. Based on these limited studies, we speculate that haplo-deficiency of *FOXC1* and, possibly *FOXF2*, may contribute to the complex heart abnormalities seen in the r6 patient.

The r6 patient also exhibited severe mental retardation and speech delay. Several studies suggest that reduced expression of genes *FOXC1*, *FOXF2* and *GMDS* which are located in the 6p25.3-pter deletion interval, affect normal brain and central nervous system (CNS) development [27–31]. In *FOXC1* null mice, significant cerebellum abnormalities were observed [27]. Brain MRI scans of mental retardation patients with known *FOXC1* gene deletions or missense mutations show a range of different cerebellum malformations including mega cisterna magna or cerebellar vermis hypoplasia [27, 28]. In other studies, FOXF2 was identified as a regulator of neural outgrowth through the modulation of nuclear active Akt [29] and FOXF1 was shown to be an important developmental regulator of the CNS [30]. Mutations in the *GMDS* gene which encodes an enzyme responsible

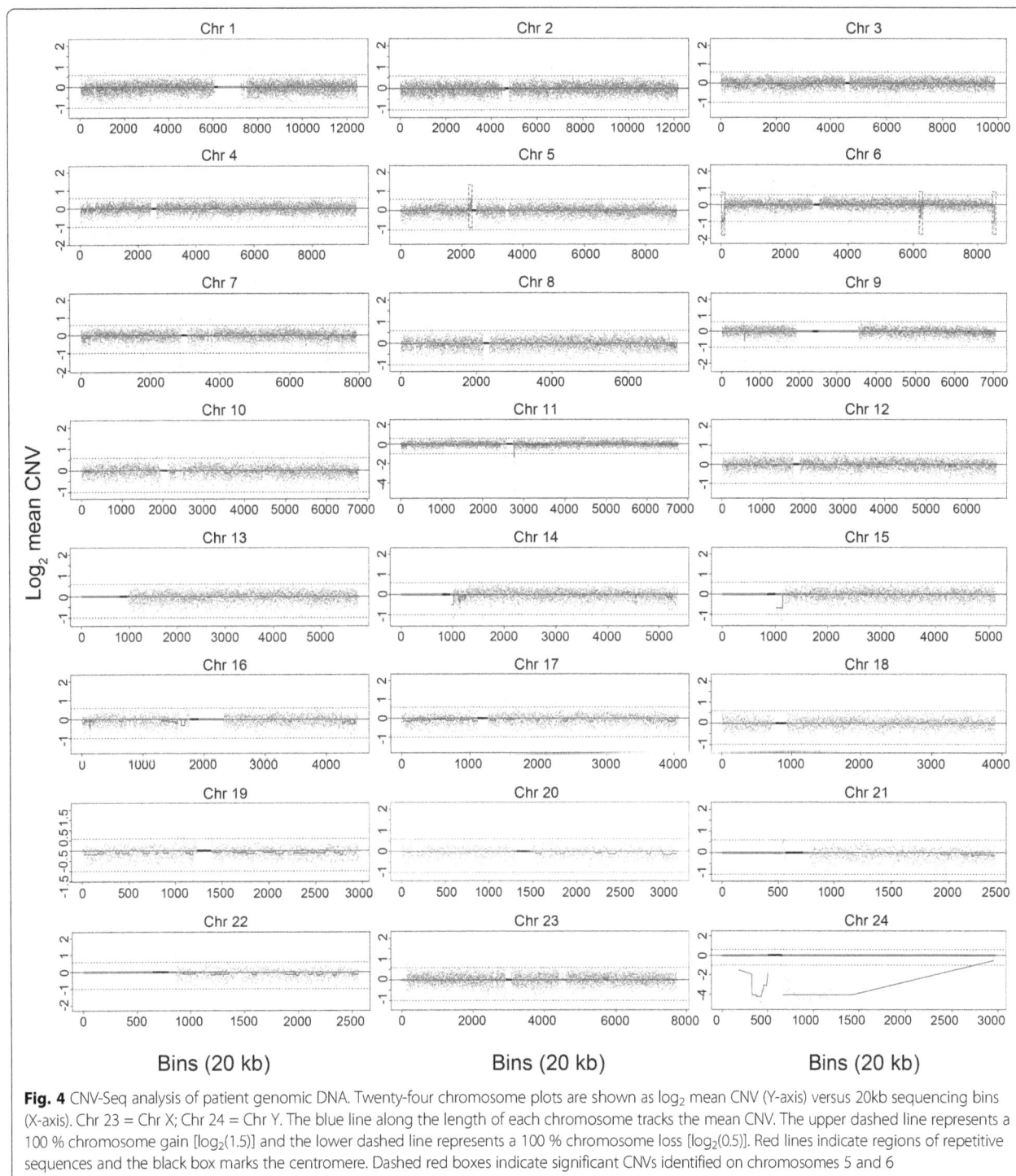

Fig. 4 CNV-Seq analysis of patient genomic DNA. Twenty-four chromosome plots are shown as log$_2$ mean CNV (Y-axis) versus 20kb sequencing bins (X-axis). Chr 23 = Chr X; Chr 24 = Chr Y. The blue line along the length of each chromosome tracks the mean CNV. The upper dashed line represents a 100 % chromosome gain [log$_2$(1.5)] and the lower dashed line represents a 100 % chromosome loss [log$_2$(0.5)]. Red lines indicate regions of repetitive sequences and the black box marks the centromere. Dashed red boxes indicate significant CNVs identified on chromosomes 5 and 6

for protein fucosylation, have also been found in a zebrafish model to cause defects in neuronal differentiation, axon branching and synapse formation [31]. In one key study, the severity of mental retardation in patients was found to be strongly associated with the size and position of *FOXC1* deletions and whether they extended further to encompass exons of the nearby *GMDS* gene [27].

Taken together, these collective studies point to haplo-deficiency of *FOXC1* and *GMDS* as the primary genes responsible for the severe mental disabilities exhibited by the r6 patient.

In regard to physical abnormalities of the patient (Fig. 1), craniofacial features were highly dysmorphic, with eye and tooth abnormalities particularly prominent.

Table 1 Genotype to phenotype associations

Main clinical findings in the patient	Gene	References
Severe mental retardation, speech delay	FOXC1	[27–29]
	FOXF2	[30]
	GMDS	[31]
Congenital heart disease, ostium secundum defect, patent ductus arteriosus, pulmonary stenosis, left superior vena cava residues and coronary sinus distention	FOXC1	[24–27]
	FOXF2	[24, 25]
Teeth agenesis	FOXF2	[30]
Leukoma	IRF4	[37, 38]
Iridogoniodysgenesis anomaly and nystagmus	FOXC1	[27]
	FOXF2	[35]

Based on several studies, *FOXC1* is believed to be the primary causative gene, although there is evidence that *FOXF2* and *IF4* genes also contribute to the phenotype. Human *FOXC1* heterozygous mutations are well known to affect eye development, causing a spectrum of ocular-associated anomalies including glaucoma and Axenfeld-Rieger syndrome [27, 32–34]. In mice, heterozygous mutations of *FOXF2* are associated with iridocorneal angle changes [35] and in one patient studied, partial iris hyperplasia was present even when the 6p deletion did not encompass the *FOXC1* gene [36]. Thus hemizygous expression of FOXC1 and FOXF2 may explain the corneal abnormalities, iridogoniodysgenesis and nystagmus observed in the patient. Further, the gene *IRF4* is important for human pigmentation of the hair skin and eyes [37, 38] and therefore loss of one copy of this gene may explain leukoma identified in the eyes of the patient. Lastly, during embryonic tooth development in rodents from the bud to differentiation stage, *FOXF2* mRNA was detected in the mesenchyme surrounding tooth germ cells, especially in the dental follicle adjacent to the outer enamel epithelium [30]. Thus, loss of one copy of the *FOXF2* gene may also be associated with the teeth agenesis exhibited by the patient. These studies suggest that while hemizygous expression of FOXC1 is probably the main cause of the craniofacial abnormalities in the patient, loss of one copy of the *FOXF2* and *IRF4* genes may have significantly exacerbated the severity of the facial abnormalities.

Based on a survey of the available literature, the evidence presented strongly points to haplodeficiency of the *FOXC1* gene as the major contributing factor to the overall phenotype of the patient and that hemizygous expression of *FOXF2*, *IRF4* and *GMDS* genes may further contribute to the phenotype. However, the phenotype of the patient was severer than that exhibited by other r6 patients reported with more extensive 6p and 6q deletions [7], in particular, growth retardation and mental development was severe. Within the 6q27 deletion

interval there were 10 genes, with only *TBP* recognized as an OMIM disease gene. Trinucleotide repeat expansion of the *TBP* gene has been shown to cause the neurological disorder spinocerebellar ataxia 17 [39]. However, since patients with r6 chromosomes involving both 6p and 6q terminal deletions exhibit a very similar phenotype to patients with r6 chromosomes involving only 6p terminal deletions [7], we argue that the 6q terminal deletion carried by the child was unlikely to have significantly contributed to the severer phenotype. This leaves the finding of r6 mosaicism in this patient as the most likely explanation. In previous studies, evidence suggests that growth and developmental delay commonly seen in patients carrying autosomal ring chromosomes is due to mosaicism caused by instability of the ring chromosome [4, 40, 41]. On this basis, we speculate that low-level r6 mosaicism, probably originating early in neonatal development, has exacerbated the severity of the symptoms exhibited by this patient, which appear to be primarily caused by the 6p25.3-pter deletion event.

Methods
Study oversight
The research study was approved by the Medical Ethics Committee of the Second Affiliated Hospital of Harbin Medical University (Approval Number KY2016-154).

Cytogenetic studies
Blood cell karyotyping was performed according to standard methods [42]. White blood cells were cultured for 72 h in PHA supplemented Serum Free Culture Medium (Guangzhou He Neng Bio Technology Co., Ltd). Skin puncture biopsies were taken from the abdominal skin, placed in PBS, cut into 0.5 mm^3 pieces, transferred into a Dispase II solution and incubated overnight at 4 °C [43]. Epidermal fibroblasts were then cultured at 37 °C under 5 % CO_2 and 90 % humidity for 12 days in PHA supplemented BIOAMFTM-3 media (Biological Industries Israel Beit Haemek Ltd). Following colcemid treatment, G banded metaphase chromosome spreads of blood and skin cells were prepared. For detection of mosaicism, a minimum of 50 cells were karyotyped.

Chromosome microarray analysis
Array CGH was performed using 8 × 60 K commercial arrays (Agilent) according to the manufacturer's recommended protocol. After DNA labeling, hybridization and washing, slides were scanned using an Agilent microarray scanner, and raw data extracted using Feature Extraction Software at the default CGH parameter settings. Putative copy number alteration intervals in each sample were identified using Agilent Genomic Workbench v6.5.0.18 software. Cy5/Cy3 ratios were converted into log2-transformed values and the Aberration Detection Method

2 algorithm applied at threshold 6.0 to identify CNVs, based on the following criteria: ≥ 5 probes per CNV interval and a minimum absolute average log2 ratio of ≥ 0.38 for the test region.

Next generation sequencing

NGS was performed by using copy number variation sequencing (CNV-Seq) as previously described [16, 44]. DNA libraries were constructed and subjected to massively parallel sequencing on the Hi Seq2500 platform (Illumina) to generate 36 bp sequencing reads. High quality reads (2.8–3.2 million) were mapped to the hg19 reference genome [45], allocated to 20 kb sequencing bins and the mean CNV plotted for each chromosome [44].

Consent

The parental guardians provided written informed consent on behalf of the child for publication of this Research Article and the accompanying image. A copy of the written consent form is available for review by the Editor-in-Chief of this journal.

Conclusions

In this study, we demonstrate molecular utility of NGS as a high resolution technology for molecular characterization of subtelomeric deletions associated with a novel r6 chromosome. Based on the defined genotype, we attributed the severe mental retardation, congenital heart disease and craniofacial abnormalities observed in the patient largely to hemizygous expression of *FOXC1*, *FOXF2* and *GMDS* genes within the 6p25.3-pter interval, although circumstantial evidence suggested that in vivo instability of the r6 chromosome exacerbated the severity of the phenotype. With ethical approval and patient consent, further tissue studies are needed to better understand the genetic basis of the variable and complex phenotypes observed in rare patients with r6 chromosomes.

Abbreviations
CMA: chromosome microarray analysis; CNV-Seq: copy number variation sequencing; NGS: next generation sequencing; r6: ring 6.

Competing interests
Authors MX and DSC are employees of Berry Genomics Corporation, Beijing and hold no stocks or bonds.

Authors' contributions
RZ, contributed to the cytogenetic studies, manuscript preparation and supervision of the study. PL, AZ, XZ, WH, contributed to the cytogenetic, array and sequencing studies. MX and DSC, contributed to data analysis and manuscript preparation. XC, participated in clinical evaluation of the patient and critically reviewed the manuscript. All authors read and approved the final manuscript.

Acknowledgments
We thank the family for their participation in this research study.

Funding
Science and Technology Research Project of Education Department of Heilongjiang Province.
Item number: 12521358.

Author details
[1]Center for Obstetrics and Prenatal Diagnosis, The Second Affiliated Hospital of Harbin Medical University, 150000 Harbin, China. [2]Department of Obstetrics and Gynaecology, The Second Affiliated Hospital of Harbin Medical University, 150000 Harbin, China. [3]Translational Medicine Center, Guangdong Women and Children's Hospital, Guangzhou 511400, China. [4]Berry Genomics Corporation, Building 9, No 6 Court Jingshun East Road, Chaoyang District, Beijing 100015, China.

References
1. Gebhart E. Ring chromosomes in human neoplasias. Cytogenet Genome Res. 2008;121(3–4):149–73.
2. Jacobs PA. Mutation rates of structural chromosome rearrangements in man. Am J Hum Genet. 1981;33(1):44–54.
3. Sigurdardottir S, Goodman BK, Rutberg J, Thomas GH, Jabs EW, Geraghty MT. Clinical, cytogenetic, and fluorescence in situ hybridization findings in two cases of "complete ring" syndrome. Am J Med Genet. 1999;87(5):384–90.
4. Guilherme RS, Meloni VF, Kim CA, Pellegrino R, Takeno SS, Spinner NB, et al. Mechanisms of ring chromosome formation, ring instability and clinical consequences. BMC Med Genet. 2011;12(2):171.
5. Vermeesch JR, Baten E, Fryns JP, Devriendt K. Ring syndrome caused by ring chromosome 7 without loss of subtelomeric sequences. Clin Genet. 2002; 62(5):415–7.
6. Le Caignec C, Boceno M, Jacquemont S, Nguyen The Tich S, Rival JM, David A. Inherited ring chromosome 8 without loss of subtelomeric sequences. Ann Genet. 2004;47(3):289–96.
7. Ahzad HA, Ramli SF, Loong TM, Salahshourifar I, Zilfalil BA, Yusoff NM. De novo ring chromosome 6 in a child with multiple congenital anomalies. Kobe J Med Sci. 2010;56(2):E79–84.
8. Urban M, Bommer C, Tennstedt C, Lehmann K, Thiel G, Wegner RD, et al. Ring chromosome 6 in three fetuses: case reports, literature review, and implications for prenatal diagnosis. Am J Med Genet. 2002;108(2):97–104.
9. Andrieux J, Devisme L, Valat AS, Robert Y, Frnka C, Savary JB. Prenatal diagnosis of ring chromosome 6 in a fetus with cerebellar hypoplasia and partial agenesis of corpus callosum: case report and review of the literature. Eur J Med Genet. 2005;48(2):199–206.
10. Wurster D, Pomeroy J, Benirschke K, Hoefnagel D. Mental deficiency and malformations in a boy with a group-C ring chromosome: 46, XY. Cr J Ment Defic Res. 1969;13(3):184–90.
11. Moore CM, Heller RH, Thomas GH. Developmental Abnormalities Associated with a Ring Chromosome 6. J Med Genet. 1973;10(3):299–303.
12. Van den Berghe H, Fryns JP, Cassiman JJ, David G. Ring chromosome 6. Karotype 46, XY, r (6)-45, XY,-6. Ann Genet. 1974;17(1):29–35.
13. Fried K, Rosenblatt M, Mundel G, Krikler R. Mental retardation and congenital malformations associated with a ring chromosome 6. Clin Genet. 1975;7(3):192–6.
14. Salamanca-Gonez F, Nava S, Armendares S. Ring chromosome 6 in a malformed boy. Clin Genet. 1975;8(5):370–5.
15. Kini KR, Van Dyke DL, Weiss L, Logan MS. Ring Chromosome 6: Case Report and Review of Literature. Hum Genet. 1979;50(2):145–9.
16. Liang D, Peng Y, Lv W, Deng L, Zhang Y, Li H, et al. Copy number variation sequencing for comprehensive diagnosis of chromosome disease syndromes. J Mol Diagn. 2014;16(5):519–26.
17. DeScipio C. The 6p subtelomere deletion syndrome. Am J Med Genet C: Semin Med Genet. 2007;145C(4):377–82.
18. Gould DB, Jaafar MS, Addison MK, Munier F, Ritch R, MacDonald IM, et al. Phenotypic and molecular assessment of seven patients with 6p25 deletion syndrome: relevance to ocular dysgenesis and hearing impairment. BMC Med Genet. 2004;5:17.
19. Delahaye A, Bitoun P, Drunat S, Gérard-Blanluet M, Chassaing N, Toutain A, et al. Genomic imbalances detected by array-CGH in patients with syndromal ocular developmental anomalies. Eur J Hum Genet. 2012;20:527–33.

20. Nakane T, Kousuke N, Sonoko H, Yuko K, Sato H, Kubota T, et al. 6p subtelomere deletion with congenital glaucoma, severe mental retardation, and growth impairment. Pediatr Int. 2013;55(3):376–81.

21. Maclean K, Smith J, St Heaps L, Chia N, Williams R, Peters GB, et al. Axenfeld-Rieger malformation and distinctive facial features: clues to a recognizable 6p25 microdeletion syndrome. Am J Med Genet A. 2005; 132A(4):381–5.

22. Bieller A, Pasche B, Frank S, Gläser B, Kunz J, Witt K, et al. Isolation and characterization of the human forkhead gene FOXQ1. DNA Cell Biol. 2001; 20(9):555–61.

23. Zhu H. Forkhead box transcription factors in embryonic heart development and congenital heart disease. Life Sci. 2015. doi:10.1016/j.lfs.2015.12.001.

24. Philip-Couderc P, Tavares NI, Roatti A, Lerch R, Montessuit C, Baertschi AJ. Forkhead transcription factors coordinate expression of myocardial KATP channel subunits and energy metabolism. Circ Res. 2008;102:e20–35.

25. Hannenhalli S, Putt ME, Gilmore JM, Wang J, Parmacek MS, Epstein JA, et al. Transcriptional genomics associates FOX transcription factors with human heart failure. Circulation. 2006;114:1269–76.

26. Seo S, Kume T. Forkhead transcription factors, Foxc1 and Foxc2, are required for the morphogenesis of the cardiac outflow tract. Dev Biol. 2006;296(2):421–36.

27. Aldinger KA, Lehmann OJ, Hudgins L, Chizhikov VV, Bassuk AG, Ades LC, et al. FOXC1 is required for normal cerebellar development and is a major contributor to chromosome 6p25.3 Dandy-Walker malformation. Nat Genet. 2009;41(9):1037–42.

28. Delahaye A, Khung-Savatovsky S, Aboura A, Guimiot F, Drunat S, Alessandri JL, et al. Pre- and postnatal phenotype of 6p25 deletions involving the FOXC1 gene. Am J Med Genet A. 2012;158A(10):2430–8.

29. Park JH, Lee SB, Lee KH, Ahn JY. Nuclear Akt promotes neurite outgrowth in the early stage of neuritogenesis. BMB Rep. 2012;45:521–5.

30. Aitola M, Carlsson P, Mahlapuu M, Enerbäck S, Pelto-Huikko M. Forkhead Transcription Factor FoxF2 Is Expressed in Mesodermal Tissues Involved in Epithelio-Mesenchymal Interactions. Dev Dyn. 2000;218:136–49.

31. Song Y, Willer JR, Scherer PC, Panzer JA, Kugath A, Skordalakes E, et al. Neural and synaptic defects in slytherin, a zebrafish model for human congenital disorders of glycosylation. PLoS ONE. 2010;5:e13743.

32. Berry FB, Lines MA, Oas JM, Footz T, Underhill DA, Gage PJ, et al. Functional interactions between FOXC1 and PITX2 underlie the sensitivity to FOXC1 gene dose in Axenfeld-Rieger syndrome and anterior segment dysgenesis. Hum Mol Genet. 2006;15:905–19.

33. Saleem RA, Murphy TC, Liebmann JM, Walter MA. Identification and Analysis of a Novel Mutation in the FOXC1 Forkhead Domain. Invest Ophthalmol Vis Sci. 2003;44:4608–12.

34. Zhang HZ, Li P, Wang D, Huff S, Nimmakayalu M, Qumsiyeh M, et al. FOXC1 gene deletion is associated with eye anomalies in ring chromosome 6. Am J Med Genet A. 2004;124A:280–7.

35. McKeone R, Vieira H, Gregory-Evans K, Gregory-Evans CY, Denny P. Foxf2: a novel locus for anterior segment dysgenesis adjacent to the Foxc1 gene. PLoS ONE. 2011;6:e25489.

36. Koolen DA, Knoers NV, Nillesen WM, Slabbers GH, Smeets D, de Leeuw N, et al. Partial iris hypoplasia in a patient with an interstitial subtelomeric 6p deletion not including the forkhead transcription factor gene FOXC1. Eur J Hum Genet. 2005;13:1169–71.

37. Han J, Kraft P, Nan H, Guo Q, Chen C, Qureshi A, et al. A genome-wide association study identifies novel alleles associated with hair color and skin pigmentation. PLoS Genet. 2008;4(5):e1000074.

38. Gathany AH, Hartge P, Davis S, Cerhan JR, Severson RK, Cozen W, et al. Relationship between interferon regulatory factor 4 genetic polymorphisms, measures of sun sensitivity and risk for non-Hodgkin lymphoma. Cancer Causes Control. 2009;20:1291–302.

39. Gao R, Matsuura T, Coolbaugh M, Zuhlke C, Nakamura K, Rasmussen A, et al. Instability of expanded CAG/CAA repeats in spinocerebellar ataxia type 17. Europ J Hum Genet. 2008;16(2):215–22.

40. Frizzley JK, Stephan MJ, Lamb AN, Jonas PP, Hinson RM, Moffitt DR, et al. Ring 22 duplication/deletion mosaicism: clinical, cytogenetic, and molecular characterisation. J Med Genet. 1999;36(3):237–41.

41. Kosztolanyi G. The Genetics and Clinical Characteristics of Constitutional Ring Chromosomes. J Assoc Genet Technol. 2009;35:44–8.

42. Carroll SG, Davies T, Kyle PM, Abdel-Fattah S, Soothill PW. Fetal karyotyping by chorionic villus sampling after the first trimester. Br J Obstet Gynaecol. 1999;106(10):1035–40.

43. Chen Y, Chen YX, Long ZG, Zhao DC, Pan Q, Dai HP, et al. Safety Assessments for Human Skin Fibroblasts Cultured in Vitro. J Chinese Physician. 2002;4(11): 1176–82.

44. Wang Y, Chen Y, Tian F, Zhang J, Song Z, Wu Y, et al. Maternal mosaicism is a significant contributor to discordant sex chromosomal aneuploidies associated with noninvasive prenatal testing. Clin Chem. 2014;60(1):251–9.

45. Li H, Durbin R. Fast and accurate short read alignment with Burrows-Wheeler transform. Bioinformatics. 2009;25:1754e1760.

19

Enrichment of small pathogenic deletions at chromosome 9p24.3 and 9q34.3 involving *DOCK8, KANK1, EHMT1* genes identified by using high-resolution oligonucleotide-single nucleotide polymorphism array analysis

Jia-Chi Wang*⃝, Loretta W. Mahon, Leslie P. Ross, Arturo Anguiano, Renius Owen and Fatih Z. Boyar

Abstract

Background: High-resolution oligo-SNP array allowed the identification of extremely small pathogenic deletions at numerous clinically relevant regions. In our clinical practice, we found that small pathogenic deletions were frequently encountered at chromosome 9p and 9q terminal regions.

Results: A review of 531 cases with reportable copy number changes on chromosome 9 revealed 142 pathogenic copy number variants (CNVs): 104 losses, 31 gains, 7 complex chromosomal rearrangements. Of 104 pathogenic losses, 57 were less than 1 Mb in size, enriched at 9p24.3 and 9q34.3 regions, involving the *DOCK8, KANK1, EHMT1* genes. The remaining 47 cases were due to interstitial or terminal deletions larger than 1 Mb or unbalanced translocations. The small pathogenic deletions of *DOCK8, KANK1* and *EHMT1* genes were more prevalent than small pathogenic deletions of *NRXN1, DMD, SHANK3* genes and were only second to the 16p11.2 deletion syndrome, 593-kb (OMIM #611913).

Conclusions: This study corroborated comprehensive genotype-phenotype large scale studies at 9p24.3 and 9q24.3 regions for a better understanding of the pathogenicity caused by haploinsufficiency of the *DOCK8, KANK1* and *EHMT1* genes.

Keywords: Small pathogenic deletions, High resolution oligonucleotide-single nucleotide polymorphism array analysis, Haploinsufficiency, Homozygous deletions

Background

Chromosomal microarray analysis (CMA) has been widely utilized for the genome-wide screening of microdeletion and microduplication syndromes [1]. The sizes of well-known microdeletion and microduplication syndromes were usually larger than 1 Mb, such as 1.4 Mb for Williams-Beuren syndrome (OMIM #194050) or 2.8 Mb for DiGeorge syndrome (OMIM #188400). Small

(<1 Mb) pathogenic deletions at regions which were not well characterized were frequently encountered during our daily clinical practice, for instance, the chromosomal regions at 9p24.3 and 9q34.3.

High-resolution oligo-SNP array is able to reveal a variety of chromosomal disorders including uniparental disomy or extremely small pathogenic deletions which would be missed by low-resolution oligonucleotide CMA. Our and other previous studies showed the cases with uniparental disomy were relatively limited in number on chromosome 9 as compared to chromosome 15, 11 and 7 [2, 3]. In contrast, small pathogenic deletions

* Correspondence: jia-chi.j.wang@questdiagnostics.com;
sjackwang1968@gmail.com
Cytogenetics Laboratory, Quest Diagnostics Nichols Institute, 33608 Ortega Highway, San Juan Capistrano, CA 92690, USA

were frequently encountered at chromosome 9p24.3 and 9q34.3 by using high-resolution oligo-SNP array in postnatal studies. Research endeavors have been significantly prioritized to specific genes such as *NRXN1* and *SHANK3* in the past [4, 5]. To the best of our knowledge, only four cases with small deletions of 192 kb, 225 kb, 465 kb and 518 kb in size at 9p24.3 involving the *DOCK8* and/or *KANK1* gene [6–8], and a case of 40 kb deletion in the *EHMT1* gene at 9q34.3 [9] have been documented.

The purpose of this study is to evaluate 1): the incidence of small (< 1 Mb) pathogenic deletions in postnatal specimens, 2): whether the small pathogenic deletions at 9p24.3 and 9q34.3 constituted a significant proportion of small deletions, 3): what proportion of deletions on chromosome 9 was caused by small pathogenic deletions at 9p24.3 and 9q34.3, 4): the efficacy of identifying extremely small homozygous pathogenic deletions using high-resolution oligo-SNP array.

Results

The incidence of small pathogenic deletions in postnatal specimens studied by high-resolution oligo-SNP array

Approximately 38,000 postnatal specimens were studied by high-resolution oligo-SNP array in our laboratory from 2011 through 2015. Of these, we reported approximately 13,000 (34 %) pathogenic variants or variants of uncertain clinical significance (VOUS). The detection rate was consistent with our previous study [2]. Of the 13,000 variants, a total of 373 recurrent (at least 3 cases) small pathogenic

losses were identified (Fig. 1). The 16p11.2 deletion syndrome, 593-kb (OMIM #611913) is the most common small pathogenic loss (107 cases). The remaining involved *NRXN1* (35 cases), *DMD* (31 cases), *DOCK8* and/or *KANK1* (30 cases), and other chromosomal regions such as 16p11.2 (OMIM #613444, 220-KB), 16p12.2 (OMIM #136570, 520-KB), 22q13.33 (OMIM #606232).

Approximately 12 % of the recurrent small pathogenic copy number losses were caused by deletions of *DOCK8* and*KANK1* at 9p24.3 and *EHMT1* at 9q34.3

The total number of deletions involving *DOCK8* and/or *KANK1* genes at 9p24.3 (30 cases, Fig. 2) and *EHMT1* gene at 9q34.3 (16 cases, Fig. 3a) constituted approximately 12 % (46/373 cases) of the recurrent small pathogenic deletions from all the chromosomes.

Small (<1 Mb) and relatively small (1–1.5 Mb) deletions constituted 59 % of pathogenic copy number losses on chromosome 9

Of 13,000 cases with reported copy number variants (CNVs), 531 cases were from chromosome 9, and 142 were pathogenic, including 104 losses, 31 gains, 7 complex chromosomal rearrangements with both losses and gains (Table 1 and Additional file 1: Figure S1). Of 104 pathogenic losses, 57 were smaller than 1 Mb in size. Of 57 cases, 46 were located at 9p24.3 and 9q34.3 regions, involving the *DOCK8, KANK1, EHMT1* genes. The size ranged from 22 kb (case 54 with *EHMT1* deletion) to

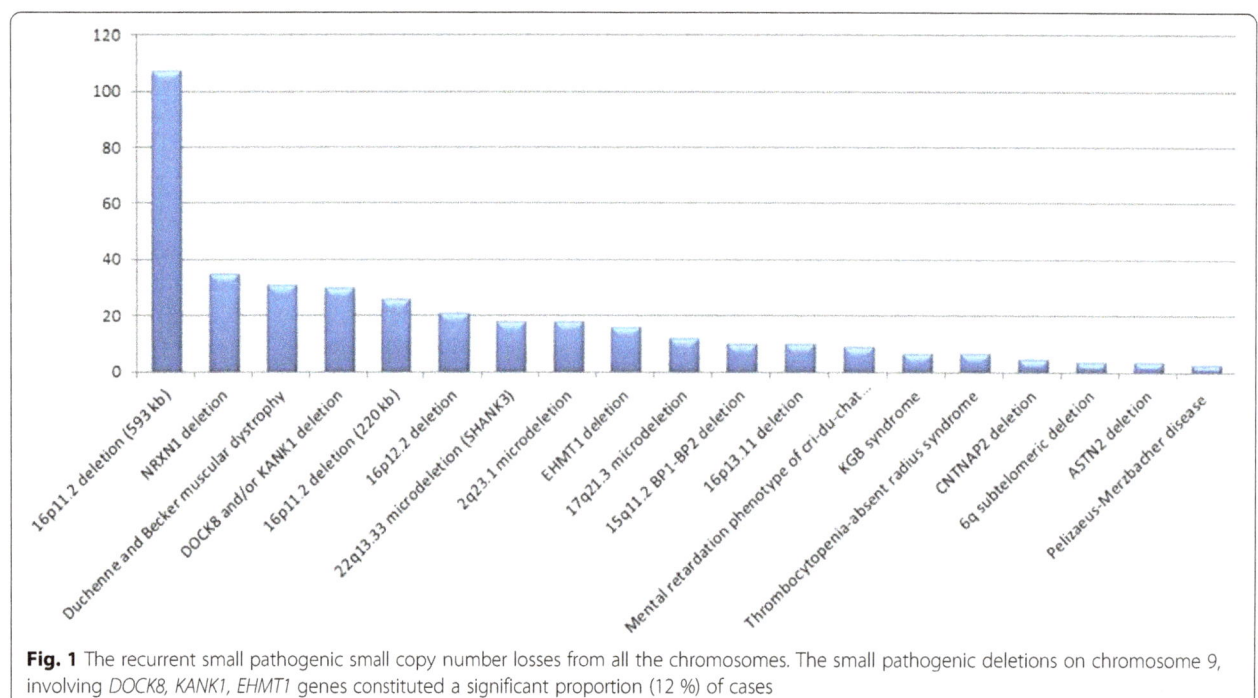

Fig. 1 The recurrent small pathogenic small copy number losses from all the chromosomes. The small pathogenic deletions on chromosome 9, involving *DOCK8, KANK1, EHMT1* genes constituted a significant proportion (12 %) of cases

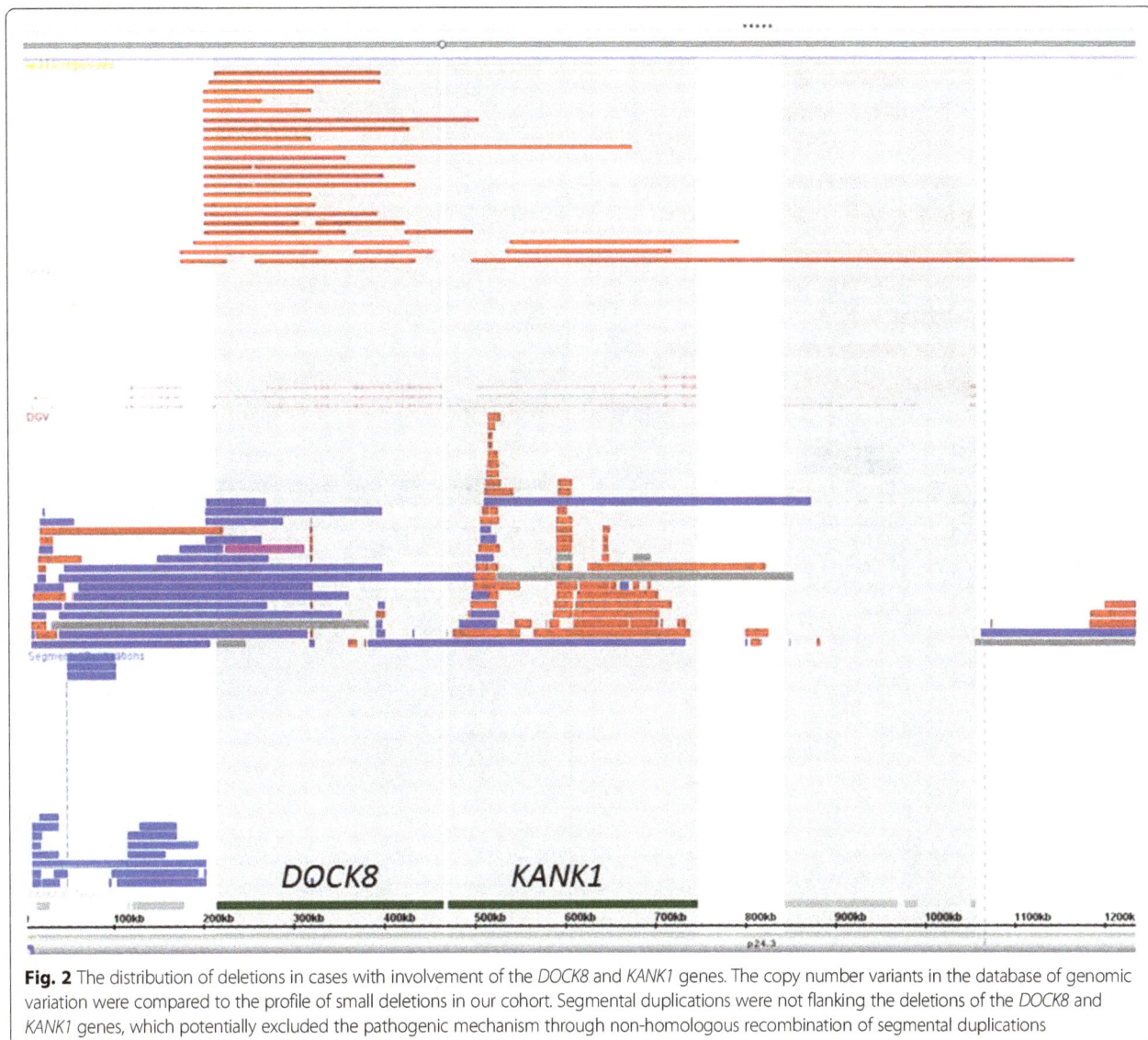

Fig. 2 The distribution of deletions in cases with involvement of the *DOCK8* and *KANK1* genes. The copy number variants in the database of genomic variation were compared to the profile of small deletions in our cohort. Segmental duplications were not flanking the deletions of the *DOCK8* and *KANK1* genes, which potentially excluded the pathogenic mechanism through non-homologous recombination of segmental duplications

790 kb (case 35), with an average of 384 kb (Table 1 and Additional file 2: Table S1). The remaining 47 cases were either resulted from interstitial deletions over 1 Mb in size (18 cases), terminal deletions over 1 Mb (14 cases), or unbalanced translocations (15 cases) that could be as small as 880 kb in size in a t(9;11)(q34.3;p15.4)(case 47, Additional file 2: Table S2). Very interestingly, of these 47 cases, four had relatively small deletions (1–1.5 Mb in size): a 1,048-kb deletion (case 10, Additional file 2: Table S2) involving the *PTCH1* gene (OMIM 601309) and diagnosis of Gorlin syndrome (OMIM #109400), a 1,349-kb deletion (case 15) involving the *STXBP1* gene and diagnosis of early infantile epileptic encephalopathy (OMIM #612164), and two 9q34.3 deletions of 1,218 kb and 1,268 kb (case 31 and 32). The small (57 cases) and relative small (4 cases) deletions

established 59 % (61/104) of pathogenic copy number losses on chromosome 9.

The 9p24.3 (0–2.2 Mb from 9p telomere) and 9q34.3 (137.4–141.2 Mb from 9p telomere) were two hot spots of pathogenic copy number losses on chromosome 9

The 9p24.3 and 9q34.3 regions were two hot spots of copy number losses on chromosome 9. A total of 35 cases majorly involved the 9p24.3 region: 30 small pathogenic deletions (case 1–30, Additional file 2: Table S1), one interstitial deletion (case 1, Additional file 2: Table S2), two terminal deletions (case 19 and 20), and two unbalanced translocations (case 33 and 35). Additionally, 26 cases were localized to 9q34.3 region: 17 small pathogenic deletions (case 41–57, Additional file 2: Table S1), one interstitial deletion (case 18, Additional file 2:

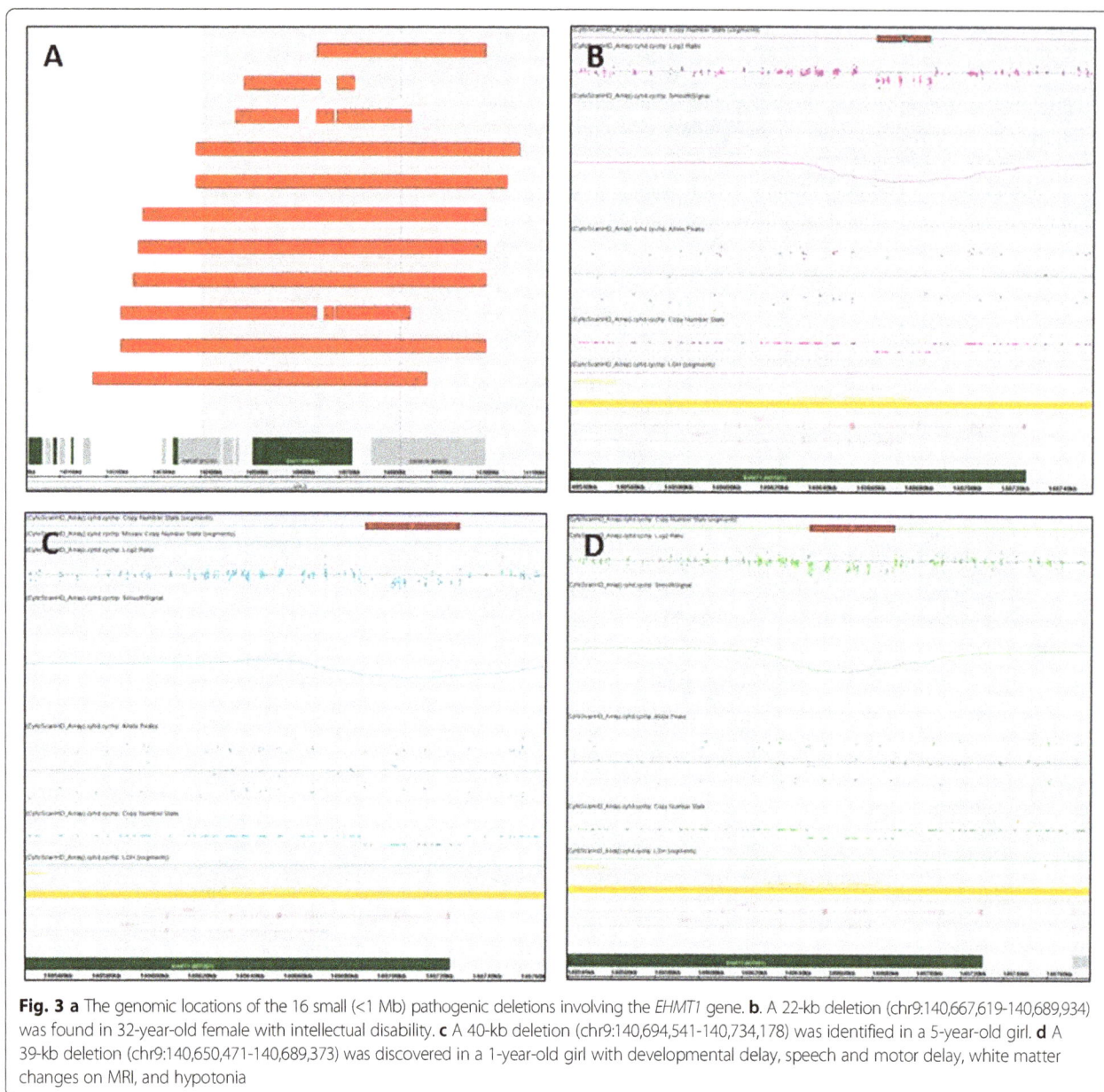

Fig. 3 a The genomic locations of the 16 small (<1 Mb) pathogenic deletions involving the *EHMT1* gene. **b**. A 22-kb deletion (chr9:140,667,619-140,689,934) was found in 32-year-old female with intellectual disability. **c** A 40-kb deletion (chr9:140,694,541-140,734,178) was identified in a 5-year-old girl. **d** A 39-kb deletion (chr9:140,650,471-140,689,373) was discovered in a 1-year-old girl with developmental delay, speech and motor delay, white matter changes on MRI, and hypotonia

Table S2), 5 large terminal deletions (case 28–32) and 3 unbalanced translocations (case 45–47). Overall, close to 60 % (61/104, 59 %) of deletions were localized to the very ends of chromosome 9 at band 9p24.3 and 9q34.3.

Rarely encountered extremely small homozygous pathogenic deletions were discovered in two cases

Extremely small homozygous pathogenic deletions were identified in two cases: 1): a new born baby girl who presented with a metabolic disorder (abnormal reflexes, hypotonia, seizures, and elevated glycine) was revealed to contain a 25-kb homozygous deletion in the *GLDC* gene, which gave rise to autosomal recessive glycine encephalopathy (nonketotic hyperglycinemia; OMIM #605899). Besides that, a 50-kb heterozygous deletion was also found in the 5′ region of the *GLDC* gene. Parental study showed the mother was a carrier of a 25-kb heterozygous deletion and the father was a carrier of a 75-kb heterozygous deletion of the *GLDC* gene. The 25-kb maternally inherited deletion was located within the 75-kb paternally inherited deletion, and therefore inheritance of abnormal allele from both parents led to a 25-kb homozygous and a 50-kb heterozygous deletion in the proband (Fig. 4); 2): a 1-year-old boy was found to have a 74-kb homozygous deletion of the *CDK5RAP2* gene in a region of homozygosity (Additional file 3: Figure S2) which

Table 1 Profile of pathogenic copy number losses and gains in chromosome 9

Type or gene involved	Number	Mean, kb	Range, kb
Copy number losses : large			
Interstitial deletion	18	5,070	1,048–16,837
Terminal deletion	14	5,273	1,218–13,593
Unbalanced translocation	15	7,053	880–17,107
Subtotal	47		
Copy number losses: small			
DOCK8	24	299	97–431
KANK1	3	369	184–670
DOCK8 and KANK1	3	419	75–676
EHMT1	16	417	22–790
ASTN2	4	150	78–271
FREM1	2	369	166–573
STXBP1	1	592	NA
COL5A1	1	370	NA
GLDC	1	50	25–75
TOPORS	1	337	NA
CDK5RAP2	1	74	NA
Subtotal	57		
Large copy number gains			
Trisomy 9p/proximal 9q	15	45,996	13,826–95,453
9q duplications	6	12,172	6,277–18,399
Unbalanced translocation	4	25,717	6,794–68,089
Tetrasomy 9q and proximal 9q due to isochromosome	3	66,477	49,843–81,113
Trisomy 9	2	140,833	NA
Triplication	1	15,972	NA
Subtotal	31		
Complex chromosomal rearrangements (CCRs)			
Inverted duplication with terminal deletion of 9p	3	Deletion: 6,377; Duplication: 32,271	
Inverted duplication with terminal deletion of 9q	1	Deletion: 161; Duplication: 3,127	
Multiple deletion and duplication	2	Losses: 1091; Gains: 12,517	
Chromothripsis	1	Loss: 134; Gains: 21,094	
Subtotal	7		
Total	142		

NA not applicable

led to autosomal recessive primary microcephaly-3 (OMIM #604804). The presence of multiple large regions of homozygosity (a total of 421 Mb) implied these two parents were closely related in blood. The proband inherited the heterozygous abnormal allele with deletion of the CDK5RAP2 gene from both parents.

Discussion

The subtelomeric region such as 1p36 is known to be gene-rich and prone to have deletions, supported by a study with a large cohort of over 5,000 cases [10]. The cases with subtelomeric rearrangements comprised of about 46 % of all the genomic abnormalities identified by CMA [10]. However, as compared to 1p36, 22q13, 4p16, 5p15, very limited cases at the ends of chromosome 9p and 9q were established [10]. When we reviewed the profile of copy number losses from our database of 38,000 postnatal cases studied by using high-resolution oligo-SNP array and sorted it based on chromosomal regions, we discovered that all the cases with 1p36 deletions were over 1 Mb: 20 cases were 1–3 Mb, eight cases were 3–5 Mb, eight cases were 5–10 Mb and five cases were 10–

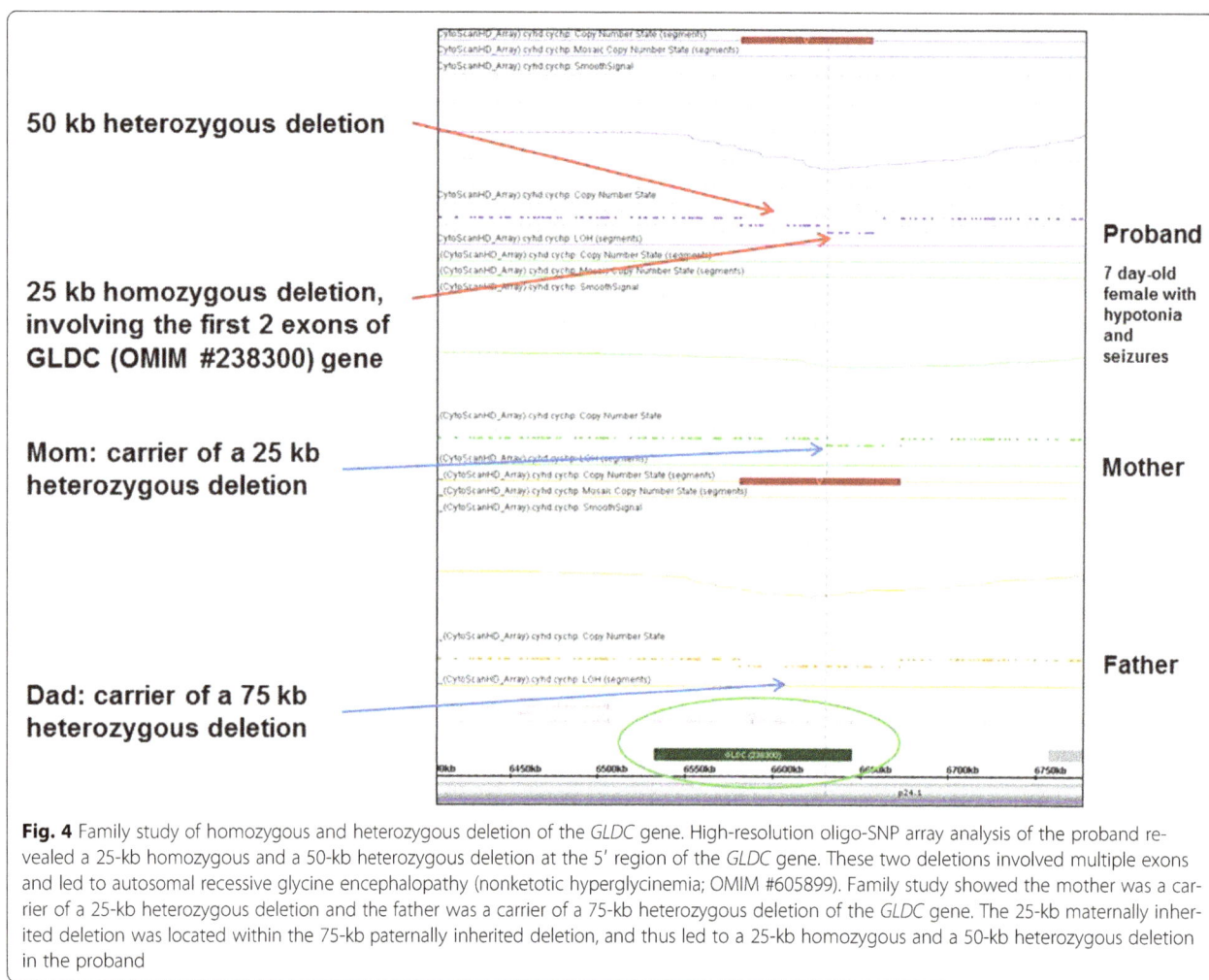

Fig. 4 Family study of homozygous and heterozygous deletion of the *GLDC* gene. High-resolution oligo-SNP array analysis of the proband revealed a 25-kb homozygous and a 50-kb heterozygous deletion at the 5′ region of the *GLDC* gene. These two deletions involved multiple exons and led to autosomal recessive glycine encephalopathy (nonketotic hyperglycinemia; OMIM #605899). Family study showed the mother was a carrier of a 25-kb heterozygous deletion and the father was a carrier of a 75-kb heterozygous deletion of the *GLDC* gene. The 25-kb maternally inherited deletion was located within the 75-kb paternally inherited deletion, and thus led to a 25-kb homozygous and a 50-kb heterozygous deletion in the proband

20 Mb in size (unpublished data). In contrast, 61 of 104 pathogenic deletions on chromosome 9 were either smaller than 1 Mb (57 cases) or between 1 and 1.5 Mb (4 cases). This finding demonstrated that the size of copy number losses conspicuously varied between chromosomal regions. In the clinical practice, the concept of vigilant selecting appropriate methods to characterize the genomic losses at different regions becomes essentially important. For instance, FISH analysis using subtelomeric or locus-specific probe may be approriate to identify 1p36 microdeletions, but may miss cases with small deletions on chromosome 9.

Extremely small intragenic deletion of the *EHMT1* gene was only reported in one case: a 40-kb intragenic deletion of the *EHMT1* gene with uncertain phenotypic consequence [9]. A more recent update on Kleefstra syndrome exhibited that the 16 newly diagnosed 9q34.3 deletions were all larger than 200 kb [11]. In our cohort, we identified a total of 24 cases with 9q34.3 deletions: 16 with small (<1 Mb) deletions involving the *EHMT1* gene (case 42–57, Additional file 2: Table S1), 5 with terminal deletion of 9q (case 28–32, Additional file 2: Table

S2), and 3 with small (880–1001 kb in size) 9q34.3 deletions due to unbalanced translocations (case 45–47, Additional file 2: Table S2). Remarkably, we brought about three extremely small (22 kb, 39 kb and 40 kb in size) intragenic deletions of the *EHMT1* gene and all were clustered at the 3′ end of the gene (Fig. 3, b-d). The 22-kb deletion (Fig. 3b) was identified in a 32-year-old female with intellectual disability; whereas, the 40-kb deletion (Fig. 3c) was found in a 5-year-old girl and the 39-kb deletion (Fig. 3d) was discovered in a 1-year-old girl with typical features of 9q34.3 deletion including developmental delay, speech and motor delay, and hypotonia [9]. In addition, a 26-year-old male with a 165-kb deletion involving *EHMT1* and CACNA1B gene (case 57, Additional file 2: Table S1) also presented clinical features which were typical for 9q34.3 deletion syndromes including mental retardation, developmental delay, speech delay, motor delay, learning disability, autism spectrum disorder, asymmetry of temporal lobe, localized polymicrogyria, loping gait and scoliosis [11].

In contrast to the *EHMT1* gene of which haploinsufficiency score was much better established by ClinGen (https://www.ncbi.nlm.nih.gov/projects/dbvar/clingen/), the sensitivity to haploinsufficiency for *DOCK8* and *KANK1* genes was not proven (Additional file 2: Table S3). There were two unrelated patients with mental retardation and developmental disability (MRD2; OMIM #614113) who were disclosed to have a heterozygous disruption of the longest isoform of the *DOCK8* gene by either deletion or a translocation of t(X;9) [12]. A recent report of another two patients with almost identical deletion involving both *DOCK8* and *KANK1* displayed two distinct phenotypes [6]. The study of a four-generation with a 225-kb deletion of the *KANK1* gene implied that an imprinting mechanism may play a role in the phenotypic variation in this family. The authors suggested *KANK1* is a maternally imprinted gene and only expressed in the paternal allele [8]. However, other report did not support this finding [7]. In our cohort, deletions of *KANK1* were found in 6 cases (case 25–30, Additional file 2: Table S1). There were not enough clinical data to determine whether *KANK1* is a maternally imprinted gene. On the other hand, *DOCK8* gene is unlikely to be maternally imprinted since the two half-brothers (a 2-year-old boy and a 7-year-old boy, case 13 and 14, Additional file 2: Table S1) both inherited the deleted *DOCK8* allele from the same mother. In addition, our patients with small deletions of the *DOCK8* gene had very strong family history (case 13/14, 17, 20/21 Additional file 2: Table S1) and shared similar clinical features, including developmental delay and intellectual disability (4 out of 5 cases), speech and motor delay (3), learning disability (2), behavior problems or autism (3), macrocephaly (2), dysmorphic or congenital anomalies (4). Our cohort provided additional pathogenic evidence for haploinsufficiency of *DOCK8* gene.

Although extremely rare, two cases with homozygous deletions of *GLDC* and *CDK5RAP2* genes were discovered in this cohort. In our previous study, we demonstrated the autosomal recessive disorders could be linked to regions of homozygosity (ROH) containing gene with point mutation which was inherited from related parents [2]. In this study, we showed additional two cases with autosomal recessive disorders which can be identified by high-resolution oligo-SNP array. The first was due to inheritance of allele with heterozygous deletion of different size from each carrier parent, which led to a homozygous deletion of *GLDC* gene (Fig. 4). The second was a homozygous deletion of the *CDK5RAP2* gene, inherited from closely related parents who carried the same heterozygous deletion (Additional file 3: Figure S2A). These two cases proved the efficacy of using high-resolution oligo-SNP array in the identification of extremely small homozygous pathogenic deletions.

Conclusions

This study demonstrated 1): the incidence of recurrent small pathogenic deletions (< 1 Mb) was approximately 3 % (373/13,000) of all reported CNVs; 2): the small pathogenic deletions at 9p24.3 and 9q34.3 constituted 12 % of small pathogenic deletions from all the chromosomes, 3): 59 % of pathogenic deletions on chromosome 9 were due to small (<1 Mb) or relatively small (1–1.5 Mb) pathogenic deletions; 4): 81 % (46/57) of small pathogenic deletions were enriched at 9p24.3 and 9q34.3 regions involving the *DOCK8, KANK1* and *EHMT1* genes; 5): high-resolution oligo-SNP array was capable of identifying homozygous deletions as small as 25 kb in size.

Methods
Patients

Patients with a broad range of clinical indications including intellectual disability, developmental delay, multiple congenital anomalies, dysmorphic features and pervasive developmental disorders were referred to our laboratory for oligo-SNP array studies. The data for this study were compiled from de-identified results of 38,000 consecutive patient specimens referred to our laboratory for constitutional oligo-SNP array study from 2011 to 2015. The patients were majorly from general population in the United States, with < 5 % from Mexico and other countries.

Oligonucleotide-single nucleotide polymorphism array analysis platforms and threshold setting

Oligo-SNP array analysis was performed on either Human SNP Array 6.0 (in 2011) or CytoScan® HD (2012–2015)(Affymetrix, Santa Clara, CA), using genomic DNA extracted from whole blood. The Human SNP Array 6.0 has 1.8 million genetic markers, including about 906,600 SNPs and 946,000 probes for the detection of CNVs. The CytoScan® HD has more than 2.67 million probes, including 1.9 million non-polymorphic copy number probes and 750,000 SNP probes. The overall resolutions are approximately 1.7 kb for Human SNP Array 6.0 and 1.15 kb for CytoScan® HD. For chromosome 9, the probes for Human SNP Array 6.0 covered: 9p(chr9:37,747-47,217,164) and 9q(chr9:65,596,318-141,091,382); for CytoScan HD®: 9p (chr9:192,129-40,784,142, chr9:43,400,082-44,900,526) and 9q (chr9:66,837,485-141,025,328). Genomic coordinates were based upon genome build 37/hg19 (2009). Hybridization, data extraction, and analysis were performed as per manufacturers' protocols. The Affymetrix® Chromosome Analysis Suite (ChAS) Software version 2.0 was used for data analysis, review, and reporting. For genome-wide screening, thresholds were set at > 200 kb for gains and > 50 kb for losses. For cytogenetically relevant regions, thresholds were set at > 100 kb for gains and > 20 kb for losses. Benign CNVs that are documented in the database of genomic variations (http://dgv.tcag.ca/dgv/app/home?-ref=GRCh37/hg19) and present in the general population were excluded from reporting.

Additional files

Additional file 1: Figure S1. Profile of abnormal CNVs and VOUS in chromosome 9 from 531 cases. A total of 142 cases with pathogenic CNVs, and 389 cases with VOUS were identified. (JPG 52 kb)

Additional file 2: Table S1. List of the cases with small (<1 Mb) pathogenic copy number loss on chromosome 9 without involvement of other chromosomes (N = 57). **Table S2.** List of the remaining cases with copy number loss on chromosome 9 (N = 47). **Table S3.** Interpretation, references and ClinGen evaluation of haploinsufficiency score of selected cytogenetically relevant genes on chromosome 9. (DOCX 43 kb)

Additional file 3: Figure S2. A. The finding of multiple large regions of homozygosity (421 Mb) was due to closely parental relatedness. B. An approximately 74-kb homozygous deletion involved multiple exons of the *CDK5RAP2* gene in a region of homozygosity at 9q33.1-q34.11 (chr9:118,503,864-132,425,233), which caused autosomal recessive primary microcephaly-3 (OMIM #604804). (JPG 60 kb)

Abbreviations

CMA: Chromosomal microarray analysis; CNV: Copy number variant; FISH: Fluorescence in situ hybridization; ISCN: International System of Cytogenetic Nomenclature; Oligo-SNP array: Oligonucleotide-single nucleotide polymorphism array; UPD: Uniparental disomy; VOUS: Variants of uncertain clinical significance

Acknowledgements

The authors acknowledge that Andrew Hellman and Jeff Radcliff provided valuable assistance in manuscript revisions.

Funding

Not applicable.

Authors' contributions

J-CW – reviewing, verification, analysis and interpretation of the data, drafting and revising the article, final approval of the version to be published. LWM – acquisition, reviewing and analysis of data. LPR - acquisition, reviewing and analysis of data. AA - conception and design, interpretation of data. RO - interpretation of data. FZB - interpretation of data. All authors read and approved the final manuscript.

Competing interests

The authors declare that they have no competing interests.

References

1. Watson CT, Marques-Bonet T, Sharp AJ, Mefford HC. The genetics of microdeletion and microduplication syndromes: an update. Annu Rev Genomics Hum Genet. 2014;15:215–44.
2. Wang JC, Ross L, Mahon LW, Owen R, Hemmat M, Wang BT, El Naggar M, Kopita KA, Randolph LM, Chase JM, Matas Aguilera MJ, Siles JL, Church JA, Hauser N, Shen JJ, Jones MC, Wierenga KJ, Jiang Z, Haddadin M, Boyar FZ, Anguiano A, Strom CM, Sahoo T. Regions of homozygosity identified by oligonucleotide SNP arrays: evaluating the incidence and clinical utility. Eur J Hum Genet. 2015;23:663–71.
3. Liehr T. Cytogenetic contribution to uniparental disomy (UPD). Mol Cytogenet. 2010;3:8.
4. Bena F, Bruno DL, Eriksson M, van Ravenswaaij-Arts C, Stark Z, Dijkhuizen T, Gerkes E, Gimelli S, Ganesamoorthy D, Thuresson AC, Labalme A, Till M, Bilan F, Pasquier L, Kitzis A, Dubourgm C, Rossi M, Bottani A, Gagnebin M, Sanlaville D, Gilbert-Dussardier B, Guipponi M, van Haeringen A, Kriek M, Ruivenkamp C, Antonarakis SE, Anderlid BM, Slater HR, Schoumans J. Molecular and clinical characterization of 25 individuals with exonic deletions of NRXN1 and comprehensive review of the literature. Am J Med Genet B Neuropsychiatr Genet. 2013;162B:388–403.
5. Soorya L, Kolevzon A, Zweifach J, Lim T, Dobry Y, Schwartz L, Frank Y, Wang AT, Cai G, Parkhomenko E, Halpern D, Grodberg D, Angarita B, Willner JP, Yang A, Canitano R, Chaplin W, Betancur C, Buxbaum JD. Prospective investigation of

autism and genotype-phenotype correlations in 22q13 deletion syndrome and SHANK3 deficiency. Mol Autism. 2013;4:18.
6. Tassano E, Accogli A, Pavanello M, Bruno C, Capra V, Gimelli G, Cuoco C. Interstitial 9p24.3 deletion involving only DOCK8 and KANK1 genes in two patients with non-overlapping phenotypic traits. Eur J Med Genet. 2016;59:20–5.
7. Vanzo RJ, Martin MM, Sdano MR, South ST. Familial KANK1 deletion that does not follow expected imprinting pattern. Eur J Med Genet. 2013;56:256–9.
8. Lerer I, Sagi M, Meiner V, Cohen T, Zlotogora J, Abeliovich D. Deletion of the ANKRD15 gene at 9p24.3 causes parent-of-origin-dependent inheritance of familial cerebral palsy. Hum Mol Genet. 2005;14:3911–20.
9. Kleefstra T, van Zelst-Stams WA, Nillesen WM, Cormier-Daire V, Houge G, Foulds N, van Dooren M, Willemsen MH, Pfundt R, Turner A, Wilson M, McGaughran J, Rauch A, Zenker M, Adam MP, Innes M, Davies C, Lopez AG, Casalone R, Weber A, Brueton LA, Navarro AD, Bralo MP, Venselaar H, Stegmann SP, Yntema HG, van Bokhoven H, Brunner HG. Further clinical and molecular delineation of the 9q subtelomeric deletion syndrome supports a major contribution of EHMT1 haploinsufficiency to the core phenotype. J Med Genet. 2009;46:598–606.
10. Shao L, Shaw CA, Lu XY, Sahoo T, Bacino CA, Lalani SR, Stankiewicz P, Yatsenko SA, Li Y, Neill S, Pursley AN, Chinault AC, Patel A, Beaudet AL, Lupski JR, Cheung SW. Identification of chromosome abnormalities in subtelomeric regions by microarray analysis: a study of 5,380 cases. Am J Med Genet A. 2008;146A:2242–51.
11. Willemsen MH, Vulto-van Silfhout AT, Nillesen WM, Wissink-Lindhout WM, van Bokhoven H, Philip N, Berry-Kravis EM, Kini U, van Ravenswaaij-Arts CM, Delle Chiaie B, Innes AM, Houge G, Kosonen T, Cremer K, Fannemel M, Stray-Pedersen A, Reardon W, Ignatius J, Lachlan K, Mircher C, van den Enden PT H, Mastebroek M, Cohn-Hokke PE, Yntema HG, Drunat S, Kleefstra T. Update on Kleefstra Syndrome. Mol Syndromol. 2012;2:202–12.
12. Griggs BL, Ladd S, Saul RA, DuPont BR, Srivastava AK. Dedicator of cytokinesis 8 is disrupted in two patients with mental retardation and developmental disabilities. Genomics. 2008;91:195–202.

20

Genomic imbalances pinpoint potential oncogenes and tumor suppressors in Wilms tumors

A. C. V. Krepischi[1,2][*][†], M. Maschietto[1,3][†], E. N. Ferreira[1], A. G. Silva[2], S. S. Costa[2], I. W. da Cunha[4], B. D. F. Barros[1], P. E. Grundy[5], C. Rosenberg[2] and D. M. Carraro[1][*]

Abstract

Background: Wilms tumor (WT) has a not completely elucidated pathogenesis. DNA copy number alterations (CNAs) are common in cancer, and often define key pathogenic events. The aim of this work was to investigate CNAs in order to disclose new candidate genes for Wilms tumorigenesis.

Results: Array-CGH of 50 primary WTs without pre-chemotherapy revealed a few recurrent CNAs not previously reported, such as 7q and 20q gains, and 7p loss. Genomic amplifications were exclusively detected in 3 cases of WTs that later relapsed, which also exhibited an increased frequency of gains affecting a 16.2 Mb 1q21.1-q23.2 region, losses at 11p, 11q distal, and 16q, and *WT1* deletions. Conversely, aneuploidies of chromosomes 13 and 19 were found only in WTs without further relapse. The 1q21.1-q23.2 gain associated with WT relapse harbours genes such as *CHD1L*, *CRABP2*, *GJA8*, *MEX3A* and *MLLT11* that were found to be over-expressed in WTs. In addition, down-regulation of genes encompassed by focal deletions highlighted new potential tumor suppressors such as *CNKSR1*, *MAN1C1*, *PAQR7* (1p36), *TWIST1*, *SOSTDC1* (7p14.1-p12.2), *BBOX* and *FIBIN* (11p13), and *PLCG2* (16q).

Conclusion: This study confirmed the presence of CNAs previously related to WT and characterized new CNAs found only in few cases. The later were found in higher frequency in relapsed cases, suggesting that they could be associated with WT progression.

Keywords: Wilms tumor, Array-CGH, Copy number alteration, CNA, Relapse, 1q21.1-q23.2 gain

Background

Wilms tumor (WT) is the most common type of malignant renal cancer in childhood, with an incidence of 7.7 in 1 million children between 0 and 14 years of age in Western populations [1, 2]. WTs exhibit a triphasic histology that recapitulates the fetal kidney development [3, 4], and similarly, gene expression profiling of isolated components mimics the ongoing process of nephrogenesis [5].

Earlier cytogenetic studies of patients with WAGR (MIM#194072), a syndrome characterized among others by susceptibility to Wilms tumor, revealed constitutional deletions on chromosome 11p13 affecting several contiguous genes (reviewed in [6]) including *WT1* [7, 8].

Latter on, cytogenetic and molecular studies of tumor material from WT sporadic cases showed the presence of somatic inactivating mutations or deletions of *WT1* in up to 15 % of the cases [9–11].

Other somatic alterations have been causally related to WT such as activating mutations in *CTNNB1* [10, 12], mutation/deletion of *WTX* [11, 13], and loss of imprinting of *IGF2* [9, 11, 14]. Recent molecular cytogenetic studies of tumoral samples have identified other genomic regions harboring genes supposedly associated with WT development, as exemplified by *HACE1* disruption at 6q21 [15], and a 2q37 deletion encompassing the *miR-562* [16]. Somatic deletions of *DIS3L2* have also been identified in a group of WT, and germline mutations of this gene results in Perlman syndrome that also presents increased WT susceptibility [17]. More recently, recurrent somatic mutations in *DROSHA*

* Correspondence: ana.krepischi@ib.usp.br; dirce.carraro@cipe.accamargo.org.br
†Equal contributors
[1]International Research Center, AC Camargo Cancer Center, São Paulo, Brazil
Full list of author information is available at the end of the article

(p.E1147K) as well as in other genes from the microRNA biogenesis machinery (*DGCR8*, *DICER1*, *XPO5* and *TARBP2*) were found in up to 12 % of WTs [18–21]. Additionally, somatic mutations in *SIX1/SIX2* were found in a subgroup of WT presenting high proliferative potential [19]. Because *SIX1* and *DROSHA* mutations were found to be heterogeneous events within primary tumors, both spatially and temporally, it was speculated if their co-occurrence were positively associated with tumor progression rather than tumor onset [22].

Somatic loss of heterozygosity (LOH) at 1p, 11q, 16q, and 22q, and deletions at 12q and 18q were correlated with an adverse outcome [23–26]. In clinical practice, combined LOH of 1p and 16q are used as markers of poor outcome for chemotherapy-naive tumors [23, 24]; however, they are detected in a very small subset of WT patients. In addition to the description of 1p, 1q, 3p, 3q, and 14q imbalances occurring at higher frequency in relapsing tumors than in other tumors [27], copy number gains at 1q have also been associated with poor prognosis in patients with favorable WT histology [28, 29]. A study reported that 1q gain has limited prognostic value for risk stratification in pre-treated WT [30]; however, it has been questioned whether the sample size was large enough and if the parameters used for defining 1q gain were validated to draw this conclusion [31].

This study was designed to assess the genomic copy number alterations profile (CNA) of WTs, aiming to identify genetic markers associated with WT, in particular those with clinical and prognostic importance.

Results

Characterization of copy number alterations in Wilms tumors

Array-CGH analysis detected a total of 350 CNAs in all 50 WT samples (mean of 7 CNAs per tumor genome), ranging from focal rearrangements (70 kb–5 Mb) to chromosome-arm alterations, and whole-chromosome aneuploidies. Full and summarized descriptions of the array-CGH data can be found in Additional file 1: Tables S1 and S2. We performed statistical analyses comparing WTs with and without relapse regarding the number, distribution and type (gain, high-copy gain, loss, homozygous loss) of CNAs. Genomic losses were more frequent in the relapse group ($p = 0.016$, Fisher exact test) than in the group without relapse, whereas high gains (>5 copies) were detected exclusively in the group of tumors from patients who relapsed (3 cases).

Typically, WTs present few alterations indicating low chromosomal instability. The $\log_2$ ratios for most alterations were in a range consistent with heterozygous losses or gains (>0.5 or <−0.5), suggestive of a low level of intra-tumor heterogeneity. As an example, Fig. 1a

shows the array-CGH results of four Wilms tumors; each lane shows the copy number profile of all chromosomes for one sample. Figure 1b summarizes the copy number findings detected in the WT cohort and their respective frequencies, showing the full cohort (upper panel) as well as tumors grouped according to the occurrence of relapse (bottom panel). Gains affecting 1q were observed in >50 % of the tumors, but frequent CNAs (>15 % of the WT group) included gains of 7q and 20q, and losses at 1p, 7p, 11q, and 16q, in addition to whole-chromosome aneuploidies of 6, 8, 12, and 20 (gains), and 22 (losses).

WTs derived from patients who later relapsed carried few genomic alterations detected in higher frequency than the group without relapse, such as 1q gain (with a peak at 1q proximal) and losses at 11p (with a peak encompassing the *WT1* gene), 11q distal, and 16q (Fig. 1b, bottom panels). Conversely, aneuploidies of chromosomes 13 and 19 (gains) were exclusively detected in the WT group without relapse.

Recurrent chromosomal alterations e minimum common regions

Table 1 describes six recurrent (frequency >15 % in the entire WT group) chromosomal rearrangements and their frequencies according to relapse status.

Focal 1q proximal gains were found in 63 % of the WT relapse group and in a significantly lower proportion in the WTs without relapse group (35.3 %). Focal losses encompassing either the *WT1* or *WTX* (*AMER1*) genes (Additional file 2: Figure S1) occurred in 12 and 6 % of WTs, respectively. The frequency of *WT1* deletions was significantly higher in WTs that later relapse than in the group without relapse (21 versus 6.4 %); one tumor from a patient who relapsed was found to carry both *WTX* and *WT1* deletions.

Twelve minimum common regions (MCRs) of chromosomal alterations detected in at least two WTs were identified and are described in Table 2.

We performed a comparative analysis of differential CNAs looking for the smallest common regions of aberrations that were more frequent in each WT group (tumors derived from patients who later presented relapse or not). In the manual curated analysis, we detected a region of 44.5 Mb at 1q21.1q31.1 (#chr1:144,053,035-188,589,610; GRCh37) that exhibited a higher frequency of gain in the relapse group than in the non-relapse group. This region encompasses the MCR of high-copy number gain at 1q21.1q23.2 (16.2 Mb), which was detected in two of the relapse WTs (*WT1104* and *WT1232*); gains of two of the affected genes, *S100A4* and *NOTCH2* were validated by qPCR in several tumors (Additional file 3: Figure S2).

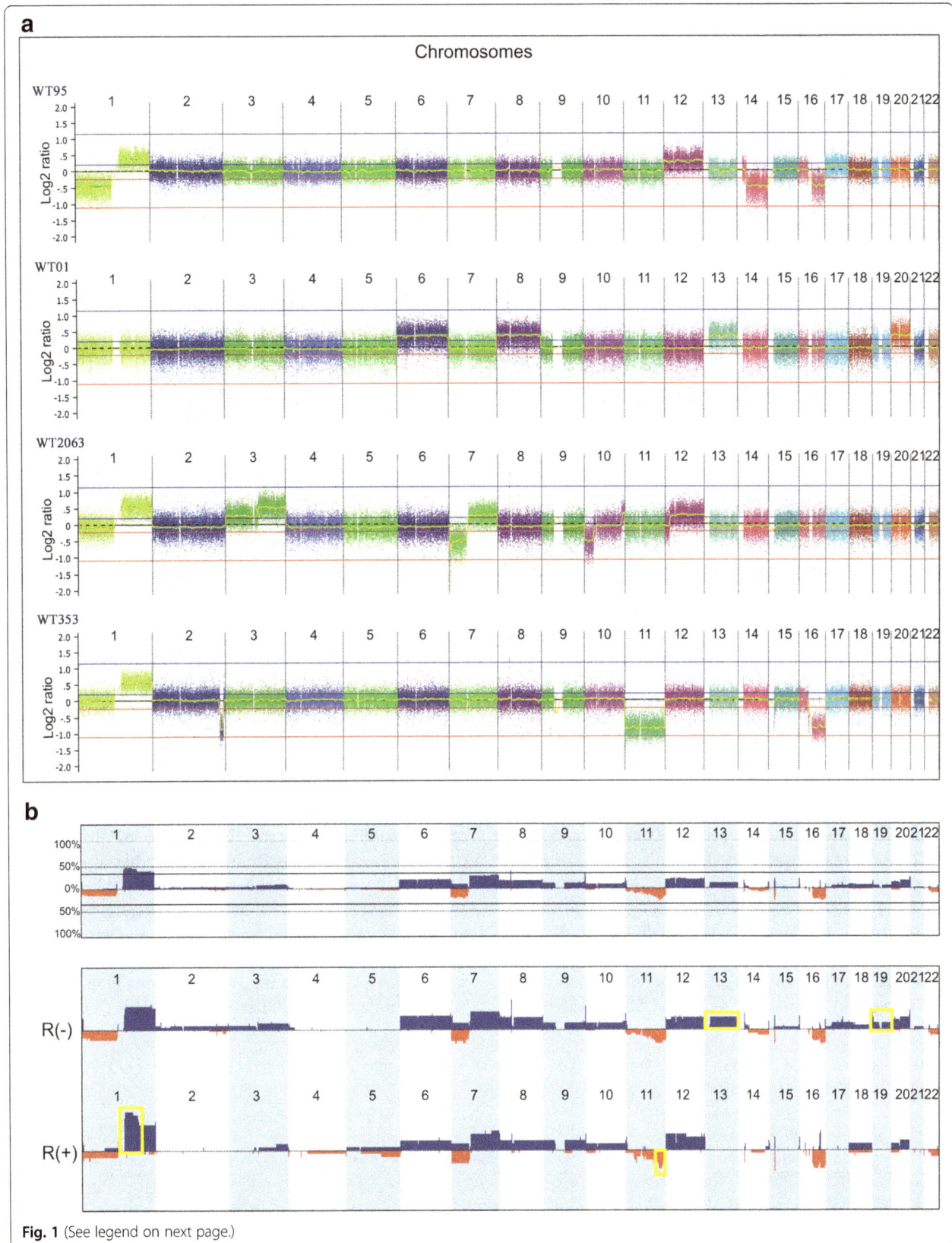

Fig. 1 (See legend on next page.)

(See figure on previous page.)
Fig. 1 Copy number profiles of sporadic Wilms tumors. All chromosomes are displayed from the short to the long arms. Images adapted from Nexus Copy Number software, Biodiscovery. **a** Array-CGH profile of four selected Wilms tumor samples. **b** Global profile of copy number alterations (CNA) and respective frequencies in the 50 WT samples (*upper panel*) and the CNA distribution according to the occurrence of relapse (*bottom panels*). Genomic gains are indicated by *blue bars*, losses by *red bars* and *yellow boxes* mark the alterations detected in higher frequency or exclusively in each group; relapsed patients (R+), non-relapsed patients (R-)

Additionally, we narrowed 14q genomic deletions to a segment at 14q24.1q32.12 common to four WTs: one relapsed tumor (*WT1232*), and three non-relapse cases (*WT095*, *WT246*, and *WT321*).

Focal chromosomal rearrangements
Two small regions exhibiting high-copy gains (log$_2$ ratio >1.4 indicating >5 copies) were detected in one relapsed WT (*WT1104*), and validated by qPCR: a 2.4 Mb 1p31.1 amplification (#chr1:80,765,303-83,606,627; GRCh37) containing only *LPHN2* (Fig. 2a, b, and c), and a 300 Kb amplification at 2q24.1 (#chr2:158,834,824-159, 135,178; GRCh37), encompassing only the *UPP2* and *CCDC148* genes (Fig. 2a, d, and e).

Regarding small genomic losses, the 1.6 Mb deletion at 6q16.3q21 (#chr6:103,820,062-105,461,750; GRCh37) encompassed only the genomic sequences of the *HACE1*, *LINC00577*, and *LIN28B* genes (Fig. 3a, b, and c), detected in two non-relapse WTs (*WT329* and *WT1070*), neither carrying *WT1* or *WTX* deletions. Another validated focal CNA detected in one tumor (*WT201*) was the 825 kb homozygous deletion at 11p14.1p14.2 (#chr11:26,688,179-27,513,817; GRCh37), harbouring *BBOX*, among others genes (*SLC5A12*, *FIBIN*, *CCDC34*, *LGR4*) (Fig. 3d, e, and f).

Gene expression analysis
To evaluate the expression of genes affected by CNAs in these WTs, we selected a set of 90 genes mapped in MCRs, focal rearrangements, and the 1q21.1q23.2 region associated with relapse. There were 35 (39 %) differentially expressed genes between WTs and differentiated kidneys (fold-change ≥|2|; p ≤0.05), with only 16 (46 %) exhibiting a concordant pattern of gene expression and type of CNA (see Table 3). Unsupervised hierarchical clustering (Additional file 4: Figure S3) based on the

expression pattern of this set of 16 genes discriminated all WT samples from all but one differentiated kidneys (DKs); however, this group of genes was not able to discriminate WT samples with or without later relapse.

Eleven genes located at genomic deletions were found to be down-regulated in WTs when compared with DKs, nine of them mapped in MCRs: *MAN1C1*, *CNKSR1*, and *PAQR7* (1p36); *INPP5D* and *ECEL1* (2q37); *SOSTDC1*, *TWIST1* and *AHR* (7p14.1p12.2); and *PLCG2* (16q22.1q24.3). The remaining two down-regulated genes, *BBOX* and *FIBIN*, were mapped in a homozygous 11p13 deletion detected in a single tumor.

Regarding those genes located at copy number gains, five of them, mapped at the 1q21.1q23.2 gain (more frequently detected in relapsed samples), were found to be over-expressed in WTs compared with DKs: *CHD1L*, *CRABP2*, *GJA8*, *MEX3A*, and *MLLT11*.

Discussion and conclusions
In this study, WTs exhibited a relatively small number of CNAs indicating low chromosomal instability, in accordance with previous reports of favourable histology WTs. Primary WTs that later relapse are supposedly more aggressive as they are resistant to chemotherapeutic treatments. The fact that these tumors displayed more chromosome alterations and higher gains is in part supported by findings of a high level CNAs found in the more aggressive diffuse anaplastic WT subtype [32]. Most of the chromosome alterations from this study has already been described by previous studies, such as 1q gain, and 11q and 16q losses [23, 27, 30] as well as alterations reported in low frequency, including the 2q37 deletion [16], and the 6q21 deletion [15]. However, a few CNAs detected in frequencies >15 % were reported here for the first time in WT, including 7q and 20q gains, and 7p loss.

Table 1 Six recurrent chromosomal rearrangements (frequency >15 % in the entire WT group) and microdeletions of *WT1* and *WTX* genes according to the relapse status

WT group	Recurrent rearrangements (chromosome arm/focal)						Whole-chromosome aneuploidies					Microdeletion of known WT genes	
	1p(−)	1q(+)	7p(−)	7q(+)	11q(−)	16q(−)	chr6	chr8	chr12	chr20(+)	chr22(−)	*WT1*	*WTX (AMER1)*
No-relapse (n = 31)	5	11	7	6	7	6	7	6	5	5	2	2	2
frequency	16.1 %	35.5 %	22.6 %	19.3 %	22.6 %	19.3 %						6.4 %	6.4 %
Relapse (n = 19)	3	12	4	5	6	6	3	3	4	2	1	4	1
frequency	15.8 %	63.2 %[a]	21.0 %	26.3 %	31.6 %	31.6 %						21.0 %[a]	5.3 %

[a]Significant differences between WTs derived from patients who later relapsed or not

Table 2 Twelve minimum common regions of chromosomal aberrations detected in Wilms tumours

Genomic coordinates (GRCh37)	Cytoband	Lenght (Mb)	Copy number type
#chr1:23,362,908-26,746,259	1p36.12p36.11	3.38	deletion
#chr1:144,824,185-161,067,947	1q21.1q23.2	16.24	amplicon
#chr2:224,323,183-236,091,182	2q37	11.77	deletion
#chr4:114,506,621-115,974,843	4q26	1.47	deletion
#chr7:39,742,350-49,836,566	7p14.1p12.2	10.10	deletion
#chr7:133548462-158674912	7q33q36.3	25.13	gain
#chr10:125,525,789-135,524,747	10q26.13q26.3	10.00	gain
#chr11:33,713,698-36,511,648	11p13p12	2.80	deletion
#chr11:111,359,499-120,743,656	11q23.1q23.3	9.38	deletion
#chr14:19,373,243-34,950,464	14q11.1q13.1	15.58	gain
#chr14:68,882,507-92,887,911	14q24.1q32.12	24.01	deletion
#chr16:71,201,074-90,294,753	16q22.1q24.3	19.09	deletion

In this study, the blastemal component of WT was micro-dissected before DNA extraction. Eventually, this procedure could minimize findings related to tumor heterogeneity that have been described in pediatric tumors [33], at least those related to cell differentiation. Unfortunately, the array-CGH platform used in this study does not allow allelic identification, impeding a careful assessment of the presence of intratumor heterogeneity at low levels.

The association between chromosomal alterations and cancer recurrence in patients with WT has been suggested by some publications, all of which share similar findings [25, 27, 34, 35]. In our samples, the 1q gain was found in 63.2 % of the tumors that later relapse in comparison with 35.5 % of the non-relapsed WTs. This higher frequency of 1q gain, compared to previous studies, can be explained by the fact that in our tumor series only the blastemal component were assessed. A specific genomic segment at 1q21.1q31.3 has been associated with WT relapse [28, 36], and in the present work this region was narrowed to a 16.2 Mb segment at 1q21.1q23.2. Five genes mapped within this 1q21.1q23.2 segment were

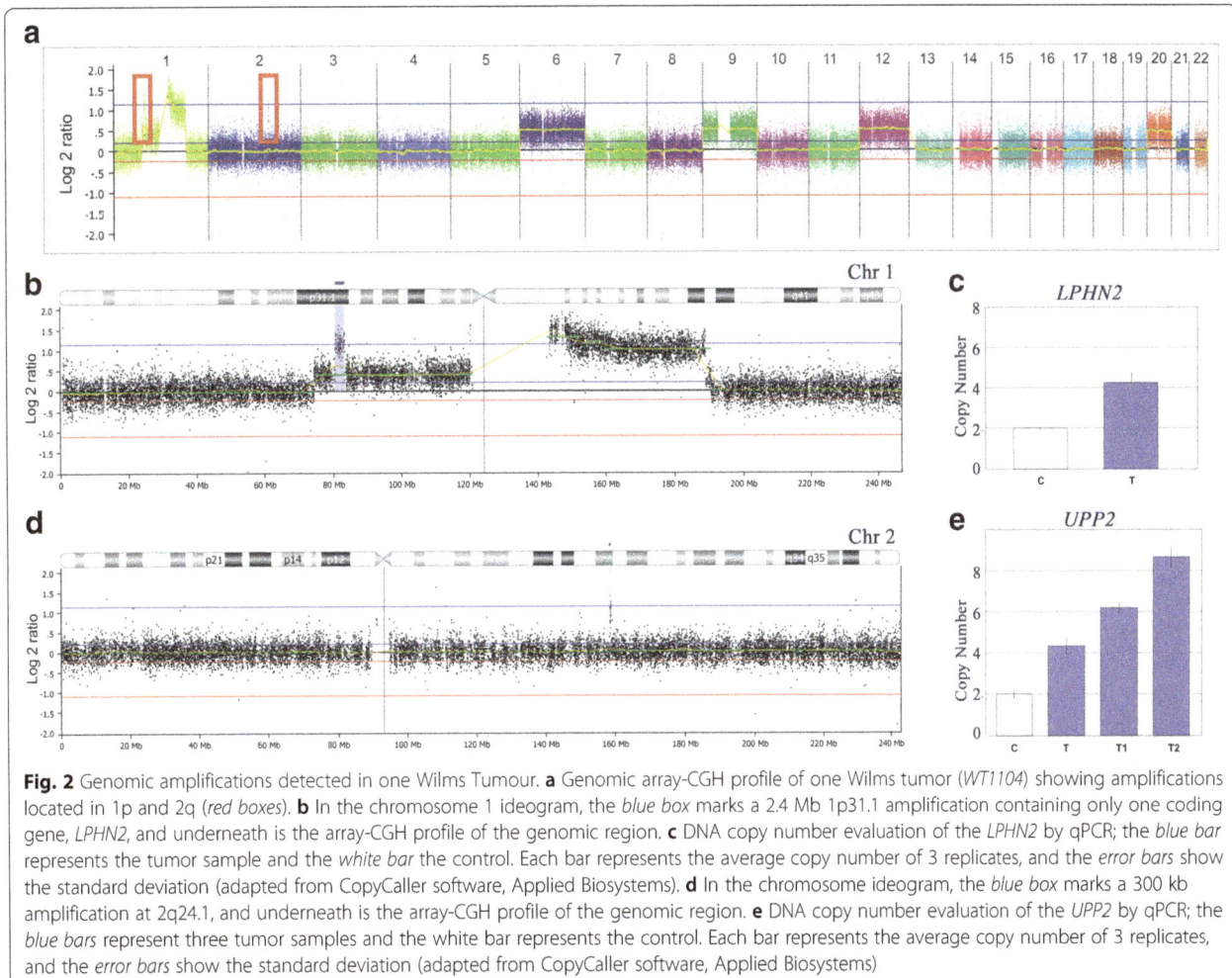

Fig. 2 Genomic amplifications detected in one Wilms Tumour. **a** Genomic array-CGH profile of one Wilms tumor (*WT1104*) showing amplifications located in 1p and 2q (*red boxes*). **b** In the chromosome 1 ideogram, the *blue box* marks a 2.4 Mb 1p31.1 amplification containing only one coding gene, *LPHN2*, and underneath is the array-CGH profile of the genomic region. **c** DNA copy number evaluation of the *LPHN2* by qPCR; the *blue bar* represents the tumor sample and the *white bar* the control. Each bar represents the average copy number of 3 replicates, and the *error bars* show the standard deviation (adapted from CopyCaller software, Applied Biosystems). **d** In the chromosome ideogram, the *blue box* marks a 300 kb amplification at 2q24.1, and underneath is the array-CGH profile of the genomic region. **e** DNA copy number evaluation of the *UPP2* by qPCR; the *blue bars* represent three tumor samples and the white bar represents the control. Each bar represents the average copy number of 3 replicates, and the *error bars* show the standard deviation (adapted from CopyCaller software, Applied Biosystems)

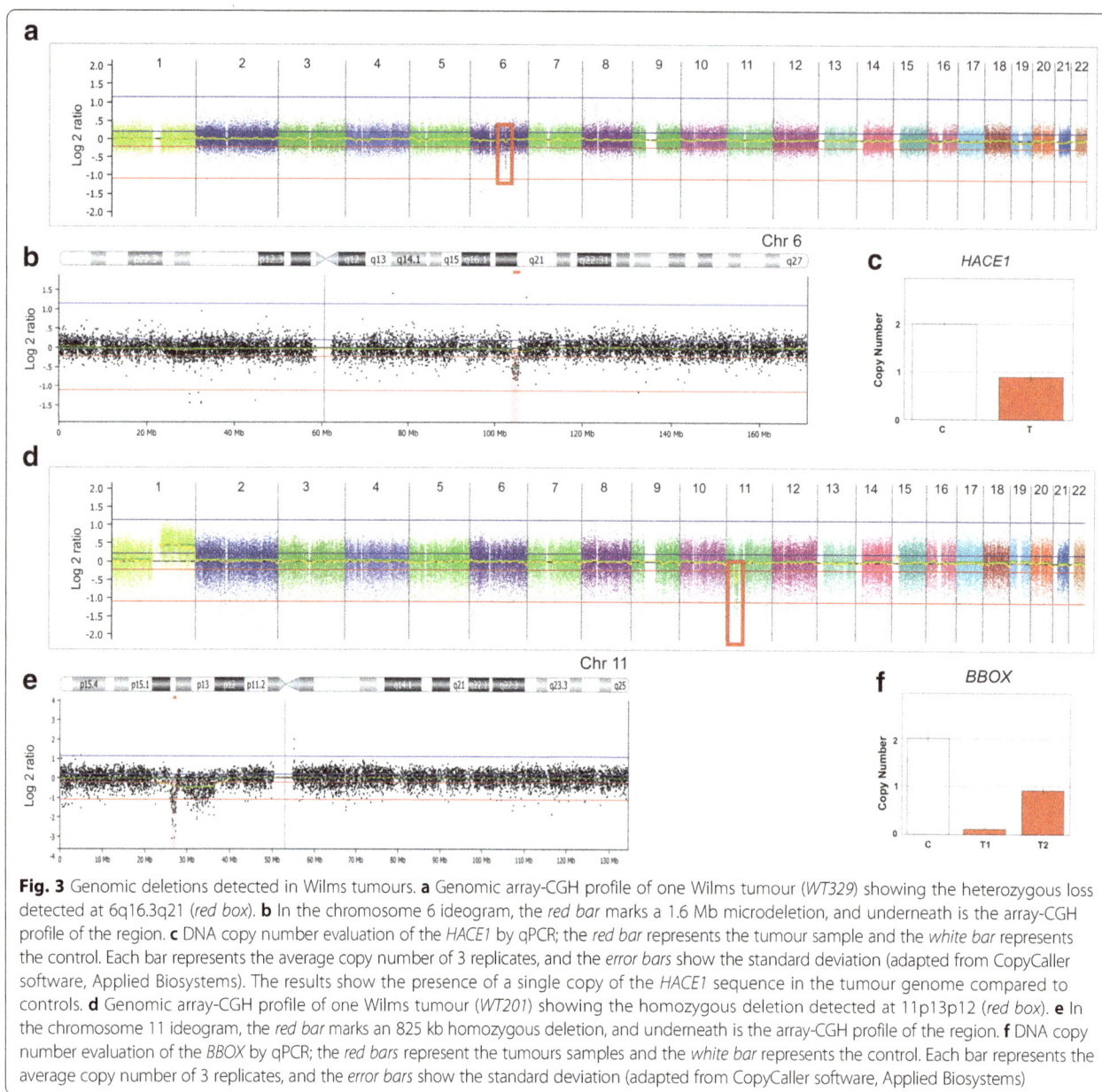

Fig. 3 Genomic deletions detected in Wilms tumours. **a** Genomic array-CGH profile of one Wilms tumour (*WT329*) showing the heterozygous loss detected at 6q16.3q21 (*red box*). **b** In the chromosome 6 ideogram, the *red bar* marks a 1.6 Mb microdeletion, and underneath is the array-CGH profile of the region. **c** DNA copy number evaluation of the *HACE1* by qPCR; the *red bar* represents the tumour sample and the *white bar* represents the control. Each bar represents the average copy number of 3 replicates, and the *error bars* show the standard deviation (adapted from CopyCaller software, Applied Biosystems). The results show the presence of a single copy of the *HACE1* sequence in the tumour genome compared to controls. **d** Genomic array-CGH profile of one Wilms tumour (*WT201*) showing the homozygous deletion detected at 11p13p12 (*red box*). **e** In the chromosome 11 ideogram, the *red bar* marks an 825 kb homozygous deletion, and underneath is the array-CGH profile of the region. **f** DNA copy number evaluation of the *BBOX* by qPCR; the *red bars* represent the tumours samples and the *white bar* represents the control. Each bar represents the average copy number of 3 replicates, and the *error bars* show the standard deviation (adapted from CopyCaller software, Applied Biosystems)

found to be up-regulated in WTs compared with DKs (*CHD1L*, *CRABP2*, *GJA8*, *MEX3A* and *MLLT11*) but not between relapse and no-relapse WT. *CRABP2* higher expression also had a weak association with high stage WTs [37]. *MLLT11* has a role with leukemogenesis [38, 39], and *CHD1L* is over-expressed in hepatocellular carcinomas [40].

Combined LOH of 16q and 1p is a known marker of poor prognosis; indeed, we found a higher frequency of 16q deletion (31.6 %) in relapsed cases when compared with non-relapsed cases (19.3 %), and narrowed to a 19 Mb segment at 16q22.1q24.3. We also found deletions affecting *WT1* in 12 % of all cases detected with a significantly higher frequency in the relapse group. Although

these genomic features could be useful as prognostic indicators for blastemal predominance, they were very infrequent events, therefore adding little to the ability to distinguish patients with different outcomes.

Losses of 14q have been shown to have a borderline association with tumor stages III and IV [27] suggesting that genes located in this chromosome region have the potential to be involved in tumor progression. WTs here studied are mostly stages III and IV tumors, and the detection of 14q deletions in four samples allowed to narrow this genomic deletion to a segment at 14q24.1q32.12 (one relapsed and three non-relapse cases).

Other MCRs of new genomic deletions highlighted few genes with a concordant profile with gene expression,

Table 3 Sixteen differentially expressed genes in the group of Wilms tumours compared to differentiated kidneys which exhibited a concordant pattern of copy number alteration (CNA)

Gene name	Fold change	Type of CNA
CNKSR1	−2.30*	1p36.12p36.11 deletion
MAN1C1	−7.37**	1p36.12p36.11 deletion
PAQR7	−10.71**	1p36.12p36.11 deletion
CHD1L	3.18**	1q21.1q23.2 gain
CRABP2	31.59**	1q21.1q23.2 gain
GJA8	25.48*	1q21.1q23.2 gain
MEX3A	10.28**	1q21.1q23.2 gain
MLLT11	14.04**	1q21.1q23.2 gain
DNMT3A	2.42**	2p25.3p11.2 gain
INPP5D	−2.56*	2q37 deletion
AHR	−9.62**	7p14.1p12.2 deletion
SOSTDC1	−21.39**	7p14.1p12.2 deletion
TWIST1	−3.26*	7p14.1p12.2 deletion
BBOX1	−39.84*	11p13p12 homozygous loss in one WT
FIBIN	−8.10*	11p13p12 homozygous loss in one WT
PLCG2	−8.96*	16q22.1q24.3 deletion

*$p < 0.05$, **$p < 0.01$

particularly *CNKSR1*, *MAN1C1* and *PAQR7* at 1p36, and *TWIST1* and *SOSTDC1* at 7p14.1p12.2, the later already suggested as tumor suppressor in WT [41]. The analysis of other small alterations of high amplitude in copy number change disclosed new candidate genes potentially associated with WT such as *LPHN2*, *UPP2*, *BBOX* and *FIBIN*. Only *BBOX* and *FIBIN*, identified in a homozygous deletion at 11p13, exhibited a concordant down-regulated pattern of gene expression when considering the entire WT group; therefore, both genes appear as candidate tumor suppressor genes for WT but need further studies to confirm their role.

We are aware that this study has limitations. The set of genes which expression were compared to differentiated kidneys, not an ideal control, came from alterations found in only one or few tumors, thus explaining the observed low level of agreement between CNAs and expression pattern. Additionally, we do not have tested other patient's tissues to exclude the possibility that part of the detected CNAs were germline alterations. However, all CNAs were checked in the Database of Genomic Variants and none of them was found to be common changes.

In summary, most of the detected CNAs in this study were described by previous works. However, the present work identified that genomic amplifications and higher number of genomic losses occur in tumors that later relapsed. Additionally, these tumors exhibited an increased frequency of a gain of a 16.2 Mb segment at 1q21.1q23.2, and losses at 11p, 11q distal, and 16q,

together with *WT1* deletions. Conversely, aneuploidies of chromosomes 13 and 19 (whole-chromosome gains) were exclusively detected in WTs without relapse, suggesting that these are good prognosis markers.

The CNAs affected the expression of few genes (overexpression of *CHD1L*, *CRABP2*, *GJA8*, *MEX3A* and *MLLT11* and down-regulation of *CNKSR1*, *MAN1C1*, *PAQR7*, *TWIST1*, *SOSTDC1*, *BBOX* and *FIBIN*) that could have an oncogene or tumor suppressor role in WT. We stress that although the studied cohort of WTs is small, most of the genomic regions here identified have been described in WT by others, reinforcing that they should be investigated in depth to disclose the possible roles of the affected genes in Wilms tumorigenesis.

While isolated genes can account for selection of specific chromosome imbalances (drivers), another alternative theory, applying an evolutionary perspective, hypothesizes that the different karyotypes with specific combinations of chromosome alterations could result in slightly different tumor subtypes. The high rate of variation within a tumor generates tumor sub-clones with different phenotypic progression, as exemplified by the acquisition of resistance to chemotherapy or the metastatic growth [42, 43]. For instance, in the case of WT, this process could also be reflected by the heterogeneous histology found within each tumor. Some preliminary data reported intra-tumor heterogeneity in 70 % of the WT cases albeit they may also share some common copy number changes [44]. Most of the alterations we found are shared by WTs from other studies, suggesting this is a relatively common route for Wilms tumorigenesis.

Methods
Material
Samples of sporadic primary WTs were obtained from 50 patients enrolled in the National Wilms tumor Study 5 (NWTS-5, Children Oncology Group). The group is enriched for WTs stages III and IV, which characteristics have been described [45]. Tumors analysed were not subjected to neoadjuvant chemotherapy; 31 of these patients exhibited no relapse after a minimum of 3 years of follow-up. All samples were obtained with informed consent. This work was conducted in accordance with the principles of the Declaration of Helsinki and was approved by the A. C. Camargo Cancer Center ethics committee under number CEP 764/06.

Comparative genome hybridization based on microarrays (array-CGH)
We performed comparative genomic hybridization based on microarrays in a commercial whole-genome 180 K platform containing 180,000 oligonucleotide

probes (Agilent Technologies; design 22060). Reference DNA was a commercially available human pool of samples from healthy donors (Promega). Briefly, samples were labelled with Cy3- or Cy5-deoxycytidine triphosphates by random priming, and purification, hybridization and washing were performed as recommended by the manufacturer. Scanned images of the arrays were processed using Feature Extraction 10.7.3.1 software (Agilent Technologies).

Array-CGH analysis was performed using Nexus Copy Number software 7.0 (Biodiscovery) with the FASST2 segmentation algorithm, according to the following settings: minimum of 5 consecutive probes (effective resolution of ~70 Kb for CNA calling), significance threshold set at 10^{-8}, and threshold $\log_2$ Cy3/Cy5 of 0.3 and 1.4 for gain or high copy gain (indicating >5 copies of the genomic sequence, and hereafter named amplification), respectively, and −0.3 and −1.1 for loss and homozygous loss, respectively. All copy number variants reported in the Database of Genomic Variants (DGV; http://dgv.tcag.ca/dgv/app/home) were excluded, as well data from sex chromosomes; the X-linked gene AMER1 (WTX) was analysed separately. The minimum common regions (MCRs) of recurrent CNAs were obtained by implementing the global frequency statistical approach of the STAC method (Significance Testing for Aberrant Copy Number [46]). Data were evaluated iregarding the total number of CNAs and the numbers of gains, losses, amplifications, and homozygous losses. Genes affected by copy number changes were annotated using the Genome browser UCSC (http://genome.ucsc.edu/). Statistical analyses were performed using the software GraphPad PRISM 5.

DNA copy number validation by real-time quantitative PCR (qPCR)

To validate 9 focal CNAs (<5 Mb), we performed qPCR using 9 TaqMan probes (see Additional file 5: Table S3) on a 7500 Fast Real-time quantitative PCR System (Applied Biosystems). Copy number determinations were performed for selected targets using TaqMan Gene Copy Number Assays (Applied Biosystems). The assays contained a FAM-labelled TaqMan probe for the target gene and a VIC-labelled TaqMan probe for the reference gene (RNaseP). The reference sample or calibrator was a commercially available human genomic DNA (Promega). The results were analysed using Copy-Caller 1.0 software (Applied Biosystems). The relative number of DNA copies for each probe was determined by the DDCt ((FAM Ct–VIC Ct) sample–(FAM Ct–VIC Ct) calibrator) method, which assumes that the calibrator DNA has two copies of the reference gene.

Gene expression analysis by reverse transcription quantitative real-time PCR (RT-qPCR)

We selected 90 genes for gene expression evaluation by RT-qPCR (Additional file 6: Table S4) that were affected by recurrent copy number changes in our cohort of WTs. Total RNA samples were enzymatically converted into first-strand cDNA using an RT^2 First Strand cDNA Kit (Qiagen). We evaluated 36 WT blastemal enriched samples and six differentiated kidneys (DK) used as controls. These control samples constituted the cortex of differentiated kidneys from nephrectomies of WT patient's macrodissected after evaluation of hematoxilin-eosin sections. We used a SYBR-green based customized array RT^2 qPCR Primer Customized Assay (Qiagen Technologies) following the manufacturer's protocol. RT-qPCR was performed in an ABI Prism 7900HT Fast Real-time Sequence Detection System (Life Technologies, Foster City, CA). ACTB, GAPDH, and HPRT1 were tested as reference genes, and the two most stable genes (as determined by geNorm [47]), namely ACTB and GAPDH, were used for normalization in the expression analysis. The array data were analysed by SDS and RQ manager (Life Technologies), and gene expression normalization was calculated using the 2ΔCq method. Genes were considered differentially expressed between groups (WTs and DKs) if the fold change was ≥|2| with p-value ≤0.05 (student t-test).

Additional files

Additional file 1: Table S1. Full CNA data identified by array-CGH in the 50 Wilms tumor samples. CNA calling was performed using the software Nexus Copy Number 7.0 (Biodiscovery). **Table S2.** Array-CGH data summary of Wilms tumor samples: total number of copy number alteration, number of each type of copy number event (gain, loss, high-copy gain, and homozygous loss), and statistical analysis. (XLS 872 kb)

Additional file 2: Figure S1. DNA copy number evaluation showing focal and homozygous losses of the WT1 (A) and WTX (B) genes by qPCR; the red bars represent tumour samples and the white bar represents the control. Each bar represents the average copy number of 3 replicates, and the error bars show the standard deviation (adapted from CopyCaller software, Applied Biosystems). (TIF 226 kb)

Additional file 3: Figure S2. DNA copy number evaluation showing amplification of S100A4 (A) and NOTCH2 (B) genes at 1q21.1-q23.2 in several tumours by qPCR; the blue bars represent tumour samples and the white bar represents the control. Each bar represents the average copy number of 3 replicates, and the error bars show the standard deviation (adapted from CopyCaller software, Applied Biosystems). (TIF 349 kb)

Additional file 4: Figure S3. Unsupervised hierarchical clustering using Pearson's correlation, and complete linkage of 36 Wilms tumour (WTs) and 6 differentiated kidney (DKs) samples based on 16 differently expressed genes (values were log2-transformed). Only genes with expression detected in more than 80 % of the samples were considered. Bootstrap resampling was performed to assess cluster reliability, and the results are represented by the coloured lines of the dendrogram (black line indicates 90–100 % reliability). Differentiated kidney samples are marked in blue, and Wilms Tumour samples are coloured pink (light pink are non-relapse samples, and dark pink are relapse samples). Columns and rows represent samples and genes, respectively; red, upregulated, and green, down-regulated genes. (TIF 425 kb)

Additional file 5: Table S3. List of genes selected for copy number validation of 9 focal rearrangements using real-time quantitative PCR (qPCR) with TaqMan Gene Copy Number assays. (DOC 34 kb)

Additional file 6: Table S4. Description of 90 genes that were selected for gene expression analysis in the group of Wilms tumors using a SYBR-green based customized array RT^2 qPCR Primer Customized Assay (Qiagen Technologies). Description of the genes selected as controls for gene expression analysis in the group of Wilms tumors using a the SYBR-green based customized array RT^2 qPCR Primer Customized Assay (Qiagen Technologies). (XLS 56 kb)

Competing interests

All authors declare no competing financial interest.

Authors' contributions

ACVK, MM, ENF, AGS, SSC, BDFB carried out the experiments. IWC characterized the morphology of the samples. PEG and DMC provided the samples. ACVK and CR participated in the design of the study. ACVK, MM and ENF performed all analyses. ACVK, CR and DMC coordinated of the study, ACVK and MM wrote the manuscript with input from all authors. All authors read and approved the final manuscript.

Acknowledgments

We thank the Children's Oncology Group for providing WT samples and the AC Camargo Cancer Center Biobank for differentiated mature kidney samples and DNA and RNA samples. MM was supported by CNPQ 400140/2014-4.

Funding

This work was supported by grants from Conselho Nacional de Pesquisa (CNPq) and Fundação de Amparo a Pesquisa do Estado de São Paulo (FAPESP 2006/00054-0, 2008/57887-9, 2009/00898-1, 2010/00223-1, 2013/08028-1).

Author details

[1]International Research Center, AC Camargo Cancer Center, São Paulo, Brazil. [2]Institute of Biosciences, University of São Paulo, São Paulo, Brazil. [3]Brazilian Biosciences National Laboratory, National Center for Research in Energy and Materials, Campinas, São Paulo, Brazil. [4]Department of Surgical and Investigative Pathology, AC Camargo Cancer Center, São Paulo, Brazil. [5]Alberta Health Services, Cancer Control Alberta, Alberta, Canada.

References

1. Stiller CA, Parkin DM. International variations in the incidence of childhood renal tumours. Br J Cancer. 1990;62:1026–30.
2. Wilms' tumor: status report, 1990. By the National Wilms' Tumor Study Committee. J Clin Oncol. 1991;9:877–87
3. Mierau GW, Beckwith JB, Weeks DA. Ultrastructure and histogenesis of the renal tumors of childhood: an overview. Ultrastruct Pathol. 1987;11:313–33.
4. Beckwith JB. Histopathological aspects of renal tumors in children. Prog Clin Biol Res. 1982;100:1–14.
5. Maschietto M, De Camargo B, Brentani H, Grundy P, Sredni ST, Torres C, Mota LD, Cunha IW, Patrão DFC, Costa CML, Soares FA, Brentani RR, Carraro DM. Molecular profiling of isolated histological components of Wilms tumor implicates a common role for the Wnt signaling pathway in kidney and tumor development. Oncology. 2008;75:81–91.
6. Dome JS, Coppes MJ. Recent advances in Wilms tumor genetics. Curr Opin Pediatr. 2002;14:5–11.
7. Gessler M, Poustka A, Cavenee W, Neve RL, Orkin SH, Bruns GA. Homozygous deletion in Wilms tumours of a zinc-finger gene identified by chromosome jumping. Nature. 1990;343:774–8.
8. Ton CC, Huff V, Call KM, Cohn S, Strong LC, Housman DE, Saunders GF. Smallest region of overlap in Wilms tumor deletions uniquely implicates an 11p13 zinc finger gene as the disease locus. Genomics. 1991;10:293–7.
9. Gadd S, Huff V, Huang C-C, Ruteshouser EC, Dome JS, Grundy PE, Breslow N, Jennings L, Green DM, Beckwith JB, Perlman EJ. Clinically relevant subsets identified by gene expression patterns support a revised ontogenic model

of Wilms tumor: a Children's Oncology Group Study. Neoplasia. 2012;14: 742–56.
10. Royer-Pokora B. Genetics of pediatric renal tumors. Pediatr Nephrol. 2013;28:13–23.
11. Scott RH, Murray A, Baskcomb L, Turnbull C, Loveday C, Al-Saadi R, Williams R, Breatnach F, Gerrard M, Hale J, Kohler J, Lapunzina P, Levitt GA, Picton S, Pizer B, Ronghe MD, Traunecker H, Williams D, Kelsey A, Vujanic GM, Sebire NJ, Grundy P, Stiller CA, Pritchard-Jones K, Douglas J, Rahman N. Stratification of Wilms tumor by genetic and epigenetic analysis. Oncotarget. 2012;3:327–35.
12. Koesters R, Ridder R, Kopp-Schneider A, Betts D, Adams V, Niggli F, Briner J, Doeberitz MVK. Mutational activation of the β-catenin proto-oncogene is a common event in the development of Wilms' tumors. Cancer Res. 1999;59:3880–2.
13. Rivera MN, Kim WJ, Wells J, Driscoll DR, Brannigan BW, Han M, Kim JC, Feinberg AP, Gerald WL, Vargas SO, Chin L, Iafrate AJ, Bell DW, Haber DA. An X chromosome gene, WTX, is commonly inactivated in Wilms tumor. Science. 2007;315:642–5.
14. Bjornsson HT, Brown LJ, Fallin MD, Rongione MA, Bibikova M, Wickham E, Fan JB, Feinberg AP. Epigenetic specificity of loss of imprinting of the IGF2 gene in wilms tumors. J Natl Cancer Inst. 2007;99:1270–3.
15. Slade I, Stephens P, Douglas J, Barker K, Stebbings L, Abbaszadeh F, Pritchard-Jones K, Cole R, Pizer B, Stiller C, Vujanic G, Scott RH, Stratton MR, Rahman N. Constitutional translocation breakpoint mapping by genome-wide paired-end sequencing identifies HACE1 as a putative Wilms tumour susceptibility gene. J Med Genet. 2010 May;47(5):342–7. doi: 10.1136/jmg.2009.072983. Epub 2009 Nov 30.
16. Drake KM, Ruteshouser EC, Natrajan R, Harbor P, Wegert J, Gessler M, Pritchard-Jones K, Grundy P, Dome J, Huff V, Jones C, Aldred MA. Loss of heterozygosity at 2q37 in sporadic Wilms' tumor: Putative role for miR-562. Clin Cancer Res. 2009;15:5985–92.
17. Astuti D, Morris MR, Cooper WN, Staals RHJ, Wake NC, Fews GA, Gill H, Gentle D, Shuib S, Ricketts CJ, Cole T, van Essen AJ, van Lingen RA, Neri G, Opitz JM, Rump P, Stolte-Dijkstra I, Müller F, Pruijn GJM, Latif F, Maher ER. Germline mutations in DIS3L2 cause the Perlman syndrome of overgrowth and Wilms tumor susceptibility. Nat Genet. 2012;277–284.
18. Torrezan GT, Ferreira EN, Nakahata AM, Barros BDF, Castro MTM, Correa BR, Krepischi ACV, Olivieri EHR, Cunha IW, Tabori U, Grundy PE, Costa CML, de Camargo B, Galante PAF, Carraro DM. Recurrent somatic mutation in DROSHA induces microRNA profile changes in Wilms tumour. Nat Commun. 2014;5(May):4039.
19. Wegert J, Ishaque N, Vardapour R, Geörg C, Gu Z, Bieg M, Ziegler B, Bausenwein S, Nourkami N, Ludwig N, Keller A, Grimm C, Kneitz S, Williams RD, Chagtai T, Pritchard-Jones K, van Sluis P, Volckmann R, Koster J, Versteeg R, Acha T, O'Sullivan MJ, Bode PK, Niggli F, Tytgat GA, van Tinteren H, van den Heuvel-Eibrink MM, Meese E, Vokuhl C, Leuschner I, et al. Mutations in the SIX1/2 Pathway and the DROSHA/DGCR8 miRNA Microprocessor Complex Underlie High-Risk Blastemal Type Wilms Tumors. Cancer Cell. 2015;27:298–311. http://siop.meetingxpert.net/SIOP_863/poster_103315/program.aspx/103315.
20. Rakheja D, Chen KS, Liu Y, Shukla AA, Schmid V, Chang T-C, Khokhar S, Wickiser JE, Karandikar NJ, Malter JS, Mendell JT, Amatruda JF. Somatic mutations in DROSHA and DICER1 impair microRNA biogenesis through distinct mechanisms in Wilms tumours. Nat Commun. 2014;2:4802.
21. Walz AL, Ooms A, Gadd S, Gerhard DS, Smith MA, Guidry Auvil JM, Meerzaman D, Chen Q-R, Hsu CH, Yan C, Nguyen C, Hu Y, Bowlby R, Brooks D, Ma Y, Mungall AJ, Moore RA, Schein J, Marra MA, Huff V, Dome JS, Chi Y-Y, Mullighan CG, Ma J, Wheeler DA, Hampton OA, Jafari N, Ross N, Gastier-Foster JM, Perlman EJ. Recurrent DGCR8, DROSHA, and SIX Homeodomain Mutations in Favorable Histology Wilms Tumors. Cancer Cell. 2015;27:286–97.
22. Spreafico F, Ciceri S, Gamba B, Torri F, Terenziani M, Collini P, Macciardi F, Radice P, Perotti D. Chromosomal anomalies at 1q, 3, 16q, and mutations of SIX1 and DROSHA genes underlieWilms tumor recurrences.Oncotarget. 2016 doi: 10.18632/oncotarget.6950.
23. Grundy PE, Breslow NE, Li S, Perlman E, Beckwith JB, Ritchey ML, Shamberger RC, Haase GM, D'Angio GJ, Donaldson M, Coppes MJ, Malogolowkin M, Shearer P, Thomas PRM, Macklis R, Tomlinson G, Huff V, Green DM. Loss of heterozygosity for chromosomes 1p and 16q is an adverse prognostic factor in favorable-histology Wilms tumor: a report from the National Wilms Tumor Study Group. J Clin Oncol. 2005;23:7312–21.
24. Messahel B, Williams R, Ridolfi A, A'Hern R, Warren W, Tinworth L, Hobson R, Al-Saadi R, Whyman G, Brundler MA, Kelsey A, Sebire N, Jones C, Vujanic G, Pritchard-Jones K. Allele loss at 16q defines poorer prognosis Wilms tumour

irrespective of treatment approach in the UKW1-3 clinical trials: a Children's Cancer and Leukaemia Group (CCLG) study. Eur J Cancer. 2009;45:819–26.

25. Natrajan R, Williams RD, Hing SN, Mackay A, Reis-Filho JS, Fenwick K, Iravani M, Valgeirsson H, Grigoriadis A, Langford CF, Dovey O, Gregory SG, Weber BL, Ashworth A, Grundy PE, Pritchard-Jones K, Jones C. Array CGH profiling of favourable histology Wilms tumours reveals novel gains and losses associated with relapse. J Pathol. 2006;210:49–58.

26. Wittmann S, Wunder C, Zirn B, Furtwängler R, Wegert J, Graf N, Gessler M. New prognostic markers revealed by evaluation of genes correlated with clinical parameters in Wilms tumors. Genes Chromosomes Cancer. 2008;47:386–95.

27. Perotti D, Spreafico F, Torri F, Gamba B, D'Adamo P, Pizzamiglio S, Terenziani M, Catania S, Collini P, Nantron M, Pession A, Bianchi M, Indolfi P, D'Angelo P, Fossati-Bellani F, Verderio P, Macciardi F, Radice P. Genomic profiling by whole-genome single nucleotide polymorphism arrays in Wilms tumor and association with relapse. Genes Chromosom Cancer. 2012;51:644–53.

28. Gratias EJ, Jennings LJ, Anderson JR, Dome JS, Grundy P, Perlman EJ. Gain of 1q is associated with inferior event-free and overall survival in patients with favorable histology Wilms tumor: a report from the Children's Oncology Group. Cancer. 2013;119:3887–94.

29. Chagtai T, Zill C, Dainese L, Williams R, Wegert J, Maschietto M, Vujanic G, Sebire N, Leuschner I, Ambros P, Kager L, O'Sullivan M, Blaise A, Bergeron C, Gisselsson D, Kool M, van den Heuvel-Eibrink M, Graf N, van Tinteren H, Coulomb A, Gessler M, Pritchard-Jones K. Gain of 1q as a biomarker in pre-treated Wilms tumour in the SIOP WT 2001 trial: a SIOP renal tumours biology consortium study. 2014.

30. Vokuhl C, Vogelgesang W, Leuschner I, Furtwängler R, Graf N, Gessler M, Dörner E, Pietsch T. 1q gain is a frequent finding in preoperatively treated Wilms tumors, but of limited prognostic value for risk stratification in the SIOP2001/GPOH trial. Genes Chromosomes Cancer. 2014;53:960–2.

31. Pritchard-Jones K, Williams R, Segers H, van den Heuvel-Eibrink M, Pieters R, van Tinteren H, Vujanic G, Bown N. Response to the letter to the editor: 1q gain is a frequent finding in preoperatively treated Wilms tumors, but of limited prognostic value for risk satisfaction in the SIOP2009/Gesellschaft für Pädiatrische Onkologie und Hämatologie (GPOH) trial. Genes Chromosomes Cancer. 2015;54:397–9.

32. Maschietto M, Williams RD, Chagtai T, Popov SD, Sebire NJ, Vujanic G, Perlman E, Anderson JR, Grundy P, Dome JS, Pritchard-Jones K. TP53 mutational status is a potential marker for risk stratification in Wilms tumour with diffuse anaplasia. PLoS One. 2014;9, e109924.

33. Mengelbier LH, Karlsson J, Lindgren D, Valind A, Lilljebjörn H, Jansson C, Bexell D, Braekeveldt N, Ameur A, Jonson T, Kultima HG, Isaksson A, Asmundsson J, Versteeg R, Rissler M, Fioretos T, Sandstedt B, Börjesson A, Backman T, Pal N, Øra I, Mayrhofer M, Gisselsson D. Intratumoral genome diversity parallels progression and predicts outcome in pediatric cancer. Nat Commun. 2015;6:6125.

34. Zin R, Pham K, Ashleigh M, Ravine D, Waring P, Charles A. SNP-based arrays complement classic cytogenetics in the detection of chromosomal aberrations in Wilms' tumor. Cancer Genet. 2012;205:80–93.

35. Williams RD, Al-Saadi R, Chagtai T, Popov S, Messahel B, Sebire N, Gessler M, Wegert J, Graf N, Leuschner I, Hubank M, Jones C, Vujanic G, Pritchard-Jones K. Subtype-specific FBXW7 mutation and MYCN copy number gain in Wilms' tumor. Clin Cancer Res. 2010;16:2036–45.

36. Segers H, van den Heuvel-Eibrink MM, Williams RD, van Tinteren H, Vujanic G, Pieters R, Pritchard-Jones K, Bown N. Gain of 1q is a marker of poor prognosis in Wilms' tumors. Genes Chromosom Cancer. 2013;52:1065–74.

37. Gupta A, Kessler P, Rawwas J, Williams BRG. Regulation of CRABP-II expression by MycN in Wilms tumor. Exp Cell Res. 2008;314:3663–8.

38. Cerveira N, Lisboa S, Correia C, Bizarro S, Santos J, Torres L, Vieira J, Barros-Silva JD, Pereira D, Moreira C, Meyer C, Oliva T, Moreira I, Martins Â, Viterbo L, Costa V, Marschalek R, Pinto A, Mariz JM, Teixeira MR. Genetic and clinical characterization of 45 acute leukemia patients with MLL gene rearrangements from a single institution. Mol Oncol. 2012;6:553–64.

39. Strunk CJ, Platzbecker U, Thiede C, Schaich M, Illmer T, Kang Z, Leahy P, Li C, Xie X, Laughlin MJ, Lazarus HM, Gerson SL, Bunting KD, Ehninger G, Tse W. Elevated AF1q expression is a poor prognostic marker for adult acute myeloid leukemia patients with normal cytogenetics. Am J Hematol. 2009;84:308–9.

40. Ma NF, Hu L, Fung JM, Xie D, Zheng BJ, Chen L, Tang DJ, Fu L, Wu Z, Chen M, Fang Y, Guan XY. Isolation and characterization of a novel oncogene, amplified in liver cancer 1, within a commonly amplified region at 1q21 in hepatocellular carcinoma. Hepatology. 2008;47:503–10.

41. Ohshima J, Haruta M, Arai Y, Kasai F, Fujiwara Y, Ariga T, Okita H, Fukuzawa M, Hata JI, Horie H, Kaneko Y. Two candidate tumor suppressor genes, MEOX2 and SOSTDC1, identified in a 7p21 homozygous deletion region in a Wilms tumor. Genes Chromosom Cancer. 2009;48:1037–50.

42. Vincent MD. The animal within: carcinogenesis and the clonal evolution of cancer cells are speciation events sensu stricto. Evolution. 2010;64:1173–83.

43. Duesberg P, Mandrioli D, McCormack A, Nicholson JM. Is carcinogenesis a form of speciation? Cell Cycle. 2011;10:2100–14.

44. Genetic heterogeneity in Wilms tumours: clonal evolution and implications for biomarker testing | NCRI Cancer Conference abstracts http://abstracts.ncri.org.uk/abstract/genetic-heterogeneity-in-wilmstumours-clonal-evolution-and-implications-for-biomarker-testing-2/. Access date: 11 Feb 2016.

45. Maschietto M, Piccoli FS, Costa CML, Camargo LP, Neves JI, Grundy PE, Brentani H, Soares FA, Camargo B De, Carraro DM. Gene expression analysis of blastemal component reveals genes associated with relapse mechanism in Wilms tumour. Eur J Cancer. 2011;47:2715–22.

46. Diskin SJ, Eck T, Greshock J, Mosse YP, Naylor T, Stoeckert CJ, Weber BL, Maris JM, Grant GR. STAC: a method for testing the significance of DNA copy number aberrations across multiple array-CGH experiments. Genome Res. 2006;16:1149–58.

47. Vandesompele J, De Preter K, Pattyn F, Poppe B, Van Roy N, De Paepe A, Speleman F. Accurate normalization of real-time quantitative RT-PCR data by geometric averaging of multiple internal control genes. Genome Biol. 2002;3:RESEARCH0034.

21

Mosaicism for structural non-centromeric autosomal rearrangements in disease-defined carriers: sex differences in the rearrangements profile and maternal age distributions

Natalia V. Kovaleva[1*] and Philip D. Cotter[2,3]

Abstract

Background: Mosaicism for an autosomal structural rearrangement (Rea) associated with clinical manifestation of chromosomal imbalance is rare. Consequently, there is a lack of basic epidemiological characterization of this kind of mosaicism, such as population rate, cytogenetic profile of Reas involved, maternal age distribution, and sex (male to female) ratio among Rea carriers. The objectives of the present study were: (i) determination of the Rea profile in clinically affected individuals, (ii) comparative analysis of the cytogenetic profile and involvement of single chromosomes to rearrangements in affected and previously reported asymptomatic carriers, (iii) analysis of the male/female ratio in carriers of various types of Rea, and, (iv) examination of parental ages distributions according to carriers' sex.

Results: Two hundred and forty six disease-defined cases of mosaicism for autosomal non-centromeric Rea with a normal cell line of known sex were identified from the literature. There was a significant difference in single chromosome involvements compared to structural rearrangements between affected and asymptomatic carriers of unbalanced Rea, $p = 0.0030$. In affected carriers, chromosome 18 was most frequently involved in structural rearrangements (12.6% of 246 instances). The least frequently rearranged were chromosomes 16 and 21 (0.8% and 1.2%, respectively). In asymptomatic carriers, the most frequently rearranged were chromosomes 5 and 21 (13% of 51 instances each). Among carriers of "loss" or "gain/loss" of genomic material, a female predominance was observed (50 M/89 F, different from population ratio of 1.06 at $p = 0.0002$). Carriers of either "gain" or balanced Rea demonstrated typical male predominance (41 M/30 F and 18 M/16 F), not different from 1.06. Maternal and paternal ages were reported in 129 and in 109 cases, respectively. There was a significant difference in maternal age distribution between male and female carriers, with mean maternal age of 25.2 years vs 28.3 years ($p = 0.032$). However, there was no difference in paternal age, with mean paternal age of 29.4 in both groups.

Conclusion: The data suggested that structural rearrangements of certain chromosomes involved in mosaicism may not be tolerated by the embryo, while others have higher survival prospects. Maternal age appears to be a risk factor for somatic mosaicism of structural Rea in female offspring or might cause an adverse effect on male embryo viability.

Keywords: Segmental somatic mosaicism, Non-centromeric autosomal rearrangement, Genomic imbalance, Sex ratio, Maternal age, Paternal age

* Correspondence: kovalevanv2007@yandex.ru
[1]Academy of Molecular Medicine, Mytniskaya str. 12/44, St. Petersburg 191144, Russian Federation
Full list of author information is available at the end of the article

Background

Somatic chromosomal mosaicism, the presence of two or more cell lines with different chromosomal constitution, is a common phenomenon in humans [1]. However, mosaicism for structural chromosomal rearrangements (N/Rea, normal line/rearrangement) is rarely reported. Consequently, there is a lack of basic epidemiological characterization of this category of mosaicism, such as population rate, cytogenetic profile of the Reas involved, maternal age distribution, and sex ratio (SR, male to female ratio) among the carriers of Reas.

Depending on factors such as the severity of genomic imbalance, the degree of mosaicism and tissue distribution, the carrier of a somatic mosaicism may be asymptomatic or may present with a variable phenotype. A recent study of patients with somatic/gonadal mosaicism described differences in cytogenetic profile among asymptomatic and affected individuals [2]. In addition, the study revealed a strong female prevalence among both affected and asymptomatic carriers of somatic/gonadal mosaicism for unbalanced Rea, unlike the typical male prevalence among carriers of balanced Rea. However, the number of affected carriers was low (2 M/10 F), not allowing for detailed evaluation of single chromosome involvement in various type of abnormalities and sex ratio among carriers of various types of Reas.

Therefore, the objectives of the present study were: (i) determination of the Rea profile in clinically affected carriers, (ii) comparative analysis of the cytogenetic profile and involvement of single chromosomes to structural rearrangements in affected and previously reported asymptomatic carriers, (iii) analysis of the sex ratio ratio in affected carriers of various types of Rea, and (iv) examination of the effect of parental ages.

Methods

We reviewed reports in the literature of mosaicism for N/Rea cases detected microscopically (up to 850-band level of resolution, i.e. ≥ 5 Mb), by conventional cytogenetics or by molecular cytogenetics. The cases were identified from various sources including PubMed. Reports of N/Rea affected carriers of unknown sex were excluded from the study. According to Barber [3], individuals were considered phenotypically affected when any type of phenotypic anomaly was reported, even if the etiological role of the chromosome abnormality in the same individual was questionable. From the sample collected, we further excluded cases of Rea with both breakpoints localized at pericentromeric regions, because of the strong female preponderance among carriers of such mosaicism [4, 5]. Cases of familial instability were also excluded from the study. The selection criteria was any rearrangement identified by cytogenetic or molecular cytogenetic techniques.

Two hundred and forty six cases of N/Rea, along with the data on their chromosome constitution, patient's's age at testing/ascertainment, parental ages at the birth of the proband, proportion of abnormal cell line(s), and the indication for testing are tabulated in Additional files 1, 2, 3, 4, 5, 6 and 7: Tables S1-S7.

Rea were classified as loss, gain, and loss/gain of genomic material. Deletions were classified as losses, duplications and additional material were classified as gains, and derivative chromosomes, isodicentrics, complex Reas, and cases with two abnormal cell lines, one of which with deletion, another one with duplication, were classified as "loss/gain". In some instances, derivatives and other rearrangements were considered as apparent or suggestive "gain" or "loss".

Data were analyzed using open access software listed in the Additional file 8: Table S8. References for Additional files 1, 2, 3, 4, 5, 6, 7 and 8 are listed in the Additional file 9: Supplemental References.

Results and discussion

N/Rea profile

A summary of the data are presented in Table 1. The prevalence of deletions over duplications in affected carriers is a well-known phenomenon. A study carried out

Table 1 Cytogenetic profile of mosaic structural rearrangements

Type of rearrangement		Sex		
		Males	Females	Total
Deletions	excluding del(13) associated with retinoblastoma	20	45	65
	del(13) associated with retinoblastoma	5	8	13
Duplications		23	16	39
Rings	apparently deleted	11	15	47
	no apparent deletion	10	10	
	uncertain	1		
Unbalanced translocations	loss	1		23
	gain	6	7	
	gain/loss	3	6	
Other unbalanced rearrangements	loss		1	29
	gain	8	5	
	gain/loss	5	10	
Apparently balanced rearrangements	inversions	2	1	13
	reciprocal translocations	5	5	
Rescued rearrangements[a]	loss	1	3	17
	gain	5	2	
	gain/loss	5	1	
Total		111	136	246

[a]including 3 deletions, 2 duplications, 2 rings, 7 unbalanced translocations, and 2 other unbalanced rearrangements

by FISH on semen samples from control donors showed similar deletion and duplication frequencies of chromosomal regions 7q11.23, 15q11q13, and 22q11 [6] while studies on affected carriers revealed a clear excess of deletions of these regions [7, 8]. Therefore, this phenomenon may be explained by phenotypic silence of some chromosomal regions when duplicated.

Balanced rearrangement carriers among 229 affected mosaic patients (excluding 17 with rescued rearrangements) were observed at a frequency of 6%, similar to rates observed in affected non-mosaic carriers. Detailed screening of microscopically balanced de novo rearrangements using high-resolution genome-wide analysis detected a chromosome imbalance in 37% of patients. In 49% of these patients, the imbalances were located in one or both breakpoint regions while the others were found elsewhere in the genome [9], being therefore just coincidental or concomitant with a balanced rearrangement.

To compare the profiles in affected and asymptomatic carriers (Table 2), we excluded one abnormality with a large cohort and specific indications from the profile analysis (13 cases of interstitial del(13) associated with retinoblastoma) and sixteen rescued rearrangements because of exclusion of such cases from the previously reported group of asymptomatic carriers. Balanced Rea (reciprocal translocations and inversions) were not included in the analysis, comprising 51% of the cases in asymptomatic carriers [2]. Of the remaining 203 cases, there were 65 deletions (32%), 39 duplications (19%), 48 rings (24%), 23 unbalanced translocations (11%), and 28 other Reas (14%). There is a significant concordance of the profile of mosaic unbalanced Reas in affected carriers with the profile found in asymptomatic carriers of somatic/gonadal mosaicism, with some prevalence of deletions in the latter group. However, it should be mentioned that among affected carriers of mosaic ring chromosomes, mosaics for deleted ring chromosomes were found more frequently compared to asymptomatic carriers (55% vs 14%). Because of the small number of samples, this difference does not reach statistical significance, and additional cases are required for a conclusion.

The distribution of single chromosome across various types of rearrangements is not uniform, as summarized in Table 3. For example, chromosome 18, being the most frequent among both deleted chromosomes and rings (12 and 10 cases, respectively), is found to have no duplications. In contrast, chromosomes 1 and 12 are more frequently found to be duplicated than deleted (6 and 7 cases vs 1 and 1). Chromosomes 21 and 16 appeared to be the least subjected to rearrangements, with only 2 and 3 of 246 instances (0.8 and 1.2%, respectively).

To compare single chromosome involvement to structural rearrangements between affected and asymptomatic carriers, we have removed balanced rearrangements (Table 4). There is a statistically significant difference between the groups at p =0.0030. Such analysis is of potential meaning for evaluation of fitness of mosaic preimplantation embryos. It might be possible that rearrangements of certain chromosomes (for example, deletion of chromosome 18) are not tolerated by the embryo while others, being involved in segmental mosaicism (for example, chromosomes 5 and 21), might have good prospects. However, again, more cases should be collected for such study. Ultimately, lethality would be a function of critical genetic content. Genotype-phenotype comparisons are more complicated in mosaic cases, compounded by the level of mosaicism and the tissue distribution.

Frequency of detection of somatic N/Rea mosaicism

The data suggests that somatic mosaicism may be more frequent than expected: 3 mosaics were detected among 32 carriers of del(5) (q14) when examining at least 125 metaphases in each individual [10]. 2 of 16 cytogenetically visible 11p13 deletions and 3 cryptic 11p13 deletions were mosaic [11]. Of 27 patients with del(16) (p11.2), two were mosaics [12], and 25 mosaics were detected among 126 del(13) (q14) reports [13]. Cytogenetic analysis showed a del(15) (q11-13) in 12 patients in whom the clinical diagnosis was certain; in two there was mosaicism, and one patient also had a t(7;15) translocation [14]. In 17 cases of monosomy of 18q12.3 one was a mosaic with a normal cell line [15]. Among 29 carriers of ring chromosomes, three had a normal cell line [16], and among six patients with a r(22), one was mosaic for a normal cell line [17]. In 1966–1991, 10 patients with r(18) were diagnosed among 82,000 patients karyotyped for constitutional reasons; three of these 10 presented with mosaicism for normal line [18].

Table 2 Cytogenetic profile of mosaicism for structural rearrangement in affected and asymptomatic patients

Group	No of carriers	Type of chromosome rearrangement, n (%)				
		Deletions[b]	Duplications	Rings	Unbalanced translocations	Other rearrangements
Affected (present study)[a]	203	65 (32%)	39 (19%)	47 (23%)[c]	23 (11%)	29 (14%)
Asymptomatic (Kovaleva, Cotter, 2016)	45	18 (40%)	9 (20%)	9 (20%)[d]	4 (9%)	5 (11%)

[a]excluding cases of apparently balanced and rescued rearrangements
[b]excluding 13 cases of del(13q) associated with retinoblastoma
[c]55% of apparently deleted rings
[d]14% of apparently deleted rings

Table 3 Distribution of single chromosomes according to type of rearrangements

Chromosome	Deletions[a]	Duplications	Rings	Unbalanced translocations	Other unbalanced rearrangements	Balanced rearrangements	Total
1	1	6	0	0	1	3	11
2	1	2	3	2	0	2	10
3	2	3	0	2	3	1	11
4	4	1	5	1	1	2	13
5	2	2	0	1	3	0	7
6	1	0	2	3	0	3	9
7	6	1	1	2	3	1	13
8	4	1	2	3	2	1	13
9	0	0	2	5	0	1	8
10	0	0	0	3	1	0	4
11	7	2	0	1	1	1	12
12	1	7	1	1	4	2	16
13	6	1	5	2	0	0	14
14	4	2	1	1	4	1	13
15	4	3	2	3	2	1	15
16	1	0	0	2	0	0	3
17	3	6	2	0	0	2	12
18	12	0	10	4	5	0	31
19	2	0	3	1	1	1	8
20	2	2	0	0	0	1	5
21	0	0	2	0	0	0	2
22	2	0	7	2	0	1	12
Total	65	39	48	39	31	24	246
Proportions	$_{0.20}0.26_{0.35}$	$_{0.11}0.16_{0.23}$	$_{0.13}0.20_{0.27}$	$_{0.11}0.16_{0.23}$	$_{0.07}0.13_{0.18}$	$_{0.06}0.10_{0.16}$	1,00
P-value	$2 \cdot 10{-}6$						

[a]excluding 13 cases of del(13q14) associated with retinoblastoma

A recent study on the frequency of mosaicism for balanced Rea, showed that mosaicism for inversions was the most common (3/103 = 2.9%) followed by mosaicism for reciprocal translocations (7/453 = 1.5%), while mosaicism for Robertsonian translocations was the least common (2/265 = 0.8%) [2]. These data obtained from the analysis of studies on a total of 56,760 patients with reproductive failures were consistent with corresponding data from a report on a constitutional chromosome analysis in 74,306 consecutive patients [19].

Diagnosis of whole chromosome or structural Rea mosaicism is likely under-reported due to low level mosaicism. Sciorra et al. [20] reported that it is the policy of most clinical genetic laboratories to count only 15 or 20 cells and to analyze 2 or 3 metaphases for work up of patients. This laboratory approach is due to various time and financial constraints, as well as *the assumption that mosaicism for a structural rearrangement, while theoretically possible, is an unlikely event*". However, the data accumulated in the literature indicated that mosaicism might be more frequent than recognized currently.

Parental and cell origin of N/Rea mosaicism

The parental origin of chromosomes involved in mosaic rearrangements was reported in few cases, being paternal in six instances [21–25] and maternal in three instances [25–27]. Additionally, the paternal origin of the abnormal chromosome was reported in two carriers of gonadal mosaicism [28, 29], yielding to cumulative figures of eight paternally derived rearrangements vs three maternally derived rearrangements. Theoretically, if mosaicism arises mostly post-zygotically, then paternally and maternally derived rearrangements are expected to have equal frequency. However, at present, there is still insufficient data to allow any certain conclusions on whether there is a bias in parental origin of postzygotic rearrangements.

The preferential paternal origin was reported for various types of *de novo* non-mosaic unbalanced structural

Table 4 Distribution of single chromosomes in affected and asymptomatic patients

Affected[a]	Asymptomatic[b]
8	
8	2
10	3
12	3
8	7 (13%)
6	1
13	
12	3
7	
4	1
11	1
14	1
14	3
12	3
14	3
3	1
11	3
31 (14%)	2 (4%)
7	1
4	3
2	7 (13%)
11	3
222	51

Difference between groups is statistically significant, $p = 0.0030$

[a]excluding balanced rearrangements (translocations and inversions)
[b]excluding 13 cases of del(13q14) associated with retinoblastoma

rearrangements: Wolf-Hirshchorn syndrome-associated rearrangements [30], del 18p- [31], del 22q13.3 [32], and a preponderance of paternally derived deletions 5p14 were reported in two studies [33, 34]. In addition, the majority of *de novo* cytogenetically balanced reciprocal translocations are of paternal origin [35]. Preferential formation in the paternal germline were detected for *de novo* balanced complex chromosome Reas [36]. High rates of *de novo* 15q11q13 inversions was found in human spermatozoa [37]. A recent study using array comparative genome hybridization confirmed a significant paternal bias for *de novo* structural variations by any mechanism in 118 individuals with intellectual disability [38].

Mosaicism with the presence of a normal cell line is commonly assumed to result from postzygotic errors. However, there is evidence that such rearrangements may originate during meiosis or may be inherited. In such cases, there should be postzygotic rescue events leading to formation of normal cell lines. Recently, Robberecht et al. [25] demonstrated that two of nine cases with mosaic segmental structural imbalances (>15%) resulted from meiotic errors, followed by multiple parallel trisomy rescue events.

Cases of proved or presumptive rescued rearrangements together with a formation of normal cell line are summarized in Additional file 7: Table S7. The majority of the mosaics for inherited Rea were not evaluated for chimerism. However, as there was sex concordance between normal and abnormal cell lines the presence of chimerism is unlikely; in chimerism some cases would be expected to be sex discordant. In addition, chimerism is an extremely rare event.

An unusual finding was the comparatively high rate of involvement of chromosome 11 in rescue events, with four cases of ten. Moreover, in one of them, the rescue appeared to be familial since the mother was a mosaic for the same abnormality with UPD for a deleted region [39]. Apparent familial tendency to rescue was reported by Juberg et al. [40] who described two sibs with mosaicism for a paternally transmitted abnormality.

All cases of mosaicism for *de novo* rearrangements had been evaluated to investigate the mechanisms of the rearrangement formation (Additional file 7: Table S7). The parental origin of the rearranged chromosome resulted from a paternal meiotic error in four cases [25, 41–43] and maternal in three cases [24, 44, 45].

Male to female ratio

The male to female ratio was analyzed across various types of rearrangements presented in Table 1 and showed significant variation depending on the type of Rea. Female predominance was observed in carriers of either "loss" or "gain/loss" Rea (50 M/89 F, different from population ratio of 1.06 at $p = 0.0002$. Carriers of either apparent "gain" or apparent balanced Rea (including rings without apparent deletion) demonstrated absence of female predominance (41 M/30 F and 18 M/16 F, respectively) not statistically different from population ratio of 1.06.

A recent study reported a strong female predominance among asymptomatic carriers of somatic/gonadal mosaicism for unbalanced Rea. Since no distortion in sex ratio was found among carriers of mosaicism for balanced Rea, a male-specific selection against abnormal cells in early embryo development was proposed [2]. However, results from the present study might indicate that selection against abnormal cells, if it exists, depends on the type of the Rea and the size of genomic imbalance. Apparently, duplications resulting in gains of chromosomal material, if not occurring more frequently in males, are not selected against in males. Similarly, both loss and gain/loss, if not occurring more frequently in females, are more tolerated in females than in males. Again, such unexpected and intriguing findings require further study.

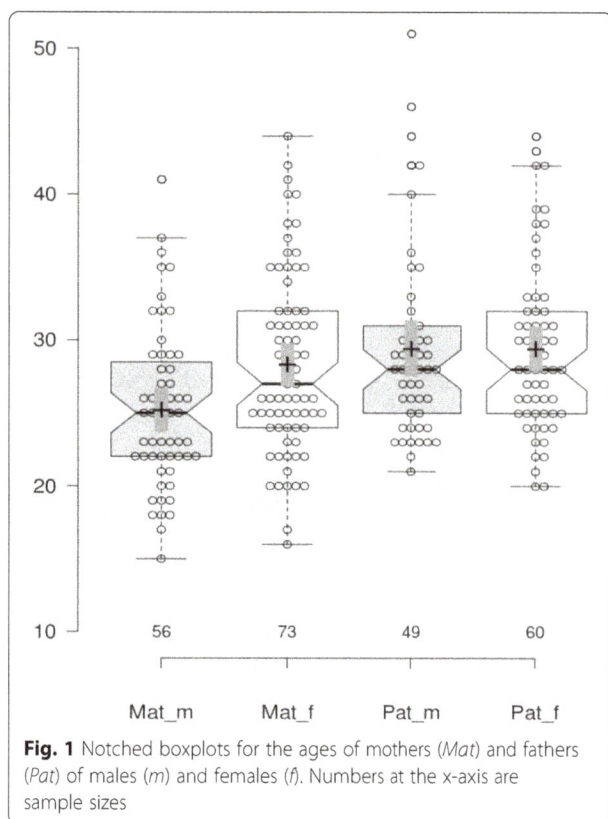

Fig. 1 Notched boxplots for the ages of mothers (*Mat*) and fathers (*Pat*) of males (*m*) and females (*f*). Numbers at the x-axis are sample sizes

Parental ages

Maternal and paternal ages were reported in 129 and 109 cases, respectively. Surprisingly we have identified a difference in maternal age distributions between male and female carriers, with mean maternal age of 25.2 years (95% CL 23.8–26.6) vs 28.3 years (95% CL 26.9–29.7), respectively, the difference is significant at $p = 0.032$. However, there is no difference in paternal age, with mean age of 29.4 years in both male and female carriers (see Figs. 1 and 2). Sex ratio displays an apparent tendency to decrease with increase of maternal age, from 4.7 in the group of <20 year to 0.3 in the group of aged 40 year and older (Table 5). No such trend was found when analyzing sex ratio according to paternal ages.

We are not aware of any previous publications reporting maternal age distribution differences between carriers of segmental mosaicism in relation to carriers' sex. This unexpected finding suggests an effect of age-related factors either on the postzygotic stability of female genomes or on intrauterine selection against affected male embryos, or on the male-specific selection against abnormal cells in early embryo development. A high intrauterine lethality of male carriers is less likely because of a lack of male predominance among abortuses with segmental mosaicism (Kovaleva, unpublished). In addition, in the group of apparently balanced carriers with no sex ratio distortion,, there is a difference between males' and females' maternal ages (23.3 years vs 30.8 years), similar to that in groups with predominance of female carriers.

Additional studies on male to female ratios in prenatally diagnosed individuals and in preimplantation embryos would clarify this issue. Further studies on the origin and mechanisms of formation of mosaicism for structural chromosomal abnormalities are indicated.

Conclusions

The cytogenetic profile of phenotype-associated Reas (responsible for abnormal clinical features) shows a predominance for deletions of genetic material. Rearrangements of certain chromosomes may not be tolerated by the embryo while others, being involved in segmental mosaicism, might have a more favorable prospects. A significant female prevalence among carriers of mosaicism for loss of genomic material, as well as among carriers of mosaicism for both loss and gain of genomic material, suggests either a male-specific selection against abnormal cell line(s) or reduced viability of male fetuses. The absence of a skewed sex ratio in carriers of mosaicism for gain of genomic material may indicate that gains, despite being disease-causing, are tolerated in proliferating cells of male embryos unlike losses of genomic material. Maternal age might be a risk factor of occurrence of somatic mosaicism for structural Rea in female offspring or might cause an

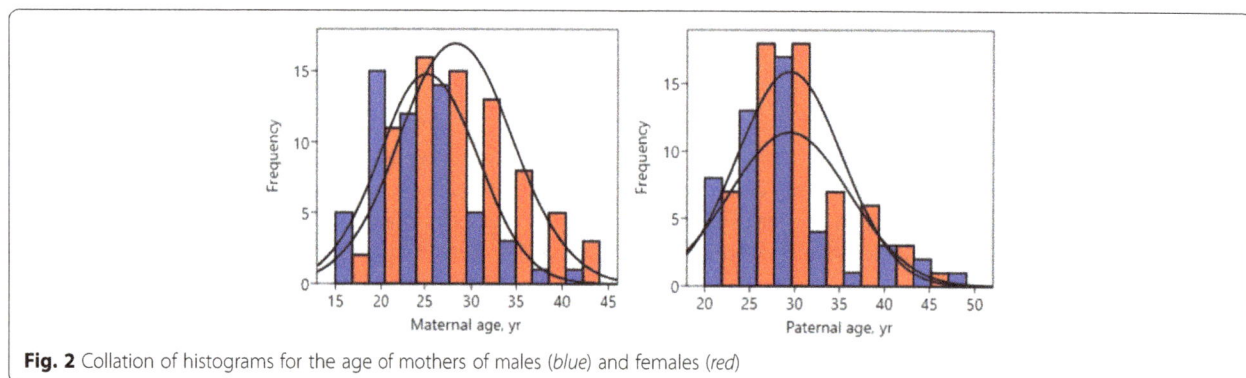

Fig. 2 Collation of histograms for the age of mothers of males (*blue*) and females (*red*)

Table 5 Sex ratio in patients with segmental mosaicism according to maternal age

Age groups, years	Males		Females		
	Number	Proportion (P1)	Number	Proportion (P2)	Sex ratio (P1/P2)
<20	8	0.14	2	0.03	4.7
20–24	19	0.34	18	0.25	1.4
25–29	19	0.34	24	0.33	1.0
30–34	5	0.09	14	0.19	0.5
35–39	4	0.07	10	0.14	0.5
≥40	1	0.02	5	0.07	0.3
Total	56	1.0	73	1.0	

adverse effect on male embryo viability. Further evaluation of parental and cell origin of mosaic Rea would be advisable for elucidation of these intriguing subjects.

Additional files

Additional file 1:Table S1. Mosaicism for deletions. Tabular data presenting details of affected carriers of mosaicism for deletion: karyotype, parental ages at patient's birth, patient's age at ascertainment/testing, proportion of abnormal cell line(s), and indications for cytogenetic testing. (XLSX 12 kb)

Additional file 2: Table S2. Mosaicism for duplications. Tabular data presenting details of affected carriers of mosaicism for duplication: karyotype, parental ages at patient's birth, patient's age at ascertainment/testing, proportion of abnormal cell line(s), and indications for cytogenetic testing. (XLSX 8 kb)

Additional file 3: Table S3. Mosaicism for ring chromosomes. Tabular data presenting details of affected carriers of mosaicism for ring chromosome: karyotype, parental ages at patient's birth, patient's age at ascertainment/testing, proportion of abnormal cell line(s), and indications for cytogenetic testing. (XLSX 10 kb)

Additional file 4: Table S4. Mosaicism for unbalanced translocations. Tabular data presenting details of affected carriers of mosaicism for unbalanced translocation: karyotype, parental ages at patient's birth, patient's age at ascertainment/testing, proportion of abnormal cell line(s), and indications for cytogenetic testing. (XLSX 9 kb)

Additional file 5: Table S5. Mosaicism for other unbalanced rearrangements. Tabular data presenting details of affected carriers of mosaicism for other unbalanced rearrangement: karyotype, parental ages at patient's birth, patient's age at ascertainment/testing, proportion of abnormal cell line(s), and indications for cytogenetic testing. (XLSX 7 kb)

Additional file 6: Table S6. Mosaicism for apparently balanced rearrangements. Tabular data presenting details of affected carriers of mosaicism for apparently balance translocation or inversion: karyotype, parental ages at patient's birth, patient's age at ascertainment/testing, proportion of abnormal cell line(s), and indications for cytogenetic testing. (XLSX 6 kb)

Additional file 7: Table S7. Mosaicism due to rescued rearrangement. Tabular data presenting details of affected carriers of mosaicism for rescued rearrangement: karyotype, parental ages at patient's birth, patient's age at ascertainment/testing, proportion of abnormal cell line(s), indications for cytogenetic testing, and description of method(s) of confirmatory study. (XLSX 7 kb)

Additional file 8: Table S8. Software used for the statistical data analysis. List of the programmes used for the data analysis, programme titles, version and/or date of release, URL, and references. (DOCX 17 kb)

Additional file 9: Reference list for Tables S1-S8. (DOCX 76 kb)

Aknowledgement
We wish to thank Dr. Nikita N. Khromov-Borisov (R.R.Vreden Russian Research Institute of Traumatology and Orthopedics) for statistical analysis of the data.

Funding
Not applicable.

Authors' contributions
NVK and PDC performed the literature search, analyzed the data and wrote the manuscript. The authors alone are responsible for the content and writing of the paper. Both authors read and approved the final manuscript.

Competing interests
The authors declare that they have no competing interests.

Author details
[1]Academy of Molecular Medicine, Mytniskaya str. 12/44, St. Petersburg 191144, Russian Federation. [2]Department of Pediatrics, University of California San Francisco, San Francisco, CA, USA. [3]ResearchDx Inc., Irvine, CA, USA.

References
1. Los FJ, Van Opstal D, van den Berg C. The development of cytogenetically normal, abnormal and mosaic embryos: a theoretical model. Hum Reprod Update. 2004;10:79–94.
2. Kovaleva NV, Cotter PD. Somatic/gonadal mosaicism for structural autosomal rearrangements: female predominance among carriers of gonadal mosaicism for unbalanced rearrangements. Mol Cytogenet. 2016;9:8.
3. Barber JCK. Directly transmitted unbalanced chromosome abnormalities and euchromatic variants. J Med Genet. 2005;42:609–29.
4. Kovaleva NV. Sex-specific chromosome instability in early human development. Am J Med Genet. 2005;36A:401–13.
5. Kovaleva NV. Nonmosaic balanced homologous translocations: some may be mosaic. Am J Med Genet. 2007;143A:2843–50.
6. Molina O, Anton E, Vidal F, Blanco J. Sperm rates of 7q11.23, 15q11q13 and 22q11.2 deletions and duplications: a FISH approach. Hum Genet. 2011;129: 35–44.
7. Thomas NS, Durkie M, Potts G, Sandford R, Van Zyl B, Youings S, Dennis NR, Jacobs PA. Parental and chromosomal origins of microdeletion and duplication syndromes involving 7q11.23, 15q11-q13 and 22q11. Eur J Hum Genet. 2006;14:831–7.
8. Sibbons C, Morris JK, Crolla JA, Jacobs PA, Thomas NS. De novo deletions and duplications detected by array CGH: a study of parental origin in relation to mechanisms of formation and size of imbalance. Eur J Hum Genet. 2012;20:155–60.
9. Feenstra I, Hanemaaijer N, Sikkema-Raddatz B, Yntema H, Dijkhuizen T, Lugtenberg D, Verheij J, Green A, Hordijk R, Reardon W, de Vries B, Brunner H, Bongers E, de Leeuw N, van Ravenswaaij-Arts C. Balanced into array: genome-wide array analysis in 54 patients with an apparently balanced de novo chromosome rearrangement and a meta-analysis. Eur J Hum Genet. 2011;19:1152–60.

10. Niebuhr E. Cytologic observations in 35 Individuals with a 5p- karyotype. Hum Genet. 1978;42:143–56.

11. Robinson DO, Howarth DJ, Williamson KA, van Heyningen V, Beal SJ, Crolla JA. Genetic analysis of chromosome 11p13 and the PAX6 gene in a series of 125 cases referred with aniridia. Am J Med Genet. 2008; 146A:558–69.

12. Shinawi M, Liu P, Kang SH, Shen J, Belmont JW, Scott DA, Probst FJ, Craigen WJ, Graham BH, Pursley A, Clark G, Lee J, Proud M, Stocco A, Rodriguez DL, Kozel BA, Sparagana S, Roeder ER, McGrew SG, Kurczynski TW, Allison LJ, Amato S, Savage S, Patel A, Stankiewicz P, Beaudet AL, Cheung SW, Lupski JR. Recurrent reciprocal 16p11.2 rearrangements associated with global developmental delay, behavioural problems, dysmorphism, epilepsy, and abnormal head size. J Med Genet. 2010;47:332–41.

13. Munier F, Pescia G, Jotterand-Bellomo M, Balmer A, Gailloud C, Thonney F. Constitutional karyotype in retinoblastoma. Case report and review of literature. Ophthalmic Paediatr Genet. 1986;10:129–50.

14. Cassidy SB, Thuline HC, Holm VA. Deletion of chromosome 15 (q11-13) in a Prader-Labhart-Willi syndrome clinic population. Am J Med Genet. 1984;17: 485–95.

15. Kotzot D, Haberlandt E, Fauth C, Baumgartner S, Scholl-Bürgi S, Utermann G. Del(18)(q12.2q21.1) caused by a paternal sister chromatid rearrangement in a developmentally delayed girl. Am J Med Genet. 2005;135A:304–7.

16. Guilherme RS, Klein E, Hamid AB, Bhatt S, Volleth M, Polityko A, Kulpanovich A, Dufke A, Albrecht B, Morlot S, Brecevic L, Petersen MB, Manolakos E, Kosyakova N, Liehr T. Human ring chromosomes – new insights for their clinical significance. Br J Med Genet. 2013;16:13–20.

17. Guilherme RS, Soares KC, Simioni M, Vieira TP, Gil-da-Silva-Lopes VL, Kim CA, Brunoni D, Spinner NB, Conlin LK, Christofolini DM, Kulikowski LD, Steiner CE, Melaragno MI. Clinical, cytogenetic, and molecular characterization of six patients with ring chromosomes 22, including one with concomitant 22q11.2 deletion. Am J Med Genet. 2014;164A:1659–65.

18. Fryns JP, Kleczkowska A, Smeets E, Van Den Berghe H. Transmission of ring chromosome 18 46, XX/46, XX, r(18) mosaicism in a mother and ring chromosome 18 syndrome in her son. Ann Genet. 1992;35:121–3.

19. Kleczkowska A, Fryns JP, Van den Berghe H. On the variable effect of mosaic normal/balanced chromosomal rearrangements in man. J Med Genet. 1990;27:505–7.

20. Sciorra LJ, Lee ML, Cuccurullo G. Translocation mosaicism in a woman having multiple miscarriages. Am J Med Genet. 1985;22:615–7.

21. Perfumo C, Cerruti Mainardi P, Cali A, Coucourde G, Zara F, Cavani S, Overhauser J, Bricarelli FD, Pierluigi M. The first three mosaic cri du chat syndrome patients with two rearranged cell lines. J Med Genet. 2000;37: 967–72.

22. Antonini S, Kim CA, Sugayama SM, Vianna-Morgante AM. Delimitation of duplicated segments and identification of their parental origin in two partial chromosome 3p duplications. Am J Med Genet. 2002;113:144–50.

23. Schluth C, Mattei MG, Mignon-Ravix C, Salman S, Alembik Y, Willig J, Ginglinger E, Jeandidier E. Intrachromosomal triplication for the distal part of chromosome 15q. Am J Med Genet. 2005;136:179–84.

24. Bonaglia MC, Giorda R, Beri S, Bigoni S, Sense A, Baroncini A, Capucci A, De Agostini I, Gwilliam R, Deloukas P, Dunham I, Zuffardi O. Mosaic 22q13 deletions: evidence for concurrent mosaic segmental isodisomy and gene conversion. Eur J Hum Genet. 2009;17:426–33.

25. Robberecht C, Voet T, Utine GE, Schinzel A, de Leeuw N, Fryns JP, Vermeesch J. Meiotic errors followed by two parallel postzygotic trisomy rescue events are a frequent cause of constitutional segmental mosaicism. Mol Cytogenet. 2012;5:19.

26. Vermeesch JR, Syrrou M, Salden I, Dhondt F, Matthijs G, Fryns JP. Mosaicism for duplication 12q (12q13→12q21.2) accompanied by a pericentric inversion in a dysmorphic female infant. J Med Genet. 2002;39:e72.

27. Melis D, Pia Sperandeo M, Perone L, Staiano A, Andria G, Sebastio G. Mosaic 13q13.2-ter deletion restricted to tissues of ectodermal and mesodermal origins. Clin Dysmorphol. 2006;15:13–8.

28. Freitas ÉL, Gribble SM, Simioni M, Vieira TP, Prigmore E, Krepischi AC, Rosenberg C, Pearson PL, Melo DG, Gil-da-Silva-Lopes VL. A familial case with interstitial 2q36 deletion: variable phenotypic expression in full and mosaic state. Eur J Med Genet. 2012;55:660–5.

29. Sánchez J, Fernández R, Madruga M, Bernabeu-Wittel J, Antiñolo G, Borrego S. Somatic and germ-line mosaicism of deletion 15q11.2-q13 in a mother of dyzigotic twins with Angelman syndrome. Am J Med Genet. 2014;164A:370–6.

30. Zollino M, Lecce R, Selicorni A, Murdolo M, Mancuso I, Marangi G, Zampino G, Garavelli L, Ferrarini A, Rocchi M, Opitz JM, Neri G. A double cryptic chromosome imbalance is an important factor to explain phenotypic variability in Wolf-Hirschhorn syndrome. Eur J Hum Genet. 2004;12:797–804.

31. Cody JD, Pierce JF, Brkanac Z, Plaetke R, Ghidoni PD, Kaye CI, Leach RJ. Preferential loss of the paternal alleles in the 18q- syndrome. Am J Med Genet. 1997;69:280–6.

32. Phelan MC. Deletion 22q13.3 syndrome. Orphanet J Rare Dis. 2008;3:14.

33. Church DM, Yang J, Bocian M, Shiang R, Wasmuth JJ. Molecular definition of deletions of different segments of distal 5p that result in distinct phenotypic features. Am J Hum Genet. 1995;56:1162–72.

34. Overhauser J, McMahon J, Oberlender S, Carlin ME, Niebuhr E, Wasmuth JJ, Lee-Chen J. Parental origin of chromosome 5 deletions in the cri-du-chat syndrome. Am J Med Genet. 1990;37:83–6.

35. Höckner M, Spreiz A, Frühmesser A, Tzschach A, Dufke A, Rittinger O, Kalscheuer V, Singer S, Erdel M, Fauth C, Grossmann V, Utermann G, Zschocke J, Kotzot D. Parental origin of de novo cytogenetically balanced reciprocal non-robertsonian translocations. Cytogenet Genome Res. 2012;136:242–5.

36. Grossmann V, Höckner M, Karmous-Benailly H, Liang D, Puttinger R, Quadrelli R, Röthlisberger B, Huber A, Wu L, Spreiz A, Fauth C, Erdel M, Zschocke J, Utermann G, Kotzot D. Parental origin of apparently balanced de novo complex chromosomal rearrangements investigated by microdissection, whole genome amplification, and microsatellite-mediated haplotype analysis. Clin Genet. 2010;78:548–53.

37. Molina O, Anton E, Vidal F, Blanco J. High rates of de novo 15q11q13 inversions in human spermatozoa. Mol Cytogenet. 2012;5:11.

38. Hehir-Kwa JY, Rodríguez-Santiago B, Vissers LE, de Leeuw N, Pfundt R, Buitelaar JK, Pérez-Jurado LA, Veltman JA. De novo copy number variants associated with intellectual disability have a paternal origin and age bias. J Med Genet. 2011;48:776–8.

39. Johnson JP, Haag M, Beischel L, McCann C, Phillips S, Tunby M, Hansen J, Schwanke C, Reynolds JF. 'Deletion rescue' by mitotic 11q uniparental disomy in a family with recurrence of 11q deletion Jacobsen syndrome. Clin Genet. 2014;85:376–80.

40. Juberg RC, Stallard R, Mowrey P, Valido CL. Dissociation of a t(12;21) resulting in a normal cell line in two trisomic 21 sons of a nonmosaic t(12; 21) father? Hum Genet. 1983;64:216–21.

41. Jobanputra V, Wilson A, Shirazi M, Feenstra H, Levy B, Anyane-Yeboa K, Warburton D. Partial uniparental disomy with mosaic deletion 13q in an infant with multiple congenital anomalies. Am J Med Genet. 2013;161A:2393–5.

42. Kotzot D, Röthlisberger B, Riegel M, Schinzel A. Maternal uniparental isodisomy 11q13qter in a dysmorphic and mentally retarded female with partial trisomy mosaicism 11q13qter. J Med Genet. 2001;38:876–81.

43. Theophile D, de Blois MC, Barth D, Gilbert B, Picq M, Delabar J, Prieur M, Vekemans M. Partial correction of monosom y 21 by a duplication of chromosome 21. Am J Hum Genet. 1993;53 Suppl 3:610.

44. Gradek GA, Kvistad PH, Houge G. Monosomy rescue gave cells with normal karyotype in a mildly affected man with 46, XY, r(8) mosaicism. Eur J Med Genet. 2006;49:292–7.

45. Blouin JL, Aurias A, Creau-Goldberg N, Apiou F, Alcaide-Loridan C, Bruel A, Prieur M, Kraus J, Delabar JM, Sinet PM. Cytogenetic and molecular analysis of a de novo tandem duplication of chromosome 21. Hum Genet. 1991;88:167–74.

22

Chromosomes in a genome-wise order: evidence for metaphase architecture

Anja Weise[1], Samarth Bhatt[1], Katja Piaszinski[1], Nadezda Kosyakova[1], Xiaobo Fan[1], Annelore Altendorf-Hofmann[2], Alongklod Tanomtong[3], Arunrat Chaveerach[3], Marcelo Bello de Cioffi[4], Edivaldo de Oliveira[5], Joachim-U. Walther[5], Thomas Liehr[1*] and Jyoti P. Chaudhuri[1,6]

Abstract

Background: One fundamental finding of the last decade is that, besides the primary DNA sequence information there are several epigenetic "information-layers" like DNA-and histone modifications, chromatin packaging and, last but not least, the position of genes in the nucleus.

Results: We postulate that the functional genomic architecture is not restricted to the interphase of the cell cycle but can also be observed in the metaphase stage, when chromosomes are most condensed and microscopically visible. If so, it offers the unique opportunity to directly analyze the functional aspects of genomic architecture in different cells, species and diseases. Another aspect not directly accessible by molecular techniques is the genome merged from two different haploid parental genomes represented by the homologous chromosome sets. Our results show that there is not only a well-known and defined nuclear architecture in interphase but also in metaphase leading to a bilateral organization of the two haploid sets of chromosomes. Moreover, evidence is provided for the parental origin of the haploid grouping.

Conclusions: From our findings we postulate an additional epigenetic information layer within the genome including the organization of homologous chromosomes and their parental origin which may now substantially change the landscape of genetics.

Keywords: Genome architecture, Parental origin, Haploid grouping, Chromosomes, Metaphase

Background

Recent studies showed that epigenetic information e.g. non-coding RNAs, DNA methylation or histone modifications are key regulators of gene expression (summarized in [1]). Besides there is another "layer" of epigenetic information on the level of higher order chromatin organization, which became more and more into the focus due to application of high resolution chromosome conformation capture assays (e.g. [2]). Nevertheless, these methods are neither able to distinguish between homologous chromosomes nor to delineate their parental origin. As apparent from chromosome territory studies by fluorescence in situ hybridization (FISH) there is a chromosome positional code which seems to be cell type and specific for time of development (e.g. [3, 4]). However, standard FISH-methods do not register the behavior of homologous chromosomes as well as their organization with respect to the parental origin, which we postulate here as an additional epigenetic "information layer".

A non-random distribution of chromosomes was suggested already in the early days of human cytogenetics [5, 6]; however, majority of cytogeneticists commonly accept that chromosomes in a metaphase spread are generally arranged completely haphazardly. Based on the observation of the bilaterally symmetric distribution of DNA and chromosome specific FISH signals in leukocytes, we demonstrated in a series of publications [7–13] a genome-wise organization of chromosomes in human and murine cells. In other words, the parental haploid chromosome sets of diploid cells are well arranged within the nucleus and also within the metaphase stage,

* Correspondence: Thomas.Liehr@med.uni-jena.de
[1]Institute of Human Genetics, Jena University Hospital, Postfach, 07740, Jena, Germany
Full list of author information is available at the end of the article

when DNA is most condensed and appears as microscopically visible chromosomes. Previously Gläss [14, 15] observed the segregation of parental haploid chromosome sets in regenerating liver cells of rats; also Pera [16] presented a hexaploid metaphase spread in vole cells, where the six sets of chromosomes were apparently lying within distinct haploid domains. Additionally, in insects and plants there are clear examples of separated parental genomes in the nuclei [17, 18].

As a rule, rather than an exception, we found this genome-wise haploid order of chromosomes in a variety of samples from different human tissues; in different species of macaque monkeys; in mice (*Mus musculus*); in aberrant human karyotypes with triploidy, tetraploidy, uniparental disomy (UPD); in human blood samples subjected to pod-FISH (parental origin determination FISH) [19] and samples with small supernumerary marker chromosomes (sSMC) [20]. The detailed analysis of three clinical cases with sSMC and UPD shed light on the functional role of this more general genome-wise order.

Our results show that there is not only a defined nuclear architecture in interphase but also in metaphase allowing bilateral organization of the two haploid sets of chromosomes. Moreover, evidence is provided for the parental origin of the haploid groupings.

Results

The homologous chromosome organization and their haploid grouping was investigated in normal human metaphase spreads of a family trio and on aberrant metaphases of different clinical cases and tissues to get hints on the functional relevance of the previously observed higher order organization of metaphases. Haploid grouping was done by drawing a symmetry line which separates the two haploid genomes in the metaphase. To demonstrate the general principle of haploid grouping in the metaphase stage of the cell cycle we explored additionally different primate species and murine samples.

Human family trio analyzed with pod-FISH

In order to analyze the organization of homologous chromosomes to each other and also with respect to their parental origin we applied pod-FISH on a family trio. Polymorphic FISH-probes, due to copy number variations which allow the distinction of homologous chromosomes, were used to draw conclusions on the parental origin of single homologous chromosomes in the child of the trio 170 metaphase spreads from peripheral blood of a normal male proband (child of a family trio) were analyzed for perfect bilateral symmetry of haploid chromosome sets, found in 51 from 170 cells (~30 %, examples are given in Additional file 1: Figure S1). 26 of these metaphases were analyzed by pod-FISH with sequential hybridizations (Fig. 1). In parallel, metaphase

spreads of each parent were also analyzed by pod-FISH to determine the parental origin of 17 autosomes, X- (and Y) chromosomes in the proband (Fig. 2). Besides the bilateral symmetry of haploid chromosome sets, a clear parental-wise grouping of the two haplosets was found in 3 out of 26 metaphase spreads analyzed (11.5 %) (exemplified in Fig. 1).

Bilateral symmetry line often reflects a mirror line dividing pairs of homologous chromosomes next to each other

The 26 metaphase spreads examined by pod-FISH were also analyzed for co-localization of homologous chromosomes, previously described as somatic pairing (Fig. 3). 85 instances of direct co-localizations were counted with a mean frequency of 3.3 per metaphase spread. The frequency per chromosome is not constant and favors predominantly chromosome 7 (31 % of cells), 19 (27 % of cells) and 13 (23 % of cells). On the other hand, a direct co-localization of both chromosomes 21 was never observed and chromosomes 2 and 22 were co-localized only in 1 out of 26 metaphase spreads (4 %).

Clinical case with aberrant bone marrow karyotype

Twenty metaphase spreads from a male patient diagnosed with acute myelogenous leukemia (AML) and trisomy 8 mosaicism in bone marrow were evaluated (47,XY,+8[15]/46,XY[5]). After grouping of haplosets the additional chromosome 8 was analyzed for affiliation to maternal or paternal haplogroup. Eleven trisomy 8 metaphases showed a location within the paternal haploset and four were assigned to the maternal haploset. Furthermore, 5 out of 15 trisomy 8 metaphases (33 %) exhibited a "next to next location" of two chromosomes 8 (Additional file 2: Figure S2).

Clinical cases with aberrant amniotic fluid and fibroblasts

Homologous chromosome haploset grouping, as well as the grouping of single chromosome combinations in a mirror-image manner and the location of homologous chromosomes along the symmetry line was also observed in tri- and tetraploid human metaphases from abortion fibroblasts and amniotic fluid cells after in situ preparation (exemplified in Fig. 4).

Clinical cases with sSMC

Twenty metaphase spreads were evaluated for each case outlined below, by drawing a line separating two haploid chromosome sets and subsequent analysis of the additional sSMC location and, in case of UPD analysis, of the affected homologous chromosomes.

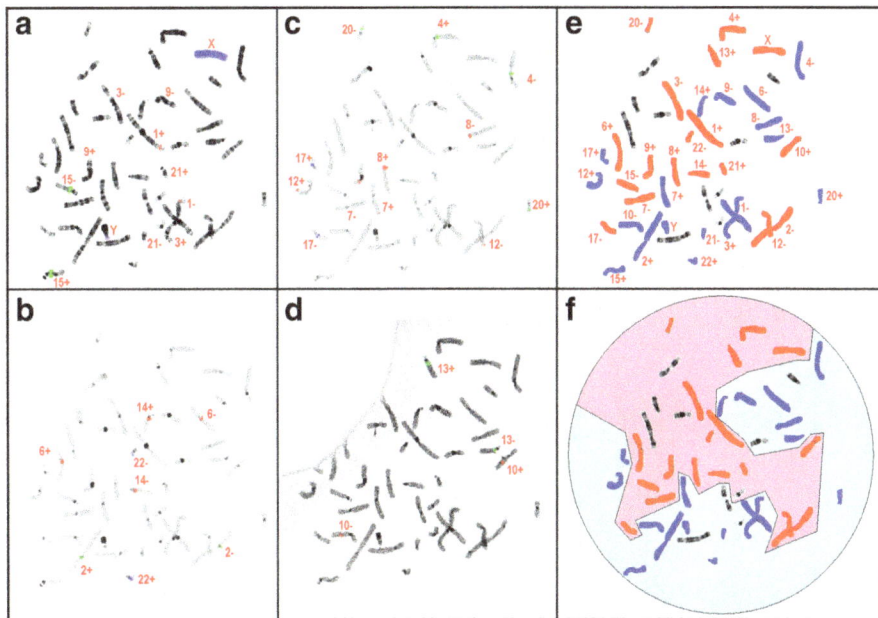

Fig. 1 Example of sequential hybridizations of informative pod-FISH probe sets on a proband metaphase spread (**a-d**). According to the parental code from Fig. 1 the chromosomes of the proband were labeled with blue for paternal origin and red for maternal origin (**e**). According to the parental origin a bilateral symmetry and a grouping of the maternal and the paternal chromosomes could be visualized in the proband metaphase (**f**)

Case 1: mos 47,XY,+min(14)(pter→ q11.1)dn, upd(14)mat heterodisomy/46,XY,upd(14)mat heterodisomy

A male patient with de novo sSMC(14) in 50 % of his cells and maternal heterodisomy 14 presented at the age of 31 with short stature and adiposity.

Bilateral symmetry line analysis showed that the sSMC was present in 11/20 metaphases and located in 6/11 on the maternal/X chromosomal haploset. Additionally, the marker chromosome was found in 7/11 metaphases next to the symmetry line, which allows also an alternative drawing of the latter (Additional file 3: Figure S3A).

Chromosomes 14 presenting maternal heterodisomy were tested with a centromere 14/21 specific probe for heteromorphisms and the chromosome 14 with a stronger centromeric signal turned out to be located in 14/20 on the paternal and in 6/20 on the maternal site (Additional file 3: Figure S3A). In 5/20 metaphases, both homologous chromosomes, and in 15/20 at least one chromosome 14 was located next to the symmetry line.

Case 2: mos 47,XY,+min(7)(:p13 → p11.1:)dn,upd(7)mat isodisomy/46,XY,upd(7)mat isodisomy

A four month old boy with a de novo sSMC(7) in 8 % of the cells and additional maternal isodisomy of the homologous chromosomes 7 showed dystrophy, developmental delay and abnormal ears.

Only 1/20 metaphases showed the sSMC located on the paternal/Y chromosomal haploset, but next to the symmetry line. Both isodisomic chromosomes 7 presented in 20/20 metaphases a clear grouping to one of the haplosets and in 14/20 metaphases both chromosomes 7 were located next to the symmetry line (Additional file 3: Figure S3B).

Case 3: 47,XY,+inv dup(22)(q11.2)mat

An additional inverted duplicated sSMC(22) inherited from the phenotypically normal mother was present in 100 % of the amniocytes in a male fetus.

In all 20 metaphase spreads the sSMC was present and located in 12/20 on the maternal/X chromosomal and in 8/20 on the paternal/Y chromosomal haploset. Furthermore, in 12/20 metaphases the sSMC was located next to the symmetry line. In 17/20 metaphases both haplosets included one of the homologous chromosomes 22 and in 10/20 metaphases both homologous were located next to the symmetry line (Additional file 3: Figure S3C).

Primate metaphases

Ten different primary primate samples, detailed in Additional file 4: Table S1, were hybridized with

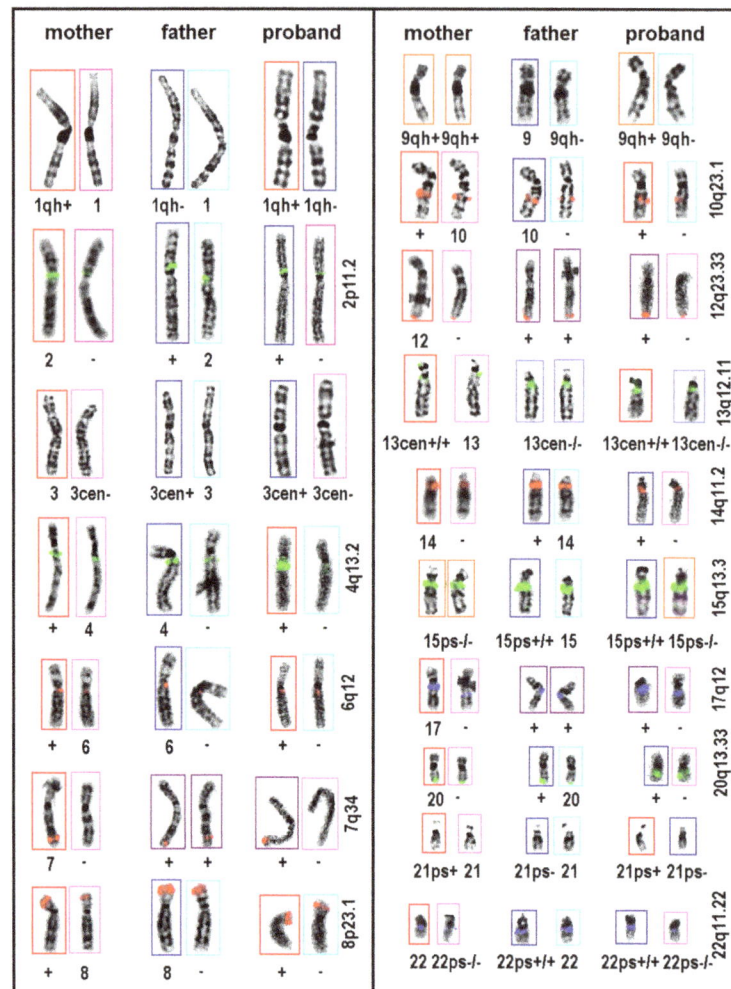

Fig. 2 Decoding parental origin for the listed chromosomes by pod-FISH probes of corresponding cytogenetic polymorphisms

human M-FISH probe sets and at least 5 metaphases were evaluated each, for bilateral symmetry, location of homologous chromosomes next to the symmetry line and chromosome grouping. With the exception of only a single chromosome, which escaped the haplotype grouping and was preferentially located on the outer area of the metaphase, all 50 metaphases analyzed from the 10 different primate species showed a bilateral grouping of chromosomes in haplosets (examples are given in Additional file 5: Figure S4).

Additionally, the metaphases showed also a chromosome grouping and a close location of homologous chromosomes next to the symmetry line as observed in human metaphases (Figs. 3 and 4).

Murine metaphases

Twelve mouse metaphase spreads from primary spleen preparation were analyzed with a mouse specific M-

FISH probe set and evaluated for bilateral symmetry, location of chromosomes next to the symmetry line and chromosome grouping.

The metaphases showed a grouping of the chromosome sets and a close location of homologous chromosomes next to the symmetry line (Additional file 6: Figure S5) as seen in the other samples before.

Discussion

The influence of preparation methods on metaphase architecture

Even though human chromosomes have been prepared uncountable times using the air drying approach for over 50 years, structure and process of chromosome spreading were not understood for a long time. Recent studies revealed that fixed lymphocytes at the metaphase stage spread after being attached to the slide surface [21] rather than "burst" their metaphase plates as suggested

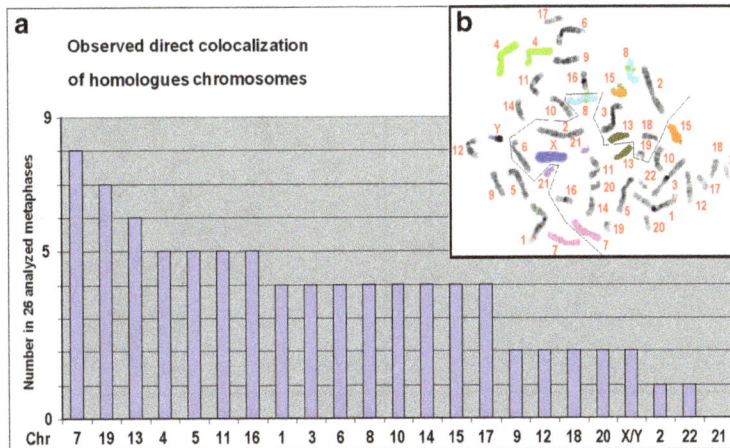

Fig. 3 a Observed direct co-localization of homologous chromosomes in 26 metaphase spreads of a normal male individual in order of observed frequencies per chromosome. **b** Example of one metaphase where chromosomes 4, 7, 8, 13, 15 and 21 labeled in different colors show direct co-localization within the metaphase plate. Further examples are given in Additional file 3: Figure S3

for years. This surprisingly slow process is humidity-dependent [22] and is driven by the evaporation of Carnoy's fixative. First methanol evaporates, followed by acetic acid. As acetic acid is hydrophilic, water is acquired from the atmosphere and the chromosomes elongate due to a stretching or swelling process [21, 23].

In earlier studies by methylation staining of mammalian spermatocytes as well as early embryonic cells the parental order and genomic separation of parental chromosome sets were detected [24]. While this parentally derived methylation pattern disappeared after the four-cell stage, the chromosomes still remained aligned during interphase (chromosome territories) and even during metaphase as suggested by us previously [7, 10–13].

Although the standard preparations were used to arrest metaphase and treat them with hypotonic shock, here large numbers of metaphase spreads were detected with clear genome-wise separation of chromosomes. Additionally, in pod-FISH sampling a distinct sorting of the maternal and paternal chromosome sets was possible, except for single chromosomes lying astray. Also human metaphase spreads from bone marrow prepared without colcemid and showed the same results. Thus, an effect of colcemid on metaphase architecture can be excluded. This was also supported by 2D and 3D chromosome territory studies with different colcemid exposure times or without colcemid treatment [25]. Furthermore, human metaphases from abortion material prepared directly on slides by in situ culture showed in principle haploid sorting of even triploid chromosome sets, as well (some single chromosomes from metaphase edge escaped due to physical forces during preparation, partially masking metaphase architecture).

Interphase architecture

In the end of the 19th century Rabl [26] and Boveri [27] suggested the occurrence of an organized domain structure in the nucleus, which are nowadays known as chromosome territories (CTs) [28]. These nuclear CTs show a functional character reflected by spatial, temporal and cell type specific organization [29].

Several models exist to explain this organization:

1. Chromosomes have a centromere-telomere orientation which is stable during anaphase and cytokinesis, with the two chromosome arms lying next to each other and the centromeres and telomeres located at opposite poles of the nucleus [26, 30]. Nevertheless, this "Rabl configuration" is said to be rarely observed in mammalian cells [29].

2. The radial model predicts central location of gene rich chromosomes (like in *Homo sapiens* = HSA #1, #17, #19, and #22) in contrast to gene poor chromosomes like HAS #4, #5, #8, #13 or #18, independent of their size [31]. Cytogenetic preparations in pre-colchicine era often had metaphase plates with smaller chromosomes located centrally.

3. Nagele [32] suggests a relative chromosome domain positioning model also for the homologous chromosomes, predicting a preferred positional relationship to each other in the interphase and prometaphase of the cell cycle. Although not stated, this model already suggests the organization of chromosomes in two haploid sets as indicated by us [7].

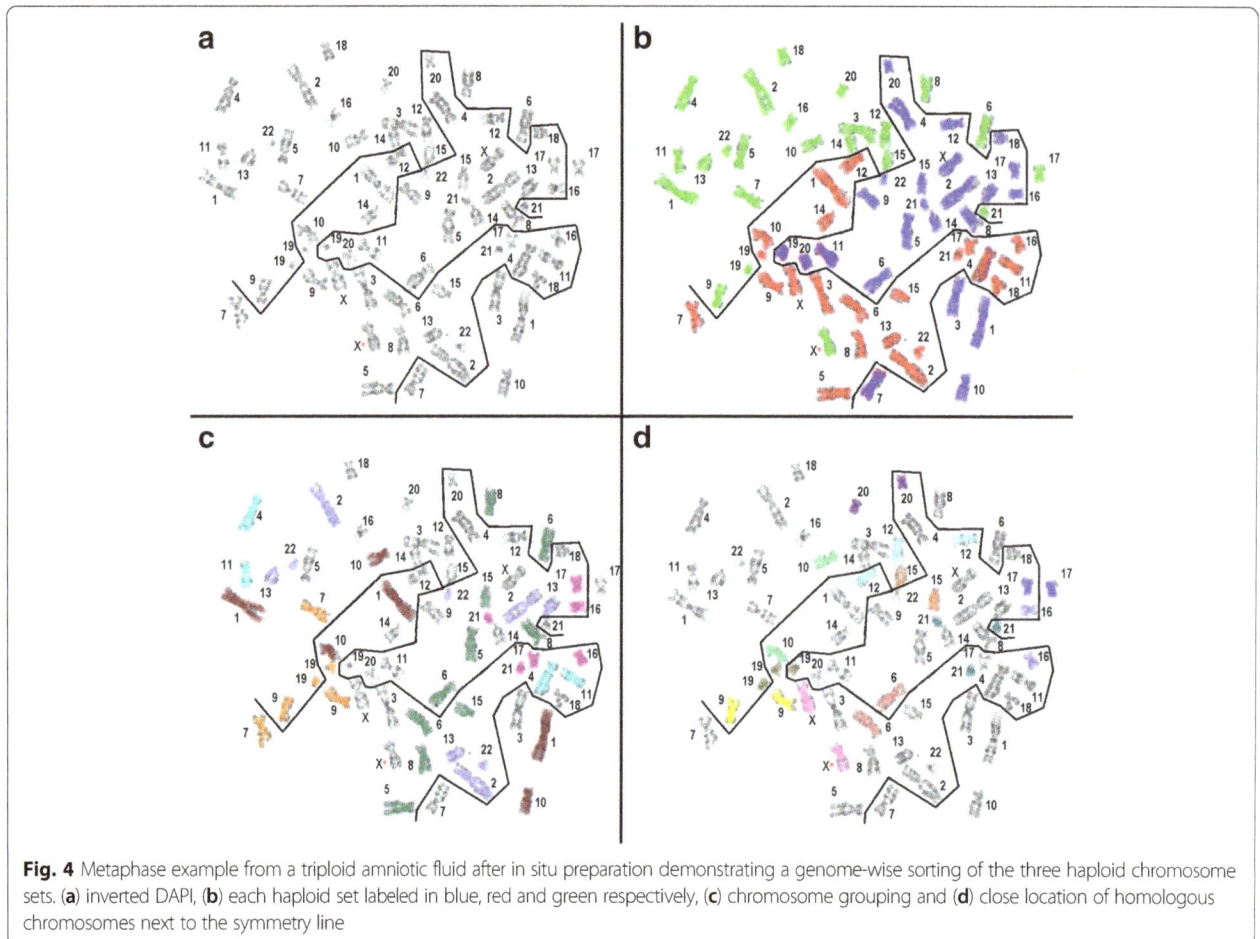

Fig. 4 Metaphase example from a triploid amniotic fluid after in situ preparation demonstrating a genome-wise sorting of the three haploid chromosome sets. (**a**) inverted DAPI, (**b**) each haploid set labeled in blue, red and green respectively, (**c**) chromosome grouping and (**d**) close location of homologous chromosomes next to the symmetry line

4. The last model also predicts the presence of a certain architecture of CTs in both interphase and metaphase in the way of a haploid grouping, which beyond human samples [7–13] was also found in plant louse cells [17], rat liver cells [14, 15] and in hexaploid vole cells [16].

Metaphase architecture and ploidy-wise bilateral sorting of chromosomes

In the present study this genome-wise haploid order of chromosomes was found as a rule, rather than an exception. From a variety of human samples, which include numerically and structurally abnormal human karyotypes and also in those derived from other species, including primates and mice the following implications can be assigned as a general model for metaphase architecture:

– Metaphase spreads show a more or less round shape similar to interphase nuclei, which in 3D represents a symmetrical distribution of the chromosomal DNA (Additional file 7: Figure S6). Interestingly, a round shape and equal DNA distribution can also be observed in so called "rosette" orientation of metaphase spreads, known classically as metaphase plates, where chromosome haplosets are arranged in a mirror wise order of homologous chromosomes [7, 11, 13]. This has already been observed in vivo and documented by the founder of cytogenetics Walther Flemming in salamander larva (Additional file 8: Figure S7) and quite recently by our group [13].

– The bilateral symmetry line often reflects a mirror line dividing two homologous chromosomes located next to each other (Figs. 3, 4; Additional file 6: Figure S5).

– This bilateral symmetry line is not always straight, since it can appear as a half circle where one haploset is surrounding the other (Additional file 1: Figure S1, Additional file 2: Figure S2, Additional file 3: Figure S3, Additional file 5: Figure S4). This might be due to metaphase chromosomes aligning in the equatorial plane of the cell (i.e. a 2D plane). Depending on the preparation and the angle of the 3D cell being fixed in 2D to the slide's surface, the ideal form of a rosette shaped metaphase spread is "lost" and the symmetry line can appear in different shapes.

- Some chromosomes escaping the bilateral symmetry are often located in the outer area of the metaphase spreads, which might be due to physical shearing forces during preparation (Additional file 5: Figure S4).
- These features of metaphase architecture are independent of the origin of material, cultivation, preparation and species, reflecting a general model for the metaphase stage of the cell cycle (Figs. 1, 2, 3, 4, Additional file 1: Figure S1, Additional file 2: Figure S2, Additional file 3: Figure S3, Additional file 4: Table S1, Additional file 5: Figure S4, Additional file 6: Figure S5, Additional file 7: Figure S6, Additional file 8: Figure S7).

Connecting interphase with metaphase architecture

Chromosomal neighborhoods seem to be dynamic within tissues and dependent on the cell cycle stage [3, 33, 34]. However, there are observations that frequent constitutional and acquired chromosomal translocation partners are located in close proximity in the nucleus and therefore more likely to interact [4, 33, 35]. Due to the molecular analysis used in Hi-C techniques, the interaction of homologous chromosomes within the two haplosets and between the two haplosets could not be analyzed. In our metaphase-directed analysis of chromosome neighborhoods we showed that homologous chromosomes are often direct neighbors separated by the bilateral symmetry line (Figs. 3, 4 and Additional file 6: Figure S5). Furthermore, certain homologous chromosomes preferentially tend to be located next to each other (chromosomes HSA #7, #19, #13, #4, #5, #11 and #16) at least in the detailed analysis of human peripheral blood cells (Fig. 3). Additionally, groups of chromosomes in a mirror-image manner, highlighting the preferred symmetry of DNA content and organization in all cell cycle stages, could be observed (Fig. 4, Additional file 6: Figure S5, Additional file 7: Figure S6 and Additional file 8: Figure S7).

One functional explanation for homologous neighborhood and mirror-image organization of chromosomes would be the advantage to minimizing connection costs in genetic networks, which is also discussed even for haploid stages in sperm that show a functional organization of genes expressed in the same tissue of an individual [36].

Parental origin of haploid sets of chromosomes

Despite the extensive investigation of metaphases of peripheral blood lymphocytes in the past, so far no approaches were available to label the chromosomes in a parental origin specific manner. Here we applied pod-FISH to study the organization of the human nucleus on metaphase-spreads.

pod-FISH has already been successfully used to identify the parental origin of individual derivative chromosomes, such as the characterization of chimerism, derivative chromosomes and uniparental disomy 15 [19, 37–41]. For the first time we applied pod-FISH to analyze the architecture and the distribution of parental chromosomes on whole metaphase spreads. In a first step, 170 lymphocyte metaphase spreads of a healthy proband were karyotyped and a bilateral distribution of the homologous chromosome pairs, as described above, was found. The statistical probability to find such sorting by chance is $1 : \binom{23}{23}$ or $1 : 8{,}388{,}607$. Then, 26 of these metaphases with a more or less perfect bilateral symmetry were subjected to sequential pod-FISH hybridizations and parental chromosome analysis (Figs. 1, 2 and Additional file 1: Figure S1). At least three of these also showed a clear parental grouping of the homologous chromosomes as shown in Fig. 1 which has a statistical chance of $1 : \frac{46!}{23!(46-23)!}$ or $1 : 8{,}233{,}430{,}727{,}600$. In other words, if this sorting would be by chance only 10–12 cells of the whole body would show such a parental grouping.

Is bilateral order more important than the parental origin?

In order to address the functional consequences of parental grouping, we analyzed clinical cases with additional marker chromosomes with known parental origin. The additional chromosome in case 1 and 3 showed a random distribution but the marker had a higher frequency than firstly expected, being located next to the symmetry line also allowing an alternative drawing of the line or a central location within the metaphase in the sense of equal symmetrical distribution of DNA. Although the homologous of the marker chromosomes in case 1 and 2 presented a UPD, reflecting only one parental origin, in both cases the uniparental origin was "ignored" and the homologous chromosomes were located in one of the two haplosets each. This may highlight that, for the metaphase architecture maintaining an equal DNA distribution is more important than the location of single chromosomes according to their parental origin.

Facilitating chromosome haplogrouping by centrioles

From a set of elegant experiments on chromosomal distribution in interspecies in vitro hybrid cells Teplitz [42] concluded that "in normal cells a mechanism (distribution control) strictly regulates movement of *a haploid set of mitotic chromosomes* into daughter cells upon cell division."

The two separate groupings of the two parental sets of chromosomes are most likely achieved by the two centrioles in the centrosome of a diploid cell. Chromosomes of each haploset are presumably tethered to one of the two centrioles [10, 13]. The relation of centrioles to two halves of bilaterally lobulated nuclei of neutrophils support this hypothesis, as demonstrated using serial electron microscopic (EM) sections and cinematographic records [43–45]. Also Lettré and Lettré [45] reported that chromosomes, spindle fibres and centrioles form a permanent structure invisible during interphase. This observation was further supported by EM studies [46]. Krioutchkova and Onishchenko [47] claimed that the number of centrioles is exactly equal to the haplosets of chromosomes in a cell. At the same time, the only centriole in a fertilized egg is provided by the sperm [48]. The paternal chromosomes appear to be bound to this centriole, which initiates the creation of a second centriole to take care of the maternal chromosomes. This step is essentially crucial to achieve the order of separation of the parental haplosets of chromosomes and to maintain it thereafter both in interphase and metaphase, i.e. during the cell cycle [10]. The maintenance of this order is also supported by the lamin-sheath that covers all of the telophase chromosomes together, forming a ring or string which subsequently gives rise to a spheroid nucleus or folds into segments to form a polymorphic nucleus [13].

We also reported that this order of genome-wise grouping in human blood cells is expressed in three distinct forms: (1) the two parental genomes side by side; (2) one genome surrounded by the other; and (3) the members of the homologous chromosomes oriented opposite to each other [13]. Following our present pod-FISH analysis we have observed that the homologous chromosomes were often next to each other divided by the line of separation of the two parental genomes (Fig. 3). This feature in the 2D projection may mean that these members of homologous are nevertheless widely apart (i.e., diametrically opposite each other) on the Z-axis of a 3D configuration. The 3-D analyses of murine and human interphase nuclei, revealing that the average distance between the homologous are larger than that between the heterologous, support this feature [49, 50].

Observations of loss of maternal chromosome 11 [51] and especially genome-wide loss of maternal alleles in Wilms' tumors [52], behavior of the three haplosets during gametogenesis in a bisexually reproducing triploid vertebrate [53] and the biphasic distribution of chromatin condensations of the two parental genomes [11] suggest that chromosomes are handled and/or addressed ploidy-wise. Maternal and paternal genomes may act alternately by opportunity or availability or necessity (cf. a mixed double tennis match). By necessity, the parental genomes do participate in harmonious cooperation, when, for example, the chromosomes bearing nucleolus-organizing-regions come together to form a nucleolus, even though they may remain tethered to their respective centrioles.

Conclusion

In summary, we found a bilateral symmetry of metaphases leading to haploid sorting of homologous chromosomes and evidence of a parental grouping of these haploid sets. This indicates i) a higher order of chromosomal topography in the cell which is caused by the parental origin of homologous chromosomes, and we hypothesize that ii) this higher order is not limited to metaphase chromosomes but also represents an inherent feature of the interphase nuclei, iii) the cell distinguishes homologous chromosomes by the parental origin and iv) besides the horizontal sorting (equatorial plane) of chromosomes during metaphase, there is a vertical sorting by parental origin.

In the last decade nuclear architecture was recognized as an independent, emerging mechanism orchestrating gene expression (reviewed in [39]. The observation that homologous chromosomes - depending on their parental origin - have a defined position in the interphase nuclei as well as in the metaphase strengthens this concept and adds the parental origin information as an additional "epigenetic layer". Architectural changes are priming events that happen before subsequent changes in gene expression and might therefore serve as future diagnostic and therapy markers e.g. in malignancys. which are well known as being associated with genetic instability and may very much be initiated by any loss of large scale chromatin order [54].

One can only speculate regarding impact and biological significance of this genome-wise order of chromosomes, however, it might be one additional mechanism leading to monoallelic expression of autosomal genes (summarized in [55]) and therefore contribute to normal phenotypic variation as well as to variable expressivity and incomplete penetrance of genetic diseases. Similarly, we may have to redefine the terms "Comparative Genomic Hybridization (CGH)" or "Loss of Heterozygosity (LOH)" by specifying the involvement of the maternal and/or paternal genomes in future or retrospective genotype phenotype correlations.

Methods

Informed consent was obtained from all individual participants included in the study; the study was approved by the Ethics Committee of Friedrich Schiller Jena University Hospital (internal code 1457-12/04).

Human and primate metaphases from peripheral blood culture and Epstein Barr virus (EBV) transformed permanent cell lines

Chromosome preparations were performed according to standard techniques [56]. An aliquot of heparinized peripheral blood (family trio and primate samples) or of frozen permanent cell lines transformed by the EBV was added to the cell culture medium, mixed with 10-20 % fetal calf serum, penicillin/streptomycin (10 mg/ml final conc.) and phytohemagglutinin (for primary blood cells, according to manufacture instruction). After 72 h of incubation at 37 °C/5 % CO_2, the cells were harvested. Thirty minutes before harvesting, colcemid (diacetyl-methylcolchicine, 0.1 μg/ml final conc.) was added to arrest the cells at metaphase stage. The "air-drying method" of chromosome preparation [57] included hypotonic treatment with 0.075 M KCl for 20 min, a fixation step and several washing steps using Carnoy's fixative (methanol/glacial acetic acid 3:1); finally, the suspension was dropped onto the slide's surface.

Primate chromosome preparations (Additional file 4: Table S1) were provided by the coauthors from Thailand and Brazil.

Permanent EBV transformed cell lines from the clinical cases mos 47,XY,+min(7)(:p13 → p11.1:),upd(7)mat isodisomy/46,XY,upd(7)mat isodisomy (EKF-#7-p12/1-m) and 46,XY,upd(14)mat heterodisomy (EKF-#14-q11/1-m) were kindly provided by the Else Kröner-Fresenius (EFK) – cellbank (Institute of Human Genetics, Jena, Germany, http://ssmc-tl.com/ekf-cellbank.html).

Human metaphases from abortion material and amniotic fluid

Chromosome preparations from abortion material and amniotic fluid material were performed according to standard techniques [56]. The primary abortion material was mechanically minced and covered with full medium mixed with penicillin/streptomycin and l-glutamate in a culture flask for 10–14 days at 37 °C/5 % CO_2. Cells were disassociated by trypsin or in the case of amniotic fluid; a sedimented aliquote was transferred to a quadriperm plate on sterile glass slides with full medium for in situ culture for 7–10 days at 37 °C/5 % CO_2. Ninety minutes before harvesting the cells colcemid (0.1 μg/ml final conc.) was added followed by hypotonic treatment (1.5 mM $MgCl_2$, 0. 1 % sodium citrate and 150 U hyalorunidase) for 10–14 min, a fixation step and several washing steps using Carnoy's fixative and final drying on the slide.

Human metaphases from bone marrow material

Chromosome preparations from heparinized bone marrow were performed according to standard techniques

[56]. An aliquot of bone marrow was added to the cell culture medium, mixed with 10–20 % fetal calf serum and penicillin/streptomycin. After 24 h of incubation at 37 °C/5 % CO_2 the cells were harvested without colcemid. Hypotonic treatment with 0.056 M KCl was performed for 20 min, a fixation step and several washing steps using Carnoy's fixative and final dropping of the suspension onto the slide's surface.

Murine metaphases from primary spleen

Mouse metaphase spreads were prepared from primary spleen and short-term culture with phytohemagglutinin. After 60 h of incubation at 37 °C/5 % CO_2 the cells were harvested. Thirty minutes before harvesting the cells, colcemid (0.1 μg/ml final conc.) was added, followed by hypotonic treatment with 0.040 M KCl for 40 min, a fixation step and several washing steps using Carnoy's fixative and final dropping of the suspension onto the slide's surface.

FISH methods

M-FISH

M-FISH (multiplex FISH using whole chromosome painting probes) was applied for the proper identification of homologous chromosomes in cross species-FISH applications on primates and mouse. For primates, a human M-FISH probe set based on glass needle dissected probes was used as described before [58]. An analog M-FISH probe set specific for mouse chromosomes was used to assign chromosomes in mouse metaphase spreads [59].

cenM-FISH

CenM-FISH (centromere multiplex FISH for all 24 human chromosomes) was applied for the proper identification of homologous chromosomes in poor quality metaphases of bone marrow preparations, according to previously published protocols [60].

pod-FISH

pod-FISH (parental origin determination FISH) was performed on metaphase spreads of a male proband and his parents (i.e. a family trio) derived from peripheral blood lymphocytes. Furthermore pod-FISH was applied on metaphase spreads of two clinical cases with karyotype mos 47,XY,+7/47,XY,+min(7),upd(7)mat isodisomy/46, XY,upd(7)mat isodisomy and 46,XY,upd(14)mat heterodisomy, respectively, derived from permanent EBV transformed cell lines. BAC clones for pod-FISH [19] were selected from CNV regions by http://projects.tcag.ca/variation/, the DNA was isolated, PCR amplified, and labeled by nick translation. Informative BAC clones that gave signal intensity differences on homologous chromosomes were further tested for parental origin. 10–25 metaphases were evaluated each. Signal differences not directly visible by eye were measured by software approaches like SCION or Axiovision software, Carl Zeiss MicroImaging GmbH, Germany.

Additional files

Additional file 1: Figure S1. Inverted DAPI images from 9 metaphase spreads of the normal proband from the family trio exemplify the bilateral grouping of haploid chromosome sets. These metaphases were also subjected to further analysis by pod FISH for determining the parental origin of the homologous chromosomes in the proband. (TIF 1521 kb)

Additional file 2: Figure S2. Bone marrow metaphases from an AML patient with mosaic trisomy 8 after cen-M-FISH. The karyotypes showing two or three times the chromosome 8, indicated with an arrow, depending on the parental location in blue (paternal) or red (maternal) haplogroups. (TIF 786 kb)

Additional file 3: Figure S3. A) Inverted DAPI images from 3 metaphases of case 1 with 47,XY,+min(14) and maternal heterodisomy 14. Due to a maternal centromere polymorphism both chromosomes 14 can be distinguished by the size of the FISH signal in cenh + and cenh-. B) Inverted DAPI images from 3 metaphases of case 2 with 46,XY,upd(7)mat. C) Inverted DAPI images from 3 metaphases of case 3 with 47,XY,+inv dup(22)mat. The karyotypes are given red and blue labels to indicate the maternal and paternal haplotypes. Arrows indicate the additional minute chromosome. (TIF 826 kb)

Additional file 4: Table S1. Primate samples used in this study. Abbreviation: PBL, peripheral blood lymphocyte. (DOCX 12 kb)

Additional file 5: Figure S4. Metaphases from ten different primate species (see also Additional file 4: Table S1) demonstrating a genome-wise sorting of the haploid chromosome sets after M-FISH showing chromosome grouping and the closer location of homologous chromosomes next to the symmetry line. (TIF 727 kb)

Additional file 6: Figure S5. Examples for observed mirror-image groups of chromosomes (left, labeled in same colors) and homologous chromosomes located next to each other along the symmetry line in HSA (A), MMU (B) and SSC (C). (TIF 359 kb)

Additional file 7: Figure S6. Round shaped metaphase spread from Silvery Langur (TCR, *Trachypithecus cristata*). Measurement of DNA content by DAPI per area resulted in ~20 % independent if the whole area is counted or a pie slice reflecting a symmetric/round shaped distribution of DNA in the metaphase state of the cell cycle. (TIF 255 kb)

Additional file 8: Figure S7. Metaphase plate from *Zellsubstanz, Kern und Zelltheilung* (1882) by Walther Flemming [13] (A) and chromosome "rosettes" from routine cytogenetic diagnostics in amniotic fluid cells after in situ culture (B) and a metaphase spread in "rosette" shape from peripheral blood lymphocytes (47,XX,+mar) after cenM-FISH (C). (TIF 876 kb)

Competing interests
The authors declare that they have no competing interests.

Authors' contributions
AW and JPC designed and coordinated the study. AW carried out the triplody, tetraploidy and M-FISH studies. SM performed the pod-FISH studies. KP contributed the sSMC and UPD FISH studies. NK carried out the murine FISH studies. XF performed the primate FISH studies. EA contributed the bone marrow FISH studies. AA-H performed statistical calculation. AT and AC prepared and karyotyped the primate samples. MBC, JUW and TL participated in drafting and critical review of the manuscript. All authors read and approved the final manuscript.

Acknowledgements
Supported by a grant from Carl Zeiss MicroImaging GmbH, Germany and by the China Scholarship Council. Competing interests. On behalf of all authors the corresponding author declares that there are no financial and non-financial competing interests.

Author details
[1]Institute of Human Genetics, Jena University Hospital, Postfach, 07740, Jena, Germany. [2]Department of General, Visceral und Vascular Surgery, Jena University Hospital, Kochstr. 2, Jena 07743, Germany. [3]Department of Biology, Faculty of Science, Khon Kaen University, 123 Moo 16 Mittapap Rd, Khon Kaen, Muang District 40002, Thailand. [4]Departamento de Genética e Evolução, Universidade Federal de São Carlos, São Carlos, SP, Brazil. [5]Instituto Evandro Chagas, Seção de Meio Ambiente, Laboratório de Cultura de Tecidos e Citogenética, Ananindeua, PA, Brazil. [6]Kinderklinik, Ludwig Maximillians Universität, 80337 Munich, Germany.

References
1. Zhang G, Pradhan S. Mammalian epigenetic mechanisms. IUBMB Life. 2014; 66:240–56.
2. Chen H, Chen J, Muir LA, Ronquist S, Meixner W, Ljungman M, Ried T, Smale S, Rajapakse I. Functional organization of the human 4D Nucleome. Proc Natl Acad Sci U S A. 2015;112:8002–7.
3. Sehgal N, Seifert B, Ding H, Chen Z, Stojkovic B, Bhattacharya S, Xu J, Berezney R. Reorganization of the interchromosomal network during keratinocyte differentiation. Chromosoma. 2015, in press.
4. Othman MAK, Lier A, Junker S, Kempf P, Dorka F, Gebhart E, Sheth FJ, Grygalewicz B, Bhatt S, Weise A, Mrasek K, Liehr T, Manvelyan M. Does positioning of chromosomes 8 and 21 in interphase drive t(8;21) in acute myelogenous leukemia? BioDiscovery. 2012;4:4.
5. Miller OJ, Mukherjee BB, Breg WR, Gamble AV. Non-random distribution of chromosomes in metaphase figures from cultured human leucocytes. I. The peripheral location of the Y chromosome. Cytogenet. 1963;2:1–14.
6. Miller OJ, Breg WR, Mukherjee BB, Gamble AV, Christakos AC. Non-random distribution of chromosomes in metaphase figures from cultured human leucocytes. II. The peripheral location of chromosomes 13, 17, 18 and 21. Cytogenet. 1963;2:152–67.
7. Chaudhuri JP, Reith A. Symmetric Chromosomal Order in Leukocytes indicated by DNA Image Cytometry and FISH. Analyt Quant Cytol Histol. 1997;19:30–6.
8. Chaudhuri JP, Fringes B, Reith A. Topographic order of chromosomes in leukocytes indicated by DNA image cytometry and mono or dual FISH with five different probes. Verhandl Dt Ges Pathol. 1997;81:689.
9. Chaudhuri JP, Walther JU. Chromosomes and Genome Organisation in Eukaryotes. Ind Scien Cruis. 2002;16:27–34.
10. Chaudhuri JP, Walther JU. Separation of parental genomes in human blood and bone marrow cells and its implications. Int J Oncol. 2003;23:1257–62.
11. Chaudhuri JP, Kasprzycki E, Battaglia M, McGill JR, Brøgger A, Walther JU, Reith A. Biphasic chromatin structure and FISH signals reflect intranuclear order. Cellular Oncol. 2005;27:327–34.
12. Chaudhuri JP, Karamanov S, Prabakaran P, McGill JR, Walther JU. Identification of Parental Chromosomes involved in Translocations BCR-ABL, t(9;22), and PML-RARA, t(15;17). Anticancer Res. 2008;28:3573–8.
13. Chaudhuri JP, Walther JU. Nuclear segmentation, compaction and bilateral symmetry in polymorphonuclear leukocytes reflect genomic order and favour immunologic function. Acta Haematol. 2013;129:159–68.
14. Gläss E. Die Identifizierung der Chromosomen im Karyotyp der Rattenleber. Chromosoma. 1956;7:655–69.
15. Gläss E. Sonderung der Chromosomen-Sätze in Rattenleberzellen. Chromosoma. 1957;8:468–92.
16. Pera F. Mechanismen der Polyploidisierung und der Somatischen Reduktion. Berlin: Springer; 1970. p. 50.
17. Brown SW, Nur U. Heterochromatic chromosomes in the Coccids. Science. 1964;145:130.
18. Leitch AR, Schwarzacher T, Mosgöller W, Bennett MD, Helsop-Harrison JS. Parental genomes are separated throughout the cell cycle in a plant hybrid. Chromosoma. 1991;101:206–13.
19. Weise A, Gross M, Mrasek K, Mkrtchyan H, Horsthemke B, Jonsrud C, Von Eggeling F, Hinreiner S, Witthuhn V, Claussen U, Liehr T. Parental-origin-determination fluorescence in situ hybridization distinguishes homologous human chromosomes on a single-cell level. Int J Mol Med. 2008;21:189–200.
20. Spittel H, Kubek F, Kreskowski K, Ziegler M, Klein E, Hamid AB, Kosyakova N, Radhakrishnan G, Junge A, Kozlowski P, Schulze B, Martin T, Huhle D, Mehnert K, Rodríguez L, Ergun MA, Sarri C, Militaru M, Stipoljev F, Tittelbach H,

Vasheghani F, de Bello Cioffi M, Hussein SS, Fan X, Volleth M, Liehr T. Mitotic stability of small supernumerary marker chromosomes: a study based on 93 immortalized cell lines. Cytogenet Genome Res. 2014;142:151–60.

21. Hliscs R, Mühlig P, Claussen U. The spreading of metaphases is a slow process which leads to a stretching of chromosomes. Cytogenet Cell Genet. 1997;76:167–71.

22. Spurbeck JL, Zinsmeister AR, Meyer KJ, Jalal SM. Dynamics of chromosome spreading. Am J Hum Genet. 1996;61:387–93.

23. Claussen U, Michel S, Mühlig P, Westermann M, Grummt UW, Kromeyer-Hauschild K, Liehr T. Demystefying chromosome preparation and the implications for the concept of chromosome condensation during mitosis. Cytogenet Genome Res. 2002;98:136–46.

24. Mayer W, Smith A, Fundele R, Haaf T. Spatial separation of parental genomes in preimplantation mouse embryos. J Cell Bio. 2000;148:629–34.

25. Mehta IS, Kulashreshtha M, Chakraborty S, Kolthur-Seetharam U, Rao BJ. Chromosome territories reposition during DNA damage-repair response. Genome Biol. 2013;14:R135.

26. Rabl C. Über Zelltheilung. Morphol Jahrb. 1885;10:214–330.

27. Boveri T, Die Befruchtung und Teilung des Eies von Ascaris megalocephala. Zellen-Studien 2. Jena, Germany: G. Fischer; 1888.

28. Cremer T, Kurz A, Zirbel R, Dietzel S, Rinke B, Schröck E, Lichter P. Role of chromosome territories in the functional compartmentalization of the cell nucleus. Cold Spring Harb Symp Quant Biol. 1993;58:777–92.

29. Parada L, Misteli T. Chromosome positioning in the interphase nucleus. Trends Cell Biol. 2002;12:425–32.

30. Cremer T, Cremer C, Baumann H, Luedtke E, Sperling K, Teuber V, Zorn C. Rabl's model of the interphase chromosome arrangement tested in Chinese hamster cells by premature chromosome condensation and laser-UV-microbeam experiments. Hum Genet. 1982;60:46–56.

31. Boyle S, Gilchrist S, Bridger JM, Mahy NL, Ellis JA, Bickmore WA. The spatial organization of human chromosomes within the nuclei of normal and emerin-mutant cells. Hum Mol Genet. 2001;10:211–9.

32. Nagele R, Freeman T, McMorrow L, Lee H. Precise spatial positioning of chromosomes during prometaphase: evidence for chromosomal order. Science. 1995;270:1831–5.

33. Bickmore WA. The spatial organization of the human genome. Annu Rev Genomics Hum Genet. 2013;14:67–84.

34. Strickfaden H, Zunhammer A, van Koningsbruggen S, Köhler D, Cremer T. 4D chromatin dynamics in cycling cells: Thedor Boveri's hypothesis revisited. Nucleus. 2010;1:284–97.

35. Engreitz JM, Agarwala V, Mirny LA. Three-dimensional genome architecture influences partner selection for chromosomal translocations in human disease. PLoS One. 2012;7:e44196.

36. Cherniak C, Rodriguez-Esteban R. Body maps on the human genome. Mol Cytogenet. 2013;6:61.

37. Weise A, Gross M, Hinreiner S, Witthuhn V, Mkrtchyan H, Liehr T. POD-FISH: a new technique for parental origin determination based on copy number variation polymorphism. Methods Mol Biol. 2010;659:291–8.

38. Polityko AD, Khurs OM, Kulpanovich AI, Mosse KA, Solntsava AV, Rumyantseva NV, Naumchik IV, Liehr T, Weise A, Mkrtchyan H. Paternally derived der(7)t(Y;7)(p11.1 approximately 11.2;p22.3)dn in a mosaic case with Turner syndrome. Eur J Med Genet. 2009;52:207–10.

39. Pombo A, Dillon N. Three-dimensional genome architecture: players and mechanisms. Nat Rev Mol Cell Biol. 2015;16:245–57.

40. Mkrtchyan H, Gross M, Hinreiner S, Polytiko A, Manvelyan M, Mrasek K, Kosyakova N, Ewers E, Nelle H, Liehr T, Volleth M, Weise A. Early embryonic chromosome instability results in stable mosaic pattern in human tissues. PLoS One. 2010;5:e9591.

41. Horsthemke B, Wawrzik M, Gross S, Lich C, Sauer B, Rost I, Krasemann E, Kosyakova N, Liehr T, Weise A, Dybowski JN, Hoffmann D, Wieczorek D. Parental origin and functional relevance of a de novo UBE3A variant. Eur J Med Genet. 2011;54:19–24.

42. Teplitz RL, Gustafson PE, Pellett OL. Chromosomal distributon in interspecies in vitro hybrid cells. Exp Cell Res. 1968;52:379–91.

43. Bessis M, Breton-Gorius J. Rapport entre noyau et centrioles dans les granulocytes étalés. Role de microtubules. Nouv Rev Fr Hematol. 1967;7:601–20.

44. Bessis M. Living blood cells and their ultrastructure. Berlin: Springer Verlag; 1973. p. 319–20.

45. Lettré M, Lettré R. Un problème cytologique: la persistence des structures du fusseau dans l'intervalle des mitoses. Rev Hématol. 1958;13:337–65.

46. Fawcett DW. An Atlas of Fine Structure, The Cell. Philadelphia: Saunders; 1966. p. 60–2.

47. Krioutchkova MM, Onishchenko GE. Structural and functional characteristics of the centrosome in gametogenesis and embryogenesis of animals. Int Rev Cytol. 1999;185:107–56.

48. Sathananthan AH. Mitosis in the human embryo: vital role of the sperm centrosome (centriole). Histol Histopathol. 1997;12:827–56.

49. Brianna Caddle L, Grant JL, Szatkiewicz J, van Hase J, Shirley BJ, Bewersdorf J, Cremer C, Arneodo A, Khalil A, Mills KD. Chromosome neighborhood composition determines translocation outcomes after exposure to high-dose radiation in primary cells. Chromosome Res. 2007;15:1061–73.

50. Heride C, Ricoul M, Kiêu K, von Hase J, Guillemot V, Cremer C, Dubrana K, Sabatier L. Distance between homologous chromosomes results from chromosome positioning constrains. J Cell Sci. 2010;123:4063–75.

51. Schroeder WT, Chao LY, Dao DD, Strong LC, Pathak S, Riccardi V, Lewis WH, Saunders GF. Nonrandom loss of maternal chromosome 11 alleles in Wilms tumors. Am J Hum Genet. 1987;40:413–20.

52. Hoban PR, Heighway J, White GRM, Baker B, Gardner J, Birch JM, Morris-Jones P, Kelsey AM. Genome-wide loss of maternal alleles in a nephrogenic rest and Wilm's tumor from a BWS patient. Hum Genet. 1995;95:651–6.

53. Stöck M, Lamatsch DK, Steinlein DK, Epplen JT, Grosse WR, Hock R, Klappenstück T, Lampert KP, Scheer U, Schmid M, Schartl M. A bisexually reproducing all-triploid vertebrate. Nat Genet. 2002;30:325–8.

54. Michor F, Iwasa Y, Vogelstein B, Lengauer C, Nowak MA. Can chromosomal instability initiate tumorigenesis? Semin Cancer Biol. 2005;15:43–9.

55. Reinius B, Sandberg R. Random monoallelic expression of autosomal genes: stochastic transcription and allele-level regulation. Nat Rev Genet. 2015;16:653–64.

56. Liehr T. Fluorescence in situ Hybridization (FISH) – Application Guide. Berlin: Springer Verlag; 2009.

57. Moorhead PS, Hsu TC. Cytologic studies of HeLa, a strain of human cervical carcinoma. III. Durations and characteristics of the mitotic phases. J Natl Cancer Inst. 1956;16:1047–66.

58. Mrasek K, Heller A, Rubtsov N, Trifonov V, Starke H, Rocchi M, Claussen U, Liehr T. Reconstruction of the female Gorilla gorilla karyotype using 25-color FISH and multicolor banding (MCB). Cytogenet Cell Genet. 2001;93:242–8.

59. Kosyakova N, Hamid AB, Chaveerach A, Pinthong K, Siripiyasing P, Supiwong W, Romanenko S, Trifonov V, Fan X. Generation of multicolor banding probes for chromosomes of different species. Mol Cytogenet. 2013;6:6.

60. Nietzel A, Rocchi M, Starke H, Heller A, Fiedler W, Wlodarska I, Loncarevic IF, Beensen V, Claussen U, Liehr T. A new multicolor-FISH approach for the characterization of marker chromosomes: centromere-specific multicolor-FISH (cenM-FISH). Hum Genet. 2001;108:199–204.

23

First insights on the retroelement *Rex1* in the cytogenetics of frogs

Juliana Nascimento[1], Diego Baldo[2] and Luciana Bolsoni Lourenço[1*]

Abstract

Background: While some transposable elements (TEs) have been found in the sequenced genomes of frog species, detailed studies of these elements have been lacking. In this work, we investigated the occurrence of the *Rex1* element, which is widespread in fish, in anurans of the genus *Physalaemus*. We isolated and characterized the reverse transcriptase (RT)-coding sequences of *Rex1* elements of five species of this genus.

Results: The amino acid sequences deduced from the nucleotide sequences of the isolated fragments allowed us to unambiguously identify regions corresponding to domains 3–7 of RT. Some of the nucleotide sequences isolated from *Physlaemus ephippifer* and *P. albonotatus* had internal deletions, suggesting that these fragments are likely not active TEs, despite being derived from a *Rex1* element. When hybridized with metaphase chromosomes, *Rex1* probes were revealed at the pericentromeric heterochromatic region of the short arm of chromosome 3 of the *P. ephippifer* karyotype. Neither other heterochromatin sites of the *P. ephippifer* karyotype nor any chromosomal regions of the karyotypes of *P. albonotatus*, *P. spiniger* and *P. albifrons* were detected with these probes.

Conclusions: *Rex1* elements were found in the genomes of five species of *Physalaemus* but clustered in only the *P. ephippifer* karyotype, in contrast to observations in some species of fish, where large chromosomal sites with *Rex1* elements are typically present.

Keywords: Repetitive DNA, in situ hybridization, Chromosome, Retrotransposon, Leptodactylidae

Background

Eukaryotic genomes contain large amounts of repetitive DNA sequences, many of which are interspersed repeats derived from transposable elements (TEs) (reviewed in [1–3]). With the ability to integrate and occupy a large portion of the eukaryotic genome, TEs greatly influence genomic architecture (reviewed in [1, 4]). TEs are also involved in karyotype evolution because these mobile sequences can induce chromosomal rearrangements, including deletions, duplications, inversions and translocations (reviewed in [1, 5]). Therefore, the identification of this type of repetitive sequence may be valuable for evolutionary cytogenetic studies.

TE sequences are grouped in two large families, class I elements (retrotransposons) and class II elements (transposons), which are characterized by the intermediate molecule used in the transposition process. Class I elements have an RNA molecule as an intermediary for transposition, while class II elements move in the genome using DNA copies as intermediates or without any intermediate [2, 6, 7]. The eukaryotic transposons are further classified as "cut-and-paste" transposons, *Helitrons* and *Politrons*, which are, respectively, non-replicative, rolling-circle replicative and self-synthesizing (reviewed in [2, 3]). Among the eukaryotic retrotransposon, two principal groups are recognized, according to the presence or absence of long terminal repeats (LTR) flanking their open ready frames (ORFs): the LTR retrotransposons and the non-LTR retrotransposons, also known as LINEs (long interspersed nucleotide element). Additionally, *Penelope* and *DIRS* (*Dictyostelium* intermediate repeat sequence) retrotransposons have been identified (reviewed in [2]).

The retrotransposons families *Rex* (Retroelement of *Xiphophorus*) *1*, *Rex2*, *Rex3* and *Rex6* are non-LTR retrotransposons, and they were first isolated from the fish genus *Xiphophorus* [8–10]. The *Rex1* element encodes a reverse transcriptase and an apurinic/apyrimidinic

---

* Correspondence: bolsoni@unicamp.br
[1]Departamento de Biologia Estrutural e Funcional, Instituto de Biologia, Universidade Estadual de Campinas, 13083-863 Campinas, São Paulo, Brazil
Full list of author information is available at the end of the article

endonuclease, which is frequently lost [9]. The 3′ untranslated region of several *Rex1* elements is followed by tandem repeat oligonucleotides that are variable in length (5–7 nt) and sequence. Based on an analysis of RT amino acid sequence, Volff and colleagues [9] reasoned that the *Rex1* sequences and *Babar* elements (for *Battrachocottus baikalensis* retrotransposon) cannot be assigned to any other known family of TE and suggested a moderately close relationship between *Rex1/ Babar* elements and members of the *CR1* family of non-LTR retrotransposons.

The *Rex* family is widespread in fishes and was already mapped to a number of fish karyotypes through in situ hybridization, providing valuable markers for karyotype comparisons (examples in [8–20]; for review, see [21]). For Anura, the only available reports on *Rex* sequences arose from studies not designed specifically for the analysis of this TE but rather from the sequencing of the whole genomes of the pipid *Xenopus tropicalis* [22, 23] and the dicroglossid *Nanorana parkeri* [24; GenBank accession number: JYOU00000000.1], which are representatives of the non-neobatrachian and Ranoidea, respectively. In addition, in contrast to fish, the karyotype organization of this or any other TE has not been explored using cytogenetic studies.

In this study, we aimed to evaluate i) whether *Rex1* is also present in Hyloidea, the Anuran superfamily that, together with Ranoidea, composes Neobatrachia and ii) whether *Rex1* sequences are sufficiently clustered in Anuran genomes to be used as chromosomal markers in Anuran cytogenetics. To assess these goals, we elected the leptodactylid genus *Physalaemus*, which comprises 46 species [25] that are currently arranged in two major clades: the *P. cuvieri* Clade with six species groups (*P. biligonigerus* group, *P. cuvieri* group, *P. gracilis* group, *P. henselii* group, *P. olfersii* group) and the *P. signifer* Clade [26]. Twenty of the species of *Physalaemus* have already been karyotyped [27–37], and the results show 2n = 22. *Physalaemus* is attractive for cytogenetic and genomic studies, particularly because of the high interspecific variation in the number and/or distribution of nucleolus organizer regions (NOR) [29, 30, 32–37]) and because heteromorphic sex chromosomes are only recognized in *P. ephippifer* [34]. We searched for sequences related to the *Rex1* family in five species belonging to different species groups of *Physalaemus* and used the isolated sequences as probes for in situ hybridization assays.

Results

Rex1 sequences of *Physalaemus* species

We obtained 23 clones containing fragments of *Rex1* isolated from genomic DNA of *Physalaemus ephippifer*, 18 from *P. albifrons*, 16 from *P. albonotatus* and one from *Physalaemus* aff. *cuvieri*. One sequence of *P.*

henselii and one of *P. spiniger* were isolated and sequenced directly without cloning.

Among the 16 fragments isolated from *Physalaemus albonotatus*, three types of sequences were found, which differed in nucleotide sequence and size. In the 339 bp sequence isolated from the *P. albonotatus* genome (Pab-Rex1C12), a 221 bp segment (positions 190–410 in Fig. 1) is missing, which was present in all of the remaining sequences isolated from the *Physalaemus* species. The first 190 bp and the last 160 bp of this sequence were highly similar to the corresponding regions of the other isolated sequences (Fig. 1). A codon analysis of this truncated sequence of *P. albonotatus* revealed an in-frame stop codon at the beginning of the isolated sequence (at positions 85–87 as shown in Fig. 1). The other two sequences isolated from *P. albonotatus* were 86 % similar to each other and were 547 bp and 571 bp in length. One segment with 6 nucleotides and another with 17 nucleotides that were present in the 571 bp fragments were absent in the 547 bp sequence (segments from positions 269–274 and from positions 421–437 as shown in Fig. 1). Two sequences that were 95 % similar to each other were also recognized among the fragments isolated from *P. ephippifer* (Fig. 1).

The *Rex1* fragments isolated from all the *Physalaemus* species, except for the 339 bp sequence of *P. albonotatus*, were very similar to each other (average similarity = 92 %) and were 68 and 73 % similar to the *Rex1/Babar* sequences already described for *Anguilla japonica* and *Battrachocottus baikalensis*, respectively (Fig. 1). We note that the sequence isolated from *Physalaemus* aff. *cuvieri* differed significantly at positions 29–52 with regard to the other sequences of *Physalaemus* (Fig. 1). When the *Rex1* sequences of *Physalaemus* (except for the 339 bp sequence of *P. albonotatus*) were compared with the sequence REX1-5_XT, which was obtained from the anuran *Xenopus tropicalis* and previously recognized as *Rex1* [22, 23] (sequence available at Repbase database http://www.girin st.org/censor/index.php), lower similarity values were found (from 54 to 58 %) (Additional file 1). Comparison of the *Rex1* sequences isolated from *Physalaemus* with the element *CR1* of *Gallus gallus*, which Volff and colleagues consider to be distantly related to *Rex1/Babar* elements [9], showed no similarity (Additional file 1).

Amino acid sequence translation of all fragments of *Rex1* (Fig. 2) allowed us to clearly identify the regions corresponding to the conserved domains 3 to 7 of the RT, as identified by Malik and colleagues [37] and Volff and colleagues [8, 9]. When compared to *Battrachocottus baikalensis* (GenBank accession number U18939.1) and *Anguilla japonica* (GenBank accession numbers AJ288466.1) sequences, the *Rex1* sequences isolated from *Physalaemus ephippifer*, *P. albifrons*, *P. henselli*, *P. spiniger*, *P. albonotatus* and *P.* aff. *cuvieri* from

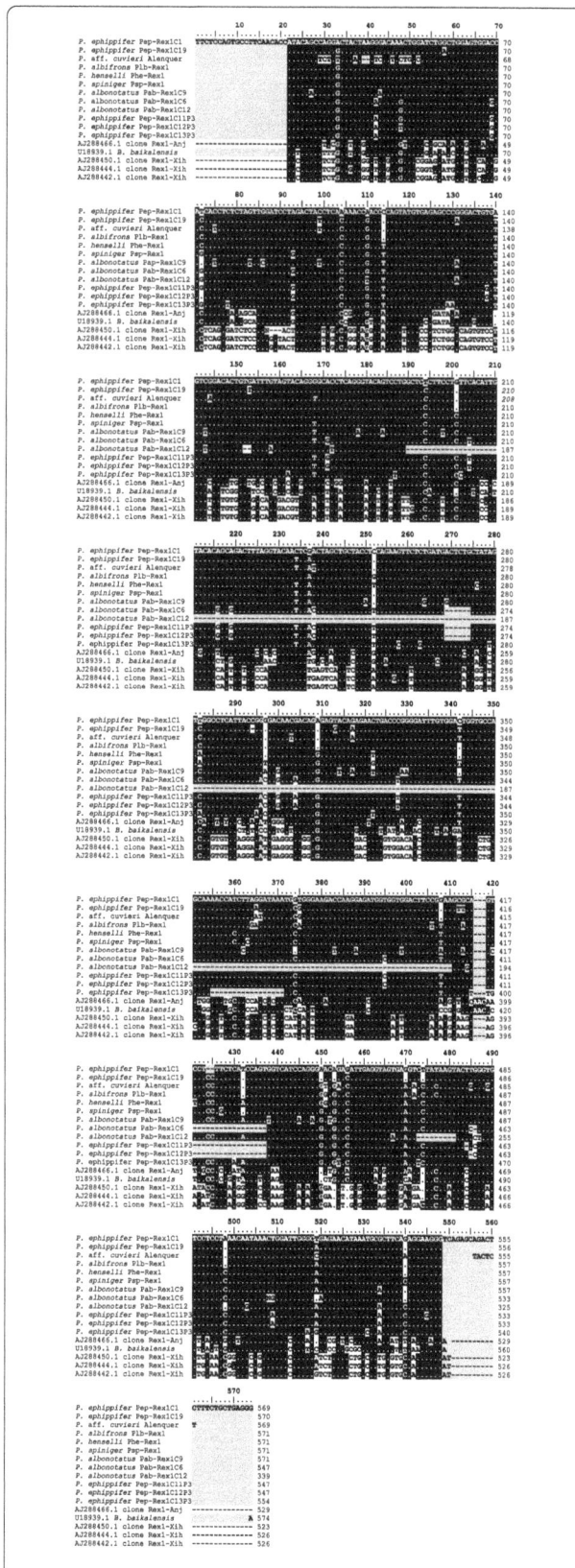

Fig. 1 Alignment of the *Rex1* fragments isolated from species of *Physalaemus* with corresponding sequences available in GenBank. The sequences *P. ephippifer* Pep-Rex1C11P3, *P. ephippifer* Pep-Rex1C12P3 and *P. ephippifer* Pep-Rex1C13P3 were obtained from the microdissected 3p *per* band. The primers used to isolate the sequences are shaded in gray at the ends of the sequences. Black areas indicate identical sites, while variable sites are colored white. Premature stop codons are shown in blue. U18939.1 is the GenBank accession number of a *Babar* sequence (a *Rex1*-related element) of *Battrachocottus baikalensis*. AJ288466.1, AJ288450.1, AJ288444.1, and AJ288462.1 are GenBank accession numbers of retroelement *Rex1* sequences isolated from *Anguilla japonica* (AJ288466.1) or *Xiphophorus helleri*

Alenquer–PA failed to show an AAC nucleotide triplet at positions 416–418 of the sequences shown in Fig. 1, as well as of the sequences isolated from *Xiphophorus helleri* [9] (GenBank accession numbers AJ288450.1, AJ288444.1 and AJ288442.1). The absence of this ACC triplet potentially affects the translation of two codons. In addition, deletions of one or two nucleotides could be detected in the fragments Pep-Rex1C1, Pep-Rex1C17 and Pep- Rex1C19 of *P. ephippifer* after comparing these sequences to the others (Fig. 1).

Mapping of *Rex1* sequences on metaphase chromosomes

When used as probes and mapped to metaphase chromosomes, the *Rex1* sequences did not reveal any chromosomal sites at all (not even small dots) in the karyotypes of *Physalaemus albonotatus*, *P. albifrons*, *P.* aff. *cuvieri* or *P. spiniger*. In contrast, the probe Pep-Rex1C17 localized to the pericentromeric region of the short arm of chromosome pair 3 (3p *per*) of *P. ephippifer* (Fig. 3), suggesting accumulation of *Rex1* sequences at this heterochromatic chromosomal region (Fig. 3 – inset). No hybridization signal was observed at any other site of this karyotype (Fig. 3), not even at regions previously revealed to be heterochromatic by Nascimento and colleagues [34]. The region at 3p *per* also hybridized with type I 5S ribosomal DNA (5S rDNA), as previously reported by Nascimento and colleagues [34].

Rex1* and 5S rDNA sequences isolated from microdissected 3p *per* of *P. ephippifer

Polymerase chain reaction (PCR) using primers for *Rex1* sequences resulted in the isolation of ~550-bp fragments from the microdissected 3p *per* band of the *Physalaemus ephippifer* karyotype, and three of these fragments were cloned and sequenced. Two cloned fragments were 547 bp (*P. ephippifer* Pep-Rex1C11P3 and *P. ephippifer* Pep-Rex1C12P3 in Fig. 1), and one was 554 bp (*P. ephippifer* Pep-Rex1C13P3 in Fig. 1). All of these fragments were very similar to the major *Rex1* sequences isolated from genomic DNA of *Physalaemus* species (Fig. 1). The 547-bp fragments and the sequence Pab-Rex1C6 of *P. albonotatus* had a deletion of two segments compared to

3   4

```
                                    10        20        30        40        50        60        70
                              ....|....|....|....|....|....|....|....|....|....|....|....|....|....|
P. ephippifer Pep-Rex1C1      FSSAFNTIQPGLLRDKLDLAGVDHHLSSWILDYLKNQPQYVRARDCESDTVICSTGAPQGTVLAFFLFTL  70
P. ephippifer Pep-Rex1C19     FSSAFNTIQPGLLRDKLDLTGVDHHLSSWILDYLTNRPQYVRAQDCVSDTVICSTGAPQGTVLAPFLFTL  70
P, aff. cuvieri Alenquer      FSSAFNTIQLCL--HYWBLAGVDHHLSSWILDYLTNRPQYVRARDCVSDTVICSTGAPQGTVLAPFLFTL  70
P. albifrons Plb-Rex1         FSSAFNTIQPGLLRDKLDLAGVDHHLSSWILDYLTNRPQYVRARDCVSDTVICSTGAPQGTVLAPFLFTL  70
P. henselli Phe-Rex1          FSSAFNTIQPGLLRDKLDLAGVDHHLSSWILDYLTNRPQYVRARDCVSDTVICSTGAPQGTVLAPFLFTL  70
P. spiniger Psp-Rex1          FSSAFNTIQPGLLRDKLDLAGVDQHLSSWILDYLTNRPQYVRARDCVSDTVICSTGAPQGTVLAPFLFTL  70
P. albonotatus Pab-Rex1C9     FSSAFNTIQPGLLRNKLDLAGVDHHLSISIILDYLTNRPQYVRAQDCVLFDTVICSTGAPQGTHLAPFLFTL 70
P. albonotatus Pab-Rex1C6     FSSAFNTIQPGLLRDKLDLAGVEQHLSSWILDYLTNRPQYVRARDCVSDTVICSTGAPQGTVLAPFLFTL  70
P. albonotatus Pab-Rex1C12    FSSAFNTIQPGLLRDKLDLAGVEQHLSIILDYLTNIPQYVRAQDCVLDTIYSTGASQGTVL-------  63
P. ephippifer Pep-Rex1C11P3   FSSAFNTIQPGLLRDKLDLAGVDHHLSSWILDYLTNRPQYVRARDWVSDTVICSTGAPQGTVLAPFLFTL  70
P. ephippifer Pep-Rex1C12P3   FSSAFNTIQPGLLRDNLDLAGVDHHLSSWILDYLTNRPQYVRARDWVSDTVICSTGAPQGTVLAPFLFTL  70
P. ephippifer Pep-Rex1C13P3   FSSAFNTIQPGLLRDKLNFQYVRARDCVSDTVICRTGAPQGTVLAPFLFTL*                    70
AJ288466.1 clone Rex1-Anj     ------IQPALLRDKLDRTGVGHHLTAWILDYLTDRPQYVRIDCDESDLVVCSTGARQGTVLAPFLFTL  63
U18939.1 B. baikalensis       FSSAFNTIQPGLLRDKLEQTGVDHHLTAWILDYLTNRPQYVRIRFCESDRVSCSTGAPAQGTVLAPFLFSI  70
AJ288450.1 clone Rex1-Xih     -------IQPLLLGEKIRRMGVNDSVIS--TDYLTGRPQFVRLGSVLSDVVVSDVGAPQGTVLSPFLFTL  62
AJ288444.1 clone Rex1-Xih     -------IQPLLLGEKIRLMGVNDSVISWTDYLTGRPQFVRLGSVLSDVVVSDVGAPQGTVLCPFLFTL  63
AJ288442.1 clone Rex1-Xih     -------IQPLLLGEKIRRMGVDDSVISW-TDYLTGRPQFVRLGSVLSDVVVSDVGAPQGTVLSPFLFTL  63
```

5   6

```
                                    80        90       100       110       120       130       140
                              ....|....|....|....|....|....|....|....|....|....|....|....|....|....|
P. ephippifer Pep-Rex1C1      YTADFRYNSTSCYLQKFSDDSAIVGLIGDNDREYRELTRGFVDWCQQNHLRINGKTKEMVVDFRRKF 140
P. ephippifer Pep-Rex1C19     YTADFRYNSTSCYLQKFSDDSAIVGLIGDNDREDKELTRGFVDWCQQNHLRINAGKTKEMVVDFRRKF 140
P. aff. cuvieri Alenquer      YTADFRYNSSSCYLQKFSDDSAIVGLITGDNDREYKELTRGFVDWCQQNHLRINAGKTKEMVVDFRRKR 140
P. albifrons Plb-Rex1         YTADFRYNSTSCYLQKFSDDSAIVGLITGDNDREYRELTRGFVDWCQQNHLRINAGKTKEMVVFGKRH 140
P. henselli Phe-Rex1          YTADFRYNSTSCYLQKFSDDSAIVGLITGDNDREYRELTRGFVDWCQQNHLRINAGKTKEMVVDFRRKR 140
P. spiniger Psp-Rex1          YTADFRYNSTSCYLQKFSDDSAIVGLITGDNDREYVTRGFVDWCQQNHLRINAGKTKEMVVDFRRKR 140
P. albonotatus Pab-Rex1C9     YTADFRYNSTYQKFSDGSAIVGLITGDNDREFKELTQGFVDWCQQNHLRINCGKTKTMVVDFRKH 140
P. albonotatus Pab-Rex1C6     YTADFRYNSPSCYLQKFSD---IVGLITDENNREYRELTGFVDWCQQNHLRINAGKTKEMAVDFRKR 139
P. albonotatus Pab-Rex1C12    YTADFRYNSPSCYLQKFSD-------------------------------------------R  67
P. ephippifer Pep-Rex1C11P3   YTADFRYNSPSCYLQKFSD---IVGLITDENNREYRELTWGFVDWCQQNHLRINAGKTKEMAVDFRKR 139
P. ephippifer Pep-Rex1C12P3   YTADFRYNSPSCYLQKFSD---IVGLITDENNREYRELTWGFVDWCQQNHLRINAGKTKEMAVDFRKR 139
P. ephippifer Pep-Rex1C13P3   YTADFRYNSPSCYLQNFQ---IVGLITSDNDREYRELTWGFVDWCQQN--------AGKTKEMVVDFRKR 135
AJ288466.1 clone Rex1-Anj     CTADFTHNSANCELQKFSDDSAIVS-ITDGDDREYRDLTQGFVDWCWNCGLQIWAGKTKEIVVDFRRCQQ 133
U18939.1 B. baikalensis       YTSDFKENSANCELQKFSDDSAIVGLISADIDNDREYRLNQDSLGWCORNRLQINSSKTKELVVDFRRGKR 140
AJ288450.1 clone Rex1-Xih     YTTDFQYNSPSCHLQKFSDDSAVVGCIGDGGEGEYRTLVDSFVEWSEQNHLRINISKTREMVIDFRRK 132
AJ288444.1 clone Rex1-Xih     YTTDFQYNSPSCHLQRFSDDSAVVGCIGDGGEGEYRTLVDSFVEWSDQNHLRLNISKTREMVIDFRRK 133
AJ288442.1 clone Rex1-Xih     YTTDFQYNSPSCHLQKFSDDSAVVGCIGDGGEGEYRALVDSFVEWSEQNHLRINICKTREMVIDFRRK 133
```

7

```
                                   150       160       170       180       190
                              ....|....|....|....|....|....|....|....|....|....|
P. ephippifer Pep-Rex1C1      P-SHPVVIQGTEIEVVRSYKYLGVLLNNKLDWAENINALQRKGQSRLFLLR 191
P. ephippifer Pep-Rex1C19     PPSHPVVIQGTDIEVVRSYKYLGVLLNNKLDWAENINALQRKGQSRLFLLR 191
P. aff. cuvieri Alenquer      PPEHPVVIQGGNIEVVKYKYWGVLLNNKLDWABNINALQRKGQVYQFLLR 191
P. albifrons Plb-Rex1         PPSHPVVIQGADIEVVKIYKYLGVLLNNKLDWAENINALQRKGQSRLFLLR 191
P. henselli Phe-Rex1          SPSQPVVIQGADIEVVKSYKYLGVLLNNKLDWAENINALQRKGQSRLFLLR 191
P. spiniger Psp-Rex1          PPAHPVVIQGTDIEVVKSYKYLGVLLNNKLDWAENINALHRKGQSRLFLLR 191
P. albonotatus Pab-Rex1C9     PPSQPVVIKRMDIEVVRSYKYLGVLLNNKLDWAENINALHRKGQSRLFLLR 191
P. albonotatus Pab-Rex1C6     ------VIQGTDIEVVKSYKY-GVLLNNK-DWARNINALQRKGQSRLFLLR 185
P. albonotatus Pab-Rex1C12    PPSQPVVIQGTDIEVEK----FCVLLNSKLDWAENINALFRKGQSRLFLLR 116
P. ephippifer Pep-Rex1C11P3   ------VIQGTDIEVVKSYKY-GVLLNNKQDWAENINALHRKGQSRLFLLR 185
P. ephippifer Pep-Rex1C12P3   ------VIQGTDIEVVKSYKY-GVLLNNKQDWAENINALHRKGQSRLFLLR 185
P. ephippifer Pep-Rex1C13P3   PPSKPVVIQGTYIEVVKYKYLGVLLNNKWTENINALHRKGQSRLFLLR 186
AJ288466.1 clone Rex1-Anj     SPPIPVNIQGMEIEWVKSYKYLGVHLNNKLDWTDDTNALYKKG------- 177
U18939.1 B. baikalensis       SPPLPLSIQGLDIE-VTSYKYLGVHLNNKLDWSDBAEALYKKGQSRLFLLR 191
AJ288450.1 clone Rex1-Xih     IPSRPLKIKGEVVEVEDYKYLGVVIGNRLDWASNTDAVCKG--------- 176
AJ288444.1 clone Rex1-Xih     TSSRPLKIKGEVVEVEDYKYLGVVIDNRLDWASNTDAVCKG--------- 177
AJ288442.1 clone Rex1-Xih     TSSRPKIKGEVVEVEDYKYLGVVIGNRLDWASNTDAVCKG--------- 177
```

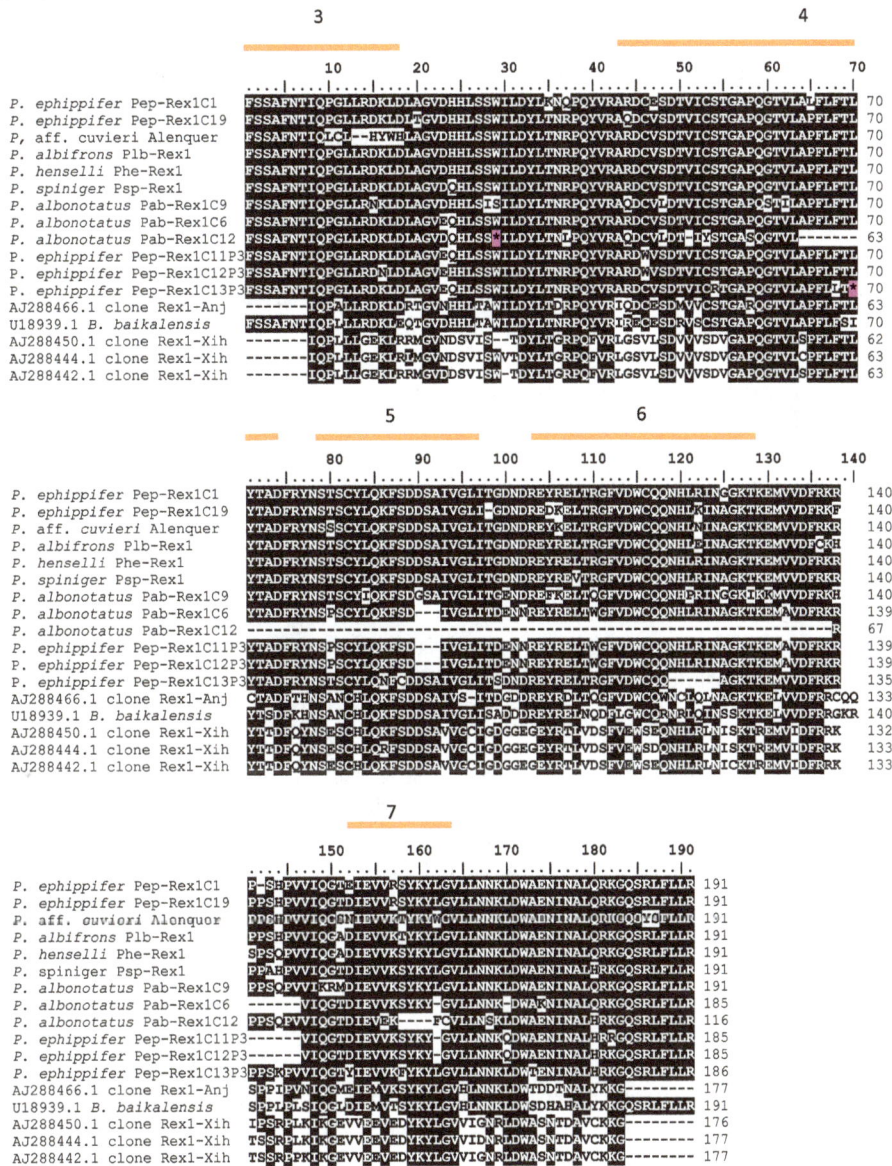

Fig. 2 Amino acid sequence inferred from the nucleotide sequences shown in Fig. 1. Black sites are conserved amino acids. Bars indicate domains 3–7 of the *Rex1* RT as determined by Volff and colleagues [8, 9] and Malik and colleagues [37]. Asterisks represent premature stop codons

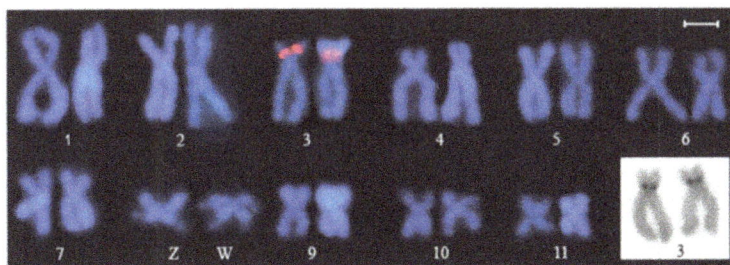

Fig. 3 Chromosome localization of the Pep-RexC17 sequence in the *Physalaemus ephippifer* karyotype. Note the hybridization signal in chromosome pair 3. The FITC-signals are shown in red for better visualization. The C-banded pair in the inset shows the band that coincides with the site detected by the *Rex1* probe and was thus microdissected for the isolation of some of the *Rex1* sequences shown in Fig. 1. Bar = 1 μm

the other sequences (from position 269 to position 274, and from position 421 to position 437 in Fig. 1).

PCR using primers for 5S rDNA resulted in the amplification of ~300-bp fragments from the microdissected 3p *per* band. Their nucleotide sequencing proved the presence of the 5S rRNA gene in this chromosome band (Fig. 4).

Discussion

The results described here suggest that the elements we isolated from the genus *Physalaemus* might represent part of the retroelement *Rex1*, or at least sequences derived from it. We have formed this hypothesize because the elements' nucleotide sequences and presumed amino acid sequences are highly similar to the previously described RT coding region sequences of *Rex1*, especially those from *Anguilla japonica* [9] and *Battrachocottus baikalensis* (GenBank accession number U18939.1 – see comment in Volff and colleagues [9]). Although Volff and colleagues [9] affirm that *Rex1/Babar* elements are somewhat related to the *CR1* element isolated from *Gallus gallus*, we could not detect any similarity between this element and the sequences isolated from species of *Physalaemus*.

The nucleotide sequences isolated from chromosome 3 of *Physalaemus ephippifer* and two of the three fragments isolated from *P. albonotatus* were similar to the RT-coding sequences of the *Rex1* elements; however, these sequences have deletions that may affect their presumed reading frame. For the sequence Pab-Rex1C12 of *P. albonotatus*, a premature stop codon was also detected. It is likely, therefore, that these sequences are no longer active retroelements. Interestingly, the truncated sequences isolated from *P. ephippifer* were isolated from the heterochromatic block at 3p per, and this chromosomal region was detected using *Rex1* probes in fluorescence in situ hybridization (FISH) assays. It is therefore reasonable to suggest that the loss of transposition ability may be related to mechanisms of accumulation of *Rex1*-derived sequences in this heterochromatic region. The accumulation of TEs in heterochromatin has been reported and

discussed by some authors [4, 19, 38–41]. Charlesworth & Langley [38] report that the suppression of heterochromatin crossing-over and gene inactivity are two factors that influence the preferential distribution of transposable sequences in such regions of the genome. For *P. ephippifer*, the molecular mechanisms involved in *Rex1*-derived sequences in 3p *per* were not investigated, but co-localization with 5S rDNA in FISH assays was an intriguing finding.

The association between TEs and rDNA sequences was already reported for many organisms. In arthropods, for example, R1 and R2 retrotransposable elements are components of the major rDNA [42, 43]. In the fish *Erythrinus erythrinus*, sequences belonging to the *Rex3* family were mapped at 5S rDNA sites and proposed to be involved in the spreading of 5S rDNA sequences in the genomes of some karyomorphs [43]. No evidence that supports the involvement of *Rex1* sequences in spreading of 5S rDNA in *Physalaemus* or any other anuran is available to date. The molecular nature of the association between these sequences (whether they are interspersed or form independent clusters that are sufficiently close to co-locate in FISH assays) as well as the evolutionary implications of this association are open questions for future studies.

Although in situ hybridization revealed a cluster of *Rex1* sequences at the heterochromatic band in the short arm of chromosome 3 of *Physalaemus ephippifer*, no other heterochromatic site in the karyotype of this species was detected by *Rex1* probes in FISH experiments. *Rex1* probes were unable to detect any chromosomal site in the karyotypes of *P. albonotatus*, *P. spiniger*, or *P. albifrons*. These findings diverge from those found for several species of fish, in which *Rex1*, *Rex3* and *Rex6* elements have been mapped to several heterochromatin sites [13, 14, 16, 19]. The FISH experiments suggest that in *Physalaemus* species, *Rex1* sequences are less abundant than those found for fish species. It is noteworthy that in the genome of anuran *Xenopus (Silurana) tropicalis*, non-LTR retrotransposons, including *Rex1*, *CR1* and *L2* elements, are estimated to correspond to only 0.6 % of the genome [23].

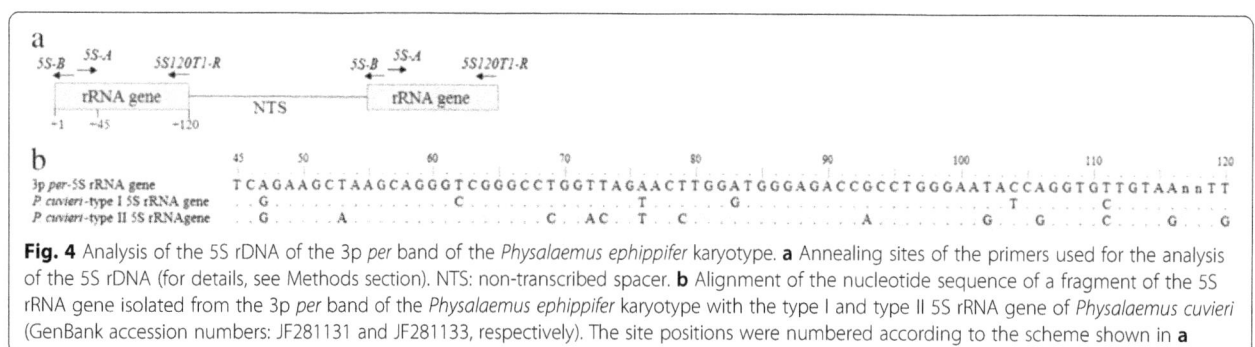

Fig. 4 Analysis of the 5S rDNA of the 3p *per* band of the *Physalaemus ephippifer* karyotype. **a** Annealing sites of the primers used for the analysis of the 5S rDNA (for details, see Methods section). NTS: non-transcribed spacer. **b** Alignment of the nucleotide sequence of a fragment of the 5S rRNA gene isolated from the 3p *per* band of the *Physalaemus ephippifer* karyotype with the type I and type II 5S rRNA gene of *Physalaemus cuvieri* (GenBank accession numbers: JF281131 and JF281133, respectively). The site positions were numbered according to the scheme shown in **a**

Conclusions

Our findings show that the *Rex1* family of retrotransposons is not restricted to *Xenopus tropicalis* and *Nanorana parkeri* but is also present in the leptodactylid genus *Physalaemus*. The occurrence of these TEs both in two basal lineages of Anura (*i.e.*, pipids and dicroglossids) and in a derived genus of Neobatrachia (*i.e.*, *Physalaemus*) suggests that this element could be largely distributed in anuran genomes. Although *Rex1* sequences were not highly clustered in the *Physalaemus* karyotypes, which differed from observations in fish species, we provided evidence for the accumulation of *Rex1* sequences in a heterochromatin site of the karyotype of *P. ephippifer* that associated with 5S rDNA sequences. Our results shed new light for further investigation into the evolutionary dynamics of both types of sequences in anuran genomes.

Methods

Samples

Individuals were used that belonged to the two major clades of *Physalaemus* (*i.e.*, *P. cuvieri* Clade and *P. signifer* Clade [26]). Samples of liver and muscle of *P. albonotatus* (*P. cuvieri* group), *P. albifrons* (*P. cuvieri* group), *P.* aff. *cuvieri* (*P. cuvieri* group), *P. ephippifer* (*P. cuvieri* group), *P. spiniger* (*P. signifer* Clade) and *P. henselii* (*P. henselii* group of the *P. cuvieri* Clade) were obtained from the tissue collection deposited at the Laboratory of Chromosomal Studies, at the Department of Structural and Functional Biology of the Institute of Biology, at the University of Campinas (UNICAMP) (Table 1). Metaphase chromosome preparations of *P. ephippifer* individuals from Belém-PA (ZUEC 13734♂; ZUEC 13740♂, ZUEC13741♀ and ZUEC 13705♂) were obtained from cell suspensions available at the same laboratory, previously obtained by Nascimento and colleagues [34]. The experiments were approved by the ethics committee CIBio/IB-UNICAMP (#2005/03).

Isolation of partial sequence of the retrotransposon Rex1 from genomic DNA

Samples of genomic DNA were isolated according to a procedure previously reported by Medeiros and colleagues [44] and subjected to PCR to isolate *Rex1* sequences. PCR assays were performed using the primers *RTX1-F1* (TTCTCCAGTGCCTTCAACACC) and *RTX1-R3* (TCCCTCAGCAGAAAGAGTCTGCTC) [9], which are specific for isolating a region of the gene encoding the RT (ORF 2) of the TE *Rex1*. The products of these reactions were analyzed after electrophoresis in a 1 % agarose gel. Bands corresponding to fragments of approximately 550 bp were observed in each case. For *Physalaemus albonotatus*, an additional band of fragments of approximately 350 bp was obtained. All of these bands were cut from the gel with sterile blades, and the DNA fragments were

Table 1 Identification, voucher number and locality of the specimens used for the isolation of the *Rex1* fragments

Species	Specimen voucher	Locality
Physalaemus albifrons (*P. cuvieri* group)	ZUEC 12361	Vassouras, Barreirinhas-MA, Brazil
Physalaemus albonotatus (*P. cuvieri* group)	ZUEC 16419	Lambari do Oeste-MT, Brazil
Physalaemus ephippifer (*P. cuvieri* group)	ZUEC 13705	Belém-PA, Brazil
Physalaemus aff. *cuvieri* (*P. cuvieri* group)	ZUEC 18191	Alenquer-PA, Brazil
Physalaemus henselii (*P. henselii* group)	MHNM 9512	Ruta 5, km 492, Pueblo Madera, Rivera, Uruguay
Physalaemus spiniger (*P. signifer* Clade)	ZUEC 14516	Reserva Salto Morato-Curitiba-PR, Brazil

ZUEC: Museu de Zoologia "Prof. Adão José Cardoso", Universidade Estadual de Campinas (UNICAMP), Campinas, São Paulo, Brasil. *MNHN*: Museo Nacional de Historia Natural de Montevideo. Uruguay. *PA*: State of Pará; *MT*: State of Mato Grosso; *MA*: State of Maranhão; *PR*: State of Paraná

purified with the GFX PCR and Gel Band DNA Purification kit (GE Healthcare).

Cloning of fragments of the retrotransposon Rex1 isolated from genomic DNA

The *Rex1* fragments amplified as described above were each inserted into the plasmid vector pGEM-T (Promega), following the manufacturer's instructions. The recombinant vectors were used to transform JM109 *Escherichia coli* competent cells using the cloning kit Transformaid Bacterial Transformation (Fermentas), following the manufacturer's directions. The positive clones were selected and used for extraction of plasmids, according to the mini-prep method described by Sambrook and colleagues [45]. For amplification of the inserts, samples of the isolated plasmids were used in PCR with T7 and SP6 universal primers. After purification with the GFX PCR and Gel Band DNA Purification kit (GE Healthcare), samples of the amplified inserts were sequenced using the BigDye Terminator kit (Applied Biosystems), according to the manufacturer's instructions. The sequences obtained were edited using BioEdit software [46], and compared to sequences available at the GenBank and Repbase databases. For comparison to sequences in the Repbase database, we used the CENSOR engine with default parameters, searching within the *Xenopus (Silurana) tropicalis* collection for *Rex1*.

Metaphase chromosome analyses

To obtain metaphase chromosome preparations of *Physalaemus ephippifer* (ZUEC 13740 and ZUEC 13741), cell suspensions available at the Laboratory of Chromosomal Studies, at the Department of Structural

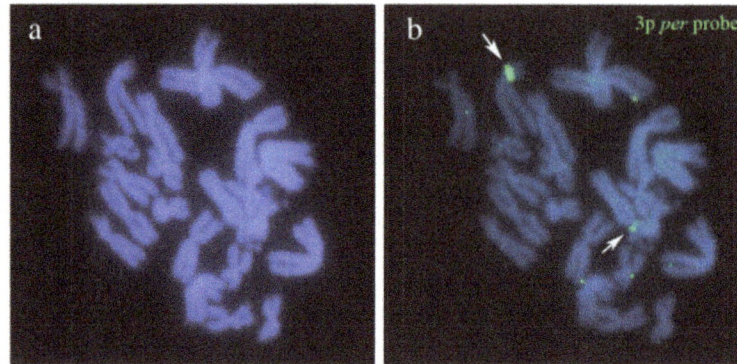

Fig. 5 *In situ* hybridization of a probe generated from the microdissection of the 3p *per* band of the karyotype of *Physalaemus ephippifer*. **a** DAPI image. **b** Merged DAPI and FISH images. Only the 3p *per* band (*arrows*) was detected

and Functional Biology of the Institute of Biology, at the University of Campinas (UNICAMP) were dropped onto clean slides. Cloned *Rex1* fragments generated from genomic DNA of *Physalaemus* species were labeled with dUTP-biotin (Roche®) by PCR and *in situ* hybridized to the karyotypes. The hybridization protocol [47] used an anti-biotin antibody (Vector) and a fluorescein isothiocyanate (FITC)-conjugated secondary antibody (Vector). The chromosomes were stained with DAPI (0.5 μg/mL).

Isolation of *Rex1* and 5S rDNA sequences from the microdissected 3p *per* band of *Physalaemus ephippifer*

To demonstrate that *Rex1* sequences are present in the pericentromeric C-band of the short arm of chromosome 3 of *Physalaemus ephippifer* (as suggested by FISH - see Results for details), which also bears 5S rDNA (as reported previously [34]), we isolated *Rex1* and 5S rDNA sequences from the microdissected 3p *per* band by PCR. For microdissection, cell suspensions of the *P. ephippifer* specimen ZUEC 13734 were dropped onto a membrane strip containing polyethylene-naphthalate (PEN) that was previously exposed to UV and incubated at −20 °C for 30 min. The material was subjected to C-banding according to a previously reported procedure [48]. The best metaphase examples were used for UV laser-microdissection of 18 copies of the heterochromatic pericentromeric region of the short arm of chromosome 3 of *P. ephippifer* with the MicroBeam 4.1 system (Zeiss). The cuts in the PEN membrane were made with UV at 0.5–0.6 μJ/pulse, and isolated regions were catapulted using a pulse of 0.2 μJ to the lid of a microtube containing 9 μL of TE buffer. The collected material was maintained in TE for at least 16 h and then subjected to PCR using the primers *RTX1-F1* and *RTX1-R3* [9] for the amplification of *Rex1* sequences and the primers *5S-A* (TACGCCCGATCTCGTCCGATC) and *5S-B* (5′-CAGGCTGGTATGGCCGTAAGC-3′) [49] for the amplification of 5S rDNA sequences. The amplified *Rex1* fragments were cloned and sequenced as

described above. Two rounds of PCR with the primers *5S-A* and *5S-B* were performed, and the amplified 5S rDNA fragments were directly sequenced using the primers *5S-A* [49] and *5S120T1-R* (AGCTTACAGCACCTGGTATTC) [50] (see the annealing sites of the primers in Fig. 4) and the BigDye Terminator kit (Applied Biosystems), according to the manufacturer's instructions.

To ensure that the microdissected regions correspond to the 3p *per* band, we used the captured DNA as probes in FISH assays. Therefore, the microdissected material was first amplified using GenomePlex Single Cell WGA4 (Sigma-Aldrich) and labeled with dUTP-biotin (Roche®) using GenomePlex Single Cell WGA3 (Sigma-Aldrich) (Fig. 5). The hybridization and probe detection protocols were the same as used with the *Rex1* probes (reported above).

Additional file

Additional file 1: Alignment of the fragments of the retroelement *Rex1* isolated from species of *Physalaemus* with corresponding sequences available in GenBank and Repbase. Note that the sequence CR1 of *Gallus gallus* (GenBank accession number U88211.1) significantly differs from all other sequences. The primers used to isolate the sequences are indicated in gray. Black areas indicate identical sites, while variable sites are colored white. Premature stop codons are shown in blue. U18939.1 is the GenBank accession number of a *Babar* sequence (a *Rex1*-related element) of *Battrachocottus baikalensis*. AJ288466.1, AJ288450.1, AJ288444.1 and AJ288442.1 are GenBank accession numbers of retroelement *Rex1* sequences isolated from *Anguilla japonica* (AJ288466.1) or *Xiphophorus helleri*. *Xenopus tropicalis* REX1-5, REX1-2 and REX1-3 are sequences isolated from *Xenopus tropicalis* and available at the Repbase database (http://www.girinst.org/censor/index.php). (DOCX 33 kb)

Competing interests

The authors declare that they have no competing interests.

Authors' contributions

JN obtained the sequences and chromosomal data and drafted the manuscript. DB collected some of the specimens and helped with the analyses. LBL designed and coordinated the study and drafted the manuscript. All authors have read and approved the final manuscript.

Acknowledgments

We thank the São Paulo Research Foundation (FAPESP) #2011/09239-0, Conselho Nacional de Desenvolvimento Científico e Tecnológico (CNPq) and Coordenadoria de Aperfeiçoamento de Pessoal de Nível Superior (CAPES/PROAP). We also thank Dr. Daniel Pacheco Bruschi for isolating and sequencing the Rex1 fragment of Physalaemus sp. from Alenquer-PA, Brazil.

Author details

[1]Departamento de Biologia Estrutural e Funcional, Instituto de Biologia, Universidade Estadual de Campinas, 13083-863 Campinas, São Paulo, Brazil. [2]Laboratorio de Genética Evolutiva, Instituto de Biología Subtropical (CONICET-UNaM), Facultad de Ciencias Exactas Químicas y Naturales, Universidad Nacional de Misiones, Félix de Azara 1552, CPA N3300LQF Posadas, Misiones, Argentina.

References

1. Frechotte C, Pritham JE. DNA transposons and evolution of eukaryotic genomics. Annu Rev Genet. 2007;41:331–69.
2. Jurka J, Kapitonov VV, Kohany O, Jurka VM. Repetitive sequences in complex genomes: structure and evolution. Annu Rev Genomics Hum Genet. 2007;8:241–59.
3. Muñoz-López M, García-Pérez JL. DNA transposon: nature and application in genome. Curr Genomics. 2010;11:115–28.
4. Kidwell MG. Transposable elements and the evolution of genome size in eukaryotes. Genetica. 2002;115:49–63.
5. González J, Petrov DA. Evolution of genome content: population dynamics of transposable elements in flies and humans. Methods Mol Biol. 2012;855:361–83.
6. Wicker T, Sabot F, Hua-van A, Bennetzen JL, Capy P, Chalhoub B, et al. A unified classification system for eukaryotic transposable elements. Nat Rev Genet. 2007;8:973–82.
7. Kapitonov VV, Jurka J. A universal classification of eukaryotic transposable elements implemented in Repbase. Nat Rev Genet. 2008;9:411–2. author reply 414.
8. Volff JN, Körting C, Sweeney K, Schartl M. The non-LTR retrotransposon Rex3 from the fish Xiphophorus is widespread among teleosts. Mol Biol Evol. 1999;16:1427–38.
9. Volff JN, Körting C, Schartl M. Multiple lineages of the non-LTR retrotransposon Rex1 with varying success in invading fish genomes. Mol Biol Evol. 2000;17:1684–4.
10. Volff JN, Körting C, Froschauer A, Sweeney K, Schartl M. Non-LTR retrotransposon encoding a restriction enzyme-like endonuclease in vertebrates. J Mol Evol. 2001;52:351–60.
11. Volff JN, Körting C, Meyer A, Schartl M. Evolution and discontinuous distribution of Rex3 retrotransposons in fish. Mol Biol Evol. 2001;18:427–31.
12. Dasilva C, Hadji H, Ozouf-Costaz C, Nicaud S, Jaillon O. Remarkable compartmentalization of transposable elements and pseudogenes in the heterochromatin of the Tetraodon nigroviridis genome. Proc Natl Acad Sci. 2002;99:13636–41.
13. Bouneau L, Fischer C, Ozouf-Costaz C, Froschauer A, Jailon O, Coutanceu JP, et al. An active Non-LTR retrotransposon with tamdem struture in the compact genome of the pufferfish Tetraodon nigroviridis. Genome Res. 2003;13:1686–95.
14. Ozouf-Costaz C, Brandt J, Körting C, Pisano E, Bonillo C, Coutanceau JP, et al. Genomes dynamics and chromosomal localization of the non-LTR retrotransposon Rex1 and Rex3 in Antartic fish. Antart Sci. 2004;16:51–7.
15. Gross MC, Schneider CH, Valente GT, Porto JIR, Martins C, Feldberg E. Comparative cytogenetic analysis of the genus of Symphysodon (discus fishes, Cichlidae): chromosomal characteristics of retrotransposons and minor ribosomal DNA. Cytogenet Genome Res. 2009;127:43–53.
16. Teixeira WG, Ferreira IA, Cabral-de-Mello DC, Mazzuchelli V, Pinhal GT, Poletto DAB, et al. Organization of the repeated DNA elements in the genome of the cichlid fish Cichla kelberi and its contributions to knowledge of fish genomes. Cytogenet Genome Res. 2009;125:224–34.
17. Mazzuchelli J, Martins C. Genomic organization of repetitive DNAs in the cichlid fish Astronotus ocellatus. Genetica. 2009;136:461–9.
18. Valente GT, Mazzucheli J, Ferreira IA, Poletto AB, Fantinatti BEA, Martins C. Cytogenetic mapping of retroelement Rex1, Rex3 and Rex6 among cichlid fish: new insights on the chromosomal distribution of transposable elements. Cytogenet Genome Res. 2011;133:34–42.
19. Schneider CH, Gross MC, Terencio ML, Do Carmo EJ, Martins C, Feldberg E. Evolutionary dynamics of retrotransposable elements Rex1, Rex3 and Rex6 in neotropical cichlid genomes. BMC Evol Biol. 2013;13:152.
20. Voltolin TP, Mendoça BB, Ferreira DC, Senhorini JA, Foresti F, Porto-Foresti F. Chromosomal localization Rex1 in the genome in five Prochilodus (Teleostei: Characiformes: Prochilodontidae) species. Mob Genet Elements. 2013;3:e25846.
21. Ferreira DC, Porto-Foresti F, Oliveira C, Foresti F. Transposable elements as potential source for understanding the fish genome. Mob Genet Elements. 2011;1:112–7.
22. Kapitonov VV, Jurka J. A family of Rex1 non-LTR retrotransposons from frogs – a consensus. Repbase Rep. 2009;9:1564–72.
23. Hellsten U, Harland RM, Gilchrist MJ, Hendrix D, Jurka J, Kapitonov V, et al. The genome of the Western clawed frog Xenopus tropicalis. Science. 2010;328:633–6.
24. Sun YB, Xiong ZJ, Xiang XY, Liu SP, Zhou WW, Tu XL, et al. Whole-genome sequence of the Tibetan frog Nanorana parkeri and the comparative evolution of tetrapod genomes. Proc Natl Acad Sci USA. 2015;2:E1257–1262.
25. Frost DR: Amphibian species of the world: an online reference. Version 6. 2015. Database accessible at http://research.amnh.org/herpetology/amphibia/index.html. American Museum of Natural History, New York, USA.
26. Lourenço LB, Targueta CP, Baldo D, Nascimento J, Garcia PCA, Andrade GA, et al. Phylogeny of Physalaemus (Anura, Leptodactylidae) inferred from mitochondrial and nuclear gene sequences. Mol Phylogenet Evol. 2015;92:204–16.
27. Beçak ML, Denaro L, Beçak W. Polyploidy and mechanisms of karyotypic diversification in Amphibia. Cytogenetics. 1970;9:225–38.
28. De Lucca EJ. Chromosomal studies in twelve species of Leptodactylidae and one Brachycephalidae. Caryologia. 1974;27:183–91.
29. Amaral MJLV, Cardoso AJ, Recco-Pimentel SM. Cytogenetic analysis of three Physalaemus species (Amphibia, Anura). Caryologia. 2000;53:283–8.
30. Silva APZ, Baldissera FA. Karyotypes and nucleolus organizer regions in four species of the genus Physalaemus (Anura, Leptodactylidae). Iheringia Ser Zool. 2000;88:159–64.
31. Quinderé YRSD, Lourenço LB, Andrade GV, Tomatis C, Baldo D, Recco-Pimentel SM. Polytypic and polymorphic cytogenetic variations in the widespread anuran Physalaemus cuvieri (Anura, Leiuperidae) with emphasis on nucleolar organizing regions. Biol Res. 2009;42:79–92.
32. Vittorazzi SE, Quinderé YRSD, Recco-Pimentel SM, Tomatis C, Baldo D, Lima JRF, et al. Comparative cytogenetics of Physalaemus albifrons and Physalaemus cuvieri species groups (Anura, Leptodactylidae). Comp Cytogenet. 2014;8:103–23.
33. Milani M, Cassini CS, Recco-Pimentel SM, Lourenço LB. Karyotypic data detect interpopulational variation in Physalemus olfersii and in first case of supernumerary chromosome in the genus. Anim Biol J. 2011;2:21–8.
34. Nascimento J, Quinderé YRSD, Recco-Pimentel SM, Lima JRF, Lourenço LB. Heterorphic Z and W sex chromosomes in Physalaemus ephippifer (Steindachner, 1864) (Anura, Leiuperidae). Genetica. 2010;138:1127–32.
35. Tomatis C, Baldo D, Kolenc F, Borteiro C. Chromosomal variation in the species of the Physalaemus henselii Group (Anura: Leiuperidae). J Herpetol. 2009;43:555–60.
36. Provete DB, Garey MV, Toledo LF, Nascimento J, Lourenço LB, Rossa-Feres DC, et al. Redescription of Physalaemus barrioi Bokermann, 1966 (Anura: Leiuperidae). Copeia. 2013;3:507–18.
37. Malik HS, Burke WD, Eickbush TH. The age and evolution of non-LTR retrotransposable elements. Mol Biol Evol. 1999;6:793–805.
38. Charlesworth B, Langley CH. The population genetics of Drosophila transposable elements. Annu Rev Genet. 1989;23:251–87.
39. Dimitri P, Junakovic N. Revising the selfish DNA hypothesis: new evidence on accumulation of transposable elements in heterochromatin. Trends Genet. 1999;15:123–4.
40. Hua-Van A, LeRouzic A, Tribaud SB, Filée J, Capy P. The struggle for life of genome's selfish architects. Biol Direct. 2011;6:19.
41. Jakubczak JL, Burke WD, Eickbush TH. Retrotransposable elements R1 and R2 interrupt the rRNA genes of most insects. Proc Natl Acad Sci. 1991;88:3295–9.
42. Zhang X, Eickbush MT, Eickbush TH. Role of recombination in the long-term retention of transposable elements in rRNA gene loci. Genetics. 2008;180:1617–26.
43. Cioffi MB, Martins C, Bertollo LAC. Chromosome spreading of associated transposable elements and ribosomal DNA in the fish Erythrinus erythrinus.

Implications for genome change and karyotype evolution in fish. BMC Evol
Biol. 2010;10:271.

44. Medeiros LR, Lourenço LB, Rossa-Feres DC, Lima AL, Andrade GV, Giaretta AA,
    et al. Comparative cytogenetic analysis of some species of the *Dendropsophus
    microcephalus* group (Anura, Hylidae) in the light of phylogenetic inferences.
    BMC Genet. 2013;14:59.

45. Sambrook J, Fritsch EF, Maniatis T: Molecular Cloning: A Laboratory Manual.
    New York: Cold Spring Harbor Press; 1989.

46. Hall TA. BioEdit: A user-friendly biological sequence alignment editor and
    analysis program for Windows 95/98/NT. Nucl Acids Symp Ser. 1999;41:95–8.

47. Viegas-Péquignot E. In situ hybridization to chromosomes with biotinylated
    probes. In: Willernson D, editor. In Situ Hybridization: A Practical Approach.
    Oxford: IRL Press; 1992. p. 137–58.

48. King M. C-banding studies on Australian hylid frogs: secondary constriction
    structure and the concept of euchromatin transformation. Chromosoma.
    1980;80:191–217.

49. Pendás AM, Morán P, Freije JP, Garcia-Vázquez E. Chromosomal mapping
    and nucleotide sequence of two tandem repeats of Atlantic salmon 5S
    rDNA. Cytogenet Cell Genet. 1994;67:31–6.

50. Rodrigues DS, Rivera M, Lourenço LB. Molecular organization and
    chromosomal localization of 5S rDNA in Amazonian Engystomops (Anura,
    Leiuperidae). BMC Genet. 2012;13:17.

24

Nucleolus-like body of mouse oocytes contains lamin A and B and TRF2 but not actin and topo II

Galina N. Pochukalina[1], Nadya V. Ilicheva[1*], Olga I. Podgornaya[1,2,3] and Alexey P. Voronin[1,2]

Abstract

Background: During the final stages of oocyte development, all chromosomes join in a limited nuclear volume for the final formation of a single complex chromatin structure – the karyosphere. In the majority of mammalian species, the chromosomes surround a round protein/fibrillar body known as the central body, or nucleolus-like body (NLB). Nothing seems to unite the inner portion of the karyosphere with the nucleolus except position at its remnants. Nevertheless, in this study we will use term NLB as the conventional one for karyosphere with the central body. At the morphological level, NLBs consist of tightly-packed fibres of 6–10 nm. The biochemical structure of this dense, compact NLB fibre centre remains uncertain.

Results: The aim of this study was to determine which proteins represent the NLB components at final stages of karyosphere formation in mouse oogenesis. To determine this, three antibodies (ABs) have been examined against different actin epitopes. Examination of both ABs against the actin N-end provided similar results: spots inside the nucleus. Double staining with AB against SC35 and actin revealed the colocalization of these proteins in IGCs (interchromatin granule clusters/nuclear speckles/SC35 domains). In contrast, examination of polyclonal AB against peptide at the C-end reveals a different result: actin is localized exclusively in connection with the chromatin. Surprisingly, no forms of actin or topoisomerase II are present as components of the NLB. It was discovered that: (1) lamin B is an NLB component from the beginning of NLB formation, and a major portion of it resides in the NLB at the end of oocyte development; (2) lamin A undergoes rapid movement into the NLB, and a majority of it remains in the NLB; (3) the telomere-binding protein TRF2 resides in the IGCs/nuclear speckles until the end of oocyte development, when significant part of it transfers to the NLB.

Conclusions: NLBs do not contain actin or topo II. Lamin B is involved from the beginning of NLB formation. Both Lamin A and TRF2 exhibit rapid movement to the NLB at the end of oogenesis. This dynamic distribution of proteins may reflect the NLB's role in future chromatin organization post-fertilisation.

Keywords: Mouse oogenesis, Morphology, Karyosphere, Nucleolus-like body, Immunofluorescence

Background

The mammalian oocyte nucleus or germinal vesicle (GV) exhibits a unique chromatin configuration that is subject to dynamic modifications during oogenesis. This process of epigenetic maturation is critical in conferring the female gamete with meiotic as well as developmental competence. In spite of its biological significance, little is known concerning the cellular and molecular mechanisms regulating large-scale chromatin structure in mammalian oocytes [1].

The epigenetic maturation morphologically appears to be the result of all chromosomes of the gametocyte joining in a limited nuclear volume with final formation of a single complex chromatin structure – the karyosphere. The karyosphere was named and first described by Blackman [2], who observed that the chromosomes in the spermatocytes of millipedes (Chilopoda) join to form a knot. The karyosphere is a form of chromosomal apparatus that sometimes exists for long periods of time within the oocytes of many animals, from hydra to higher

* Correspondence: nad9009@yandex.ru
[1]Institute of Cytology, Russian Academy of Sciences, St Petersburg 194064, Russia
Full list of author information is available at the end of the article

vertebrates [3]. The term "karyosphere" has been suggested to designate the complex of a former nucleolus (also referred to as NLB), adjacent chromatin, and the adjacent nuclear bodies (including IGCs) in human GV oocytes [4]. However, although lampbrush chromosomes (which often precede karyosphere formation) have been discussed in numerous studies, karyosphere formation has received considerably less attention. The active state of the nucleus is succeeded by a decrease in the transcriptional activity of chromosomes and nucleoli, and the accumulation of chromosomes into a karyosphere. It is thought that karyosphere formation is the result of chromosomal inactivation in respect of RNA synthesis [5]. The morphological appearance of the karyosphere varies in the animal kingdom, though two main plans become evident: (1) karyosphere formation is paralleled by the appearance of newly-formed capsule-shaped structure around the chromosomes – karyosphere capsule (KC); (2) the chromosomes surround the round protein/fibrillar body – the central body [6] or nucleolus like body (NLB) [3]. It is generally assumed that the KC represents a specialized component of the oocyte nuclear matrix (NM) supporting the chromosomes of large GVs [5].

Sequential changes occurring in chromatin organization during folliculogenesis in mice has been described as the formation of a perinucleolar chromatin rim in the GV [7]. In the case of mouse oogenesis, other terms have been utilised to describe the changes. Chromatin in developing mouse oocytes is initially found decondensed, in a configuration termed the non-surrounded nucleolus (NSN). Subsequent growth leads to chromatin becoming progressively condensed, forming a heterochromatin rim in close apposition with the nucleolus remnants – thus acquiring a configuration termed surrounded nucleolus (SN) [3].

The oocytes' transcriptional reduction is followed by the transformation of the nucleolar structure; the nucleolus gradually loses all of its classical components [8, 9], transforming into the structure known as a NLB. The NLB with chromatin surrounding the central body represents feature of many mammalians, including humans [3, 4, 8, 10]. Recently, several reviews of large-scale chromatin organization in mammalian oocytes have been published [11, 12].

Nothing seems to unite the inner portion of the karyosphere with the nucleolus except position at its remnants. NLB does not exhibit an argentophilic reaction [13]. The fibrillar component of the NLB central body consists of acid proteins. At the morphological level, NLB consists of tightly-packed fibres of 6-10 nm [3]. Some nucleolar proteins have been observed to move from the NLB into tiny granules at its periphery, and then in the nucleoplasm [3]. Few proteins, which are considered markers for the different nuclear compartments,

have been found at the NLB periphery or in its vacuole: coilin, polymerase II, and splicing factors [3, 9]. Recently, the following nucleolar proteins have been discovered in the dense fibre centre of NLB, under special treatments: UBF, fibrillarin, NPM1, C23 [14, 15], NPM2 [16], and RPL26 [15]. This study investigates the presence of alternate protein components of the NLB.

The antibodies used were based on the assumption that the NLB could be a specialized component of the oocyte NM in the same manner as the karyosphere capsule. F-actin was revealed as a basic component of the KC in several insects [17–19] and also in frogs [20]. It has been shown that actin also has a crucial role in the maintenance of oocyte nuclear architectonics, and its depolymerization leads to a collapse of nuclear structures [21, 22].

One of the best-characterized extrachromasomal protein bodies, IGCs, often abut the mouse NLB [23]. IGCs are suggested as one of the most universal and evolutionarily-conserved nuclear domains [24, 25]. They primarily represent nuclear storage sites for pre-mRNA splicing factors [3, 26, 27], though extensive studies conducted during the past two decades have introduced the notion that IGC functions are broader than initially thought; these domains are involved in many other nuclear processes directly connected with gene expression and nuclear architecture [3, 25], and could participate in NLB formation.

Topoisomerase II (topo II) was one of the first NM proteins to be identified [28, 29]. Type II topoisomerases are archetypal nucleic acid remodelling enzymes that, using ATP as a cofactor, can varyingly add or remove DNA supercoils and either form or unlink DNA tangles [30]. Several studies on vertebrate systems indicate that this enzyme plays a role in the shaping of mitotic chromatin: topo II is the main factor in chromosome condensation, and represents a component of the chromosome core [31]. Topo II could be involved in the condensation process when chromatin is highly condensed around the NLB.

The nuclear lamina consists of lamins, which belong to type V intermediate filament proteins [32]. Lamins are categorized into two types, A and B, based on their biochemical and sequence characteristics. Small, yet significant fractions of both A- and B-type lamins are also present throughout the nuclear interior during interphase. Some of these internal lamins may be nascent proteins that were recently transported from the cytoplasm and in preparation for assembly into the lamina [33]. Several independent lines of experiments suggest that the A- and B-type lamins form separate filamentous networks in the lamina of somatic cells. High resolution confocal microscopy suggests that each type of lamin forms a distinct meshwork structure with a relatively small number of points of colocalization in somatic cells [34]. The same is true for oocytes. Based on electron microscopy, it is evident that overexpressed lamin A and lamin B2 form different types of filaments in separate intranuclear compartments of Xenopus oocyte nuclei. Lamin B2 formed irregular, wavy filaments associated with intranuclear membrane structures induced by the expression of lamin B2. In contrast, lamin A formed thick, multi-layered assemblies of filaments closely associated with the endogenous lamina formed by lamin B3 [35]. This was the reason for the utilisation of antibodies against both lamin A and lamin B.

The nuclear lamina and the internal nuclear matrix (NM) are two parts of the NM preparations [36]. The NM is a network dispersed throughout the nucleus, which is operationally defined as being resistant to high salt or detergents, i.e. insoluble [37]. Since it is associated with protein machinery for transcription, RNA splicing, and DNA replication, NM is believed to play a fundamental role in the organization of these processes [36, 38]. We will use term "nuclear matrix" (NM) in the current paper, as a NM preparation was initially used for mouse TRF2 isolation.

Telomeric binding factor 2 (TRF2) was discovered in the outer fraction of the NM, i.e. nuclear lamina [39], and was originally isolated from the nuclear envelope of frog oocytes [40]. The attachment of telomeres to the nuclear envelope in meiosis, and the resulting "bouquet" formation are thought to promote proper chromosome pairing via the concentration of chromosome attachment sites within a limited region of the nucleus [41]. This attachment undoubtedly occurs in germ cells during the central meiotic phases [42], though latter frog oocyte chromosomes are packed into a tight karyosphere with KC. Oocytes were collected at the stage when chromosomes are separated from the envelope, but it was assumed that the protein of interest remained associated with it. As a result, a membrane-associated telomere-binding protein (MTBP) was discovered. The protein exhibited binding specificity to telomeric DNA, and anti-MTBP antibodies (AB) were raised in guinea pig [40, 43, 44].

Two vertebrate proteins which bind to double-stranded telomeric DNA have been described: TRF1 [45, 46] and TRF2 [47, 48]. Six core proteins: TRF1, TRF2, TIN2, POT1, TPP1 and Rap1, form the telosome or shelterin complex, regulating telomere structure and function [49]. Both TRF1 and 2 contain a specific Myb-related protein motif - telobox peptide [47]. It is assumed that TRF2's main role is to protect telomeres from DNA repair activities, which would prevent chromosomal aberrations involving chromosome ends such as end-to-end fusion [50, 51].

TRF2 is tightly bound to the nuclear membrane in frog oocyte nuclei [43], in the nuclear envelope and its remnants in mouse cells [39]. Lamin B was used as the protein marking the nuclear envelope remnant. Lamin B (a protein associated with the nuclear envelope remnants during mitosis) [52], and TRF2 colocalised as demonstrated by the double AB labelling. TRF2 antibodies were used to check protein position with respect to the NLB.

The aim of this study was to determine which proteins compose the NLB's central body during the final stages of karyosphere formation in mouse oogenesis.

Methods

Oocytes

Female Balb/C mice were purchased from the Rappolovo Breeding Centre of the Russian Academy of Medical Sciences (Rappolvo, Russia). Preovulatory oocytes from the antral follicles of sexually mature mice (one to two months of postnatal development) were used. The cumulus-enclosed oocytes were collected from ovaries by gentle puncturing of antral follicles with a needle in 4 % formaldehyde, freshly-prepared from paraformaldehyde in a phosphate-buffered saline (PBS) solution to prevent the resumption of meiosis. Oocytes were subsequently incubated in 0.1 % Triton X-100 in phosphate-buffered saline (PBS) for 10 min. Overall, approximately 300 oocytes were used in this study, and 10 oocytes were used for each treatment. All experimental treatments contained oocytes from three to five different mice. All experiments were repeated at least three times.

Antibodies

The following primary antibodies (ABs) were utilized in this study: mouse monoclonal antibody (mAb) against non-snRNP splicing factor SC35 (Sigma; cat. no. S4045; dilution for immunofluorescence (IF) 1:50); mouse mAb against lamin A (Abcam; cat. no. ab8980; dilution for IF 1:100, for Western blot (WB) 1:500); rabbit polyclonal antibody (pAb) against TRF2 (Abcam; cat. no. ab 4182; dilution for IF 1:100, for WB 1:2000); rabbit pAb against topo II (Sigma; cat. no. AV04007; dilution for IF 1:200); rabbit pAb against a synthetic peptide conjugated to KLH derived from within residues 400 - 500 of Mouse lamin B1 (Abcam; cat. no. ab16048; dilution for IF 1:100, for WB 1:3000). ABs against different actin parts: mouse mAb against actin N-end (amino acid residues 50-70) (Millipore; cat. no. MAB1501R; dilution for IF 1:50); rabbit pAb against actin N-end (the first nine amino acid residues of the N-terminal region of actin) (Sigma; cat. no. A2103; dilution for IF 1:200); rabbit pAb against actin C-end (peptide of 11 amino acid residues AGP-SIVHRKCF) (Sigma, cat. no. A2066, dilution for IF 1:200). It is known that AB MAB1501R reacts with all actin isoforms on immunoblot [53] and AB PAB A2066 was successfully used in immunoblot and immune-gold electron microscopy [21].

The antibody mixture was used for double staining of oocyte preparations [54]. Secondary antibodies were the Alexa-488 or Alexa-568 conjugated goat anti-mouse, goat anti-rabbit, rabbit anti-mouse immunoglobulins (IgGs) (Molecular probes; dilution 1:200). Secondary antibodies for Western blot were the anti-mouse IgG (whole molecule)-alkaline phosphatase antibody produced in goat (Sigma, cat. no. A3562) and the anti-rabbit IgG (whole molecule)-alkaline phosphatase antibody produced in goat (Sigma, cat. no. A3687; dilution 1:10000).

Immunoblotting

The method for mouse liver nuclei isolation has already been described [55, 56]. Briefly, liver tissue was homogenised in ten volumes of pH 7.5 solution containing 0.32 M sucrose, 25 mM Tris-HCl, 5 mM $MgCl_2$, and 1 mM PMSF. After centrifugation at 1000 rpm, raw nuclei were loaded onto a 2 M sucrose cushion and pelleted at 100,000 g ($+4^0$ C) for 40 min. The preparations were checked for purity by phase-contrast microscopy, and the pure nuclei were used for Western blot to inspect the ABs. SDS-PAGE was conducted as described in a previous study [57]. The products were transferred to immobilon polyvinylidene fluoride transfer membrane (Millipore, Hertfordshire, UK) by Electroblot (BioRad Lab Ltd, Hertfordshire, UK) at 50 mA in an electrophoresis buffer containing 10 % ethanol. Blocking was conducted using 5 % skimmed milk for 1 hr in PBS (137 mM NaCl, 2.7 mM KCl, 10 mM Na_2HPO_4, 1.76 mM KH_2PO_4, pH 7.4) with 0.05 % Tween 20 (Sigma). This basic solution was used for all AB experiments. The first ABs, appropriately diluted in PBS-Tween buffer, were applied overnight at +4 °C. After washing with PBS-Tween, the blots were incubated with either anti-rabbit or anti-mouse alkaline phosphatase for 1 hr at room temperature, then stained with NBT-BCIP in a solution of 50 mM Tris-HCl (pH 9.5), 5 mM MgCl2, and 100 mM NaCl for around 30 min. Alkaline phosphatase added without first AB gave no staining.

Immunofluorescence/confocal microscopy

Indirect immunofluorescent cytochemistry was conducted on total preparations of isolated oocytes using the method described in detail in previous papers [9, 58]. The incubation of the first antibody solution was conducted overnight in a moist chamber at 4 °C. After rinsing in PBS, the preparations were incubated with secondary antibodies for 1.5 h at room temperature. After rinsing in PBS, the preparations were additionally stained for 1 min with DAPI (Molecular probes; dilution 1:1000) to reveal DNA, and mounted in Vectashield medium (Vector Laboratories). Preparations were analysed in a Leica TCS SP5 confocal microscope equipped with argon (488 nm) and heliumneon (543 and 633 nm) lasers at 40x objective (NA 1.25).

Merged images were obtained using ImageJ 1.37a software (National Institutes of Health).

Immuno-gold electron microscopy

Oocyte fixation and embedding for electron microscopy were performed using a routine technique [4]. Oocytes were prefixed for 1.5 h in a solution containing 4 % formaldehyde (Ted Pella, Redding, Calif., USA) and 0.5 % glutaraldehyde in PBS, then fixed overnight in 2 % formaldehyde at 4 °C. After rinsing in PBS containing 0.05 M NH_4Cl (Sigma) and subsequent dehydration in an ethanol series, oocytes were embedded in medium grade LR White resin (Polyscience, Warrington, Pa., USA). Ultrathin sections were incubated for 10 min in a blocking buffer containing 0.5 % fish gelatin (Sigma) and 0.02 % Tween-20 (Sigma) in PBS (pH 7.4). Sections were then incubated in the primary antibody solution overnight in a moist chamber at 4 °C. After rinsing in PBS containing 0.1 % fish gelatin and 0.05 % Tween-20, the sections were incubated with secondary goat anti-mouse and goat anti-rabbit IgGs conjugated with 10 nm gold particles (Electron Microscopy Sciences, USA). As a control, additional sections were incubated only in secondary antibodies. Ultrathin sections were contrasted with 1 % uranyl acetate-water solution and examined in a Carl Zeiss Libra 120 electron microscope operated at 80 kV. Magnification was inserted to the images automatically. The figures were prepared in Adobe Photoshop (Adobe Systems).

Results
Immunoblotting

The main antibodies (ABs) used in this study were examined using Western blot (Fig. 1). ABs against TRF2 do not have cross-reactivity with TRF1. The band correspond to the apparent molecular mass (Mr) of 70 kDa while TRF1 Mr is 60 kDa [43, 59]. ABs against Lamin A and Lamin B also do not react with the opposite type. Therefore, these ABs could be used to trace their corresponding proteins. AB (mAb) against splicing factor SC35 was successfully utilized in previous studies to trace IGCs in somatic mouse cells [60]. All three ABs against actin stain one band of ~42 kDa on Westernblot, though their advantage is the possibility to recognize different actin epitopes, which is beyond Western blot's resolution. Western blot could not distinguish which domain is stained on immunoblot. Therefore, reliance existed upon commercial descriptions or the existing literature published (see Material and Methods).

Cumulus cells

Mouse oocytes grow in multilayer follicles composed of cumulus cells, which could always be found in preparations. Cumulus cells were used as an example in order to trace the typical staining of somatic cells. It is evident

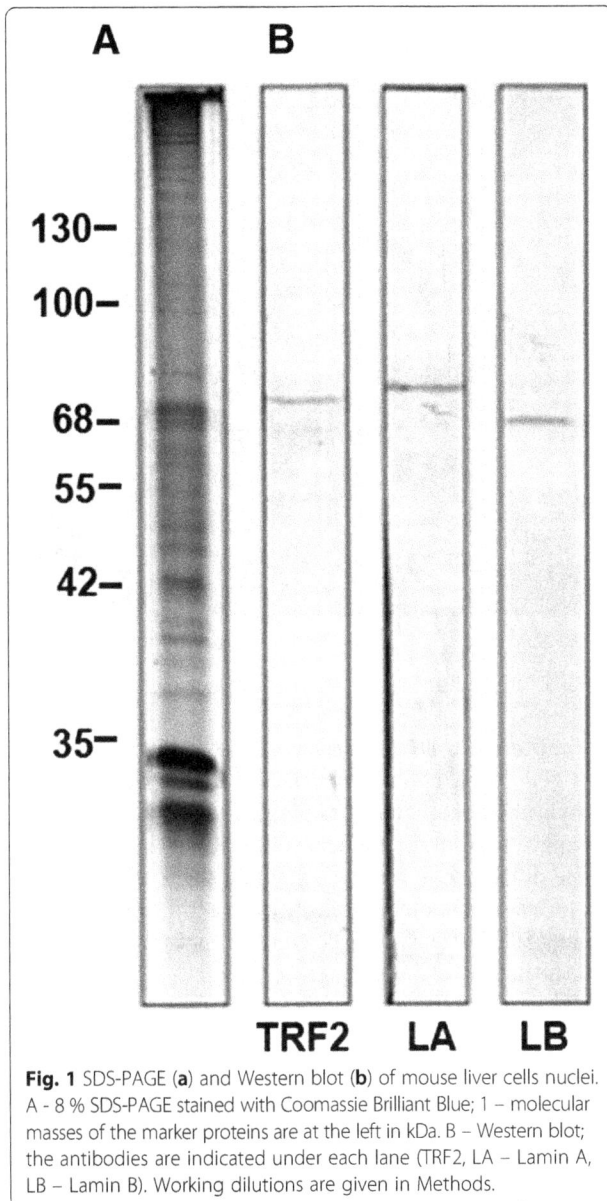

Fig. 1 SDS-PAGE (**a**) and Western blot (**b**) of mouse liver cells nuclei. A - 8 % SDS-PAGE stained with Coomassie Brilliant Blue; 1 – molecular masses of the marker proteins are at the left in kDa. B – Western blot; the antibodies are indicated under each lane (TRF2, LA – Lamin A, LB – Lamin B). Working dilutions are given in Methods.

input in gene silencing [63], but lamin B1 is mainly immobile. This suggests that the internal B-type lamins are tightly associated with other relatively immobile structures such as heterochromatin [34].

TRF2 locations in somatic [44] and spermatogenic [64, 65] cells have been determined. It has been suggested that TRF2 possesses intimate connections with the nuclear envelope [66]. Mouse chromosomes are telocentric, with the centromere located adjacently to one of the two telomeres. The telomeric and centromeric regions of chromosomes form the heterochromatic material, and are therefore involved in chromocentre formation. The TRF2 location in cumulus cells corresponds to the one previously observed: a portion of the TRF2 label is at the NE and another portion is at the rim of the inner chromocentres (Fig. 2, TRF2).

As a result, it is evident that ABs work at immunoblot and exhibit the expected positions in somatic cells.

Oocytes' stages classification

The oocyte nucleus is subjected to important and relatively rapid nuclear architecture modifications during late growth stages. Chromatin is visible on the DAPI stained images, and stages of oocyte development could be determined from the NLB position – being central at the stage 1 (Fig. 3, 1). The characteristic feature of oocyte development, the karyosphere traced by the NLB moves toward the NE at stage 3 from its central position at stage 1 (Fig. 3). The final steps of the karyosphere formation are divided into 3 stages for descriptive purposes, and follow the classification published [67, 68]. In 1st stage oocytes, euchromatin exhibits a decondensed configuration, with heterochromatin aggregates distinguished as chromocentres (Fig. 3, 1). In intermediate stage 2 (Fig. 3, 2) the karyosphere displays a mixed configuration in between the 1st and 3rd stages, with decondensed chromatin in the nucleoplasm and only a partial ring of chromatin around the NLB. At stage 3 (Fig. 3, 3), chromatin is highly-condensed and forms a ring around the NLB.

Nuclear actin

In somatic cells, actin filaments form part of a large, viscoelastic structure in the nucleoplasm, and may act as scaffolds which help to organize nuclear contents [69]. It is reasonable to assume that structural proteins could be NLB components. Therefore, three types of ABs against actins' different domains were used to trace the different forms of actin which can exist within the oocyte nucleus.

During all stages of oocyte development, both ABs against actin N-end exhibited similar results: spots inside nucleus (GV). Double staining with AB against SC35 and actin revealed the colocalization of these proteins in IGCs (Fig. 4 a, b). This perfect correspondence is visible

that cumulus cells' nuclei possess prominent chromocentres, as is characteristic for somatic mouse cells [61]. DNA staining highlighted the alignment of chromocentres mainly at the border of the nuclei, and a number of them were located in the nuclei interior. Chromatin arranged into distinct radial zones which could be determined after DAPI staining. Ordered radial alignment of chromocentres has been observed for chickens [62], and similar arrangement could be traced on some of our images (Fig. 2, DNA).

Lamins A and B represent necessary components of the somatic cells' nuclear envelope (NE), though staining with ABs is different. Lamin A mostly underlines the NE (Fig. 2, LA), while lamin B gravitates toward chromocentres (Fig. 2, LB). Both lamin types are known for their

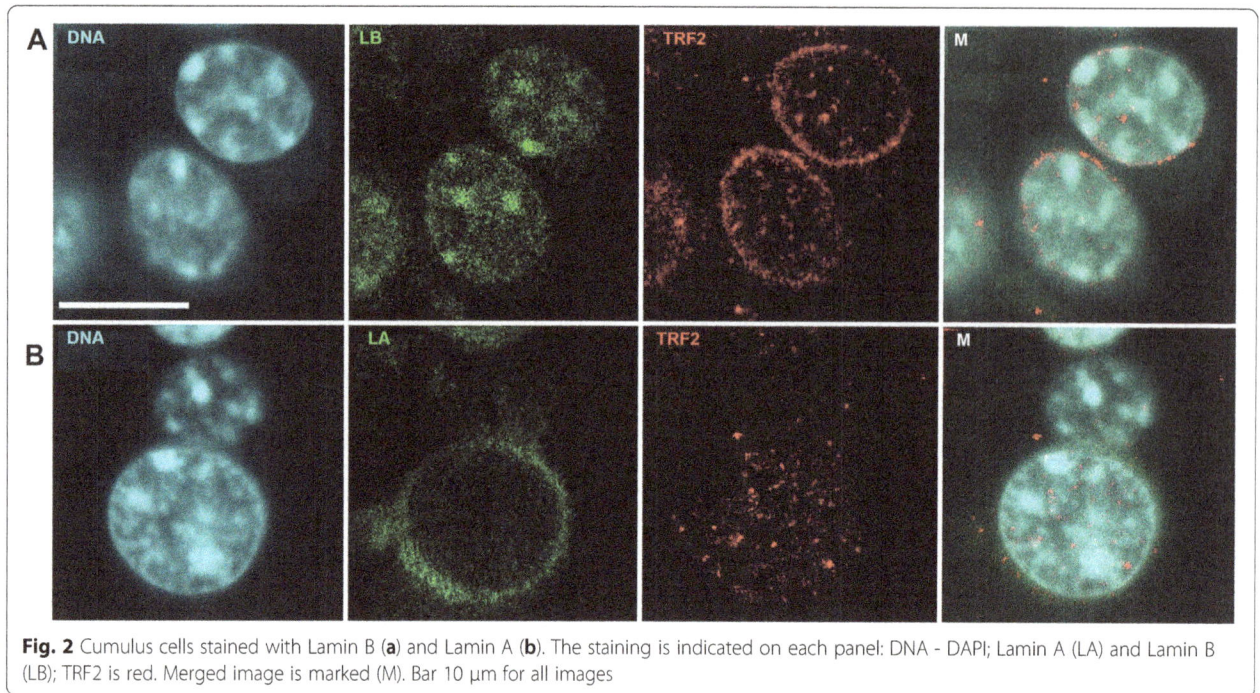

Fig. 2 Cumulus cells stained with Lamin B (**a**) and Lamin A (**b**). The staining is indicated on each panel: DNA - DAPI; Lamin A (LA) and Lamin B (LB); TRF2 is red. Merged image is marked (M). Bar 10 μm for all images

in the case of AB MAB1501R against 20 amino acid residues at actin N end (Fig. 4, a). Polyclonal AB against the first 9 amino acid residues at the actin N-end also reveals actin in IGCs, though nuclear envelope is also underlined (Fig. 4, b). Some diffuse staining around the nucleus in the cytoplasm was also observed. In contrast, polyclonal AB against peptide at the C-end reveals a different result: actin exclusively followed chromatin detected by DAPI staining. IGCs contain only the marker protein SC35. AB A2066 reveals only the actin colocalized with the chromatin. Both types of the chromatin are stained: the diffuse part and the one parked in

chromocentres. This is clearly visible in the merged images (Fig. 4, c, M). These ABs recognize nuclear actin exclusively, without any staining in the cytoplasm or in the space surrounding nuclei (Fig. 4, C vs. B).

The difference in actin AB staining suggests that different forms of monomeric (oligomeric) actin exist in oocyte nuclei [70], but not a single form of actin is involved in NLB formation.

Topo II

Topo II was identified within the chromosome scaffold fraction. Immunostaining of unextracted chromosomes

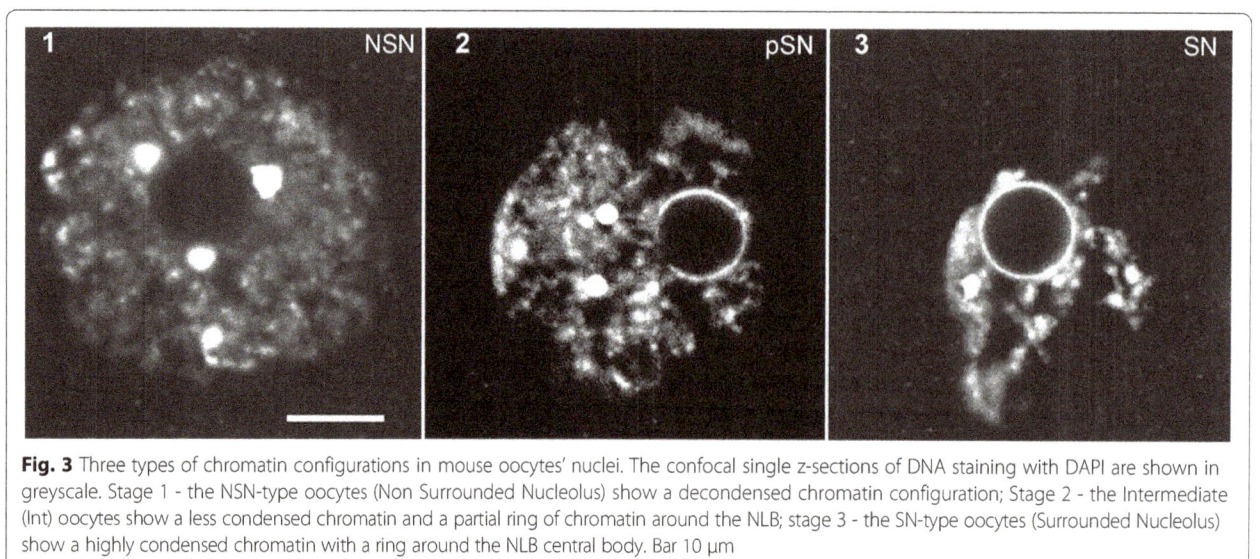

Fig. 3 Three types of chromatin configurations in mouse oocytes' nuclei. The confocal single z-sections of DNA staining with DAPI are shown in greyscale. Stage 1 - the NSN-type oocytes (Non Surrounded Nucleolus) show a decondensed chromatin configuration; Stage 2 - the Intermediate (Int) oocytes show a less condensed chromatin and a partial ring of chromatin around the NLB; stage 3 - the SN-type oocytes (Surrounded Nucleolus) show a highly condensed chromatin with a ring around the NLB central body. Bar 10 μm

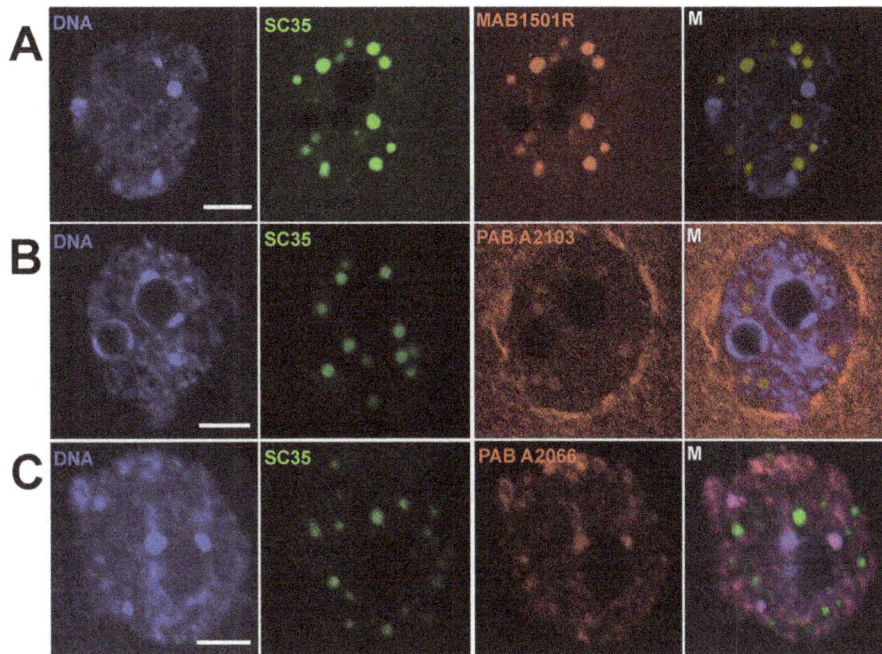

Fig. 4 Double immunofluorescence of oocytes' nuclei with SC35 AB (green) and three ABs against actin (red). **a** – 1st stage oocyte stained with MAB1501R (amino acids residues 50-70 at N-end); (**b**) – 2nd stage oocyte stained with PAB A2103 (the first 9 amino acids residues at N-end); (**c**) - 1st stage oocyte stained with PAB A2066 (11 amino acids residues at C-end). M – merged images. DAPI staining is in blue (DNA). Bar 10 μm for all images

and in-vivo observations have confirmed the existence of an axial core distribution in native metaphase chromosomes for topo II [71].

AB against topo II (Topo2A) were used to check its position in the oocyte GV. In spite of chromatin being highly condensed in the late oocytes' nuclei, Topo II distribution differs from mitotic chromosomes in that no recruitment of Topo II to chromatin exists at the rim of NLBs (Fig. 5, DNA). Topo II displays a dotted pattern throughout the nucleoplasm with unlabelled IGCs. Additionally, NLB does not contain topo II at all stages; Fig. 5

represents the 3rd stage oocyte, and staining of 1st and 2nd stage oocytes appears similar. The enrichment of the label rather follows the condensed chromatin, yet does not coincide with it (Fig. 5).

Lamins

Lamins were the subsequent proteins to be traced. Lamins represent the main proteinaceous components of the nuclear envelope. Lamin B is present in the NLB from the 1st stage though it always marks the chromocentres remnants (pointed by arrows, Fig. 6, b; Fig. 7,

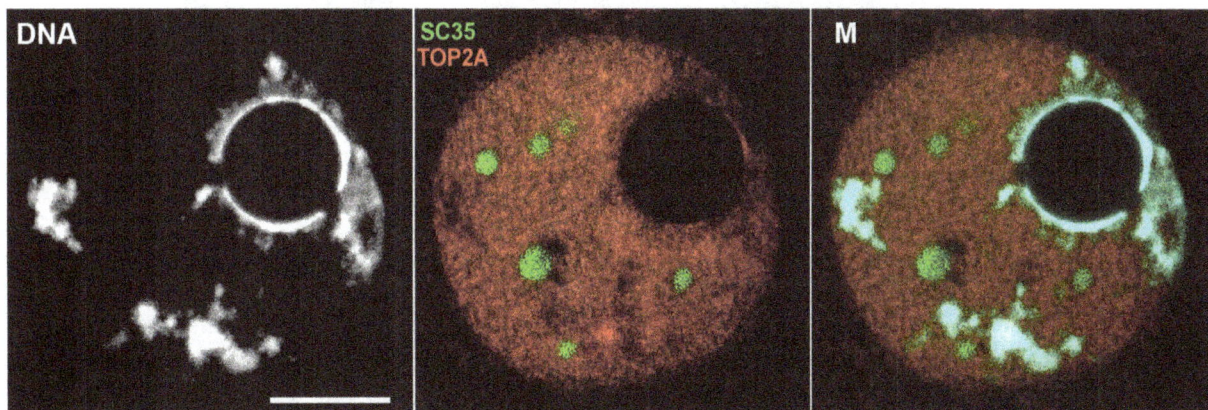

Fig. 5 Stage 3 oocyte nucleus double stained with AB against SC35 (green) and Topo II (red). DAPI staining is in grayscale (DNA); M – merged image. Bar 10 μm

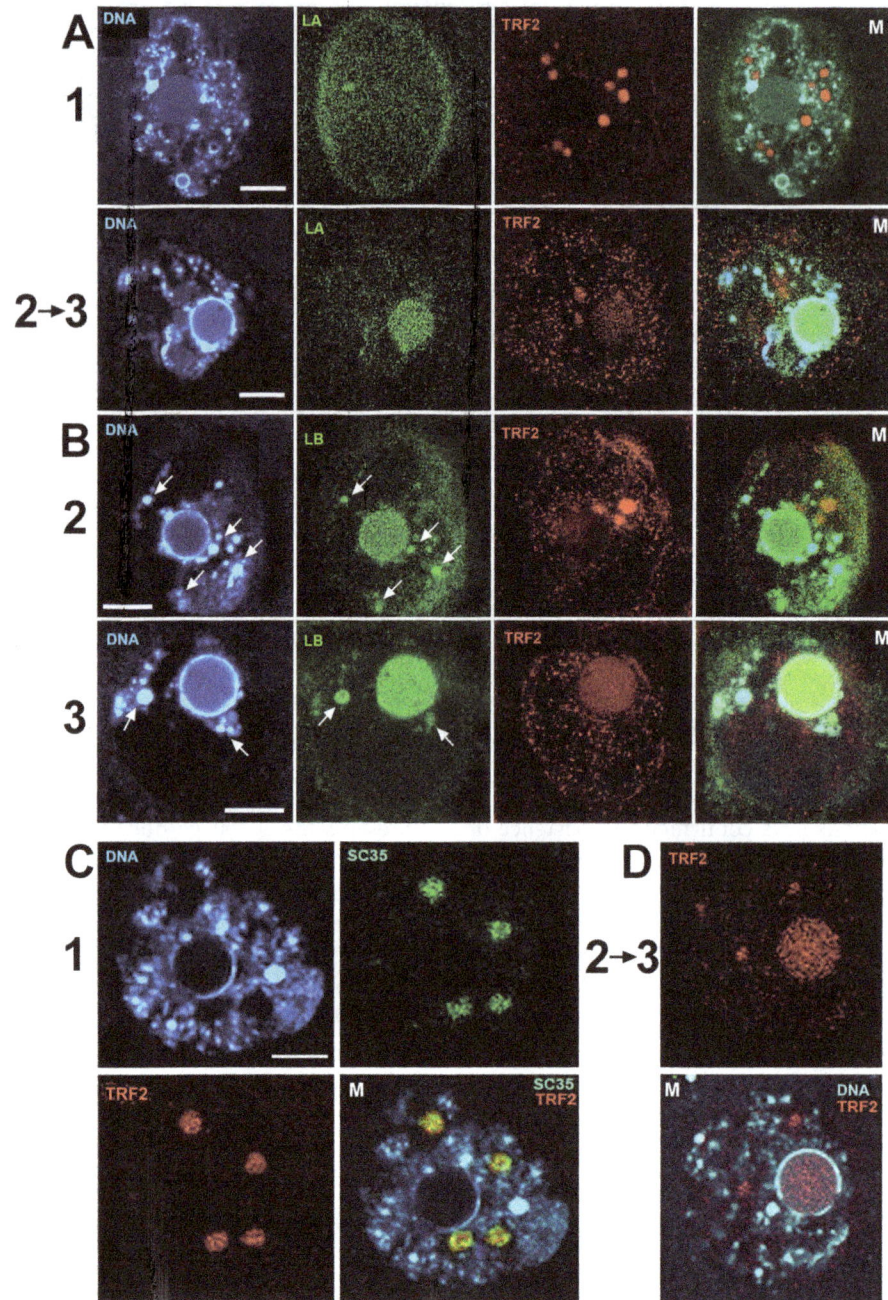

Fig. 6 Double immunofluorescence of oocytes nuclei with TRF2 AB (red) and other ABs (green). Oocyte stages are indicated at the left for each panel (**a**, **b**, **c**, **d**). A – AB against Lamin A; B - AB against Lamin B. 1st image in each row – DAPI (DNA), M – merged images. C – staining is indicated on each image; D – TRF2 and DAPI staining of the nucleus progressing from stage 2 to stage 3. Bar 10 µm for all images

Lamin B). Lamin A also comes to the NLB from 1st to 3rd stage (Fig. 6, a). It appears as though a higher level of lamin B than lamin A remains at the NE. The NE should retain its integrity, and lamin B better suits this purpose. There are cells without lamin A, but no cells without lamin B type. T-cells and B-cells express only B-type lamins; undifferentiated human and mouse embryonic stem (ES) cells lack lamins A/C, but express lamins B1 and B2

[72]. B-type lamin is expressed throughout embryogenesis, whereas lamin A and lamin C are not expressed until the tissue differentiation stage of development [33]. It is visible that some of lamin A is stored in the NLB to be used, likely in early embryogenesis (Fig. 6, a).

Chromocentres with low transcriptional activity are visible by intensive DAPI staining (Fig. 2, DNA). Namely, the chromocentres are stained with lamin B AB in cumulus

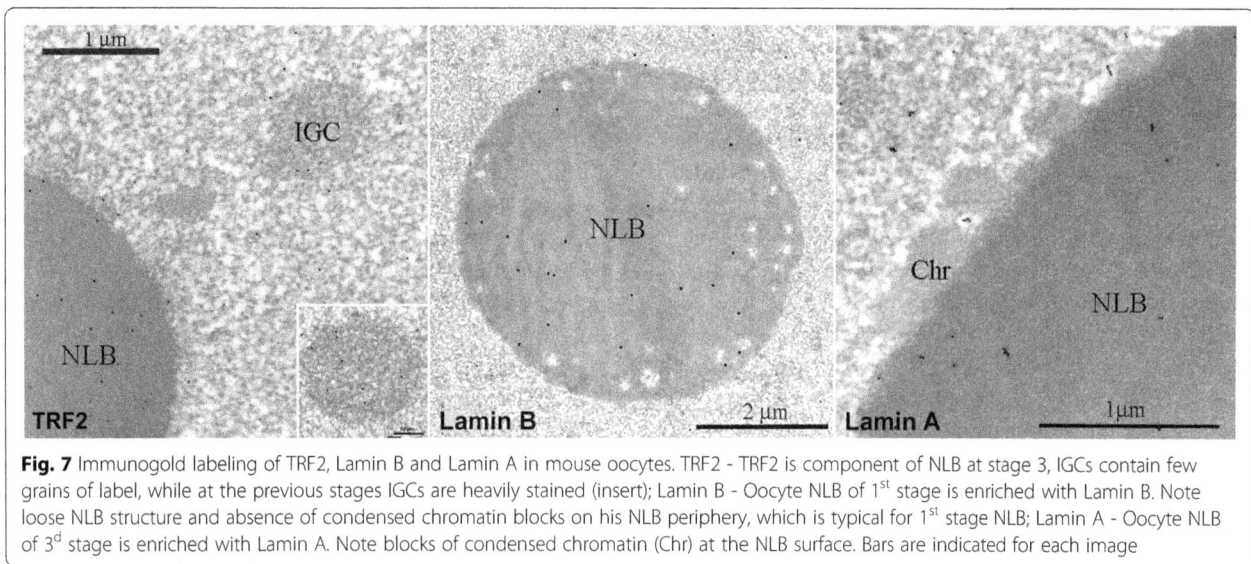

Fig. 7 Immunogold labeling of TRF2, Lamin B and Lamin A in mouse oocytes. TRF2 - TRF2 is component of NLB at stage 3, IGCs contain few grains of label, while at the previous stages IGCs are heavily stained (insert); Lamin B - Oocyte NLB of 1st stage is enriched with Lamin B. Note loose NLB structure and absence of condensed chromatin blocks on his NLB periphery, which is typical for 1st stage NLB; Lamin A - Oocyte NLB of 3^d stage is enriched with Lamin A. Note blocks of condensed chromatin (Chr) at the NLB surface. Bars are indicated for each image

cells (Fig. 2, a). The same tendency is visible in oocytes: lamin B gravitates toward chromocentres, while lamin A never marks them (Fig. 6, a, b). Together, these images suggest a difference in lamin type distribution, and the involvement of lamin B in chromocentres formation. Both lamin types are involved in NLB formation (Fig. 6, a, b; Fig. 7). Lamin A exhibits rapid migration from the NE to the NLB between the 1st and 3rd stages of oocyte development.

TRF2

TRF2 is not connected with telomeres during all 3 final stages of oogenesis. It is established that most heterochromatic regions with telomeres and centromeres move to the rim of the karyosphere and NLB at stage 3, and coincide with chromocentres at previous stages [68]. TRF2 was not observed to coincide with chromocentres (Fig. 6). This result is unsurprising, as TRF2 is known to be separated from telomeres, and attached to the nuclear envelope in frog oocytes. In the diplotene stage, TRF1 remains connected with telomeres in chromatin, whereas TRF2/MTBP does not [43]. Its membrane location has been established by biochemical and morphological observations in mouse cells as well [44, 64]. In mouse oocytes, TRF2 at stages 1 and 2 resides in SC35 domains (Fig. 6, c, d) and moves rapidly to the NLB at stage 3 (Fig. 6).

It was discovered that TRF2 is an IGCs resident at certain stages of oocyte maturation. The correspondence of TRF2 and SC35 labels inside IGCs is not perfect (Fig. 6, c, d); both present in a dotted pattern, though dots abut to each other rather than overlay. SC35 domains are the last TRF2-containing compartment prior to its relocation to the protein central body (Fig. 6, d). Thus, the behaviour of some proteins remains highly dynamic even during last stages of oocyte maturation. Y14, the core protein of the exon junction complex, was the first to

have its transient position in IGCs confirmed by the gene engineering approach [73]. Now, TRF2 exhibits the same tendency: it moves quickly from IGCs to NLBs.

Immuno-gold electron microscopy (EM) has been conducted to confirm proteins' presence in NLB (Fig. 7). Lamin A is included in the NLB at stage 3 (Fig. 7, Lamin A), and lamin B is the NLB component from the beginning of its formation (Fig. 7, Lamin B). The TRF2 AB also exhibits heavy NLB labelling, and few grains are present in IGCs – though IGCs did contain TRF2 at previous stages (Fig. 7, TRF2, insert). Mouse oocyte IGCs have been described at the EM level [23]. Large mouse preovulatory oocytes contain 10–20 roundish bodies, which are clearly defined morphologically (1–4 μm in diameter), scattered throughout the nucleoplasm. Mouse oocyte IGCs display several ultrastructural peculiarities. Their granules are 10–15 nm, which is slightly smaller than the typical 20-25-nm interchromatin granules of somatic cells [3]. It is likely that the increase in size and acquisition of a IGC's roundish form in karyosphere and NLB-containing oocyte nuclei is the consequence of oocyte transcription inactivation. Similar morphological changes occur in somatic cells treated with transcription inhibitors [3]. TRF2 belongs to the fibrillar IGCs' component when included in these structures. As a result, immune-gold labelling confirms TRF2 movement from IGCs to the NLB, and the involvement of lamin A and lamin B in NLB formation.

Discussion

Proteins absent in the NLB

Actin

The function and form (monomer, filament, or noncanonical oligomer) of nuclear actin is highly-contested, and its localization and dynamics are largely unknown.

However, a break-through occurred using the gene engineering approach [69]. A set of fluorescent nuclear actin probes have been designed, constructed, and validated to visualize nuclear actin monomers and filaments in live somatic cells (human U2OS osteosarcoma). The probes' construction allows the distinguishing of monomeric from polymeric actin. It is shown that probes which bind to monomeric actin are concentrated in IGCs. Filamentous actin forms a set of punctate structures of uniform size. These structures are scattered throughout the interchromatin space, and are excluded from chromatin-rich regions. These observations argue against direct participation of the majority of canonical actin filaments in gene regulation or chromatin remodelling [69].

Filamentous actin exists in oocyte nuclei [21, 22], though it is hardly the only form of actin present. With the set of ABs used, the position of actins' various forms were traced, and an attempt was made to determine the mechanism by which nuclear monomeric actin is contained in a unique microenvironment to regulate chromatin interaction – instead of supporting actin polymerization.

Actin consists of four subdomains labelled S1–S4. Subdomains S2 and S4 make up the pointed (-) end of actin, and subdomains S1 and S3 represent the barbed (+) end [74]. In classical actin polymerization, filament grows from its barbed end to where the pointed end of the next monomer attached. Both N-end and C-ends included in the S1 subdomain and epitope C4 (MAB1501R) are embedded in S1. S2 subdomain is involved in interactions with DNA-binding proteins [74].

Spontaneous actin polymerisation is inhibited by proteins that sequester actin monomers, such as profilin and thymosin b4 [70, 75, 76]. Profilin is the SC35 domain component in the mouse oocyte [77]. C-end is directly involved in profilin binding; therefore it could be expected that only the N-end is available for the interaction, and consequently, only ABs against N-end recognize the actin-profilin complex (Fig. 4, a, b). AB against the first nine amino acid residues of the N-terminal region of actin (PAB A2103) also recognizes short actin oligomers surrounding the nuclear envelope (Fig. 4, b). The first amino acids of actin N-end are not involved in interactions with other proteins, and could be free in oligomerization. In somatic cells, nuclear actin filaments form short scaffolds that interact with a viscoelastic structure abutting the nuclei membrane [69]. It is also possible that the same type of structure is recognized in the oocyte by A2103 AB (Fig. 4, b).

The opposite end of the actin monomer, S2 subdomain, is involved in interaction with DNAse and components of the chromatin remodelling complex. Actin alone was unable to bind DNA, while the INO80 chromatin remodelling complex with its actin–Arp module can bind DNA [70, 77]. In the context of the chromatin remodelling complex, nuclear actin has gained the ability to either interact directly with chromatin or regulate chromatin binding indirectly through conformational changes [78]. Antibody against the C-end (A2066) reveals that actin is in tight association with the oocytes' chromatin. Staining does not depend on the chromatin state - whether it packed in chromocentres or relatively dispersed (Fig. 4, c). Similar results have been obtained on NPB (nucleolus precursor bodies) of early mouse embryos. Actin is not a component of NPB in either male or female pronucleus [79]. AB against actin C-end (A 2066, Sigma) reveals one of the actin forms in association with the rim of NPB while AB against actin N-end (A2103, Sigma) stain actin outside the nucleus [80]. The NPB and NLB are considered to be related; the content of these structures could be dynamic, especially after fertilisation. Nevertheless, actin is not found within these bodies.

TopoII

Topo II and SMC2, components of the condensing complex, were the first proteins identified in the mitotic chromosome scaffold. The main representatives within the scaffold fraction are Topo II [28, 31], condensins [31], and KIF4A [81, 82].

Previous studies have analysed the dynamic behaviour of major scaffold proteins in somatic cells, suggesting that several scaffold proteins are in fact very dynamic in relation to their presence on chromosomal structure. The most dynamic scaffold component is KIF4A (t. 2.5 s) [82], followed by topo II (t. 15 s) [83]. The expression of topo II-isoform increases during the late S phase, decreases at the end of the M phase, and is dramatically reduced in the G1/G0 phase of the cell cycle [84]. Then, an anti-Topo II-α antibody labels cells in the S, G2, and M phases of the cell cycle [71]. An oocyte, with its long diplotena, is at meiosis 1st prophase when karyosphere formation occurs. Therefore, relatively prominent Topo2A staining can be observed. However, it is evident that topo II is not involved in chromatin condensation in this case (Fig. 5). No dramatic changes were observed in topo II location during oocyte maturation from the 1st to 3rd stages.

As a result, actin and Topo II do not represent protein components of the NLB.

NLB proteins are dynamic at last stages of oocyte maturation: IGC versus NLB

The very term nucleolus like body (NLB) reflects its' relation to nucleolus, so the ribosomal proteins were the first to check. While no nucleolar protein has been detected within the NLB mass by conventional immunocytochemistry, a protease digestion assay was applied to find putative presence of the nucleolar proteins in the NLB interior. The dynamic distribution of some of the proteins have been noticed. The ribosomal RPL26 protein was detected within the NLBs of NSN-type oocytes (1st stage) but is virtually absent from NLBs of SN-type oocytes (3d stage). Same is true for the ribosomal RNA (rRNA). Fluorescence in situ hybridization with oligonucleotide probes targeting 18S and 28S rRNAs shows that, in contrast to active nucleoli, NLBs of fully-grown oocytes are impoverished for the rRNAs, which is consistent with the absence of transcribed ribosomal genes in the NLB interior. Authors conclude that NLBs of fully-grown mammalian oocytes serve for storing major nucleolar proteins but not rRNA [15]. Even major nucleolar proteins such as UBF, fibrillarin, NPM1/nucleophosmin/B23, nucleolin revealed after proteinase K treatment show clear redistribution inside NLB between NSN-type (1st stage) and SN-type (3d stage) oocytes [15]. In the current study we discovered that lamin A, lamin B and TRF2 also exhibit dynamic distribution during last stages of oocyte development.

Lamins

In recent years, evidence has begun to accumulate regarding the association of A- and B-type lamins with different types of chromatin. It was assumed that A-type lamins are preferentially associated with gene-rich regions of active chromatin [34]. In somatic cells, lamin-A was discovered proximal to the nuclear membrane (Fig. 2, b). No active chromatin was present in the oocyte nucleus, and the staining with AB against lamin A belongs mainly to the nuclear envelope at stage 1 (Fig. 6, a). Lamin B1 appears to be primarily associated with the borders of regions with low gene density and low transcriptional activity. Genomic domains of 50 kb to 10 Mb in size are bounded by regions that are enriched in interactions with lamin B1 [85]. These domains, called lamin-associated domains (LADs), may represent the heterochromatin frequently observed as being closely opposed to the inner NE in many somatic cells. The morphological approach does not allow for the distinguishing of LADs, though chromocentres with low transcriptional activity are visible by intensive DAPI staining (Fig. 2, DNA). Namely, the chromocentres are stained with lamin B AB in cumulus cells (Fig. 2, 2) as well as in oocytes: lamin B gravitates toward chromocentres, while lamin A never marks them (Fig. 6, a, b). So, lamin B is involved in chromocentres' formation in both cell types. Both lamin types are involved in NLB formation (Fig. 6, a, b; Fig. 7). The rapid migration of lamin A from the NE to the NLB between the 1st and 3rd stages of oocyte development coincides with the TRF2 movement.

TRF2

Telomere-membrane associations are often observed in morphological studies [86], and TRF2 is the good candidate for the responsibility of attaching the telomere-protein complex to the nuclear envelope, though its relationship to the lamins remains to be elucidated in detail. A-type lamins certainly affect both nuclear membrane and telomere dynamics [87].

In mice pachytene spermatocytes, membrane structures which abut the synaptonemal complex attachment sites contain TRF2. During spermiogenesis and in fully formed spermatozoa, TRF2 unexpectedly localized at the acrosomal membrane that is adjacent to the nucleus – apart from the expected TRF2 position at the nuclear periphery. Telomere distribution is not static in cultured cells throughout the cell cycle or during spermatogenesis. When telomeres are attached to the nuclear envelope, such as during synaptonemal complex formation, TRF2 is the member of the protein complex which appears to be responsible for telomere attachment [64].

The direct biochemical interaction between lamin A and TRF2 has been established [88]. A-type lamins have been widely discussed since the discovery that LMNA mutations or defective posttranslational processing of pre–lamin A causes the majority of human diseases (termed laminopathies) that are accompanied with shortened telomere lengths [89, 90]. A shift in telomere localization was observed in the absence of A-type lamins, suggesting an active role of A-type lamins in the positioning of telomeres. A-type lamins play a role in the maintenance of telomeres, though the molecular mechanisms remain unknown [91]. The findings of the current study contribute to the existing evidence of connection between lamin A and telomeres.

TRF2's position in the oocyte NLB leads to the suggestion that TRF2 location could reflect preparation for fertilisation events. After fertilisation, the chromatin-surrounded NLB proceeds into second prophase mitosis, and should be assembled quickly in chromosomes. Chromosomes are not distinguished in the chromatin rim surrounding the NLB (Fig. 3; [68]). Likely, the NLB is a storage place for the proteins involved in chromatin orientation. NLB dissolved in 2nd mitotic division helps to arrange the ring of chromosomes. The NLB's important post-fertilisation role in future chromatin organization has been recently confirmed [14].

NLB structural role

Protein composition of the karyosphere central body, often referred to as NLB, especially of its' dense fibrillar component, was obscure for a long time. Some nucleolar components were found in vesicles at the NLB periphery [9] or revealed after special treatments [14, 15]. The central body is formed at the former nucleolus place and some of its components can be captured, but they cannot be the major components. Nucleolar activity is absolutely suppressed in the NLB and de novo nucleolus activity is established while zygote NPB discarded [92]. Karyosphere central body is rather essential for proper chromosomes organization before fertilization. Lamins are one of the main components organizing high-order chromatin structures and were first to be found in the NLB, which seems to be consistent with the central body structural role. Fast move of TRF2 to the central body was unexpected; however, recently discovered direct interaction between TRF2 and lamin A explains the mechanism. TRF2 as the structural protein responsible for telomere-membrane attachment fits into the picture. Identification of lamins as one of the main fibrillar NLB components supports the idea that the NLB central body organizes chromatin before fertilization.

Conclusions

It was discovered that: (1) Lamin B is a component of the NLB from the very beginning of its formation and major portion of it collected in NLB at the end of oocyte development; (2) lamin A undergoes rapid movement into the NLB, where the majority of it remains; (3) TRF2 resides in the IGCs up until the final stages of oocyte development, when a significant portion of it relocates to the NLB. Surprisingly, no forms of actin or topo II represented components of the NLB. Other proteins critical to chromatin organization are expected in NLB; this study reports the first findings of those present.

Abbreviations

AB, antibody; BCIP, 5-bromo-4-chloro-3′indolylphosphate; DAPI, 4,6-diamidino-2-phenylindole; EM, electron microscopy; ES, embryonic stem cells; GV, germinal vesicle; IF, immunofluorescence; IGCs, interchromatin granule clusters; IgGs, immunoglobulins; KC, karyosphere capsule; LADs, lamin-associated domains; mAb, monoclonal antibody; Mr, molecular mass; MTBP, membrane-associated telomere-binding protein; NBT, nitro blue tetrazolium; NE, nuclear envelope; NLB, nucleolus-like body; NM, nuclear matrix; NPB, nucleolus precursor bodies; NSN, non-surrounded nucleolus; pAb, polyclonal antibody; PBS, phosphate-buffered saline; SN, surrounded nucleolus; TRF2, telomeric binding factor 2; WB, Western blot

Acknowledgements

We are indebted to V.N. Parfenov, who sadly recently passed away, for the initiation of this work. We also thank Y.I. Gukina for her technical assistance.

Funding

This work was supported by the Russian Foundation for Basic Research (grant no.15-04-01857, 16-34-00714), Russian Science Foundation (grant no.15-15-20026) and the granting program for "Molecular and Cell Biology" of the Russian Academy of Sciences. Editing and publishing costs have been paid for by a grant from the Russian Science Foundation (grant no.15-15-20026).

Authors' contribution

GNP and APV conceived the project and designed experiments. GNP and NVI completed all the experimental work, including microscopic and biochemical analysis. OIP and APV coordinated the work. OIP and NVI are responsible for the manuscript preparation. All authors read and approved the final manuscript.

Competing interests

The authors declare that they have no competing interests.

Author details

[1]Institute of Cytology, Russian Academy of Sciences, St Petersburg 194064, Russia. [2]Saint Petersburg State University, St Petersburg 199034, Russia. [3]Far Eastern Federal University, Vladivostok 690950, Russia.

References

1. De La Fuente R. Chromatin modifications in the germinal vesicle (GV) of mammalian oocytes. Dev Biol. 2006;292:1–12.
2. Blackman MW. The spermatogenesis of the Myriapods. I. Notes on the spermatocytes and spermatids of Scolopendra. Kansas Univ Quart. 1901;10:61–76.
3. Bogolyubova IO, Bogolyubov DS. Oocyte nuclear structure during mammalian oogenesis. In: Perrotte A, editor. Recent Adv Germ Cells Research. New York: Nova Science Publishers, Inc.; 2013. p. 105–33.
4. Parfenov V, Potchukalina G, Dudina L, Kostyuchek D, Gruzova M. Human antral follicles: oocyte nucleus and the karyosphere formation (electron microscopic and autoradiographic data). Gamete Res. 1989;22:219–31.
5. Gruzova MN, Parfenov VN. Karyosphere in oogenesis and intranuclear morphogenesis. Int Rev Cytol. 1993;144:1–52.
6. Gruzova MN, Parfenov VN. Ultrastructure of late oocyte nuclei in Rana temporaria. J Cell Sci. 1977;28:1–13.
7. Mattson BA, Albertini DF. Oogenesis: chromatin and microtubule dynamics during meiotic prophase. Mol Reprod Dev. 1990;25:374–83.
8. Zybina EV, Zybina TG. Changes in the arrangement of chromosomes and nucleoli related to functional peculiarities of developing mammalian oocytes during meiotic prophase. Tsitologiia. 1992;34:3–23.
9. Pochukalina GN, Parfenov VN. Nucleolus transformation in mouse antral follicles: Distribution of coilin and components of RNA-polymerase I complex. Cell Tissue Biol. 2008;2:522–30.
10. Zybina EV, Grishchenko TA, Semenov VM. Ultrastructure of the fibrillar center in oocyte nucleoli at the diplonema stage in the golden hamster. Tsitologiia. 1984;26:1246–9.
11. Tan JH, Wang HL, Sun XS, Liu Y, Sui HS, Zhang J. Chromatin configurations in the germinal vesicle of mammalian oocytes. Mol Hum Reprod. 2009;15:1–9.
12. Luciano AM, Franciosi F, Dieci C, Tessaro I, Terzaghi L, Modina SC, et al. Large-scale chromatin structure and function changes during oogenesis : the interplay between oocyte and companion cumulus cells. Anim Reprod. 2014;11:141–9.
13. Antoine N, Lepoint A, Baeckeland E, Goessens G. Ultrastructural cytochemistry of the nucleolus in rat oocytes at the end of the folliculogenesis. Histochemistry. 1988;89:221–6.
14. Fulka H, Langerova A. The maternal nucleolus plays a key role in centromere satellite maintenance during the oocyte to embryo transition. Development. 2014;141:1694–704.
15. Shishova KV, Lavrentyeva EA, Dobrucki JW, Zatsepina OV. Nucleolus-like bodies of fully-grown mouse oocytes contain key nucleolar proteins but are impoverished for rRNA. Dev Biol. 2015;397(2):267–81.
16. Burns KH, Viveiros MM, Ren Y, Wang P, DeMayo FJ, Frail DE, et al. Roles of NPM2 in chromatin and nucleolar organization in oocytes and embryos. Science. 2003;300(5619):633–6.
17. Swiatek P. Formation of the karyosome in developing oocytes of weevils (Coleoptera, Curculionidae). Tissue Cell. 1999;31:587–93.
18. Rübsam R, Büning J. F-actin is a component of the karyosome in neuropteran oocyte nuclei. Arthropod Struct Dev. 2001;30:125–33.
19. Bogolyubov DS, Batalova FM, Kiselyov AM, Stepanova IS. Nuclear structures in Tribolium castaneum oocytes. Cell Biol Int. 2013;37:1061–79.

20. Parfenov VN, Davis DS, Pochukalina GN, Sample CE, Bugaeva EA, Murti KG. Nuclear actin filaments and their topological changes in frog oocytes. Exp Cell Res. 1995;217:385–94.

21. Kiseleva E, Drummond SP, Goldberg MW, Rutherford SA, Allen TD, Wilson KL. Actin- and protein-4.1-containing filaments link nuclear pore complexes to subnuclear organelles in Xenopus oocyte nuclei. J Cell Sci. 2004;117:2481–90.

22. Maslova A, Krasikova A. Nuclear actin depolymerization in transcriptionally active avian and amphibian oocytes leads to collapse of intranuclear structures. Nucleus. 2012;3:300–11.

23. Pochukalina GN, Bogolyubov DS, Parfenov VN. Interchromatin Granule Clusters of Mouse Preovulatory Oocytes: Organization Molecular Composition, and Possible Functions Cell and Tissue Biology. Cell Tissue Biol. 2010;4:167–76.

24. Bogolyubov D, Stepanova I, Parfenov V. Universal nuclear domains of somatic and germ cells: some lessons from oocyte interchromatin granule cluster and Cajal body structure and molecular composition. Bioessays. 2009;31:400–9.

25. Spector DL, Lamond AI. Nuclear Speckles. Cold Spring Harb Perspect Biol. 2011;3:a000646.

26. Misteli T, Spector DL. The cellular organization of gene expression. Curr Opin Cell Biol. 1998;10:323–31.

27. Dundr M, Misteli T. Functional architecture in the cell nucleus. Biochem J. 2001;356:297–310.

28. Earnshaw WC, Halligan B, Cooke CA, Heck MM, Liu LF. Topoisomerase II is a structural component of mitotic chromosome scaffolds. J Cell Biol. 1985;100:1706–15.

29. Gasser SM. Laroche T, Falquet J, Boy de la Tour E, Laemmli UK. Metaphase chromosome structure. Involvement of topoisomerase II. J Mol Biol. 1986; 188:613–29.

30. Schoeffler AJ, Berger JM. DNA topoisomerases: harnessing and constraining energy to govern chromosome topology. Q Rev Biophys. 2008;41:41–101.

31. Maeshima K, Laemmli UK. A two-step scaffolding model for mitotic chromosome assembly. Dev Cell. 2003;4:467–80.

32. Dechat T, Pfleghaar K, Sengupta K, Shimi T, Shumaker DK, Solimando L, et al. Nuclear lamins: major factors in the structural organization and function of the nucleus and chromatin. Genes Dev. 2008;22:832–53.

33. Adam SA, Goldman RD. Insights into the Differences between the A- and B-Type Nuclear Lamins. Adv Biol Regul. 2012;52:108–13.

34. Shimi T, Pfleghaar K, Kojima S, Pack CG, Solovei I, Goldman AE, et al. The A- and B-type nuclear lamin networks: microdomains involved in chromatin organization and transcription. Genes Dev. 2008;22:3409–21.

35. Goldberg MW, Huttenlauch I, Hutchison CJ, Stick R. Filaments made from A- and B-type lamins differ in structure and organization. J Cell Sci. 2008;121:215–25.

36. Nickerson J. Experimental observations of a nuclear matrix. J Cell Sci. 2001;114:463–74.

37. Berezney R, Mortillaro MJ, Ma H, Wei X, Samarabandu J. The nuclear matrix: a structural milieu for genomic function. Int Rev Cytol. 1995;162A:1–65.

38. Malyavantham KS, Bhattacharya S, Barbeitos M, Mukherjee L, Xu J, Fackelmayer FO, et al. Identifying functional neighborhoods within the cell nucleus: proximity analysis of early S-phase replicating chromatin domains to sites of transcription, RNA polymerase II, HP1gamma, matrin 3 and SAF-A. J Cell Biochem. 2008;105:391–403.

39. Podgornaya OI, Voronin AP, Enukashvily NI, Matveev IV, Lobov IB. Structure-specific DNA-binding proteins as the foundation for three-dimensional chromatin organization. Int Rev Cytol. 2003;224:227–96.

40. Bugaeva EA, Podgornaya OI. Telomere-binding protein from the nuclear envelope of oocytes of the frog Rana temporaria. Biochemistry (Mosc). 1997;62:1311–22.

41. Lima-de-Faria A. Molecular evolution and organization of chromosomes. New York: Elsevier Science Press; 1983.

42. Dernburg AF, Sedat JW, Cande WZ, Bass HW. Cytology of Telomeres. In: Telomeres, vol. 29. New York: Cold Spring Harbor Laboratory Press; 1995. p. 295–338.

43. Podgornaya OI, Bugaeva EA, Voronin AP, Gilson E, Mitchell AR. Nuclear envelope associated protein that binds telomeric DNAs. Mol Reprod Dev. 2000;57:16–25.

44. Voronin AP, Lobov IB, Gilson E, Podgornaia OI. A telomere-binding protein (TRF2/MTBP) from mouse nuclear matrix with motives of an intermediate filament-type rod domain. J Anti Aging Med. 2003;6:205–18.

45. Chong L, van Steensel B, Broccoli D, Erdjument-Bromage H, Hanish J, Tempst P, et al. A human telomeric protein. Science. 1995;270:1663–7.

46. Broccoli D, Chong L, Oelmann S, Fernald AA, Marziliano N, van Steensel B, et al. Comparison of the human and mouse genes encoding the telomeric protein, TRF1: chromosomal localization, expression and conserved protein domains. Hum Mol Genet. 1997;6:69–76.

47. Bilaud T, Koering CE, Binet-Brasselet E, Ancelin K, Pollice A, Gasser SM, et al. The telobox, a Myb-related telomeric DNA binding motif found in proteins from yeast, plants and human. Nucleic Acids Res. 1996;24:1294–303.

48. Bilaud T, Brun C, Ancelin K, Koering CE, Laroche T, Gilson E. Telomeric localization of TRF2, a novel human telobox protein. Nat Genet. 1997;17:236–9.

49. Palm W, de Lange T. How shelterin protects mammalian telomeres. Annu Rev Genet. 2008;42:301–34.

50. Van Steensel B, Smogorzewska A, de Lange T. TRF2 protects human telomeres from end-to-end fusions. Cell. 1998;92:401–13.

51. Muñoz P, Blanco R, Blasco MA. Role of the TRF2 telomeric protein in cancer and ageing. Cell Cycle. 2006;5:718–21.

52. Glass JR, Gerace L. Lamins A and C bind and assemble at the surface of mitotic chromosomes. J Cell Biol. 1990;111:1047–57.

53. Lessard JL. Two monoclonal antibodies to actin: one muscle selective and one generally reactive. Cell Motil Cytoskeleton. 1988;10:349–62.

54. Cmarko D, Verschure PJ, Martin TE, Dahmus ME, Krause S, Fu X-D, et al. Ultrastructural Analysis of Transcription and Splicing in the Cell Nucleus after Bromo-UTP Microinjection. Mol Biol Cell. 1999;10:211–23.

55. Belgrader P, Siegel AJ, Berezney R. A comprehensive study on the isolation and characterisation of the HeLa S3 nuclear matrix. J Cell Sci. 1991;98:281–91.

56. Lobov IB, Tsutsui K, Mitchell AR, Podgornaya OI. Specific interaction of mouse major satellite with MAR-binding protein SAF-A. Eur J Cell Biol. 2000;79:839–49.

57. Laemmli UK. Cleavage of structural proteins during the assembly of the head of bacteriophage T4. Nature. 1970;227:680–5.

58. Pochukalina GN, Parfenov VN. Nucleolus in multilayer follicles oocytes of mouse (fibrillarin and RNA polymerase I topography, their association with coilin). Tsitologiia. 2006;8:674–83.

59. Ilicheva NV, Podgornaya OI, Voronin AP. Telomere repeat factor 2 (TRF2) is responsible for the telomere attachment to the nuclear membrane. Adv Prot Chem Struct Biol. 2015;101:67–96.

60. Enukashvily N, Donev R, Sheer D, Podgornaya O. Satellite DNA binding and cellular localisation of RNA helicase P68. J Cell Sci. 2005;118:611–22.

61. Zatsepina OV, Zharskaya OO, Prusov AN. Isolation of the constitutive heterochromatin from mouse liver nuclei. Methods Mol Biol. 2008;463:169–80.

62. Berchtold D, Fesser S, Bachmann G, Kaiser A, Eilert JC, Frohns F, et al. Nuclei of chicken neurons in tissues and three-dimensional cell cultures are organized into distinct radial zones. Chromosome Res. 2011;19:165–82.

63. Solovei I, Wang AS, Thanisch K, Schmidt CS, Krebs S, Zwerger M, et al. LBR and lamin A/C sequentially tether peripheral heterochromatin and inversely regulate differentiation. Cell. 2013;152:584–98.

64. Dolnik AV, Kuznetsova IS, Voronin AP, Podgornaia OI. Telomere-binding TRF2/MTBP localization during mouse spermatogenesis and cell cycle of the mouse cells L929. J Anti Aging Med. 2003;6:107–21.

65. Dolnik AV, Pochukalina GN, Parfenov VN, Karpushev AV, Podgornaia OI, Voronin AP. Dynamics of satellite binding protein CENP-B and telomere binding protein TRF2/MTBP in the nuclei of mouse spermatogenic line. Cell Biol Int. 2007;31:316–29.

66. Kuznetsova IS, Voronin AP, Podgornaya OI. Telomere and TRF2/MTBP localization in respect to satellite DNA during the cell cycle of mouse cell line L929. Rejuvenation Res. 2006;9:391–401.

67. Bouniol-Baly C, Hamraoui L, Guibert J, Beaujean N, Szöllösi MS, Debey P. Differential transcriptional activity associated with chromatin configuration in fully grown mouse germinal vesicle oocytes. Biol Reprod. 1999;3:580–7.

68. Bonnet-Garnier A, Feuerstein P, Chebrout M, Fleurot R, Jan HU, Debey P, et al. Genome organization and epigenetic marks in mouse germinal vesicle oocytes. Int J Dev Biol. 2012;56:877–87.

69. Belin BJ, Cimini BA, Blackburn EH, Mullins RD. Visualization of actin filaments and monomers in somatic cell nuclei. Mol Biol Cell. 2013;24:982–94.

70. Weston L, Coutts AS, La Thangue NB. Actin nucleators in the nucleus: an emerging theme. J Cell Sci. 2012;125:3519–27.

71. Vagnarelli P. Chromatin reorganization through mitosis. Adv Protein Chem Struct Biol. 2013;90:179–224.

72. Constantinescu D, Gray HL, Sammak PJ, Schatten GP, Csoka AB. Lamin A/C expression is a marker of mouse and human embryonic stem cell differentiation. Stem Cells. 2006;24:177–85.

73. Kiselev A, Stepanova I, Adonin L, Batalova F, Parfenov V, Bogolyubov D, et al. Characterization of Tribolium castaneum oocyte nuclear structures

using microinjection of a fusion nuclear porotein mRNA. Mol Repod & Dev. 2015;82:628–9.

74. Bartholomew B. Monomeric actin required for INO80 remodeling. Nat Stuct Mol Biol. 2013;20:405–7.

75. Safer D, Golla R, Nachmias VT. Isolation of a 5-kilodalton actin-sequestering peptide from human blood platelets. Proc Natl Acad Sci U S A. 1990;87:2536–40.

76. Shlüter K, Jockusch BM, Rothkegel M. Profilins as regulators of actin dynamics. Biochim Biophys Acta. 1997;1359:97–109.

77. Pochukalina GN, Parfenov VN. Localization of actin and mRNA export factors in the nucleus of murine preovulatory oocytes. Cell Tissue Biol. 2012;6:423–34.

78. Kapoor P, Chen M, Winkler DD, Luger K, Shen X. Evidence for monomeric actin function in INO80 chromatin remodeling. Nat Struct Mol Biol. 2013;20:426–32.

79. Bogolyubova I, Stein G, Bogolyubov D. FRET analysis of interactions between actin and exon-exon-junction complex proteins in early mouse embryos. Cell Tissue Biol. 2013;7:37–42.

80. Bogolyubova IO, Parfenov VN. Immunofluorescence detection of nuclear actin in early mouse embryos. Cell Tissue Biol. 2012;6:458–64.

81. Mazumdar M, Sundareshan S, Misteli T. Human chromokinesin KIF4A functions in chromosome condensation and segregation. J Cell Biol. 2004;166:613–20.

82. Samejima K, Samejima I, Vagnarelli P, Ogawa H, Vargiu G, Kelly DA, et al. Mitotic chromosomes are compacted laterally by KIF4 and condensin and axially by topoisomerase IIα. J Cell Biol. 2012;199:755–70.

83. Tavormina PA, Côme MG, Hudson JR, Mo YY, Beck WT, Gorbsky GJ. Rapid exchange of mammalian topoisomerase II alpha at kinetochores and chromosome arms in mitosis. J Cell Biol. 2002;158:23–9.

84. Taniguchi K, Wakabayashi T, Yoshida T, Mizuno M, Yoshikawa K, Kikuchi A, et al. Immunohistochemical staining of DNA topoisomerase IIalpha in human gliomas. J Neurosurg. 1999;91:477–82.

85. Guelen L, Pagie L, Brasset E, Meuleman W, Faza MB, Talhout W, et al. Domain organization of human chromosomes revealed by mapping of nuclear lamina interactions. Nature. 2008;453:948–51.

86. Comings DE. Arrangement of chromatin in the nucleus. Hum Genet. 1980;53:131–43.

87. De Vos WH, Houben F, Hoebe RA, Hennekam R, van Engelen B, Manders EM, et al. Increased plasticity of the nuclear envelope and hypermobility of telomeres due to the loss of A-type lamins. Biochim Biophys Acta. 1800;2010:448–58.

88. Wood AM, Rendtlew Danielsen JM, Lucas CA, Rice EL, Scalzo D, et al. TRF2 and lamin A/C interact to facilitate the functional organization of chromosome ends. Nat Commun. 2014;5:5467.

89. Andrés V, González JM. Role of A-type lamins in signaling, transcription, and chromatin organization. J Cell Biol. 2009;187:945–57.

90. Decker ML, Chavez E, Vulto I, Lansdorp PM. Telomere length in Hutchinson-Gilford progeria syndrome. Mech Ageing Dev. 2009;130:377–83.

91. Gonzalez-Suarez I, Redwood AB, Perkins SM, Vermolen B, Lichtensztejin D, Grotsky DA, et al. Novel roles for A-type lamins in telomere biology and the DNA damage response pathway. EMBO J. 2009;28:2414–27.

92. Kyogoku H, Fulka Jr J, Wakayama T, Miyano T. De novo formation of nucleoli in developing mouse embryos originating from enucleolated zygotes. Development. 2014;141:2255–9.

Permissions

All chapters in this book were first published in MC, by BioMed Central; hereby published with permission under the Creative Commons Attribution License or equivalent. Every chapter published in this book has been scrutinized by our experts. Their significance has been extensively debated. The topics covered herein carry significant findings which will fuel the growth of the discipline. They may even be implemented as practical applications or may be referred to as a beginning point for another development.

The contributors of this book come from diverse backgrounds, making this book a truly international effort. This book will bring forth new frontiers with its revolutionizing research information and detailed analysis of the nascent developments around the world.

We would like to thank all the contributing authors for lending their expertise to make the book truly unique. They have played a crucial role in the development of this book. Without their invaluable contributions this book wouldn't have been possible. They have made vital efforts to compile up to date information on the varied aspects of this subject to make this book a valuable addition to the collection of many professionals and students.

This book was conceptualized with the vision of imparting up-to-date information and advanced data in this field. To ensure the same, a matchless editorial board was set up. Every individual on the board went through rigorous rounds of assessment to prove their worth. After which they invested a large part of their time researching and compiling the most relevant data for our readers.

The editorial board has been involved in producing this book since its inception. They have spent rigorous hours researching and exploring the diverse topics which have resulted in the successful publishing of this book. They have passed on their knowledge of decades through this book. To expedite this challenging task, the publisher supported the team at every step. A small team of assistant editors was also appointed to further simplify the editing procedure and attain best results for the readers.

Apart from the editorial board, the designing team has also invested a significant amount of their time in understanding the subject and creating the most relevant covers. They scrutinized every image to scout for the most suitable representation of the subject and create an appropriate cover for the book.

The publishing team has been an ardent support to the editorial, designing and production team. Their endless efforts to recruit the best for this project, has resulted in the accomplishment of this book. They are a veteran in the field of academics and their pool of knowledge is as vast as their experience in printing. Their expertise and guidance has proved useful at every step. Their uncompromising quality standards have made this book an exceptional effort. Their encouragement from time to time has been an inspiration for everyone.

The publisher and the editorial board hope that this book will prove to be a valuable piece of knowledge for researchers, students, practitioners and scholars across the globe.

List of Contributors

Carla Sustek D'Angelo, Monica Castro Varela, Claudia Irene Emílio de Castro, Paulo Alberto Otto and Celia Priszkulnik Koiffmann
Human Genome and Stem Cell Research Center (HUG-CELL), Department of Genetics and Evolutionary Biology, Institute of Biosciences, University of Sao Paulo, Rua do Matao no 277, Cidade Universitaria-Butanta, Sao Paulo, SP 05508-090, Brazil

Ana Beatriz Alvarez Perez and Luis Garcia-Alonso
Department of Morphology and Genetics, Paulista School of Medicine, Federal University of Sao Paulo (UNIFESP), Sao Paulo, SP, Brazil

Charles Marques Lourenço
Neurogenetics Unit, Clinics Hospital of Ribeirao Preto, Faculty of Medicine, University of Sao Paulo, FMRP-USP, Ribeirao Preto, SP, Brazil

Chong Ae Kim and Debora Romeo Bertola
Genetic Unit, Children's Institute, Faculty of Medicine, University of Sao Paulo, FMUSP, Sao Paulo, SP, Brazil

Fernando Kok
Department of Neurology, Faculty of Medicine, University of Sao Paulo, FMUSP, Sao Paulo, SP, Brazil

Fan Yu, Ping Wang, Xueting Li, Yongji Huang, Ling Luo, Yongqing Yang, Rukai Chen and Liangnian Xu
National Engineering Research Center for Sugarcane, Fujian Agriculture and Forestry University, Fuzhou, China

Zuhu Deng
National Engineering Research Center for Sugarcane, Fujian Agriculture and Forestry University, Fuzhou, China
Guangxi Collaborative Innovation Center of Sugar Industries, Guangxi University, Nanning, China

Qinnan Wang and Jiayun Wu
Guangdong Provincial Bioengineering Institute, Guangzhou Sugarcane Industry Research Institute, Guangzhou, China

Yanfen Jing and Xinlong Liu
Sugarcane Research Institute of Yunnan Agriculture Science Academy, Kaiyuan, China

Muqing Zhang
Guangxi Collaborative Innovation Center of Sugar Industries, Guangxi University, Nanning, China

Wenfu Li, Xianfu Wang and Shibo Li
Genetics Laboratory, University of Oklahoma Health Sciences Center, 1122 NE 13th Street, Suite 1400, Oklahoma City, OK 73104, USA

Wei Shu
Department of Cell Biology and Genetics, School of Pre-Clinical Medicine, Guangxi Medical University, Nanning, Guangxi 530021, China

Qiping Hu
Department of Cell Biology and Genetics, School of Pre-Clinical Medicine, Guangxi Medical University, Nanning, Guangxi 530021, China
Laboratory of Clinical Cytogenetics and Genomics, Department of Genetics, Yale School of Medicine, New Haven, CT 06520, USA

Peining Li and Hongyan Chai
Laboratory of Clinical Cytogenetics and Genomics, Department of Genetics, Yale School of Medicine, New Haven, CT 06520, USA

Senol Citli
Trabzon Kanuni Training and Research Hospital, Medical Genetics Unit, Trabzon, Turkey

Ahmet Cevdet Ceylan
Trabzon Kanuni Training and Research Hospital, Medical Genetics Unit, Trabzon, Turkey
Ankara Yıldırım Beyazıt University, Ankara Atatürk Training and Research Hospital, Department of Medical Genetics, Ankara, Turkey

Haktan Bagis Erdem and Ibrahim Sahin
Ankara Diskapi Yildirim Beyazit Training and Research Hospital, Medical Genetics Unit, Ankara, Turkey

Elif Acar Arslan
Karadeniz Technical University, School of Medicine, Department of Child Neurology, Trabzon, Turkey

Murat Erdogan
Kayseri Training and Research Hospital, Department of Medical Genetics, Kayseri, Turkey

Christine J. Ye
The Division of Hematology/Oncology, Department of Internal Medicine, University of Michigan, Ann Arbor, MI 48109, USA

Sarah Regan, Guo Liu and Sarah Alemara
Center for Molecular Medicine and Genomics, Wayne State University School of Medicine, Detroit, MI 48201, USA

Henry H. Heng
Center for Molecular Medicine and Genomics, Wayne State University School of Medicine, Detroit, MI 48201, USA
Department of Pathology, Wayne State University School of Medicine, Detroit, MI 48201, USA

Renata Woroniecka, Jolanta Rygier, Klaudia Borkowska, Iwona Rzepecka, Martyna Łukasik, Agnieszka Budziłowska and Barbara Pieńkowska-Grela
Cancer Genetic Laboratory, Pathology and Laboratory Diagnostics Department, Centre of Oncology, M. Skłodowska-Curie Memorial Institute, Warsaw, Poland

Beata Grygalewicz
Cancer Genetic Laboratory, Pathology and Laboratory Diagnostics Department, Centre of Oncology, M. Skłodowska-Curie Memorial Institute, Warsaw, Poland
Department of Pathology and Laboratory Diagnostics, Maria Skłodowska-Curie Memorial Cancer Center and Institute of Oncology, 15B Wawelska Str, 02-034, Warsaw, Poland

Grzegorz Rymkiewicz and Katarzyna Błachnio
Flow Cytometry Laboratory, Pathology and Laboratory Diagnostics Department, Centre of Oncology, M. Skłodowska-Curie Memorial Institute, Warsaw, Poland

Beata Nowakowska, Magdalena Bartnik and Monika Gos
Department of Medical Genetics, Mother and Child Institute, Warsaw, Poland

Thomas Liehr
Jena University Hospital, Friedrich Schiller University, Institute of Human Genetics, Kollegiengasse 10, D-07743 Jena, Germany

Ruen Yao, Tingting Yu, Niu Li and Jian Wang
Department of Medical Genetics and Molecular Diagnostic Laboratory, Shanghai Children's Medical Center, Shanghai Jiaotong University School of Medicine, Shanghai 200127, China

Xuyun Hu and Yiping Shen
Department of Medical Genetics and Molecular Diagnostic Laboratory, Shanghai Children's Medical Center, Shanghai Jiaotong University School of Medicine, Shanghai 200127, China
Boston Children's Hospital, Boston, MA 02115, USA

Cheng Zhang
Boston Children's Hospital, Boston, MA 02115, USA

Xiumin Wang
Department of Endocrinology and Metabolism, Shanghai Children's Medical Center, Shanghai Jiaotong University School of Medicine, Shanghai 200127, China

Yanru Pei and Yu Cui
State Key Laboratory of Crop Biology, Shandong Agriculture University, Tai'an 271018, Shandong, China

Honggang Wang and Xingfeng Li
State Key Laboratory of Crop Biology, Shandong Agriculture University, Tai'an 271018, Shandong, China
College of Agronomy, Shandong Agriculture University, Tai'an 271018, Shandong, China

Yanping Zhang and Yinguang Bao
College of Agronomy, Shandong Agriculture University, Tai'an 271018, Shandong, China

Chung-Er Huang
International College of Semiconductor Technology, National Chiao-Tung University, Hsinchu, Taiwan
Cytoaurora Biotechnologies, Inc. Hsinchu Science Park, Hsinchu, Taiwan

Wen-Hsiang Lin and Dong-Jay Lee
Department of Genomic Medicine and Center for Medical Genetics, Changhua Christian Hospital, Changhua, Taiwan
Department of Genomic Science and Technology, Changhua Christian Hospital Healthcare System, Changhua, Taiwan

Gwo-Chin Ma
Department of Genomic Medicine and Center for Medical Genetics, Changhua Christian Hospital, Changhua, Taiwan
Department of Genomic Science and Technology, Changhua Christian Hospital Healthcare System, Changhua, Taiwan
Institute of Biochemistry, Microbiology and Immunology, Chung-Shan Medical University, Taichung, Taiwan
Department of Medical Laboratory Science and Biotechnology, Central Taiwan University of Science and Technology, Taichung, Taiwan

Ming Chen
Department of Genomic Medicine and Center for Medical Genetics, Changhua Christian Hospital, Changhua, Taiwan

Department of Genomic Science and Technology, Changhua Christian Hospital Healthcare System, Changhua, Taiwan
Department of Obstetrics and Gynecology, College of Medicine, National Taiwan University, Taipei, Taiwan
National Chiao-Tung University, Hsinchu, Taiwan
Department of Obstetrics and Gynecology, Changhua Christian Hospital, Changhua, Taiwan
Department of Medical Genetics, National Taiwan University Hospital, Taipei, Taiwan
Department of Life Science, Tunghai University, Taichung, Taiwan

Hei-Jen Jou
Department of Obstetrics and Gynecology, Taiwan Adventist Hospital, Taipei, Taiwan
Department of Obstetrics and Gynecology, College of Medicine, National Taiwan University, Taipei, Taiwan

Hsin-Fu Chen
Department of Obstetrics and Gynecology, College of Medicine, National Taiwan University, Taipei, Taiwan
Graduate Institute of Medical Genomics and Proteomics, College of Medicine, National Taiwan University, Taipei, Taiwan

Yi-Shing Lin
Welgene Biotechnology Company, Nangang Business Park, Taipei, Taiwan

Norman A. Ginsberg
Department of Obstetrics and Gynecology, Feinberg School of Medicine, Northwestern University Medical Center, Chicago, IL, USA

Frank Mau-Chung Chang
Department of Electrical Engineering, University of California Los Angeles, Los Angeles, CA, USA
National Chiao-Tung University, Hsinchu, Taiwan
Department of Obstetrics and Gynecology, Changhua Christian Hospital, Changhua, Taiwan

Daiyan Li, Dan Long, Tinghui Li, Yanli Wu, Yi Wang, Lili Xu, Xing Fan, Lina Sha, Haiqin Zhang, Yonghong Zhou and Houyang Kang
Triticeae Research Institute, Sichuan Agricultural University, 211 Huimin Road, Wenjiang, Chengdu, Sichuan 611130, China

Jian Zeng
College of Resources, Sichuan Agricultural University, 211 Huimin Road, Wenjiang, Chengdu, Sichuan 611130, China

Frédéric Brioude and Irène Netchine
INSERM, UMR_S 938, CDR Saint-Antoine, F-75012 Paris, France

UMR_S 938, CDR Saint-Antoine, Sorbonne Universities, UPMC Univ Paris, 06 Paris, France
APHP, Armand Trousseau Hospital, Pediatric Endocrinology, Paris, France

Sandra Chantot-Bastaraud
INSERM, UMR_S 938, CDR Saint-Antoine, F-75012 Paris, France
UMR_S 938, CDR Saint-Antoine, Sorbonne Universities, UPMC Univ Paris, 06 Paris, France
APHP, Armand Trousseau Hospital, Pediatric Endocrinology, Paris, France
APHP, Hôpital Armand-Trousseau, Département de Génétique, UF de Génétique Chromosomique, Paris, France

Svea Stratmann, Matthias Begemann, Miriam Elbracht and Thomas Eggermann
Institute of Human Genetics, RWTH University Hospital Aachen, Pauwelsstr 30, D-52074 Aachen, Germany

Luitgard Graul-Neumann
Institute of Human Genetics, Charité University Hospital, Berlin, Germany

Madeleine Harbison
Department of Pediatrics, Icahn School of Medicine at Mount Sinai, New York, NY, USA

Nataliya Huleyuk and Iryna Tkach
Institute of Hereditary Pathology, NAMS of Ukraine, Lysenko Str. 31a, Lviv 79008, Ukraine

Danuta Zastavna
Institute of Hereditary Pathology, NAMS of Ukraine, Lysenko Str. 31a, Lviv 79008, Ukraine
Department of Biotechnology and Bioinformatics, Faculty of Chemistry, Rzeszow University of Technology, Al. Powstańców Warszawy 6, 35-959 Rzeszow, Poland

Miroslaw Tyrka
Department of Biotechnology and Bioinformatics, Faculty of Chemistry, Rzeszow University of Technology, Al. Powstańców Warszawy 6, 35-959 Rzeszow, Poland

Nils Mandahl, Linda Magnusson, Jenny Nilsson, Elsa Arbajian and Fredrik Mertens
Division of Clinical Genetics, Department of Laboratory Medicine, Lund University, SE-221 84 Lund, Sweden

Anders Isaksson and Björn Viklund
Array and Analysis Facility, Uppsala University, Uppsala, Sweden

Fredrik Vult von Steyern
Department of Orthopedics, Clinical Sciences, Lund University and Skåne University Hospital, Lund, Sweden

Anna I. Solovyeva, Vera N. Stefanova and Serghei Iu. Demin
Institute of Cytology RAS, St. Petersburg 194064, Russia

Olga I. Podgornaya
Institute of Cytology RAS, St. Petersburg 194064, Russia
Saint Petersburg State University, St. Petersburg 199034, Russia
Far Eastern Federal University, Vladivostok 690922, Russia

Hong-Guo Zhang, Rui-Xue Wang, Yuan Pan, Han Zhang, Lei-Lei Li, Hai-Bo Zhu and Rui-Zhi Liu
Center for Reproductive Medicine and Center for Prenatal Diagnosis, First Hospital, Jilin University, 71 Xinmin Street, Chaoyang District, Changchun, Jilin Province 130021, China

Rui Zhang, Xuan Chen, Xiumin Lu, Yu Liu and Yan Li
Center for Obstetrics and Prenatal Diagnosis, The Second Affiliated Hospital of Harbin Medical University, 150000 Harbin, China

Peiling Li
Department of Obstetrics and Gynaecology, The Second Affiliated Hospital of Harbin Medical University, 150000 Harbin, China

Liang Zhang
Translational Medicine Center, Guangdong Women and Children's Hospital, Guangzhou 511400, China

Mengnan Xu and David S. Cram
Berry Genomics Corporation, Building 9, No 6 Court Jingshun East Road, Chaoyang District, Beijing 100015, China

Jia-Chi Wang, Loretta W. Mahon, Leslie P. Ross, Arturo Anguiano, Renius Owen and Fatih Z. Boyar
Cytogenetics Laboratory, Quest Diagnostics Nichols Institute, 33608 Ortega Highway, San Juan Capistrano, CA 92690, USA

E. N. Ferreira, B. D. F. Barros and D. M. Carraro
International Research Center, AC Camargo Cancer Center, São Paulo, Brazil

A. C. V. Krepischi
International Research Center, AC Camargo Cancer Center, São Paulo, Brazil

Institute of Biosciences, University of São Paulo, São Paulo, Brazil

M. Maschietto
International Research Center, AC Camargo Cancer Center, São Paulo, Brazil
Brazilian Biosciences National Laboratory, National Center for Research in Energy and Materials, Campinas, São Paulo, Brazil

A. G. Silva, S. S. Costa and C. Rosenberg
Institute of Biosciences, University of São Paulo, São Paulo, Brazil

I. W. da Cunha
Department of Surgical and Investigative Pathology, AC Camargo Cancer Center, São Paulo, Brazil

P. E. Grundy
Alberta Health Services, Cancer Control Alberta, Alberta, Canada

Natalia V. Kovaleva
Academy of Molecular Medicine, Mytniskaya str. 12/44, St. Petersburg 191144, Russian Federation

Philip D. Cotter
Department of Pediatrics, University of California San Francisco, San Francisco, CA, USA
ResearchDx Inc., Irvine, CA, USA

Anja Weise, Samarth Bhatt, Katja Piaszinski, Nadezda Kosyakova, Xiaobo Fan and Thomas Liehr
Institute of Human Genetics, Jena University Hospital, Postfach, 07740, Jena, Germany

Jyoti P. Chaudhuri
Institute of Human Genetics, Jena University Hospital, Postfach, 07740, Jena, Germany
Kinderklinik, Ludwig Maximillians Universität, 80337 Munich, Germany

Annelore Altendorf-Hofmann
Department of General, Visceral und Vascular Surgery, Jena University Hospital, Kochstr 2, Jena 07743, Germany

Alongklod Tanomtong and Arunrat Chaveerach
Department of Biology, Faculty of Science, Khon Kaen University, 123 Moo 16 Mittapap Rd, Khon Kaen, Muang District 40002, Thailand

Marcelo Bello de Cioffi
Departamento de Genética e Evolução, Universidade Federal de São Carlos, São Carlos, SP, Brazil

Edivaldo de Oliveira and Joachim-U. Walther
Instituto Evandro Chagas, Seção de Meio Ambiente, Laboratório de Cultura de Tecidos e Citogenética, Ananindeua, PA, Brazil

Juliana Nascimento and Luciana Bolsoni Lourenço
Departamento de Biologia Estrutural e Funcional, Instituto de Biologia, Universidade Estadual de Campinas, 13083-863 Campinas, São Paulo, Brazil

Diego Baldo
Laboratorio de Genética Evolutiva, Instituto de Biología Subtropical (CONICET-UNaM), Facultad de Ciencias Exactas Químicas y Naturales, Universidad Nacional de Misiones, Félix de Azara 1552, CPA N3300LQF Posadas, Misiones, Argentina

Galina N. Pochukalina and Nadya V. Ilicheva
Institute of Cytology, Russian Academy of Sciences, St Petersburg 194064, Russia

Alexey P. Voronin
Institute of Cytology, Russian Academy of Sciences, St Petersburg 194064, Russia
Saint Petersburg State University, St Petersburg 199034, Russia

Olga I. Podgornaya
Institute of Cytology, Russian Academy of Sciences, St Petersburg 194064, Russia
Saint Petersburg State University, St Petersburg 199034, Russia
Far Eastern Federal University, Vladivostok 690950, Russia

Index

www.ingramcontent.com/pod-product-compliance
Lightning Source LLC
Chambersburg PA
CBHW080508200326
41458CB00012B/4125